Diagnostic Radiology in Emergency Medicine

Editors

Peter Rosen, M.D.
Adjunct Professor, Departments of Medicine and Surgery;
Director of Education, Emergency Department
University of California School of Medicine
San Diego, California

Peter E. Doris, M.D.
Clinical Associate Professor of Radiology and Medicine
University of Chicago Hospitals
Chicago, Illinois;
Medical Director, Department of Radiology
St. Anthony Medical Center
Crown Point, Indiana

Roger M. Barkin, M.D.
Chairman, Department of Pediatrics and Newborn Medicine
Rose Medical Center;
Professor of Surgery
University of Colorado Health Sciences Center
Denver, Colorado

Suzanne Z. Barkin, M.D.
Assistant Professor of Radiology
University of Colorado Health Sciences Center;
Staff Radiologist
Denver General Hospital
Denver, Colorado

Vincent J. Markovchick, M.D.
Associate Professor, Division of Emergency Medicine
University of Colorado Health Sciences Center;
Director, Emergency Medical Services
Denver General Hospital
Denver, Colorado

with 792 illustrations

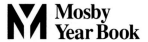
Mosby
Year Book

St. Louis Baltimore Boston Chicago London Philadelphia Sydney Toronto

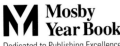
Mosby
Year Book
Dedicated to Publishing Excellence

Editor: Anne S. Patterson
Senior Developmental Editor: Kathryn H. Falk
Project Manager: John A. Rogers
Senior Production Editor: Helen C. Hudlin
Manuscript Editors: Kathy Lumpkin, Roger McWilliams
Production: Suzanne Fannin, Kathy Weigand
Book Design: Jeanne Wolfgeher

Mosby–Year Book, Inc., Company
11830 Westline Industrial Drive
St. Louis, Missouri 63146

Library of Congress Cataloging-in-Publication Data
Diagnostic radiology in emergency medicine / [edited by] Peter Rosen,
   et al.
       p. cm.
    Includes bibliographical references and index.
    ISBN 0-8016-6267-2
    1. Diagnosis, Radioscopic. 2. Emergency medicine. I. Rosen,
Peter.
    [DNLM: 1. Emergencies. 2. Emergency Medical Services.
3. Radiography--methods.   WN 200 D5365]
RC78.D48   1991
616.07'57--dc20
DLC
for Library of Congress   91-33719
                                                           CIP

00 99 98 C/MY 9 8 7

To my wife, Ann, whose patience in the production of this book considerably surpassed my own lack thereof.
Peter Rosen, **M.D.**

To the three persons who are my life: Carole, Tim, and Nancy, for always being there, and to my parents and Carole's parents.
Peter E. Doris, **M.D.**

To our children, Adam and Michael. for their tolerance and encouragement and to the continued collegiality of emergency physicians and radiologists in the care of patients on the front lines.
Roger M. Barkin, **M.D.**
Suzanne Z. Barkin, **M.D.**

To my wife, Leslie, and my children, Nicole, Tasha, and Nadia, for their continued love and support.
Vincent J. Markovchick, **M.D.**

CONTRIBUTORS

Jean Abbott, M.D.
Assistant Professor, Department of Surgery,
Section of Emergency Medicine,
University of Colorado School of Medicine,
Denver, Colorado

Richard V. Aghababian, M.D.
Associate Professor of Medicine;
Director, Division of Emergency Medicine,
University of Massachusetts Medical School,
Worcester, Massachusetts

Robert A. Barish, M.D.
Director, Emergency Medical Services;
Assistant Professor of Surgery,
University of Maryland Medical System/Hospital,
Baltimore, Maryland

Suzanne Z. Barkin, M.D.
Assistant Professor of Radiology,
University of Colorado Health Sciences Center;
Staff Radiologist,
Denver General Hospital,
Denver, Colorado

Steven M. Barrett, M.D.
Associate Professor of Surgery;
Chief, Section of Emergency Medicine,
University of Oklahoma Health Sciences Center,
Oklahoma City, Oklahoma

Robert P. Cavallino, M.D.
Clinical Associate Professor of Radiology,
University of Illinois College of Medicine;
Chairman, Department of Radiology,
Illinois Masonic Medical Center,
Chicago, Illinois

David Cohen, M.D.
Attending Physician,
Department of Emergency Medicine,
Good Samaritan Hospital,
Phoenix, Arizona

Douglas G. Connell, M.D., F.R.C.P.(C.)
Head, General Radiology and CT Scanning,
Department of Radiology,
Vancouver General Hospital;
Assistant Professor, Department of Radiology,
University of British Columbia,
Vancouver, British Columbia, Canada

Richard H. Daffner, M.D.
Professor of Radiologic Sciences,
Medical College of Pennsylvania;
Head, Section of Skeletal and Trauma Radiology,
Allegheny General Hospital;
Clinical Professor of Radiology, University of Pittsburgh,
Pittsburgh, Pennsylvania

Terrence C. Demos, M.D.
Professor of Radiology,
Loyola University Medical Center,
Maywood, Illinois

Peter E. Doris, M.D.
Clinical Associate Professor of Radiology and Medicine,
University of Chicago Hospitals,
Chicago, Illinois;
Medical Director, Department of Radiology,
St. Anthony Medical Center,
Crown Point, Indiana;
Consultant Radiologist,
St. James Hospital and Health Centers,
Chicago Heights, Illinois

Mary L. Dunne, M.D.
Attending Physician, Department of Emergency Medicine,
St. Francis Hospital,
Poughkeepsie, New York

Pat Dunne, M.D.
Attending Physician,
Department of Radiology, Cook County Hospital,
Chicago, Illinois

Michael P. Earnest, M.D.
Professor of Neurology and Preventive Medicine,
University of Colorado Health Sciences Center;
Director of Neurology, Denver General Hospital,
Denver, Colorado

Elizabeth A. Eelkema, M.D.
Staff Radiologist,
St. Clair Memorial Hospital,
Pittsburgh, Pennsylvania

Thomas Falvo, D.O.
Attending Physician,
Department of Emergency Medicine,
Jefferson Hospital,
Pittsburgh, Pennsylvania

Constance S. Greene, M.D.
Residency Director, Department of Emergency Medicine,
Cook County Hospital,
Chicago, Illinois

Wolfgang Goy, M.D.
Associate Chairman,
Department of Radiology and Diagnostic Imaging,
Maricopa Medical Center,
Phoenix, Arizona

Ann L. Harwood-Nuss, M.D.
Professor, Division of Emergency Medicine,
University of Florida Health Sciences Center,
Jacksonville, Florida

Marsha J. Heinig, M.D., Ph.D.
Assistant Professor of Radiology,
Department of Radiology,
University of Colorado Health Sciences Center;
Staff Radiologist,
Department of Radiology,
Denver General Hospital,
Denver, Colorado

Leo Hochhauser, M.D., F.R.C.P.(C.)
Assistant Professor, Department of Radiology,
S.U.N.Y. Health Science Center,
Syracuse, New York

Brian R. Holroyd, M.D., F.R.C.P.(C.)
Assistant Chief, Department of Emergency Medicine,
Valley Medical Center, Fresno, California;
Assistant Clinical Professor of Family and Community
    Medicine,
University of California School of Medicine,
San Francisco, California

D. Michael Hunt, M.D.
Assistant Professor, Department of Emergency Medicine,
George Washington University Medical Center,
Washington, D.C.

Kenneth C. Jackimczyk, M.D.
Program Director, Emergency Medicine Residency Program,
Department of Emergency Medicine,
Maricopa Medical Center,
Phoenix, Arizona

Thomas H. Johnson, M.D.
Professor, Department of Radiological Sciences,
University of Oklahoma Health Sciences Center,
Oklahoma City, Oklahoma

John G. Keene, M.D.
Director, Department of Emergency Medicine,
St. Francis Hospital,
Poughkeepsie, New York

Kevin J. Kirshenbaum, M.D.
Resident, Department of Radiology,
Illinois Masonic Medical Center,
Chicago, Illinois

Ron W. Lee, M.D.
Assistant Professor of Medicine;
Director, Section of Emergency Medicine,
Loyola University Medical Center,
Maywood, Illinois

Richard R. Lesperance, M.D.
Chief of Radiology,
Valley Medical Center, Fresno, California;
Associate Clinical Professor of Radiology,
University of California School of Medicine,
San Francisco, California

Louis J. Ling, M.D.
Senior Associate Physician,
Department of Emergency Medicine;
Associate Medical Director for Academic Affairs,
Hennepin County Medical Center,
Minneapolis, Minnesota

Neal Little, M.D.
Clinical Instructor, Department of Surgery,
University of Michigan Medical School;

Emergency Physician, St. Joseph Mercy Hospital,
Ann Arbor, Michigan

Vesna Martich, M.D.
Chief Resident, Department of Radiology,
University of Chicago Hospitals,
Chicago, Illinois

James J. Mathews, M.D.
Chief, Division of Emergency Medicine;
Associate Professor of Clinical Medicine,
Northwestern University Medical School,
Chicago, Illinois

Harold J. Matthies, M.D.
Assistant Professor of Radiology,
Northwestern University Medical School,
Chicago, Illinois

John B. McCabe, M.D.
Professor and Chairman, Department of Emergency Medicine,
S.U.N.Y. Health Science Center,
Syracuse, New York

John McGill, M.D.
Associate Physician,
Department of Emergency Medicine,
Hennepin County Medical Center,
Minneapolis, Minnesota

Steven M. Montner, M.D.
Assistant Professor of Radiology,
University of Chicago Hospitals,
Chicago, Illinois

Edward J. Newton, M.D., F.R.C.P.(C.)
Assistant Professor of Emergency Medicine,
University of Southern California Medical Center,
Los Angeles, California

Yuri R. Parisky, M.D.
Assistant Professor of Radiology,
University of Southern California Medical Center,
Los Angeles, California

Peter T. Pons, M.D.
Assistant Professor of Emergency Medicine,
Department of Surgery,
University of Colorado Health Sciences Center;
Associate Director, Emergency Department,
Denver General Hospital,
Denver, Colorado

Beatrice D. Probst, M.D.
Assistant Professor of Medicine,
Section of Emergency Medicine,
Loyola University Medical Center,
Maywood, Illinois

Peter Rosen, M.D.
Adjunct Professor, Departments of Medicine and Surgery;
Director of Education, Emergency Department,
University of California School of Medicine,
San Diego, California

Carl M. Sandler, M.D.
Professor of Radiology and Surgery (Urology);
Chief, Genitourinary Radiology,
The University of Texas Health Science Center at Houston,
Houston, Texas

Jeffrey J. Schaider, M.D.
Assistant Professor of Clinical Emergency Medicine,
University of Illinois College of Medicine;
Attending Physician, Department of Emergency Medicine,
Cook County Hospital,
Chicago, Illinois

Frederick J. Schwab, M.D.
Assistant Professor, Department of Radiology,
George Washington University Medical Center,
Washington, D.C.

George L. Sternbach, M.D.
Clinical Associate Professor of Surgery,
Emergency Medicine Service,
Stanford University Medical Center,
Stanford, California;
Emergency Physician, Seton Medical Center,
Daly City, California

David L. Symonds, M.D.
Assistant Professor of Radiology,
University of Colorado Health Sciences Center;
Attending Staff Radiologist, Denver General Hospital,
Denver, Colorado

Ellen Taliafero, M.D.
Staff Physician, San Francisco General Hospital,
San Francisco, California

Saul Taylor, M.D.
Assistant Professor of Radiology,
University of Minnesota Medical School;
Staff Radiologist,
Department of Radiology,
Hennepin County Medical Center,
Minneapolis, Minnesota

David Thickman, M.D.
Associate Professor and Chief, Division of Ultrasound,
Department of Radiology,
University of Colorado Health Sciences Center,
Denver, Colorado

Cynthia B. Umali, M.D.
Associate Professor of Radiology,
University of Massachusetts Medical School,
Worcester, Massachusetts

Ron M. Walls, M.D.
Head, Department of Emergency Medicine,
Vancouver General Hospital;
Head, Division of Emergency Medicine,
University of British Columbia,
Vancouver, British Columbia, Canada

James J. Walter, M.D.
Associate Professor and Chief,
Section of Emergency Medicine,
University of Chicago Hospitals,
Chicago, Illinois

DePriest Whye, Jr., M.D.
Assistant Professor,
Division of Emergency Medicine,
Department of Surgery,
University of Maryland Medical System/Hospital,
Baltimore, Maryland

Jeremy Young, M.D.
Associate Professor,
Department of Diagnostic Radiology,
University of Maryland Medical System/Hospital,
Baltimore, Maryland

PREFACE

A strong alliance exists between emergency medicine and radiology. With an average of 30% of imaging orders originating from the Emergency Medicine Department, not only is there a mutual need to understand each others' disciplines, there is also a need for effective communication between the two specialities to avoid errors in interpretation and in subsequent patient management. What is the value of a technically "perfect" imaging study when it is not indicated in the first place, no one can interpret it accurately in the second, and the reading is not timely?

This text is an attempt to address the mutual vision of the emergency physician and radiologist. The entire text has been written and edited by physicians representing both specialities. With this unique foundation, we have attempted to cover the important diagnostic steps in the evaluation of the emergency patient. The text is not intended as an atlas of every imaging study but rather as a guide to the radiographic approach in evaluating the emergency patient. The authors address the proper sequencing of radiographic studies and make recommendations concerning which studies provide optimal information based on national standards and on the various institutional philosophies as substantiated by the literature. If the radiographic approach to a clinical problem has not been standardized by clinical consensus, an equally acceptable alternative is presented with discussion of when either would be preferable. When no published data are available, the practice preferences of the individual authors are recommended.

There will, of course, be disagreement with the philosophies and management sequences that are recommended. The editors of this text make no pretense to represent the final word on all clinical dilemmas. Our intent is to recommend a prudent and acceptable practice that makes logistic as well as clinical sense. This intent is based on the real and extensive clinical experience of the editors and authors. The text is intended not only for the emergency physician in training or practice but also for the radiologist in training or practice. In addition, hopefully, this text will assist both the physician who may practice in a setting where only an occasional major emergency arises as well as the physician who practices in a major trauma center. It is our hope that by creating a road map for effective clinical interaction, there will be an improved alliance and congeniality between the two specialities. Finally, we have been most fortunate to have had the benefit of mutual interaction between our two specialities in writing this text, and it is the expressed hope of the editors that this experience will benefit all of our colleagues and, of course, the patient.

Peter Rosen
Peter E. Doris
Roger M. Barkin
Suzanne Z. Barkin
Vincent J. Markovchick

ACKNOWLEDGEMENTS

With gratitude, we acknowledge the following individuals who have helped make this text a reality:

The authors, for the selfless sharing of their time, effort and knowledge; Helen Hudlin, Kathryn Falk, Kathi Thompson, Anne Patterson and the Mosby team, for their unfailing attention to detail and for making all the pieces come together in a timely fashion;

Marty Martell, for her tremendous assistance;

The St. Anthony radiologists and St. James radiologists and the members of the Departments of Radiology and the medical staffs at St. Anthony and St. James Hospital Medical Centers, who have participated in this, a team effort; Sister Antoinette Marie Vanderwerf, O.S.F, Stephen Leurck, and John Douglas, for their confidence; Janet Maginot and Pat Meyer, for their patience and understanding; Raphael Wilson, Chien-Tai Lu, David Levin, and Martin Hochhauser, for their guidance and inspiration; the Mayo consultants, James Greene and Martha Mechei, for their clinical focus on the patient; and Peter Rosen, who has remembered a conversation in 1972 about Emergency Radiology for twenty years;

The members of the Department of Pediatrics and Newborn Medicine at Rose Medical Center, the members of the Departments of Surgery and Radiology at the University of Colorado Health Sciences Centers, and the members of the Department of Radiology at Denver General Hospital, for their instrumental support in bringing this book to fruition;

And Linda Schearer, for her patience and outstanding support.

Our sincerest appreciation.

CONTENTS

Diagnostic Radiology in
Emergency Medicine

General Principles

General Principles

George L. Sternbach
Peter E. Doris
Peter Rosen

Few scientific developments have influenced the clinical practice of medicine as profoundly as did the discovery by Wilhelm Conrad Roentgen of "a new kind of rays" in 1895. Roentgen named the phenomena "x-rays" because of their then unknown character. Even the initial communication describing his investigations presaged a medical use: "If the hand be held between the discharge-tube and the screen, the darker shadow of the bones is seen within the slightly dark shadow-image of the hand itself."[1]

A remarkable aspect of the subsequent development of radiography was the rapid acceptance it achieved as a standard medical diagnostic method. Almost immediately after Roentgen had produced the photographic image of his hand, the popular press was filled with extravagant projections of what the new mystery rays could reveal. Experimentation began that promptly entered radiographs into the diagnostic armamentarium. This process subsequently led to the development of adjunctive techniques such as conventional tomography, contrast urography, angiography, and computed tomography. However, plain radiography still forms much of the basis of diagnostic medicine today.

The emergency physician makes extensive use of radiography, and progress in the field has been reflected as strongly in the practice of emergency medicine as in any area of clinical medicine. Emergency medicine requires the regular utilization of x-ray studies. In fact, other than the radiologist no other medical specialist is required to possess familiarity with as wide a gamut of radiographic subjects as is the emergency physician. In no other field is the practitioner required to order and interpret so great an array of radiographs: studies of the head, neck, face, spine, thorax, abdomen, pelvis, and all aspects of the extremities. The interpretive knowledge required ranges from appreciation of subtle findings that may be the harbingers of important but noncritical pathology to the interpretation of difficult radiographs on whose correct reading the patient's life or function may depend.

For each emergency patient, a decision must be made regarding treatment and disposition. This decision is based on conclusions about the nature and severity of the illness and may affect whether a patient receives a given form of treatment, hospitalization, or referral. Deferral of this decision is sometimes an option, but most often it is deleterious to delay. Radiographic studies may form the crux of the diagnostic investigation that enables the emergency physician to formulate a correct and prudent decision. At times it will be possible to involve a radiology consultant to aid in this process, but frequently the emergency physician will have to make the decision alone.

The emergency physician must, therefore, develop a philosophy about the use of diagnostic radiography. It should be a flexible approach so that the management of each patient is individual. However, there has to be some basis for ordering and interpreting x-ray studies, and this philosophy should be integrated into the overall principles of emergency medicine.

CARE OF THE CRITICALLY ILL PATIENT

In no other area is a coherent philosophy of radiographic use more essential than in the resuscitation of the critically ill patient. In this setting the philosophy will reflect a certain ambivalence. For the patient who is not critically ill, the timing of a radiographic study in the assessment sequence is straightforward. However, in dealing with the critically ill patient, timing of studies represents a two-edged sword: on the one hand, it may provide the key for making or excluding a diagnosis in a situation in which there may be no other easy way for this to be done. On the other hand, obtaining a necessary radiograph may obstruct the expeditious resuscitation, stabilization, monitoring, and management of the patient.

No matter how valuable the radiographic proof of any condition might be, it must be secondary to patient stability. For example, having the patient sit up for a chest x-ray study may provide more accurate information about intrathoracic pathology but might cause a hypovolemic patient to sustain a fatal dysrhythmia.

Therefore, it has long been our dictum that no procedure of a purely diagnostic nature should be instituted until stabilization of the patient has been achieved. There should be no radiographic study employed until the airway has been established, and respiratory and circulatory integrity have been assured. The critically ill patient's first requirement is not radiographic proof of a given pathology; it is the rapid assessment and support of vital life functions.

In fact, there are a number of instances in which obtaining a radiograph is actually contraindicated. For example, the physician who deems it necessary to obtain a chest radiograph depicting a suspected case of tension pneumothorax may later be called on to explain why the diagnosis of this life-threatening condition was not made on clinical grounds and why the patient was allowed to undergo the delay inherent in the radiography process, a delay that could only exacerbate the condition.

Even after patient stabilization has been initiated, optimal information may be difficult to elicit without having the patient positioned in a way that may not be desirable. There is no question, for example, that a great deal more information about the presence and size of a hemothorax can be obtained from an upright rather than a supine chest radiograph. However, it is often contraindicated to place the patient in this position because of the risk of injury to the cervical spine. Radiographic assessment of pneumoperitoneum also strongly depends on positioning the patient. A considerable amount of free air can be present without any abnormality being noted on a supine abdominal radiograph. On the other hand, even a few cubic centimeters of air can be detected beneath the diaphragm if the patient is positioned properly. Unfortunately, this may involve an upright position before exposing the film, which is something a very ill patient may not be able to tolerate. A similar difficulty arises regarding assessment of a chest radiograph for evidence of a great vessel injury. The information provided by a portable supine chest radiograph is certainly limited. Even if the radiograph is of good quality (which the exigency of performing the procedure may pre-

vent), the mediastinum will inevitably be widened, its borders indistinct, and a small hemothorax can be obscured.

An important decision, then, involves when (if ever) a patient is sufficiently stable to assume a position in which the radiograph will yield the most useful information. A related decision involves whether a patient is stable enough to transfer from the emergency department to a special studies suite to undergo further evaluation. In the case of plain radiographs, a compromise may involve accepting the limitations of the portable technique. However, in instances of special studies that cannot be performed portably, this is not an option.

The difficulty of transferring the patient is compounded by the fact that the special studies suite is frequently an undesirable place to deal with the possibility of cardiac arrest or substantial patient deterioration. As an area, it may be physically remote from the emergency department and be lacking in space, access to the patient, and suitable personnel to conduct an optimal resuscitation.

Even routine monitoring or nursing functions become difficult or impossible when the patient is placed in a CT scanner gantry. Moreover, patients may become confused or combative from the sensory deprivation of a darkened radiologic room. There are no side rails on x-ray tables, and many confused patients have been put at risk of falling during radiographic examination.

ORDERING RADIOGRAPHIC STUDIES

The emergency physician should establish principles to guide the ordering of studies. Intelligent ordering and use of studies require knowledge of the nature of an illness or the mechanism of an injury. Although radiographic evaluation constitutes an important part of the overall evaluation of many conditions, it should be seen as augmenting rather than supplanting thorough physical evaluation. Neither should the radiograph be viewed before the patient is examined (though it is recognized that in many institutions a triage officer will order studies before the physician has contact with the patient). The practitioner must request the most appropriate radiographic views for various situations. This can only be accomplished on the basis of examination of the patient. In a patient with an injury to the shoulder, for example, it must be determined whether diagnosis will best be served by a view of the glenohumeral joint, clavicle, scapula, or the acromioclavicular joint (with or without weight bearing).

Recognizing the place of adjunctive views available to complement standard projections is also useful. For example, in addition to a standard series of the knee, special views may be necessary. Examples of these are the axial or "sunrise" view to visualize the patella, the intercondylar or "tunnel" projection to delineate the tibial tubercles, and stress views to reflect the degree of stability of the collateral ligaments. In fact, whenever an extremity view is obtained, especially in dealing with trauma, it is good policy to be sure that the entire extremity involved appears on the radiograph, including both the proximal and distal joints. There may be injuries in the contiguous skeleton or soft tissue away from the site of maximal trauma that may be missed if the radiographic focus is too narrow.

Although it is generally best to limit radiographs to the area involved and avoid indiscriminate ordering, there are times when a wide range of radiographic evaluation is in order. For example, localizing a bullet is often difficult. The path that a bullet may take in the body is often unpredictable. The localization of a bullet below the diaphragm in a patient who is shot in the chest may entirely change the course of treatment. Consequently, all the potential paths that a bullet might take in the body must be considered, and studies ordered accordingly.

In addition, the physician must be cognizant of common injury associations. For example, fracture of the calcaneus suffered in a fall should call to mind the possibility of associated spinal fracture. Clinical presentation may not be an infallible guide to the presence of such concurrently sustained injuries. For instance, the patient may not be simultaneously aware of two foci of pain because of the phenomenon of extinction of simultaneous afferent sensory inputs.

One should also be aware of the relatively low yield of certain studies. For example, the lumbosacral spine series in most cases of back pain is often ordered for other than strictly medical indications but rarely shows any pathology. Another example is the plain film abdominal study in appendicitis, which rarely provides a diagnosis that was not suspected before it was ordered.

It is sometimes necessary to have radiographs repeated after therapeutic intervention has occurred or to follow changes in the patient's status. The postreduction radiograph after a bone fracture has been manipulated is an obvious example. Also, studies need to be obtained after central venous lines are inserted to ensure that no pneumothorax has been induced and to ascertain proper position of the catheter.

RADIOGRAPHIC INTERPRETATION

The first rule of radiographic interpretation is that it must take place. The physician ordering a study is responsible for its evaluation. (The requirement in the case of special studies is somewhat different and will be discussed later.) It is not prudent to blindly accept the reading of a consultant, though we by no means wish to discourage obtaining appropriate consultation.

In evaluating the radiograph, one must first ascertain that the technical quality of the study is adequate, the degree of exposure is appropriate, and the entire area of concern has, in fact, been included on the radiograph. Every physician has had the experience of being handed a chest radiograph with a costophrenic sulcus "cut off" or with a patient identification plate that overlies a crucial area of interest. Such studies must be augmented or repeated.

Once a study has been performed, the entire radiograph must be evaluated for abnormalities. Findings in addition to the one anticipated should be noted. In a chest radiograph ordered for assessment of possible pneumonia, one must still evaluate other areas such as the cardiac silhouette, the mediastinum, and the soft tissues.

The presence of a particularly dramatic abnormality will often divert the viewer's attention from other findings. It may in fact be wise to literally cover an area of overt abnormality (or at least to consciously disregard it) while the remainder of the radiograph is evaluated. It is prudent to follow the dictum: "look in the corners of the film." Such a systematic assessment of the entire radiograph will minimize the chances of overlooking important but subtle abnormalities.

Comparison views are sometimes extremely important as an aid in evaluating a finding of unclear significance. Obtaining views of the contralateral extremity in a child is an obvious example. The comparison of the epiphyseal pattern may be instrumental in determining whether a lucent line viewed on the radiograph represents a fracture or the cartilaginous portion of an epiphysis. There are also instances in adults in which viewing the opposite side may be helpful in diagnosis. A number of congenital variations have a tendency toward bilaterality. For example, bipartite patella, which may at times be confused with patellar fracture, is frequently present bilaterally. The presence of such a variant on the uninvolved side may be extremely reassuring evidence against a fracture.

In the category of comparison radiographs, which is most important and often overlooked, one may need to look no further than the radiographic file room. Previous radiographic studies can be compared, and clarification can often be made on the basis of this comparison. At times the patient may be saved an extensive evaluation when it can be determined that abnormalities are pre-existing rather than acute.

SPECIAL STUDIES

It is often necessary to use adjunctive radiographic studies, such as computed tomography (CT scan), ultrasonography, angiography, magnetic resonance imaging (MRI), or contrast urography. The emergency physician must, of course, have a clear idea of which studies are indicated for the diagnosis of various conditions. However, the role of the radiology consultant must also be considered. Frequently, a consultant must be called on to perform or interpret the study. Consequently, the proper coordination of such studies with the consultant is important, and communication of precisely which findings are being sought and other particulars regarding the patient is essential.

In determining which special studies should be done, it is important that the emergency physician remain informed about technologic advances. Thus the CT scan has dramatically changed diagnostic assessment of patients with head injury and other intracranial processes. In the emergency situation, as elsewhere, use of a head CT scan has become standard in the assessment of a number of clinical entities and has displaced or entirely eliminated a number of other procedures from the diagnostic queue.

Unfortunately, the availability of certain technologies also introduces a risk of overuse or inappropriate timing. When a patient has developed a herniation syndrome, obtaining a CT scan to document the presence of an epidural hematoma may prevent patient salvage or may increase morbidity because what the patient needs is a cranial decompression not a diagnostic procedure.

Moreover, it is insufficient merely to throw technology at a clinical problem. There is not much unanimity, for example, about the place of abdominal CT scans in emergency evaluation, especially regarding their place in assessment of blunt abdominal injury. The advantages and disadvantages of abdominal CT scans vs. diagnostic peritoneal lavage are highly controversial, and the relative sensitivities of these procedures have been vigorously debated in the medical literature.[2-8]

The extent to which special studies are used is quite variable from institution to institution. The emergency physician must make note of the preference and expertise of the consultant, as this will influence the quality of information a special study will provide. With regard to the controversy surrounding the abdominal CT scan, for example, it may be that the main variable is not the sensitivity of the study itself so much as the capability of interpreting the scan—that is, the ability and experience of the radiologist.[2]

The emergency physician must know the contraindications and precautions to performing various special studies. This particularly involves problems of administering radiographic contrast material. In addition, it is the emergency physician who is most likely to be called on if an adverse reaction to radiographic contrast occurs and he must be adept at management of the various complications that may arise.

The emergency physician should, furthermore, be cognizant of precisely the degree of diagnostic investigation necessary to be undertaken in the emergency department and should resist the pursuit of additional studies if patient management will not be influenced by the results.

DISPOSITION

Although it is obvious that radiographs frequently play a substantial role in the formulation of a prudent patient disposition, it is well to recall that one must treat the patient rather than the radiograph. When radiographic evidence differs from that garnered by evaluation of the patient, a conservative approach must be pursued. Therefore, for example, if a fracture is strongly suspected clinically

but there is no radiographic confirmation, the patient must be treated as though a fracture exists. The clinical suspicion may be confirmed or excluded at a later time with follow-up radiographs or other studies. For instance, fracture of the carpal navicular is a well-recognized entity for which immobilization is recommended on clinical grounds irrespective of the lack of abnormal radiographic findings. Application of this philosophy is especially important in treating trauma to the lower extremities because of continued damage that weight bearing may cause to a limb in which a fracture was mistakenly thought to have been excluded.

ADDITIONAL CONSIDERATIONS

There are certain limitations to the information radiographs provide and these must be recognized. The appearance of a Salter V epiphyseal fracture may be quite benign. The presence of a normal chest radiograph is compatible with (in fact is the rule in) acute pulmonary embolism, and the presence of negative radiographs should by no means be reassuring with respect to the absence of pathology in such clinical possibilities. When the radiograph is not diagnostic, additional studies may be required.

Radiographic studies will, at times, be ordered for medico-legal or medicopsychologic rather than strictly medical indications. Many patients harbor a magical faith in the capabilities of x-rays, one that is frequently not justified. Such patients may come to the emergency department with the expectation that radiographic assessment will form a portion of their evaluation, and they may be more readily reassured (sometimes unreasonably so) by a set of negative radiographs than by an opinion based on clinical judgment. Currently we do not recommend that radiographic studies be ordered without a sound reason but rather believe that the place of such studies should be considered within the overall sphere of the patient's expectations.

REFERENCES

1. Glasser O: *Wilhelm Conrad Roentgen and the early history of the roentgen rays,* Springfield, Ill, 1934, Charles C Thomas.
2. Bresler MJ: Computed tomography vs peritoneal lavage in blunt abdominal trauma, *Topics Emerg Med* 10:59, 1988.
3. Goldstein AS, Sclafani SJA, Kupferstein NH et al: The diagnostic superiority of computed tomography, *J Trauma* 25:938, 1985.
4. Marx JA, Moore EE, Jorden RC et al: Limitations of computed tomography in the evaluation of acute abdominal trauma: a prospective comparison with diagnostic peritoneal lavage, *J Trauma* 25:933, 1985.
5. Pietzman AB, Makaroun MS, Slasky BS et al: Prospective study of computed tomography in initial management of blunt abdominal trauma, *J Trauma* 26:585, 1986.
6. Fabian TC, Mangiante EC, White TJ et al: A prospective study of 91 patients undergoing both computed tomography and peritoneal lavage following blunt abdominal trauma, *J Trauma* 26:602, 1986.
7. Bresler MJ: Computed tomography of the abdomen, *Ann Emerg Med* 15:280, 1986.
8. Henneman PL, Marx JA: Diagnostic peritoneal lavage vs CT, *Ann Emerg Med* 15:1509, 1986.

PART TWO

Trauma

2

Multiple Trauma

Ron M. Walls
Douglas G. Connell

Timely and correct management of the patient who has been subjected to multisystem trauma requires the highest level of integrated emergency department functioning. This chapter outlines an organized approach to the multiple trauma patient, including patients with multisystem trauma as well as those with isolated trauma accompanied by shock. In either circumstance, optimal patient management depends on the establishment of a sound plan for dealing with the patient and activation of such a plan long before the patient arrives in the emergency department. In major trauma hospitals, trauma response is accomplished by a multidisciplinary team under the directorship of a captain and includes many personnel in addition to physicians and nurses. In the small rural hospital, initial trauma response may consist solely of a single attending physician with the assistance of one or more nurses and extremely limited ancillary and diagnostic services. In either case, the overall response to trauma must be planned, delineated, and documented, and all personnel responding to

trauma must be intimately familiar with their specific tasks and their role within this framework.

The principal issues involved in the radiographic assessment of the multiple trauma patient are:

- Choice and sequence of appropriate radiographic studies and the interplay between these studies and general trauma resuscitation, including the role of radiography in the primary hospital when early transfer to a regional trauma center is inevitable.
- Physical, configurational, and technical responsibilities of individual patient evaluations.
- Role of the radiologist as a consultant.

SELECTION AND SEQUENCING OF RADIOGRAPHIC ASSESSMENT
ABCs of trauma radiology

The issues of appropriate sequence, ordering of priorities, and the integration of radiographic assessment into the overall management of the trauma patient can perhaps best be addressed by considering the ABCs of trauma resuscitation and relating these to the ABCs of trauma radiology.[1] The widely known ABCs of trauma resuscitation are:

- **A** irway
- **B** reathing
- **C** irculation

Addition of **D** for disability, representing a screening neurologic examination, and **E** for exposure, representing complete removal of the patient's garments, completes the primary survey advocated by the American College of Surgeons.[1] *There is no role for radiographic assessment of the multiple trauma patient during the performance of the primary survey.* In general, the entire primary survey is completed within minutes of the patient's arrival. Essential radiographic assessment is performed as early as possible during the secondary survey phase of trauma resuscitation.

Although guidelines may be used to represent general principles and approach, radiographic assessment of the multiple trauma patient must be individualized, and flexibility and minute-by-minute modification are essential. With this proviso, one can recommend specific ABCs of trauma radiology (see box opposite).

Adaptation of this basic framework will facilitate an appropriate sequence of radiographic assessment and will prevent omission of essential studies.

Axial skeleton (cervical spine radiography). All victims of blunt multisystem trauma must be assumed to have a cervical or other spinal injury until this is excluded by a combination of clinical examination and radiographic study.[1-4] Therefore all patients should be immobilized on a long spine board or equivalent device until it is known to be safe to remove these precautions. In the context of multiple trauma, it is essential to know early in the course of the resuscitation whether spinal column injury has occurred. Injury to the cervical, thoracic, or lumbar spine may substantially alter management decisions.

The nature and timing of radiographic assessment of the spine depends on the management philosophy of the physician or institution. In a center where nasotracheal intubation is the initial airway maneuver of choice, cervical spine radiography may be deferred until later in the course of resuscitation because the radiographic findings may have little impact on management of the airway.[1,4,5] If the airway maneuver of choice, however, is orotracheal intubation with in-line immobilization, knowledge of a potentially unstable cervical spine injury may be of paramount importance.[6-9] Similarly, early cervical spine radiography is essential in those centers that use cricothyrotomy rather than orotracheal intubation with in-line immobilization as the initial procedure in the patient with a potentially unstable cervical spine.[10-12] These centers do not consider oral intubation with in-line immobilization to be safe until, as a minimum, a lateral radiograph, showing all seven cervical vertebrae and the cervicothoracic junction, demonstrates absence of injury.[13-16] It will be left to the reader to modify the suggested approach to ensure optimal management in each individual institution and situation and as philosophy of traumatic airway management evolves.

The question arises: does *every* multiple trauma patient require radiography of the cervical spine? In order to exclude cervical spine injury on the basis of clinical examination alone and without the use of cervical spine radiography, all of the conditions listed in the box above must be met[17-20] (see Chapter 3).

It is readily apparent that it is essentially futile to attempt to exclude cervical spine injury on clinical grounds in the context of multisystem trauma because the likelihood of meeting all of these conditions is exceedingly remote in this patient population. *Therefore all victims of blunt multisystem trauma require cervical spine radiography early in the course of their resuscitation.*

ABCs of trauma radiology

A xial skeleton (cervical spine radiography)
B reathing (chest radiography)
C irculation (pelvic radiography)
D efinitive diagnostic studies (including computed tomography, intravenous pyelography, angiography, etc.)
E xtremities

Clinical exclusion of cervical spine injury

- The patient has a normal mental status, unclouded by head injury, drug or ethanol intoxication, excessive anxiety, and psychiatric or medical conditions.
- The patient is able to understand and communicate well with the examiner.
- The patient has had no complaints of neck pain of any kind at any time since the traumatic incident.
- There is no significant injury that might distract the patient's attention sufficiently to obscure nominal cervical pain (e.g., fractured femur, chest wall contusion).
- There is no tenderness to palpation of the cervical spine.
- There is no neurologic disorder of the trunk or extremities evident by history or physical examination.

However, patients with isolated single-system trauma with shock, such as those with traumatic amputation of an arm or leg by industrial machinery, can be assumed to be free of spinal injury if it is known that there was no mechanism for such injury to have occurred. In other cases, spinal radiography should be considered. Paradoxically, victims of penetrating trauma present a somewhat more complex situation. In these cases, radiography of the spine is indicated only if the injury is suspected to have directly involved the spine, or if there was associated blunt trauma accompanying the penetrating trauma, such as a patient who was stabbed in the chest and then fell down a flight of stairs. In any case, where doubt exists, spinal radiography should be considered (see Chapters 3 and 9).

Until recently, radiographic evaluation of the cervical spine was performed in the vast majority of trauma patients, while radiography of the thoracic and lumbar spine was reserved only for those cases in which there was significant likelihood of injury to these areas. Recently, however, there has been an increasing weight of opinion that lateral in place radiographs of the thoracic and lumbar vertebrae should be part of the diagnostic evaluation of any patient who has sustained significant blunt trauma and in whom the conditions outlined in the box above cannot be met.[21-25] For instance, patients who formerly died of massive motor vehicle injuries are surviving because of seat belt use, improved vehicle design, additional safety features such as airbags, and improved prehospital care.[26,27] Therefore, the frequency of identification of thoracic and lumbar spine fractures is increasing.[21,22,26] Thus, if any doubt exists as to the presence of injury, it is appropriate to obtain lateral radiographs of the cervical, thoracic, and lumbar spine as part of the evaluation of the patient who has suffered blunt multiple trauma. Of these areas, a lateral radiograph of the cervical spine should be obtained first because of the importance of cervical spine radiography in active airway management. In general, the thoracic and lumbar spine studies can be obtained along with studies of the extremities in the secondary radiographic survey, unless there is a clinical indication to proceed on a more urgent basis (see Chapter 9). Until radiographic evaluation of the entire spine is complete, the patient should remain immobilized on a long spine board.

Breathing (chest radiography). As in the case with the cervical spine, occult injury to the thoracic cavity or its contents can substantially alter the patient's course and the sequence of management decisions. Therefore a chest radiograph should be obtained early in the course of the secondary survey for all multiply injured patients.[1,21] Absence of chest crepitus, subcutaneous emphysema, or objective evidence of pneumothorax, bony thoracic injury, or other intrathoracic pathology does not lessen the need for a chest radiograph although it may allow the radiograph to be deferred to slightly later during the resuscitative sequence. Just as the absence of clinical evidence of chest injury does not preclude the need for chest radiography, treatment of obvious or strongly suspected thoracic injuries should not be delayed pending radiographic confirmation. For example, the hypotensive blunt trauma patient with obvious thoracic cage injury and subcutaneous emphysema requires immediate tube thoracostomy; this should not be delayed until there is radiographic confirmation of pneumothorax (see Chapter 5).

Circulation (pelvic radiography). It is most important to obtain an anteroposterior (AP) view of the pelvis in all cases of major multisystem trauma.[1,21,28] The absence of apparent injury on physical examination is often unreliable and is clouded by the patient's altered mental status or the presence of other injuries. Early identification of pelvic fracture is essential to permit appropriate stabilization, management, and preparation for the often enormous number of transfusions that such a patient may require.[29-33] Interpretation of clinical findings, such as hematuria, or diagnostic tests, such as peritoneal lavage, will also be influenced by pelvic fracture.[34] Finally, angiography with or without embolization may be indicated for severe, on-going hemorrhage in the patient with pelvic fracture[29,30,32-37] (see Chapters 7 and 8).

Definitive diagnostic studies. The decision to undertake definitive diagnostic studies, such as computed tomography (CT scan) or contrast studies, is primarily influenced by the patient's condition and by the physical con-

figuration and characteristics of the hospital. A patient who has suffered catastrophic injury, such as massive intra-abdominal hemorrhage, requires immediate operative treatment and it is unlikely that definitive diagnostic studies can be undertaken preoperatively. In these cases, a "one-shot" intravenous pyelogram (IVP) might be the only study indicated.

The availability of diagnostic radiography facilities may also influence the decision to undertake further studies. For example, if the CT scanner is adjacent to the trauma resuscitation suite, then CT scans will be readily accessible. If, on the other hand, the scanner is located a substantial distance from the emergency department, it may be considered unwise to expose the patient to the risk of a long transport and a substantial period of time outside the safe confines of the resuscitation area.

Similarly, there is a tendency to obtain too many radiographic studies on patients who require transfer to a regional trauma center. In fact, if there is clear indication for transfer following the completion of the ABC part of the trauma radiology sequence, it is probably unwise to proceed with additional radiographic studies unless these can be done without any attendant delay in the patient's transfer. It is a tragedy when patients arrive at the regional trauma center in traumatic arrest with innumerable extremity radiographs and other unnecessary and time-consuming diagnostic studies accompanying them.

The decision to undertake definitive diagnostic studies must be carefully coordinated. The vascular surgeon who has been consulted may want to proceed immediately with aortic arch angiography, and the trauma surgeon or general surgeon may want an abdominal CT scan, with intravenous and gastrointestinal contrast. Proper coordination of these studies is essential to prevent excessive administration of contrast material. The role of the radiologist as a consultant is particularly important during this phase.

Extremities. In general, radiographic examination of the extremities should be the final study undertaken during the course of trauma resuscitation. Exception to this may occur when there is a dislocation with obvious vascular compromise and an immediate radiographic study is indicated. Radiographs of the thoracic and lumbar spine generally will be obtained at this point in the resuscitative sequence if they were not obtained earlier. It is important that this phase of the radiographic evaluation of the patient not be omitted or conducted in a superficial manner. A significant number of injuries are not diagnosed in the multiply injured patient because of inadequate examination of available radiographs and also because appropriate radiographs have not been obtained.[38-41]

Obtaining appropriate radiographic studies

The expertise and facilities available within the hospital and the physical configuration of the trauma area will profoundly influence decisions concerning radiographic studies.

In the community hospital with limited trauma response and only basic radiographic capability, patient assessment and stabilization should focus on the Advanced Trauma Life Support (ATLS) primary and secondary surveys in conjunction with the ABCs of trauma radiology outlined previously. Studies falling under category *D* or *E* in trauma radiology should be undertaken in the community hospital only when (1) information from these studies is essential in order to make a decision regarding transfer of the patient, (2) information is considered important for patient management and patient transfer will not be delayed, or (3) patient transfer is not anticipated.

In all other cases, realization that the patient requires definitive care in another hospital should stimulate prompt initiation of transfer procedures and curtailment of further diagnostic radiographic studies that can be later undertaken in the trauma-receiving hospital.

In larger hospitals, of course, a wider range of radiographic services is available. These services can be divided into basic radiology and special diagnostic studies.

Basic radiology. Basic radiology refers to plain film radiography and simple contrast studies such as intravenous pyelography and urethrography. Most of these studies should be obtained in the trauma resuscitation area during the phase of patient care when it is not safe to allow the patient to leave the emergency department to go to the radiology suite. It is not appropriate that the patient be taken to another part of the hospital, no matter how proximate, to obtain radiographs that are needed during the early phases of resuscitation. Development of such films must be prompt, and there must be a mechanism for returning them immediately to the trauma resuscitation area to be viewed by the physician caring for the patient. Ideally, a film processor should be located near the trauma resuscitation area. Similar considerations apply to the location of the radiology facility that is used by the emergency department. It is strongly advisable to have an emergency radiology area that is dedicated to the service of emergency patients located in, or immediately adjacent to, the emergency department. This has the advantage of close proximity and also fosters the spirit of communication and cooperation that results in optimal patient assessment and safety. A well equipped radiology facility adjacent to the emergency department will provide complete radiographic service for the vast majority of emergency patients and will permit prompt and safe evaluation of multiple trauma patients.

Special diagnostic studies. Although desirable, it is rarely possible to locate the angiography and computed tomography suites in close proximity to the emergency department. In modern teaching hospitals, what is often considered "close" to the emergency department may require a transfer of several hundred yards down a corridor from the emergency department trauma area to the diagnostic radiology suite. Such a transfer represents a highly vulnerable period for the patient, and exposure to this unsafe environ-

ment should be minimized. Although it is recognized that "high-tech" radiology services, which are used predominantly by inpatients, cannot necessarily be located adjacent to the emergency department, their location should be such that critically ill patients can undergo these essential diagnostic studies in a timely fashion. There must be policies adopted regarding the safe transport of patients to and from the radiology facility and a requirement that a physician or other personnel should be in continuous attendance who is capable of monitoring and undertaking resuscitative measures should the patient suddenly deteriorate.

Portable vs. radiology department radiographs. It is often difficult to decide whether to undertake radiographic studies using a portable or built-in technique in the trauma area as opposed to sending the patient to the emergency radiology facility. As outlined previously, the location of the emergency radiology facility may influence this decision substantially. In any case, there are three prime considerations when deciding to obtain portable films: (1) exposure of emergency department personnel to ionizing radiation, (2) technical inferiority of portable radiographs, and (3) patient safety.

Exposure of emergency department personnel to ionizing radiation. Exposure to radiation during portable imaging is caused by deflected (scatter) radiation. When an x-ray photon is deflected or scattered by the patient, it retains most of its original energy. In standard x-rays, 50% to 90% of the total number of photons emerging from the patient are scatter radiation. With thick regions, such as the abdomen, only 1% of the photons from the initial beam reach the x-ray film. The remainder are scattered.[42] All ionizing radiation is harmful and exposure to such radiation must be minimized. Radiation may cause harm to an individual by two mechanisms: the somatic effect and the genetic effect. The possibility of inducing carcinoma in an individual is called the somatic effect. Leukemia is the most common neoplasm that may be induced. Although the risk is small, there is no doubt that low doses of radiation can cause neoplasms usually after long latent periods, ranging from 5 to 20 years. The second harmful effect of radiation is the genetic effect on future generations. This effect is more complex and depends more on exposure of large segments of the population to radiation than on exposure of a few individuals. Nevertheless it remains a concern.

Exposure to radiation may be controlled by three factors: time, distance, and barriers. By limiting the time portable equipment is used, exposure is minimized. Only portable radiographs that are essential should be obtained when emergency staff are in an unprotected area. Also, during x-ray exposure, whenever possible, staff should remove themselves from the immediate area and stand behind protective shields.

One of the most effective means of reducing radiation exposure is by distancing oneself from the patient. This is an extremely effective way of limiting exposure since radiation exposure diminishes inversely with the square of distance. For example, for a field size (exposed area of the patient) of 400 cm^2, scatter radiation is reduced by a factor of 1000 at a distance of 1 m.

The final way of diminishing radiation is to use barriers. The most effective are fixed barriers that may be in close proximity to the resuscitation area and behind which staff may momentarily step during an exposure. In the event that one cannot step aside even for a few brief seconds (which in most instances should prove possible), a lead apron may be worn. In almost all instances, by combining the three methods, exposure of staff to radiation can be kept to an acceptable minimum. Radiation exposure monitors may be used by staff in unprotected areas and will confirm that the methods are, in fact, effective.[43,44]

Technical inferiority of portable radiographs. In general, radiographs obtained in the radiology department will be superior to those obtained by portable technique (see later discussion).

Patient safety. Despite the preceding considerations, the patient's condition may mandate portable radiographs. The patient often will not be "stable" enough to permit safe transfer to the radiology department to obtain the studies, no matter how stable and uninjured the patient might initially appear. Trauma patients are often young and well compensated initially but rapidly deteriorate once the compensatory mechanisms are exceeded. Therefore all initial radiographs (the ABCs of trauma radiology) should be obtained in the emergency department using portable equipment or fixed equipment that is built into the resuscitation area. Once these have been obtained, however, and the patient has exhibited substantial stability in respiratory, hemodynamic, and CNS function, more sophisticated radiographic studies can be obtained in the radiology department.

ANATOMIC AND PHYSICAL CONSIDERATIONS
Patient and facility considerations

The decision to obtain radiographs using portable technique as opposed to transporting the patient to the radiology department is of primary importance when designing the trauma unit. The volume and nature of trauma patients, location of the emergency radiology suite, existence of an emergency radiology suite distinct from the main radiology department, availability of consultative service within the hospital, and numerous other factors will affect the decision to obtain portable radiographs. Certain specific limitations on performing various radiographic studies on the emergency patient will be discussed in detail in the chapters that follow. However, there are particular difficulties encountered in the general evaluation of the multiple trauma patient.

Virtually every multiple trauma patient will be immobilized on a long spine board with a semi-rigid cervical collar and varying use of tape, sandbags, belts, straps, and other immobilization devices applied. Although this im-

mobilization is of paramount importance to protect the patient from spinal cord injury, such devices present significant obstacles to the radiographic assessment of the patient. Most important of these obstacles is the inability of the patient to be placed in an upright position, either sitting or standing, to facilitate proper chest radiography. Similarly, cervical spine radiography would be substantially simplified if it were possible to place the patient in the upright position. This would result in a natural lowering of the shoulders and easier visualization of the cervical thoracic junction. However, because of injuries, simple maneuvers, such as gentle wrist traction to draw the shoulders down and permit cervical spine radiography, are rendered more difficult. The following paragraphs deal with a few general guidelines in evaluating the immobilized multiple trauma patient.

The first study obtained on the multiple trauma patient is often of the lateral cervical spine using a combination of simple cross-table and swimmer's techniques. Obtaining an adequate lateral radiograph down to the C7/T1 junction is often greatly facilitated by prior explanation to the patient. Unless the patient is head injured, intoxicated, or otherwise rendered incapable of understanding an explanation and receiving reassurance, it is extremely worthwhile to explain what the procedure involves and what it is for in order to enlist the patient's help in achieving the desired goal. For instance, calmly explaining to the patient that the shoulders are interfering with an adequate study of the neck and briefly demonstrating the technique of lowering the shoulders into a "slouched" position, accompanied by the examiner aiding the patient by applying gentle traction to the patient's wrists, may greatly facilitate the radiograph. When traction is to be applied to the arms, it is very important that the person applying the traction continue to talk to the patient while gently pulling down on first one arm and then the other in a step-wise fashion in order to produce a smooth downward traction without jerking. Similarly, the patient's cervical spine immobilization must be monitored to ensure that excessive amounts of traction are not being applied to the as yet undiagnosed cervical spine.[8,9] If the patient is in a cervical collar and taped or strapped firmly to the spine board, it may be possible for the arm traction to produce enormous amounts of traction and distraction of the cervical spine. Therefore it is essential that the traction applied be meticulously controlled. The best way to achieve this is to ensure that the "counterweight" opposing the traction is simply the weight of the patient's head; the forehead and chin tape should be removed briefly while the patient's cervical spine immobilization is continually supervised. Thus, when the traction applied to the patient's arms begins to slide the patient's body down toward the person applying the traction, the only weight resisting the movement is the weight of the head. If the cervical spine were to remain completely immobilized and taped to the board, it would be possible for the person applying the traction to apply 35 or more pounds of traction to the spine with potentially catastrophic consequences.[8] If the patient is uncooperative and, therefore, removal of the tape immobilization is felt to be unwise, a physician knowledgeable in such techniques ought to be the one applying the arm traction. Blind application of brute force in these circumstances may aggravate injury.

Radiographic "clearance" of the cervical spine is not achieved through simple lateral radiography (see Chapter 3). In the multiply injured patient, at least three radiographic views are required to assess the cervical spine.[45-47] These views must be interpreted in the context of a reliable examination of the patient for neurologic deficit. If any fracture is identified in this initial radiographic assessment, additional evaluation is usually necessary. In one large series, 53% of fractures detected on CT scan were missed on standard radiography. Most of these were immediately adjacent to identified fractures.[39] In addition, the thoracic spine and lumbar spine must be cleared either clinically or by a combination of clinical and radiographic evaluation before the patient is allowed to sit up.[21-23]

Patients who are in four-point restraints because of combative behavior due to head injury, intoxication, or both, will be difficult to evaluate radiographically until their combative behavior is controlled. In addition, combative behavior and the act of struggling against restraints may aggravate an unstable spine injury. In these circumstances, judicious use of sedation or active airway management with neuromuscular blockade is indicated. After immediately correctable causes of combative behavior,

such as hypoglycemia, have been excluded, sedation using an intravenous agent such as haloperidol in dosage increments of 0.15 mg/kg may greatly facilitate both patient management and radiographic study.[48-53]

The design of the trauma area itself and the number of personnel present may also interfere with radiographic study. Too often, individual personnel assisting in trauma resuscitation consider their task more important than the obtaining of radiographic studies. This may, in fact, not be the case, and it is essential that the trauma captain maintain discipline to ensure that radiographic studies are carried out in a timely and orderly fashion.

Physics-related considerations

The superiority of radiographs obtained with fixed radiologic as opposed to portable equipment relates to the basic physics involved in obtaining a radiographic image. Visibility of structures on plain film studies depends on using x-rays of sufficient energy so that they are able to adequately penetrate the body. Also, a sufficient number of x-ray photons of optimal energy must be produced.

Image formation depends on the differential attenuation of x-ray photons by various tissues. The energy of the x-ray photon plays a primary role in this. One must have an adequate number of photons of optimal energy so that contrast between tissues is maximized. Portable equipment uses, by necessity, a portable x-ray generator, which is less powerful and efficient than those available on fixed equipment. Thus portable equipment is not able to produce the same quality of studies that can be obtained from fixed

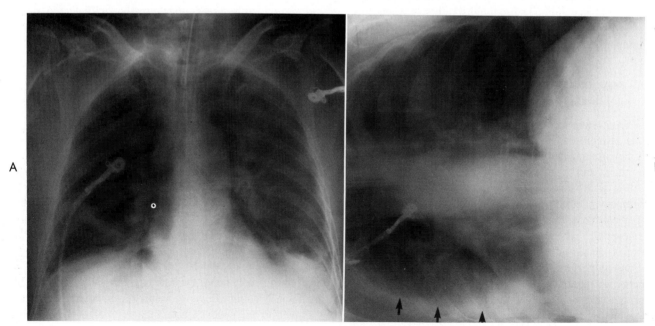

Fig. 2-1. A, Supine AP chest radiograph of an intubated multiple trauma patient. Although there is a suggestion of generally increased opacity of the left lung field compared to the right, it is impossible to determine whether this is due to hemothorax or parenchymal injury. **B,** Left lateral decubitus chest radiograph of the same patient. Note the layering of the left hemothorax *(arrows),* which is now clearly visible.

units. For instance, it is virtually impossible to combine on a single portable film proper exposure of the lungs and adequate penetration of the mediastinum.[54,55]

Clear visibility of structures depends not only on an adequate number of x-ray photons of sufficient energy to create an image but also on excluding deflected x-ray photons (scatter radiation), which degrade the quality of the radiographic image. The exclusion of deflected x-rays is crudely accomplished by placing collimators on the exiting side of the patient immediately adjacent to the film. These collimators eliminate the deflected x-ray photons. In fixed equipment, specially designed moving grids accomplish this task. In portable units, this effect can only be obtained by using portable grids. Portable grids are not as effective

as moving grids, and, therefore, an inferior quality image is produced. It is not possible to use the more closely spaced moving grids for portable studies because the portable x-ray generator limits the number of photons available to produce an image. This filtering would further reduce the number of photons such that a satisfactory image could not be obtained. Furthermore, if the grid is not perfectly lined up with the x-ray tube, fewer x-rays penetrate the grid to expose the film. This phenomenon, called "grid cutoff," further reduces the ability of portable equipment to adequately expose the film and is greater the more collimated the grid.

The ability to produce a correctly exposed x-ray (film latitude) is reduced as the energy is reduced. It is, there-

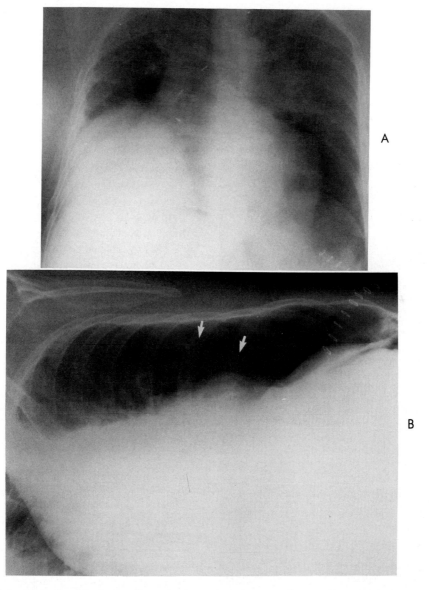

Fig. 2-2. A, Supine AP chest radiograph of a patient demonstrating an elevated right hemidiaphragm but no evidence of pneumothorax. (Surgical clips are from recently performed operation.) **B,** Right lateral decubitus chest radiograph of the same patient. Note the large left pneumothorax now visible in the left hemithorax *(arrows)* and the absence of lung markings at the left base.

fore, technically more difficult to obtain a satisfactory film exposure. Additional techniques to optimize exposure, such as photo timers, are also not available with portable equipment. In simple terms, portable equipment may not only inadequately penetrate the patient but may also produce images of inferior quality.

Positional compromises are also necessary in the evaluation of the multiple trauma patient. A portable supine chest radiograph, which is obtained with a short focal-film distance, has numerous disadvantages. Supine positioning may make it difficult to recognize intrathoracic fluid or an anterior pneumothorax (Figs. 2-1 and 2-2). The magnification inherent in these portable films makes assessment of the mediastinum difficult. Without a lateral radiograph, subtle, but crucial, pathology such as a sternal fracture may be easily missed (Fig. 2-3).

In dealing with the abdomen, similar considerations apply. Free air or fluid is not easily seen without an upright or decubitus study.

In the cervical spine, it is often impossible to adequately visualize the C7/T1 region with portable equipment (Fig. 2-4). In patients in whom there is neurologic compromise or clinical concern, it is essential that further imaging using fixed equipment or CT scans be done.

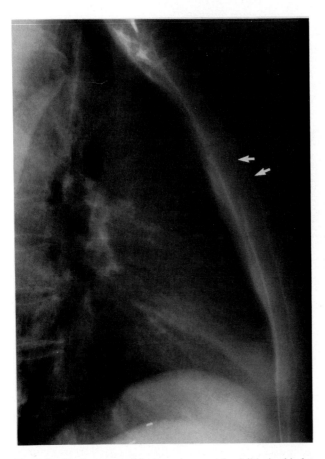

Fig. 2-3. Obvious sternal fracture *(arrows)* is visible in this lateral chest radiograph. The sternum is not seen in standard AP or PA views.

Life-threatening conditions, such as pneumothorax, free air, hemothorax or hemoperitoneum, aortic injuries or significant cervical spine fractures, may all be missed on initial portable supine films. If significant injuries are not to be missed, further imaging with fixed equipment and optimal positioning, as well as evaluation with other modalities such as computed tomography, must be undertaken following stabilization of the patient.

Pitfalls in the early radiographic evaluation of the trauma patient

As outlined previously, radiographic study of the trauma patient is often limited by factors beyond one's control. The patient's precise injuries, the location of the radiology facility, immobilization of the patient, behavior of the patient, availability of personnel, and the physics of radiology all combine to render evaluation of the multiple trauma patient more difficult than would normally be the case for evaluation of a specific injury or system. A number of these difficulties have been discussed. Further problems occur in choosing the type of views to be taken and in sequencing those views.

Supine chest radiography. The initial chest radiograph obtained in the evaluation of the multiple trauma patient is performed using supine anteroposterior (AP) technique, whereas a standard chest radiograph is obtained using upright posteroanterior (PA) technique (see Chapter 5). The resultant change in projection of the various intrathoracic structures and the change in location of intrapleural fluid or air as compared with the upright or decubitus technique render diagnosis more difficult.

These problems are exemplified by plain film assessment of the mediastinum for suspected aortic injury. Fig. 2-5, *A* shows a supine AP chest radiograph of a multiple trauma patient demonstrating a wide, poorly defined mediastinum and, therefore, suspicious for traumatic rupture of the aorta. Fig. 2-5, *B* is a repeat of the supine AP radiograph with a nasogastric tube in place. The additional appearance of the deviated nasogastric tube adds to the suspicion of aortic injury. Fig. 2-5, *C* is the upright, 72-inch, AP radiograph of the identical patient, still with the nasogastric tube in place. The upper mediastinum is now normal in appearance, the aortic contour is clearly visualized, and the nasogastric tube is not deviated. If one were not able to obtain an upright film using this technique, unnecessary aortography might be undertaken.

Similarly, differentiation between hemothorax and pulmonary contusion may be difficult in the supine study and extremely straightforward in an upright or decubitus radiograph (see Fig. 2-1).

Pneumothorax may also be subtle or impossible to diagnose on the supine radiograph because of the anterior location of the air in relation to the lungs. In the upright or decubitus study, the air will rise to the superior extent of the pleural cavity and the pneumothorax will assume a traditional appearance (see Fig. 2-2).

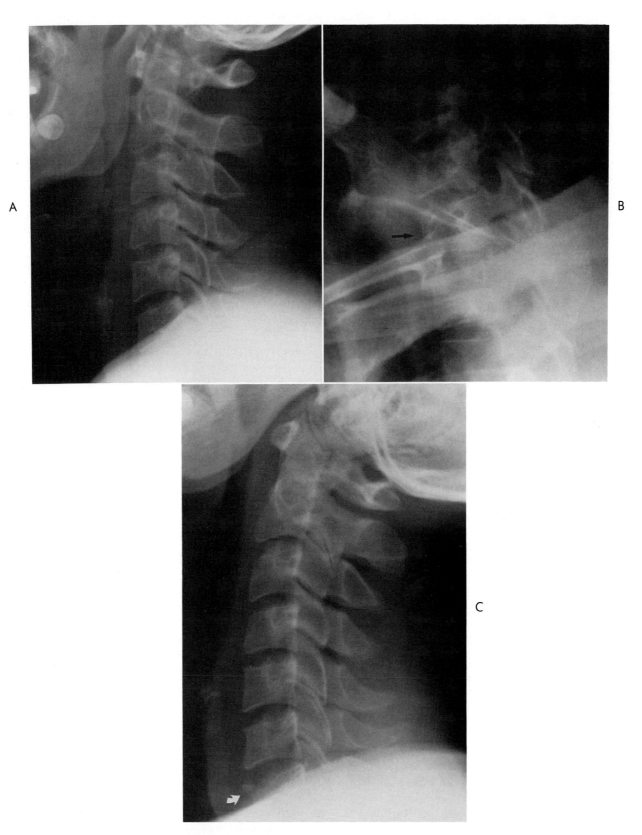

Fig. 2-4. Cross-table lateral (**A**) and swimmer's view (**B**) of the cervical spine showing only the first six vertebrae in the cross-table lateral radiograph but normal alignment C6/C7 without evidence of fracture of C7 *(arrow)* on swimmer's view. **C,** Repeat lateral cervical spine radiograph of the same patient. Note the superior tear-drop fracture *(arrow)* of C7.

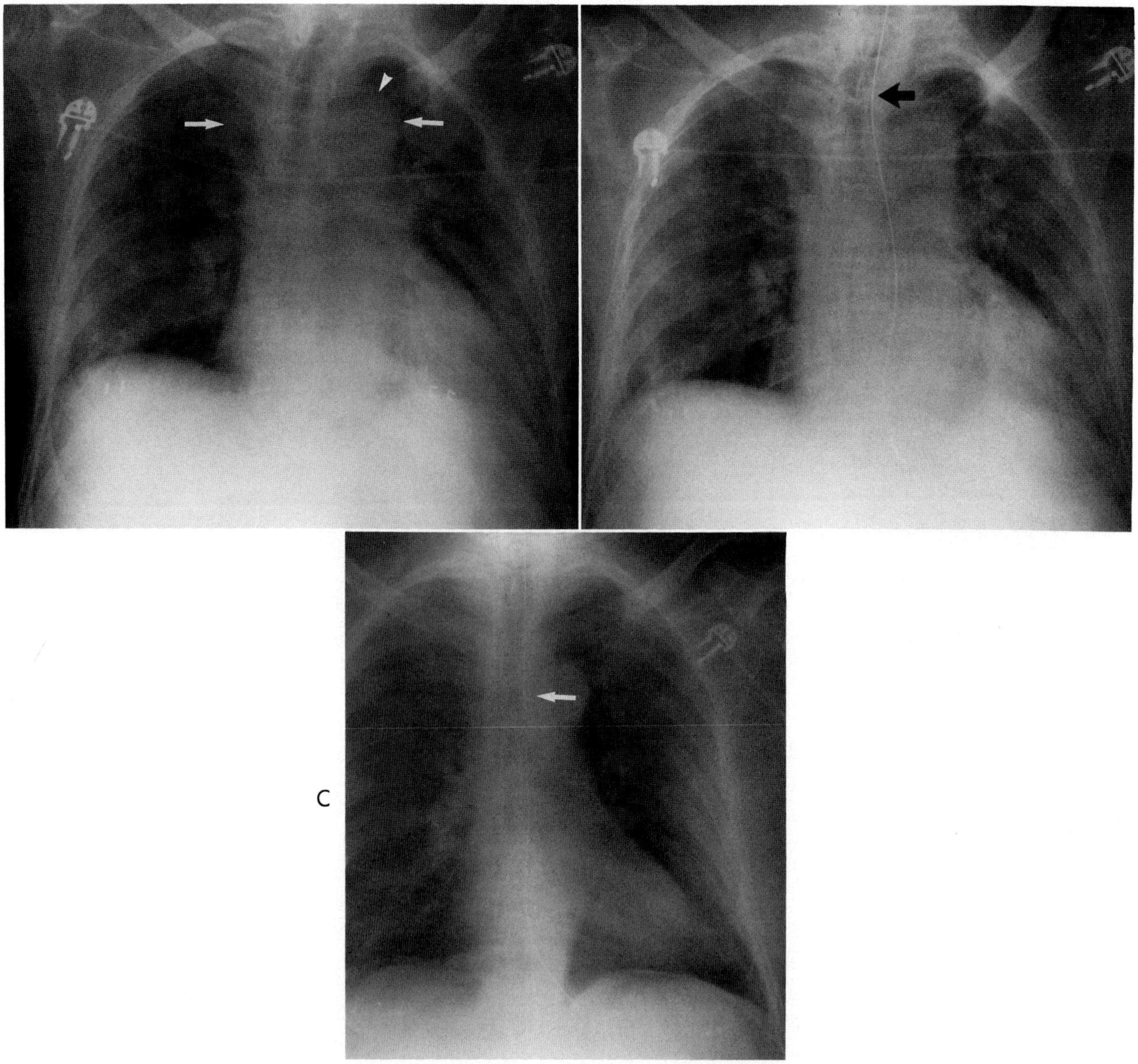

Fig. 2-5. A, Supine AP chest radiograph of a multiple trauma patient showing poor aortic definition *(arrowhead)* and wide mediastinum *(arrows)* suggestive of aortic injury. **B,** Repeat supine
AP chest radiograph of the same patient, now with nasogastric tube in place. Note the apparent
deviation of the nasogastric tube *(arrow)* from left to right. **C,** Upright, 72-inch, AP chest radiograph of the same patient as in **A** and **B.** The mediastinum now appears completely normal, the
aorta is well defined, and the nasogastric tube *(arrow)* is not deviated.

Finally, supine chest radiography that is performed in
the trauma unit consists of an AP film without a concomitant lateral view. The absence of the lateral view may conceal important diagnostic information (see Figs. 2-3 and
2-6).

**Cross-table radiography of the lumbar and thoracic
spine.** Cross-table radiographs of the lumbar and thoracic
spine are difficult to obtain using portable equipment. The

upper thoracic vertebrae cannot be visualized in the standard lateral projection because of the superimposition of
the shoulders. In large individuals it may not be possible
to adequately penetrate the lower lumbar region. In certain
fracture types, such as burst fractures, it is not possible to
properly assess the integrity of the spinal canal.[56] These
fractures are commonly unstable and are frequently associated with fractures at other levels (see Chapter 9). A CT

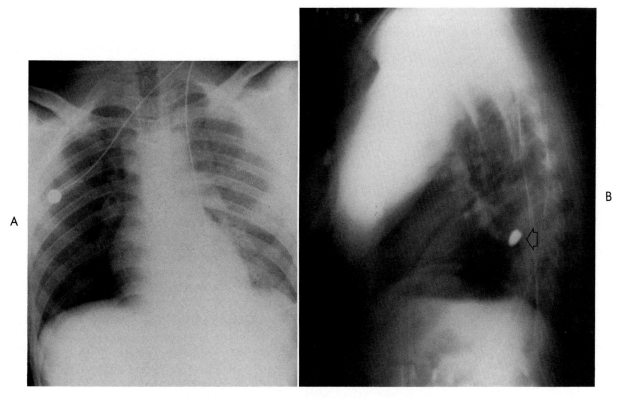

Fig. 2-6. A, Supine AP chest radiograph of an assault victim with obvious increase in opacity of the left hemithorax, representing hemothorax or pulmonary parenchymal injury. **B,** Upright right lateral chest radiograph of the same patient, following insertion of a left chest tube. A bullet *(arrow)* is now clearly visible behind the heart.

scan or conventional tomography is required to fully assess these injuries and to exclude cord compromise.[57]

Sequencing of special radiographic studies. Timing of the administration of intravenous contrast material is worthy of special discussion in the multiple trauma patient. Planning these studies to avoid premature administration of a contrast material before another study (which might require additional contrast) is essential. For example, an abdominal CT scan in a trauma patient requires administration of both oral and intravenous contrast material (see Chapter 6). Early administration of intravenous contrast material for intravenous pyelography in the trauma unit is not only unnecessary but increases the hazard to the patient. Investigation of the patient's most significant and pressing injuries may be seriously compromised by the prior administration of contrast material. For example, if intravenous contrast material has been administered, intracranial hemorrhage may not be visualized on a CT scan.

In a patient with exsanguinating pelvic arterial bleeding, the presence of contrast material from a ruptured bladder or urethra may seriously compromise recognition of pelvic bleeding and may inhibit selective vessel catheterization and embolization.[29] Furthermore there is a limit to

the amount of contrast material that can be safely given to a patient who is hypotensive. Intravenous or intra-arterial contrast material may compromise renal function in a kidney that is predisposed to renal damage by factors such as hypovolemia, pre-existing renal disease, or underlying medical conditions such as diabetes mellitus or multiple myeloma. One must be careful to arrange studies so that administration of contrast material is minimized and particularly so that a more essential study is not obscured or compromised by previous contrast material administration.[58-60]

One-shot intravenous pyelogram. Plain abdominal radiography is virtually never indicated in blunt, multiple trauma (see Chapter 6). However, administration of a single dose of intravenous contrast, such as 50 ml of nonionic contrast material[24] can facilitate visualization of both kidneys and often the renal pelvis in a very expeditious fashion. This information may be essential when taking the blunt trauma patient directly to the operating room, both from the standpoint of identifying the presence of bilaterally functioning kidneys and, in limited fashion, delineating the presence of extensive proximal injury. Renal vascular injury may be identified using this technique and knowledge that a functioning kidney is present on the contralateral side may be invaluable when making a decision to perform a nephrectomy vs. attempted preservation of the organ.

However, because of the considerations discussed previously in the section on sequencing of studies, a one-shot intravenous pyelogram should not be done unless the patient is proceeding directly to the operating room, and further diagnostic studies are neither indicated nor possible.

RADIOLOGIST AS CONSULTANT

The radiologist plays a central role in the management of the acutely traumatized patient. This role comprises three main areas of expertise: (1) selection of the most effective examinations in the most appropriate sequence, (2) interpretation of examinations, and (3) performance of indicated special procedures.

Selection of the most effective examinations in the most appropriate sequence

In recent years, the availability of computed tomography, ultrasonography, conventional tomography, and angiography has added to the complexity of choosing the most appropriate examination for the injured patient. The "right test at the right time" depends not only on what equipment is available but on where it is located. The multiplicity of injuries in a patient with massive blunt trauma creates a problem since a serious and unsuspected injury may be overlooked while attention is diverted to another less severe, although more obvious, injury.[61,62]

An immediate CT scan has its indications, but it always depends on the location of the equipment and the stability of the patient.

If a dedicated CT scanner is present in the emergency department, a CT scan may be the test of choice for a traumatized patient with suspected intra-abdominal injury,[63] whereas if a CT scanner is some distance away or unavailable, diagnostic peritoneal lavage may be preferable. For example, in a stable patient with hematuria, a CT scan would be preferable to excretory urography. Not only would the CT scan allow assessment of free intraperitoneal blood, but it would also exclude unrecognized injuries to other organs. Often so-called delayed splenic rupture is, in fact, really a case of delayed diagnosis.[36] The CT scan of the kidney is more accurate than excretory urography in evaluating renal parenchymal injury, perirenal hemor-

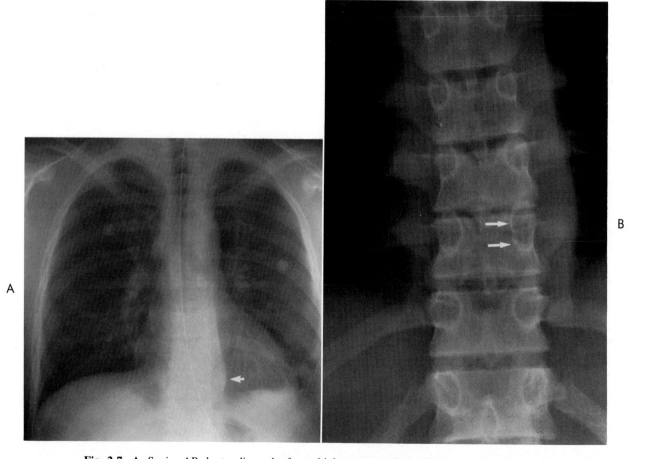

Fig. 2-7. A, Supine AP chest radiograph of a multiple trauma patient. Note the subtle bulging of the mediastinal soft tissue contour adjacent to T10 *(arrow).* **B,** Cone-down AP view of the lower thoracic spine of the same patient. A left pedicle fracture *(arrows)* is now clearly demonstrated.

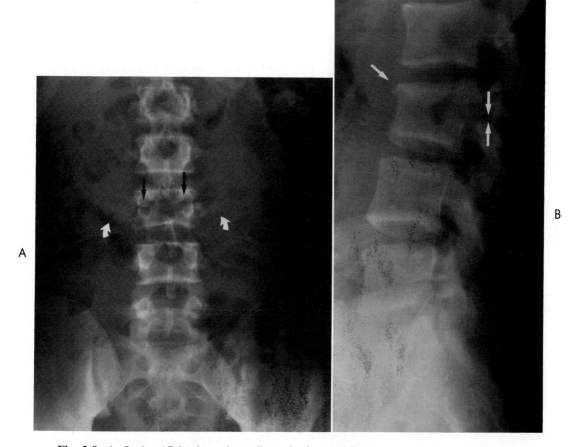

rhage, and the presence or absence of urine extravasation. These three criteria are the crucial clinical factors in deciding between surgical and nonsurgical management.[63]

Interpretation of examinations

Interpretation of a radiographic examination clearly is an area in which the radiologist, with specific training and experience in the interpretation of plain radiographs, plays an important role. Significant injuries may be extremely subtle on portable supine radiographs or even on properly obtained standard studies. The radiologist's training and methodic approach to the interpretation of radiographic studies will lead to a higher rate of identification of these injuries (Figs. 2-7 to 2-9). When there is any suspicion of significant injury, definitive studies must be obtained. When an abnormality is noted on cervical spine radiography, further evaluation with a CT scan or conventional tomography is indicated. If significant injury is suspected and standard plain radiographs demonstrate no evidence of unstable injury, conventional tomography or flexion and extension views (Fig. 2-10) may be indicated (see Chapter 9).

Whenever possible, patients who are potential surgical candidates and who have severe pelvic fractures should undergo a CT scan before surgery. Pearson and Hargadon[64] demonstrated that 29% of acetabular fractures were missed on plain radiographs. Griffiths et al.[65] demonstrated that a CT scan of pelvic fractures resulted in a change of management in as many as one third of cases. The addition of multiplanar and three-dimensional reconstruction allows the surgeon to fully appreciate the extent of these complex injuries.

Appropriate evaluation of stable patients with abdominal injuries may allow the surgeon to consider conservative therapy. In a study of CT evaluation of patients with hepatic lacerations, Federle[63] demonstrated that 60% of these injuries could be managed without surgery if appropriate clinical and CT assessment was used. Kuhn and Berger[66] reported similar experiences in pediatric patients

Fig. 2-8. A, Supine AP lumbar spine radiograph of a multiple trauma patient. The Chance fracture through the L3 transverse processes *(white arrows)* and pedicles *(black arrows)* is extremely subtle in this view. **B,** Lateral lumbar spine radiograph of the same patient. The L3 fracture with loss of height of the anterior aspect of the vertebral body *(single arrow)* and extension of the fracture through the posterior elements bilaterally *(paired arrows)* is now clearly demonstrated. The increase in height of the posterior aspect of the vertebral body is evidence of the distraction mechanism of this fracture.

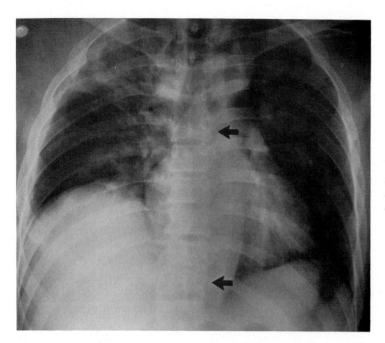

Fig. 2-9. Supine AP chest radiograph of a multiple trauma patient demonstrating a widened left paraspinal mass with subtle fractures of T5 and T10 *(arrows)* that can easily be overlooked if a methodical approach to evaluation of the radiograph is not used. The fractures were subsequently demonstrated by conventional tomography.

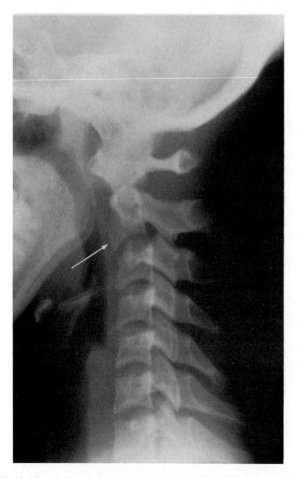

Fig. 2-10. Flexion lateral cervical spine radiograph of a multiple trauma patient demonstrating significant anterior subluxation of C2 on C3 *(arrow).* The cross-table lateral cervical spine radiograph was completely normal, but the patient's persistent complaints of severe neck pain led to the flexion/extension studies. Note the absence of soft tissue swelling anterior to the injury.

with splenic injuries; 79% of their patients were managed nonoperatively using early CT scans combined with careful ongoing observation.[62,66]

Performance of indicated special procedures

A third area of involvement of the radiologist is in the performance of indicated special procedures. These include urethrography; cystography; intravenous, oral, and rectal contrast material administration; and angiography.

An example that emphasizes the importance of radiologic consultation is the patient with exsanguinating pelvic hemorrhage. It is undesirable for a hemodynamically unstable patient with a pelvic fracture to undergo an unnecessary laparotomy. If the tamponading effect of the peritoneum is lost, the extraperitoneal pelvic hemorrhage may extend into the abdomen and the surgeon is then unable to control this exsanguinating hemorrhage. The only option in such a circumstance may be proximal ligation of both iliac vessels, which may be ineffective. It has been shown experimentally that bilateral internal iliac occlusion diminishes pelvic blood flow by only 48%.[33]

An immediate CT scan might exclude a significant intraperitoneal cause for blood loss and confirm the blood accumulation to be extraperitoneal within the pelvis. Selective angiographic embolization of the bleeding vessels could then be undertaken. It is essential that this evaluation be undertaken concomitantly with patient stabilization, but with exsanguinating pelvic hemorrhage it is often impossible to stabilize the patient until the site of hemorrhage is controlled.[36]

PEDIATRIC PATIENT

General trauma resuscitation of the pediatric patient follows the same basic principles as resuscitation of the adult patient, with appropriate modification for the psychologic and anatomic differences between children and adults.

PREGNANT PATIENT

Caution should be exercised in radiographic study of any pregnant or potentially pregnant patient, especially in the first trimester of pregnancy. Nevertheless, in the context of multisystem trauma, all indicated studies should be performed, including pelvic radiography. Careful planning to avoid redundant or unnecessary studies and appropriate shielding of the gonadal area and gravid uterus will further reduce the small risk to the unborn child.[67]

SUMMARY

Few areas of emergency medicine demonstrate as many difficulties and challenges as does management of the multiple trauma victim. Appropriate planning of facilities and resources, training of personnel, and close cooperation between emergency physicians, radiologists, and other specialists will ensure optimal patient outcome.[36,62]

I wish to acknowledge the assistance of Jennifer Johnson, whose hard work and attention to detail were invaluable during the production of this chapter. R.M.W.

REFERENCES

1. American College of Surgeons: *Advanced trauma life support instructor's manual,* 1988, ACS.
2. Jorden RC: Multiple trauma. In Rosen P, Baker FJ II, Barkin R et al, eds: *Emergency medicine: concepts and clinical practice,* ed 2, St Louis, 1988, CV Mosby.
3. Collicott PE: Initial assessment of the trauma patient. In Mattox KL, Moore EE, and Feliciano DV, eds: *Trauma,* East Norwalk, 1988, Appleton and Lange.
4. Walls RM: Airway management in the blunt trauma patient: how important is the cervical spine? *Can J Surg,* 1991 (in press).
5. Aprahamian C, Thompson BM, Finger WA et al: Experimental cervical spine injury model: evaluation of airway management and splinting techniques. *Ann Emerg Med* 13:584, 1984.
6. Rhee KJ, Green W, Holcroft JW et al: Oral intubation in the multiply injured patient: the risk of exacerbating spinal cord damage, *Ann Emerg Med* 19:511, 1990.
7. Holley J, Jorden RC: Airway management in patients with unstable cervical spine fractures, *Ann Emerg Med* 18:151, 1989.
8. Bivens HG, Ford S, Bezmalinovic Z et al: The effect of axial traction during orotracheal intubation of the trauma victim with an unstable cervical spine, *Ann Emerg Med* 17:53, 1988.
9. Kaufman HH, Harris JH, Spencer JA et al: Danger of traction during radiography for cervical spine trauma, *JAMA* 247:2369, 1982.
10. McGill J, Clinton JE, and Ruiz E: Cricothyroidotomy in the emergency department, *Ann Emerg Med* 11:361, 1982.
11. Erlandson MJ, Clinton JE, Ruiz E et al: Cricothyroidotomy in the emergency department revisited, *J Emerg Med* 7:115, 1989.
12. Walls RM: Cricothyroidotomy. In Campbell WH, ed: Airway management and anesthesia in the emergency department, *Emerg Med Clin North Am* 6:725, 1988.
13. Knopp RK: The safety of orotracheal intubation in patients with suspected cervical-spine injury, *Ann Emerg Med* 19:603, 1990.
14. Joyce SM: Cervical immobilization during orotracheal intubation in trauma victims, *Ann Emerg Med* 17:145, 1988.
15. Turner LM: Cervical spine immobilization with axial traction: a practice to be discouraged, *J Emerg Med* 7:385, 1989.
16. VandenHoek T, Propp D: Cervicothoracic junction injury, *Am J Emerg Med* 8:30, 1990.
17. Bachulis BL, Long WB, Hynes GD et al: Clinical indications for cervical spine radiographs in the traumatized patient, *Am J Surg* 153:473, 1987.
18. Fischer RP: Cervical radiographic evaluation of alert patients following blunt trauma, *Ann Emerg Med* 13:905, 1984.
19. Cadoux CG, White JD: High-yield radiographic considerations for cervical spine injuries, *Ann Emerg Med* 15:236, 1986.
20. Ringenberg BJ, Fisher AK, Urdaneta LF et al: Rational ordering of cervical spine radiographs following trauma, *Ann Emerg Med* 17:792, 1988.
21. Mackersie RC, Shackford SR, Garfin SR et al: Major skeletal injuries in the obtunded blunt trauma patient: a case for routine radiologic survey, *J Trauma* 28:1450, 1988.
22. Pal JM, Mulder DS, Brown RA et al: Assessing multiple trauma: is the cervical spine enough? *J Trauma* 28:1282, 1988.
23. Powell JN, Waddell JP, Tucker WS et al: Multiple-level noncontiguous spinal fractures, *J Trauma* 29:1146, 1989.
24. Reid DC, Henderson R, Saboe L et al: Etiology and clinical course of missed spine fractures, *J Trauma* 27:980, 1987.
25. Kopferschmid JP, Weaver ML, Raves JJ et al: Thoracic spine injuries in victims of motorcycle accidents, *J Trauma* 29:593, 1989.
26. Bohlin NI: A statistical analysis of 28,000 accident cases with emphasis on occupant restraint value (Passenger Car Engineering Department, AB Volvo), Eleventh Stapp Car Crash Conference Proceedings, New York, 1967, Society of Automotive Engineers.
27. Orsay EM, Dunne M, Turnbull TL et al: Prospective study of the effect of safety belts in motor vehicle crashes, *Ann Emerg Med* 19:258, 1990.
28. Gillott A, Rhodes M, and Lucke J: Utility of routine pelvic x-ray during blunt trauma resuscitation, *J Trauma* 28:1570, 1988.
29. Kam J, Jackson H, and Ben-Menachem Y: Vascular injuries in blunt pelvic trauma, *Radiol Clin North Am* 19:171, 1981.
30. Stock JR, Harris WH, and Athanasoulis CA: The role of diagnostic and therapeutic angiography in trauma to the pelvis, *Clin Orthop* 151:31, 1980.
31. Young JWR, Burgess AR, Brumback RJ et al: Pelvic fractures: value of plain radiography in early assessment and management, *Radiology* 160:445, 1986.
32. Patterson FP, Morton KS: The cause of death in fracture of the pelvis, *J Trauma* 13:849, 1973.
33. Burchel RC: Physiology of internal iliac artery ligation, *J Obstet Gynaecol Br Comm* 75:642, 1968.
34. Hubbard SG, Brivins BA, Sachatello CR et al: Diagnostic errors with peritoneal lavage in patients with pelvic fractures, *Arch Surg* 114:844, 1979.
35. Reynolds BM, Balsano NA: Venography in pelvic fractures, *Ann Surg* 173:104, 1971.
36. Ben-Menachem Y: Logic and logistics of radiography, angiography, and angiographic intervention in massive blunt trauma, *Radiol Clin North Am* 19:9, 1981.
37. Matalon TSA, Athanasoulis CA, Margolies MN et al: Hemorrhage with pelvic fractures: efficacy of transcatheter embolization, *AJR* 133:859, 1979.
38. Harley JD, Mack LA, and Winquist RA: CT of acetabular fractures: comparison with conventional radiography, *AJR* 138:413, 1982.
39. Acheson MB, Livingston RR, Richardson ML et al: High-resolution CT scanning in the evaluation of cervical spine fractures: comparison with plain film examinations, *AJR* 148:1179, 1987.
40. Ross SE, Schwab CW, David ET et al: Clearing the cervical spine: initial radiologic evaluation, *J Trauma* 27:1055, 1987.
41. Griffiths HJ, Standertskjold-Nordenstam CG, Burke J et al: Computed tomography in the management of acetabular fractures, *Skeletal Radiol* 11:22, 1984.
42. Christensen EE, Curry TS III, and Dowdey JE: *An introduction to the physics of diagnostic radiology,* ed 3, Philadelphia, Lea & Febiger.

43. Singer CM, Baraff LJ, Benedict SH et al: Exposure of emergency medicine personnel to ionizing radiation during cervical spine radiography, *Ann Emerg Med* 18:822, 1989.

44. Weiss EL, Singer CM, Benedict SH et al: Physician exposure to ionizing radiation during trauma resuscitation: a prospective clinical study, *Ann Emerg Med* 19:134, 1990.

45. Macdonald RL, Schwarz ML, Mirich D et al: Diagnosis of cervical spine injury in motor vehicle crash victims: how many x-rays are enough? *J Trauma* 30:392, 1990.

46. Shaffer MA, Doris PE: Limitation of the cross table lateral view in detecting cervical spine injuries: a retrospective analysis, *Ann Emerg Med* 10:508, 1981.

47. Mace SE: Emergency evaluation of cervical spine injuries: CT versus plain radiographs, *Ann Emerg Med* 14:973, 1985.

48. Walls RM: The combative trauma patient: a paradigm of trauma leadership, *J Emerg Med,* 1991 (in press).

49. Silverstein S, Frommer DA, Marx JA et al: Parenteral haloperidol in combative patients: a prospective study, *UAEMS,* 1986 (abstract).

50. Ayd FJ: Haloperidol: twenty years clinical experience, *J Clin Psychiatry* 39:807, 1978.

51. Tesar GE, Murray GB, and Cassem NH: Use of high-dose intravenous haloperidol in the treatment of agitated cardiac patients, *J Clin Psychopharmacol* 5:344, 1985.

52. Adams F: Emergency intravenous sedation of the delirious, medically ill patient, *J Clin Psychiatry* 49(suppl):22, 1988.

53. Clinton JE, Sterner S, Steimachers A et al: Haloperidol for sedation of disruptive emergency patients, *Ann Emerg Med* 16:319, 1987.

54. Mirvis SE, Fritz SL, Siegel JH et al: A radiographic system for use in emergency and intensive care units, *AJR* 150:691, 1988.

55. Fraser RG, Paré JAP: *Diagnosis of diseases of the chest,* ed 2, vol 1, Philadelphia, 1977, WB Saunders.

56. Harris JH, Harris WH: *The radiology of emergency medicine,* Baltimore, 1975, Williams & Wilkins.

57. Dalinka MK, Boorstein JM, and Zlatkin MB: Computed tomography of musculoskeletal trauma, *Radiol Clin North Am* 27:933, 1989.

58. Cohan RH, Dunnick NR, and Bashore TM: Treatment of reactions to radiographic contrast material, *AJR* 151:263, 1988.

59. Miller DL, Chang R, Wells WT et al: Intravascular contrast media: effect of dose on renal function, *Radiology* 167:607, 1988.

60. vanSonnenberg E, Neff CC, and Pfister RC: Life-threatening hypotensive reactions to contrast media administration: comparison of pharmacologic and fluid therapy, *Radiology* 162:15, 1987.

61. Ward RE: Study and management of blunt trauma in the immediate post-impact period, *Radiol Clin North Am* 19:3, 1981.

62. McCort JJ: Caring for the major trauma victim: the role for radiology, *Radiology* 161:1, 1987.

63. Federle MP: Computed tomography of blunt abdominal trauma, *Radiol Clin North Am* 21:461, 1983.

64. Pearson JB, Hargadon EJ: Fractures of the pelvis involving the floor of the acetabulum, *J Bone Joint Surg* 44(B):550, 1986.

65. Griffiths HJ, Standertskjold-Nordenstein CG, Burk J et al: Computed tomography in the management of acetabular fractures, *Skeletal Radiol* 11:22, 1984.

66. Kuhn JP, Berger PE: Computed tomography in the evaluation of blunt abdominal trauma in children, *Radiol Clin North Am* 19:503, 1981.

67. Esposito TJ, Gens DR, Smith LG et al: Evaluation of blunt abdominal trauma occurring during pregnancy, *J Trauma* 29:1628, 1989.

Head and Neck Trauma

Jeffrey J. Schaider
Pat Dunne

Treating injuries of the head and neck is one of the most difficult and challenging problems that the emergency physician faces in trauma care. Immediate decisions must be made regarding airway management, surgical intervention, and evaluation using radiographic diagnostic techniques. This chapter will define the various radiographic techniques that are used in the diagnosis and management of blunt and penetrating trauma to the soft tissue areas of the neck, the cranium, and their contents.

SOFT TISSUE NECK TRAUMA

Injuries to the soft tissue area of the neck are increasing given the greater availability of firearms and the rising number of motor vehicle accidents. The lack of bony protection in the anterior neck makes this area especially vulnerable to severe, life-threatening injuries.

Rapid identification of neck injuries with early intervention is the key to treatment. Because of the large number of anatomic structures contained in the neck (Fig. 3-1), multiple organ systems may be injured concurrently. A thorough, but rapid, investigation must be made to prevent airway compromise from laryngeal trauma, neurologic and bleeding complications from vascular damage, or the spread of infection from occult esophageal injuries. This section will evaluate and define the radiographic approach to non-bony cervical injuries.

Penetrating neck trauma

The initial management of the patient with penetrating neck trauma should include a rapid assessment of the patient's ABCs, followed by a secondary survey to determine the extent of the patient's neck injury and to search for any other evidence of trauma. Early airway management must often be initiated even before there is any evidence of airway compromise. Bleeding in the neck should be controlled by direct pressure, rather than the use of blind clamping.[1,2] Once the patient is stable, soft tissue cervical and chest radiographs should be obtained expeditiously.

Soft tissue lateral (Fig. 3-2) and anteroposterior (AP) cervical radiographs aid in the detection of subcutaneous emphysema and prevertebral air (Fig. 3-3). The presence of subcutaneous emphysema or prevertebral air should not be assumed to be secondary to a knife or bullet track[3] but rather may be an indication for immediate surgical exploration.[1,2,4,5] Soft tissue cervical radiographs can also determine the location and trajectory of missile fragments.

Chest radiographs aid in the detection of a pneumothorax or hemothorax that may necessitate the insertion of a chest tube. Pneumomediastinum (Fig. 3-4) signifies violation of the airway or esophagus. Widened mediastinal structures may result from injury to the great vessels. Missile fragments that enter the neck may burrow directly into the chest and travel via the venous system to the heart and into the pulmonary arteries or may embolize directly to the head. In one study of 110 bullet wounds to the neck, 48 patients had positive chest x-ray findings, including six cases of hemothorax, nine of pneumothorax, and four combined.[4]

Prior to 1940, penetrating neck wounds were handled nonoperatively unless major hemorrhage mandated intervention. However, aggressive mandatory surgical exploration for all wounds that penetrate the platysma helped re-

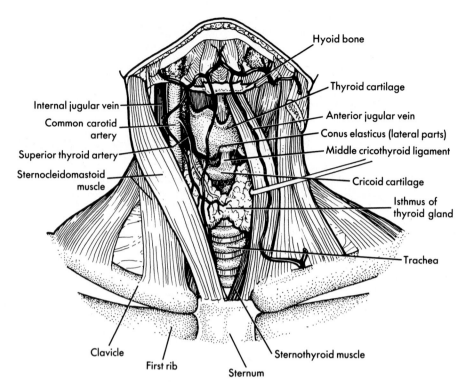

Fig. 3-1. Illustration of the major structures of the neck. (From Rosen P, Baker FJ II, Barkin R et al: *Emergency medicine: concepts and clinical practice,* ed 2, vol 1, St Louis, 1988, CV Mosby.)

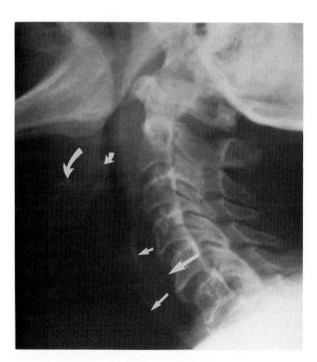

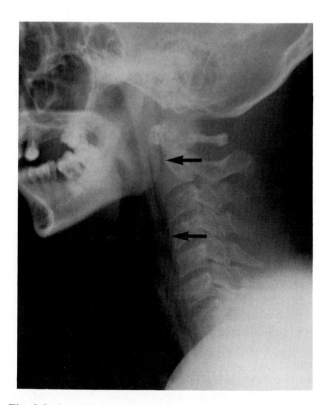

Fig. 3-2. Normal endolateral neck. Epiglottis *(short curved arrow),* hyoid bone *(large curved arrow),* laryngeal cartilage *(short arrow),* trachea *(medium arrow), and* prevertebral soft tissues *(large arrow).*

Fig. 3-3. Lateral view of the neck in a patient after a stab wound to that area reveals linear collections of prevertebral air *(arrows).*

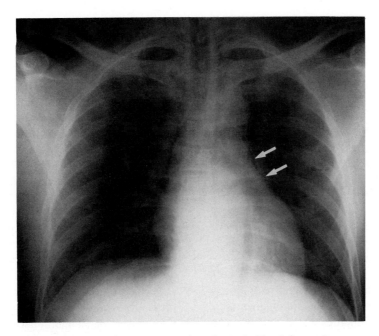

Fig. 3-4. PA view of the chest in the same patient shown in Fig. 3-3 reveals a pneumomediastinum *(arrows)*.

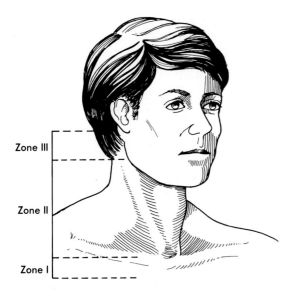

Fig. 3-5. Illustration defining the three zones of the neck. (From Rosen P, Baker FJ II, Barkin R et al: *Emergency medicine: concepts and clinical practice,* ed 2, vol 1, St Louis, 1988, CV Mosby.)

duce mortality from 18% in the Spanish-American War to 7% in World War II[6] and to 4% to 7% in the Vietnam War.[7] Proponents of such mandatory neck exploration warn of disastrous complications from delayed surgical treatment[8-13] while others question the accuracy of nonoperative clinical and radiographic assessment.[14] Recently, however, there has been a growing consensus that selective conservative management of penetrating neck wounds is both safe and helps to avoid the 50% negative exploration rate found in the mandatory exploration policy.[1,2,4-6,15-20]

Indications for surgical exploration of anterior neck wounds include the following:

Vascular system
  History of substantial blood loss
  Persistent bleeding
  Enlarging hematoma
Respiratory system
  Hemoptysis
  Crepitus
  Dysphonia
Digestive tract
  Hematemesis
  Dysphagia
  Crepitus
Nervous system
  Neurologic deficit
Non-evaluative patient
  Intoxication
  Lack of cooperation
  Associated injury

Diagnostic radiographic imaging (angiography, esophagography, and computed tomography) is essential to exclude occult injuries when practicing a selective surgical exploration policy.

Radiographic imaging for suspected vascular injury. To determine the need for angiography in patients with penetrating neck injuries, the neck is subdivided into three zones[21] (Fig. 3-5):

• Zone I: the area below the sternal notch.
• Zone II: the area between the sternal notch and the angle of the mandible.
• Zone III: the area above the angle of the mandible.

In asymptomatic stable patients with penetrating

wounds to the neck that violate the platysma but do not meet the criteria for immediate surgery listed previously, the general recommendations for dealing with zone I and II injuries are well accepted while there is controversy regarding the management of zone III injuries (Fig. 3-6).

For zone I injuries, all patients require angiography to determine the integrity of the thoracic outlet vessels.[1,2,15,17,22] Those with a negative angiogram can be safely observed. For zone II injuries, patients can be observed for expanding hematoma, respiratory distress, or the development of neurologic symptoms without the use of angiography.[1,2,15,22,23] For zone III injuries, most authors advocate[2,15,17,24] angiography to assess the status of the internal carotid artery and the intracerebral circulation while Narrod and Moore[1] feel that angiography is unnecessary in asymptomatic patients.

In symptomatic patients with criteria for formal neck exploration who can be stabilized, preoperative angiography is indicated for the following type of injuries (Fig. 3-7). All patients with zone I injuries whose condition permits the study should undergo angiography since positive angiographic findings necessitate a thoracotomy before neck exploration to repair the thoracic outlet vessels.[1,15,17,22] In patients with multiple injuries in zone II, angiography should be strongly considered before surgical exploration.[1] All patients with zone III injuries should undergo angiography since high internal carotid artery injuries are difficult to visualize at surgery.[24] In addition, high internal ca-

rotid artery injuries may require carotid artery ligation and concomitant extracranial/intracranial bypass[1] (Figs. 3-8 to 3-11).

In addition to diagnosis, angiography also has a therapeutic role in the treatment of vascular injuries of the neck. Therapeutic arterial embolization has been shown to be effective in arterial neck trauma.[24] Embolization is sometimes used as an alternative method of therapy whenever arterial ligation is anticipated or a direct surgical approach is difficult or impossible. Examples of zone III injuries that can be treated by embolization include: (1) expendable vessels, such as the external carotid artery whose rich collateral flow makes embolization a safe alternative to ligation, and (2) poorly accessible vessels, such as the vertebral artery and the internal maxillary artery, for which repair is rarely possible and ligation is usually performed.[24,25]

Radiographic imaging for suspected esophageal injury. Recognition of esophageal injury is very difficult since it is an uncommon injury[26] and associated injuries to the vascular and respiratory systems often mask esophageal trauma.[26,27] Delayed surgical repair of the esophagus results in a very high morbidity and mortality due to early contamination of the paraesophageal space with saliva and bacteria following esophageal injury.[28] Because of the high morbidity and mortality from unrecognized and untreated injuries, an aggressive approach to the diagnosis of esophageal injury from penetrating trauma is warranted.

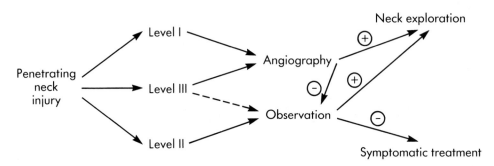

Fig. 3-6. Management of asymptomatic stable patients with penetrating neck injury. (From Narrod JA, Moore EE: *J Emerg Med* 2:14, 1984, Pergamon Press.)

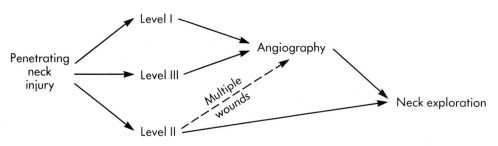

Fig. 3-7. Management of symptomatic stable patients with penetrating neck injury. (From Narrod JA, Moore EE: *J Emerg Med* 2:14, 1984, Pergamon Press.)

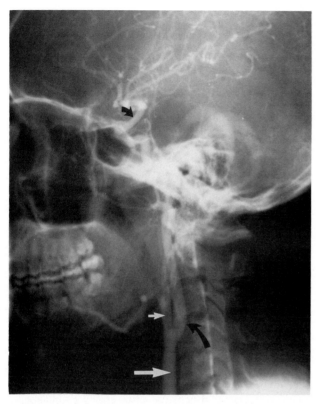

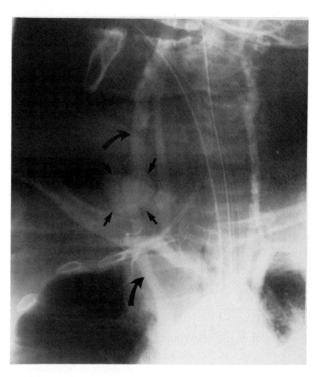

Fig. 3-8. Lateral left carotid angiogram demonstrates normal common *(long arrow)*, internal *(curved arrows)*, and external *(short arrow)* carotid arteries.

Fig. 3-10. Arch aortogram following a gunshot wound reveals a large lobulated common carotid pseudoaneurysm *(short arrows)* and a carotid jugular fistula *(curved arrows)*, zone II injury.

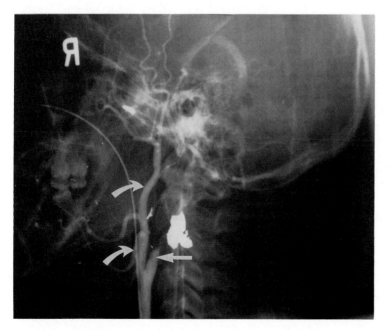

Fig. 3-9. Lateral right carotid angiogram reveals complete occlusion of the internal carotid artery *(arrow)* in zone II. Note the patent external carotid artery *(curved arrows)* and multiple bullet fragments.

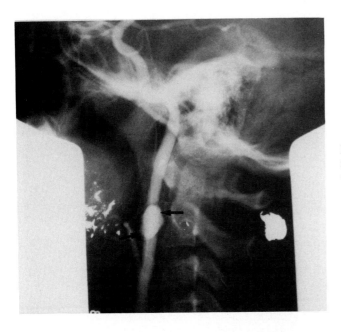

Fig. 3-11. Lateral right carotid angiogram reveals a pseudoaneurysm of the internal carotid artery *(arrows)*, zone III injury. (Courtesy Elizabeth Eelkema, MD.)

Any penetrating injury in proximity to the esophagus should be assumed to have penetrated this organ until proved otherwise.

Physical signs of esophageal disruption include pain and tenderness in the neck, resistance of the neck to passive motion, crepitus, dyspnea, dysphagia, and bleeding from the mouth or nasogastric tube.[28] Physical signs, however, are often nondiagnostic.[27]

Radiographic imaging to diagnose esophageal injury is difficult because of the high false negative rate. No one study should be relied on to exclude esophageal perforation, but rather a combination of physical signs, plain chest and neck radiographs, and contrast esophagograms should be used to confirm the diagnosis.[26]

In any patient with a suspected cervical esophageal injury, soft tissue AP and lateral cervical radiographs and chest radiographs should be obtained. The presence of subcutaneous emphysema,[27,28] increased prevertebral shadow, and widening of the superior mediastinum are signs of possible esophageal injury. Radiographic evidence of esophageal disruption on chest radiographs include pleural effusion, pneumothorax, pneumomediastinum,[28] and mediastinal widening.[27] Normal chest radiographs do not exclude the possibility of esophageal injury. In one study,[28] 6 of 17 patients with penetrating esophageal trauma had normal cervical and chest radiographs.

Esophageal contrast studies may be helpful in the diagnosis of esophageal injury but should not be relied on solely to exclude trauma to the esophagus. Esophagography should be used frequently due to the nonspecific nature of the physical examination and the high incidence of concomitant injuries.[27] Esophagography should be performed: (1) on patients with positive physical findings, (2) when the projectile is in proximity to[27,28] or crosses the midline,[27] (3) if the missile has traveled beyond the limits of surgical exploration,[28] and (4) in the presence of subcutaneous air on cervical and chest radiographs.[26]

Gastrograffin should be used initially as a contrast agent since it is water soluble and less contaminating than barium when extravasated. A negative gastrograffin esophagogram should be followed by consultation with an endoscopist in the event that endoscopy is recommended before the use of barium in order to increase diagnostic accuracy.

Esophagography has a 30% to 50% false negative rate* and should be followed by esophagoscopy in patients with suspected esophageal perforation. Some authors[1,2] surgically explore all patients with abnormal soft tissue air, without performing esophagography or esophagoscopy because of the low sensitivity of these tests. They only perform esophageal contrast studies and endoscopy on zone I penetrating injuries if the wound approaches the mediastinum. These authors do not perform esophagography on asymptomatic patients with zone II and zone III injuries due to overlying bony shadows and contractions of the cricopharyngeus muscle that make the study technically difficult.[1,2]

Radiographic imaging for suspected laryngeal injury. The incidence of laryngeal injury in penetrating neck trauma varies from less than 10% to about 30%.[30] The signs and symptoms of penetrating laryngeal injury include voice alteration, airway compromise, subcutaneous emphysema, crepitus, and hemoptysis.[30] Some patients may be asymptomatic. Early active airway management is essential for patients with significant injury.

The diagnosis of laryngeal injury rests mainly on visualization of the endolarynx via indirect or direct laryngos-

---

*References 1, 3, 22, 26, 28, 29.

copy.[30] Visualization of the hypopharynx and larynx should be a standard part of the evaluation of patients with penetrating neck injury.[30]

Radiographic evaluation serves an adjunctive role. Soft tissue cervical radiographs may demonstrate subcutaneous emphysema or prevertebral air. Visualization with plain radiographs of a fractured larynx is possible in some patients, but a CT scan of the larynx very accurately identifies the location and extent of laryngeal fracture.[30] A CT scan should be performed when diagnosis of laryngeal fracture is suspected even in the presence of a negative examination of the endolarynx. In addition, a CT scan is helpful to diagnose laryngeal fracture when the endolarynx cannot be visualized, such as in an intubated patient.

Prompt diagnosis of laryngeal fracture and immediate surgical repair when indicated provides optimal management of such injuries.

Blunt neck trauma

Blunt trauma of the soft tissue of the neck may produce life-threatening emergencies similar to those of penetrating neck trauma. The injuries may be more subtle, however, because of the nonspecific nature of their initial presentation and the multitude of concomitant injuries. Rapid evaluation and treatment is the key to a successful outcome. Early airway management is mandatory for any signs of potential or incipient airway compromise.

Radiographic imaging for suspected vascular injury. Blunt trauma accounts for 3% to 10% of cervical vessel injuries.[31] The diagnosis of blunt carotid injury is very difficult. Twenty-five to 50% of patients have no external signs of cervical trauma.[32-34] Delayed neurologic deficits are the rule rather than the exception. Only 10% of patients have symptoms of transient ischemic attacks or strokes within 1 hour of their injury.[34] Most patients develop some symptoms within the first 24 hours after injury, but 17% develop symptomatology only days or weeks after.[34,35-37]

Crissey and Bernstein[38] have described four types of craniocervical injury that may produce traumatic thrombosis of the carotid artery: (1) a direct blow to the anteromedial neck with compression of the carotid artery; this occurs in about 50% of the patients and is most common in the elderly due to fracture of an atheromatous plaque at the carotid bifurcation;[36,38] (2) a blow to the side of the head or face causing rotation and hyperextension of the head and neck; this stretches the carotid artery across the bodies of the first and second cervical vertebrae or the transverse process of the third cervical vertebra, resulting in the rupture of the intima and media (most common in young patients who are victims of violent assaults or motorcycle accidents)[36]; (3) blunt or penetrating oral trauma, which are rare causes and more common in children, usually occurring when they fall on objects that are thrust in the open mouth; and (4) basilar skull fractures that may cause thrombosis of the intrapetrous portion of the internal carotid artery.

Fracture and disruption of the intima and sometimes the media, is the pathologic lesion responsible for the symptoms seen in blunt carotid trauma[33] (Fig. 3-12). Ninety-three percent of the lesions found in blunt cervical vessel injury are found at the bifurcation of the carotid arteries or higher.[31]

Angiography is not only the key to diagnosing blunt cervical vessel injuries but is also a necessity before surgical repair.[31,35,39] As previously mentioned, the signs of carotid artery injury may be delayed and extremely subtle. Carotid angiography is safe and should be employed in any patient strongly suspected of having sustained blunt carotid trauma,[35] or in any patient with the following signs and symptoms of cervical vessel injury:

- Hematoma in the lateral neck, particularly in the anterior triangle of the neck.[32,35]
- Bruit over the carotid circulation.[39]
- Horner's syndrome (ptosis, myosis, and anhydrosis) due to stretching or compression of the sympathetic ganglia.[32,33,38]
- Transient ischemic attacks.[32,33,38]
- Neurologic findings incongruent with head CT scan findings.[31]
- Basilar skull fracture in a patient with focal neurologic signs and a normal CT scan of the brain.[31]
- Lucid interval between the trauma and development of focal neurologic symptoms with a normal CT scan of the head.[33,34,38]

Complete four-vessel angiographic evaluation should be employed since multiple vessel injuries occur in approximately 40% of cases.[7,35,39,40] Angiography must be done early in the diagnostic work-up when symptomatology suggests injury. Angiographic visualization of the intracranial circulation is necessary, especially if neurologic deficits are present or if extracranial or intracranial bypass grafts are being considered as an operative repair.

Surgical repair improves outcome in patients with continuing antegrade flow, mild neurologic deficits,[35] and accessible lesions of recent onset.[31] There is as yet no reported experience with thrombolytic therapy for these lesions.

Radiographic imaging for suspected esophageal injury. Esophageal perforation from blunt cervical trauma is exceedingly rare.[41] The classic findings of esophageal perforation, such as subcutaneous emphysema, pneumomediastinum, severe chest or abdominal pain, are symptoms that are also found in more common injuries resulting from blunt cervical trauma.[28,41] In one study,[41] 78% of patients had symptoms, signs, or radiographic findings consistent with esophageal injury.

Diagnostic imaging. Plain radiographs, including soft tissue cervical radiographs and chest radiographs, should be performed on all patients with significant blunt cervical trauma. The presence of cervical subcutaneous emphysema, pneumomediastinum, pneumothorax, or pleural effusion should suggest esophageal injury.[41]

Esophagography should be performed on patients with

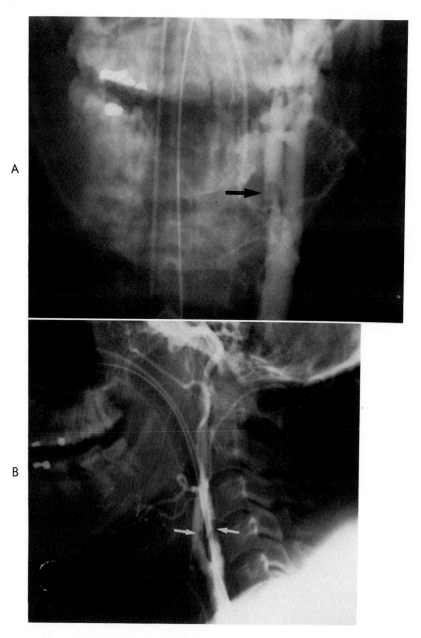

Fig. 3-12. A, AP projection reveals a filling defect in the proximal left internal carotid artery *(arrow)* following a direct blow to the neck, zone II injury. **B,** Lateral view of the same patient shows the previously demonstrated filling defect in the internal carotid artery as well as a second defect in the external carotid artery *(arrows)*. Surgical exploration revealed intimal tears with overlying thrombus.

suspected esophageal perforation. In one study[41] of 43 reported esophagograms, there were six false negatives. Esophagograms should initially be performed with a water-soluble contrast material such as gastrograffin and, if negative, should be repeated using barium to increase diagnostic yield.[41,42] A positive result confirms injury, but a negative esophagogram does not exclude esophageal trauma. Endoscopy should be performed on all patients with a high probability of injury, even with a negative esophagogram.

Radiographic imaging for suspected laryngeal injury.
Laryngeal injury usually results from a direct blow to the anterior neck that compresses the thyroid and cricoid cartilages against the cervical spine.[43] The "padded dash syndrome"[44] is a common mechanism for laryngeal trauma and occurs when a person's head strikes the windshield, causing hyperextension of the neck. The exposed anterior neck then strikes the narrow edge of the dash causing injury to the larynx.

Clinical findings. The classic signs and symptoms of

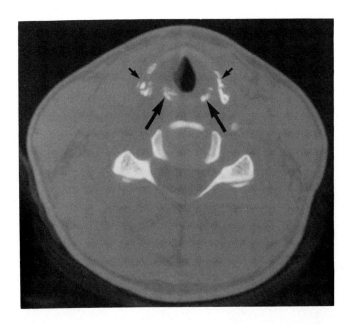

Fig. 3-13. Nonenhanced CT scan of the neck reveals multiple fractures of the thyroid cartilage *(small arrows)* and cricoid cartilages *(large arrows)*. (Courtesy Hugh D Curtin, MD.)

laryngeal injury include voice change, difficulty swallowing, hemoptysis, inability to tolerate a supine position, subcutaneous emphysema, and abrasions over the anterior neck.[43,45] However, few or no signs of laryngotracheal damage may be present.[45]

Diagnostic imaging. All patients with suspected laryngeal damage should initially undergo soft tissue lateral cervical radiographs and chest radiographs. The presence of subcutaneous emphysema, pneumomediastinum, or pneumothorax is suggestive of airway injury. Soft tissue lateral cervical radiographs may aid in the confirmation of airway distortion, but they usually provide inadequate visualization of cartilaginous damage.[43,46] Direct fiberoptic laryngoscopy provides accurate information on the status of the mucosa. The cartilage, however, is best evaluated with a CT scan. Both a CT scan and direct laryngoscopy are required in the evaluation of patients with suspected blunt upper airway injury.[47-50]

Patients with minor endolaryngeal hematomas or lacerations without detectable fracture on laryngoscopy should undergo a CT scan to confirm the integrity of the larynx[47,50] (Fig. 3-13). Some authors[50] recommend observation alone, without the use of CT scans, for patients who exhibit only mild vocal cord edema or small endolaryngeal hematomas with normal vocal cord movement.

Treatment. Patients with edema, hematoma, and minor mucosal disruptions without exposed cartilage noted on laryngoscopy require a CT scan. Those patients with nondisplaced fractures can be managed nonoperatively.[47,50] The use of CT scans in more significant laryngeal injuries is controversial. Some groups[47,48] feel that patients with massive edema, mucosal tears, exposed cartilage, and vocal cord immobility require immediate surgical intervention and that CT scans are redundant. Others feel that such scans are useful in preoperative planning since computed

tomographic images yield information not clearly visible on clinical examination.[49] In intubated patients, CT scans are useful to determine the need for open exploration since laryngoscopy cannot be performed.

Early airway management is the key for patients with signs of either potential for or actual airway compromise. Several authors[48,51] feel that endotracheal intubation is safe for airway control, while others[47,50] advocate tracheostomy. Cricothyrotomy is relatively contraindicated. Patients with an adequate airway, but with edematous or ecchymotic vocal cords, should be admitted for observation. Those patients with a displaced fracture or dislocated cartilage should be taken directly to the operating room.

Radiographic imaging in strangulation injury. Strangulation results from pressure on the neck and causes a broad spectrum of blunt neck trauma. Generally, the force required to cause laryngeal injury is usually immediately lethal.[52] For this reason, strangulation injuries with significant trauma are usually viewed by the pathologist rather than the emergency physician.

The method of strangulation is generally the most important determinant of type of injury. Most suicide hanging victims either place the ligature too high on the neck to damage the larynx or jump from heights too low to create high-velocity compressive forces that will seriously disrupt it.[52] Manual strangulation and ligature strangulation are most often associated with laryngeal and hyoid bone fractures.[52-54] Manual and ligature strangulations both involve a force that is static, similar to those created by Travis et al.[54] in their Static Force Tests.[52] These tests show that low-velocity forces can cause serious thyroid and cricoid cartilage fractures without causing gross crepitus, internal mucosal tears, or compromise of the airway. Forensic studies have found that the transverse intimal tears at the bifurcation of the common carotid arteries seen in judicial hangings are rare in nonjudicial hangings.[53] The traction injury, reported in about 5% of nonjudicial hangings, involves only slight bleeding into the walls of the carotid artery or minimal tears in the intima at the level of the ligature.[53]

Strangulation injuries should be evaluated cautiously not only because of the possible life-threatening nature of the injuries but also because of the psychologic and legal ramifications. Although injuries that will lead to chronic laryngeal stenosis are unlikely to occur, some survivors may suffer injuries that will cause permanent voice changes if left unrepaired. An aggressive approach to the diagnosis of laryngeal fractures is warranted.[52]

Soft tissue lateral cervical radiographs may demonstrate the presence of a laryngeal fracture, hyoid fracture (Fig. 3-14), prevertebral air, or subcutaneous emphysema. As previously mentioned, a CT scan should be performed in patients who have a significant mechanism for laryngeal injury and who demonstrate more than very mild edema of the endolarynx on indirect examination.[52]

The use of angiography for the diagnosis of vascular injuries should be used in a similar fashion as described for blunt trauma to the neck.

HEAD TRAUMA

Radiographic imaging of the cranium is essential in the management of head-injured patients. This section will investigate the roles of skull radiographs, computed tomography, and magnetic resonance imaging (MRI) in the evaluation of cranial trauma.

Blunt cranial trauma

The initial management of the severely head-injured patient should consist of a rapid assessment of the patient's stability, followed by a primary and secondary survey, including a thorough neurologic examination. Early airway intervention is essential. A CT scan of the brain without intravenous contrast will detect neurosurgically correctable lesions and will determine the need for craniotomy.

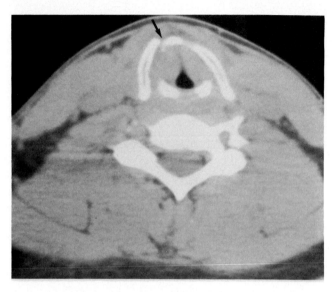

Fig. 3-14. Nonenhanced CT scan of neck showing fracture of the hyoid bone *(arrow)* following strangulation. (Courtesy Hugh D Curtin, MD.)

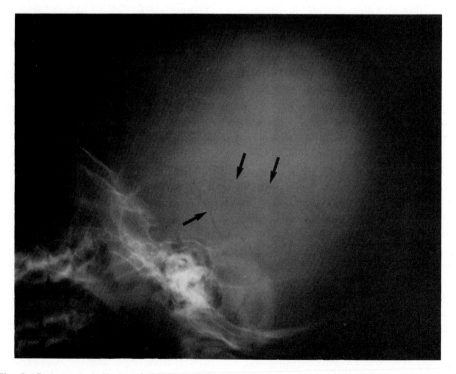

Fig. 3-15. Lateral skull view following a fall reveals nondisplaced linear fractures of the parietal and temporal bones *(arrows)*.

This section will discuss the radiographic approach to blunt cranial trauma. Emphasis will be placed on determining the correct radiographic procedure for the patient's level of cranial trauma and the time since injury.

Skull radiographs for blunt head injury. Since 1970, there has been decreasing use of skull radiographs in the evaluation of blunt cranial trauma. The discovery of a skull fracture (Fig. 3-15) as an isolated finding rarely warrants intervention.[55-58] It is the intracranial injuries resulting from head trauma that necessitate medical or surgical intervention to ensure a satisfactory outcome.[56,59] CT scans have replaced skull radiographs as the procedure of choice to detect intracranial injuries.

The controversy over whether skull radiographs are beneficial has not been completely resolved.[56,59-66] There has been a trend toward the use of high-yield criteria that can help identify patients whose management will be altered by the use of these studies (see criteria box).[56,59,64] Skull radiographs are not indicated in a large group of patients with minor (low-risk for intracranial injuries) or major (high-risk for intracranial injuries) head injuries (see risk box) but may be

beneficial in a select group of patients with certain clinical findings.[61]

The low-risk group, in particular, does not benefit from skull radiographs. In one study,[59] of a total of 9765 patients undergoing skull radiographs and meeting the criteria for the low-risk group, there were no intracranial injuries detected. The key to treatment of these patients was close observation.[59,67] There was no benefit or alteration of management based on information from skull radiographs.[59,62,67] Likewise, skull radiographs are not indicated in the high-risk group since an immediate CT scan is indicated.[59,67]

However, skull radiographs may alter the management of a select group of patients. Patients who possibly have a depressed skull fracture should undergo this test. The classic mechanism causing a depressed skull fracture is a large force directed over a small area. Fragments driven 5 mm or more below the inner skull table are likely to lacerate the dura or cortex.[68] Depressed skull fractures may be diagnosed via plain skull radiographs (Fig. 3-16). Tangential views of the fracture site (Fig. 3-17), however, are a more

---

Criteria for conventional skull radiographic studies

Potential for depressed skull fracture
Potential for penetrating injury
Missile penetration of the skull
Age less than 2 years
Potential for management alteration

From Health and Human Services: *The selection of patients for x-ray examination: skull x-ray for trauma,* Publication FDA 86-8263, 1986.

Risk for intracranial injury with head trauma

Low-risk group
  No symptoms
  Headache
  Dizziness
  Scalp hematoma
  Scalp laceration
  Scalp contusion or abrasion
High-risk group
  Depressed level of consciousness not clearly due to other causes
  Focal neurologic signs
  Decreasing level of consciousness
  Palpable depressed fracture
  Open wounds with exposed brain or CSF leak
  Post-traumatic seizures
  Prolonged unconsciousness following head trauma
  Abnormal mental status
  Progressive post-traumatic headache
  Progressive post-traumatic vomiting

Modified from Health and Human Services: *The selection of patients for x-ray examination: skull x-ray for trauma,* Publication FDA 86-8263, 1986.

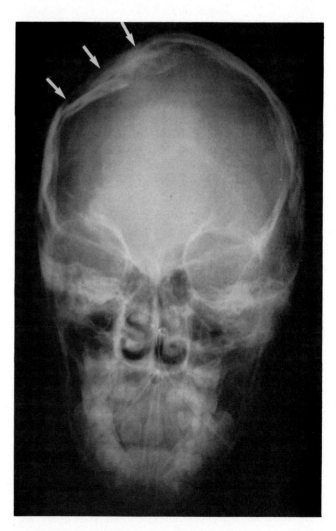

Fig. 3-16. AP view of the skull shows a depressed comminuted fracture of the parietal bone *(arrows)*, following a blow with a blunt object.

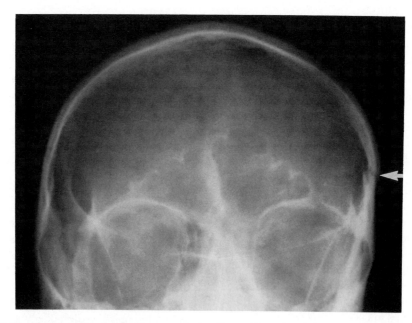

Fig. 3-17. Skull fracture visualized on standard radiographic series. A left tangential view, which was obtained to rule out a depressed fracture, shows several millimeters of depression in this parietal fracture *(arrow)*. (Courtesy Elizabeth Eelkema, MD.)

accurate method for detecting such skull fractures and measuring the degree of depression. Patients with depressed skull fractures should also undergo CT scans of the head to further define the amount of bony impingement on the intracranial cavity or the presence of associated bleeding or an intracranial foreign body (Figs. 3-18 and 3-19).

An open skull fracture is associated with an overlying laceration or one that extends into the paranasal sinuses, mastoid air cells, or the middle ear. Open skull fractures predispose the patient to infection. The fractures can usually be diagnosed clinically by direct palpation and visualization of the skull through the laceration. Skull radiographs may be indicated if there is a question as to whether or not a fracture is present, or if there is the potential for penetration of the cranial vault as might occur with a stab wound of the head.

Acute craniocerebral trauma in children differs from that found in adults. Open sutures (Fig. 3-20) with relative elasticity of the skull and incomplete myelinization with increased plasticity of the hemispheres permit severe distortions between the skull, underlying vessels, and brain.[59] Hematomas, tentorial and dural tears, and shearing injuries are much more common in young children (less than 2 years old) than in adults.[58] Depressed skull fractures in children are associated with an increased incidence of subsequent epilepsy. Diastatic fractures are associated with leptomeningeal cysts and hemorrhagic infarcts.

In children, the circumstances of the head injury are sometimes not clear. Nonaccidental trauma (NAT) is a major problem in infancy and childhood. Due to differ-

ences between child and adult head injury and because of the potential for NAT, some clinicians obtain skull radiographs in children with suspected skull fractures. In two studies[55,69] the incidence of skull fractures in children were 8.6% and 27% of those undergoing radiographic evaluation. In both studies, the presence of a simple skull fracture, without associated clinical abnormalities of the central nervous system, had no impact on the child's clinical course. However, depressed or compound fractures did alter the course of some of these children.

In one study,[55] the incidence of serious intracranial sequelae in children without skull fracture was 8%. In children with a skull fracture, it was 12%. The use of skull radiographs in children should be limited to children with suspected depressed or compound fractures or to those in whom radiographs would help in overall care because of parental concerns and to help in identifying NAT.

Intoxicated patients with head injuries are a final group of patients who might benefit from skull radiographs. Since altered mental status is presumed to be the result of alcohol, a prolonged period of observation is required before discharge. In several studies,[59,61,62,70] the presence of skull fracture in such patients is associated with a higher incidence of intracranial injuries in head trauma. Detection of a skull fracture early in the diagnostic work-up may expedite the search for intracranial injuries. Any patient with an altered mental status out of proportion to the alcohol level or with a deteriorating level of consciousness should undergo a CT scan immediately.

Computed tomography for blunt head injury. Since its introduction in 1972, computed tomography (CT scan)

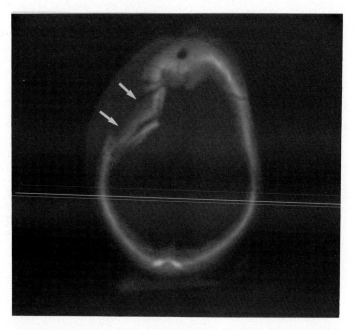

Fig. 3-18. CT scan at bone window settings revealing a severely depressed comminuted skull fracture *(arrows)* following a blow with a hammer.

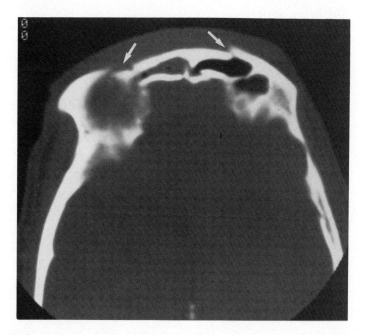

Fig. 3-19. CT scan at bone window settings showing a depressed fracture through inner and outer tables of the frontal sinuses *(arrows)*.

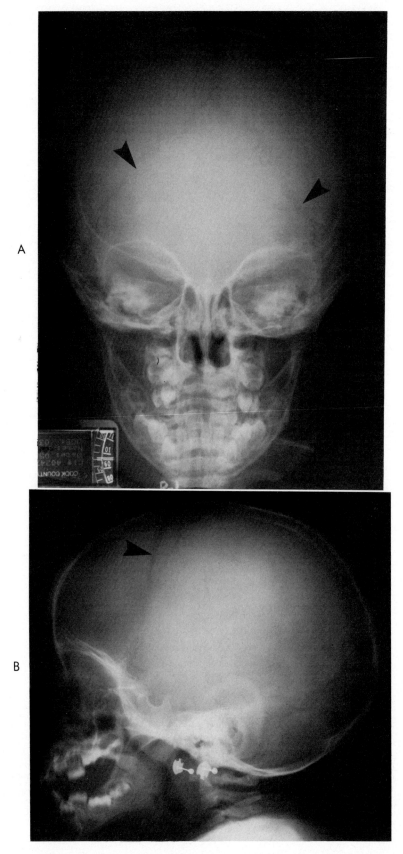

Fig. 3-20. Normal AP **(A)** and lateral **(B)** views of the skull in an infant demonstrating normal open sutures *(arrowheads)*.

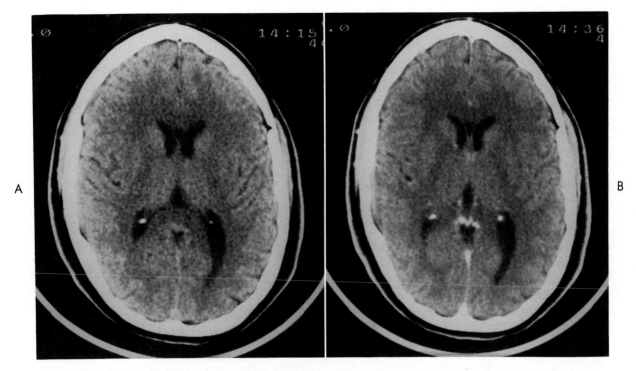

Fig. 3-21. Normal nonenhanced (**A**) and enhanced (**B**) CT scans at the level of the lateral ventricles.

Table 3-1. Glasgow coma scale

Eye opening	Talking	Motor	Score
Does not open eyes	Makes no noise	No motor response to pain	1
Opens eyes with pain	Moans, makes unintelligible sounds	Extensor response (decerebrate)	2
Opens eyes at loud verbal command	Talks, but nonsensical	Flexor response (decorticate)	3
Opens eyes on own	Seems confused, disoriented	Moves part of body but does not remove noxious stimulus	4
	Carries on conversation	Pushes away noxious stimulus	5
	Alert and oriented	Follows simple motor commands	6

From Rosen P, Baker FJ II, Barkin R et al, eds: *Emergency medicine: concepts and clinical practice,* ed 2, St Louis, 1988, CV Mosby.

has revolutionized the diagnosis and treatment of head injury. The CT scan is recognized as superior to skull radiography for detecting brain injury. It differentiates various tissue densities and can detect acute hemorrhage (Fig. 3-21). A CT scan is noninvasive, requires very little positioning, is rapid, and can be completed in less than 5 minutes. Linear skull fractures may be missed on a CT scan; however, these fractures are not clinically significant unless there is associated intracranial injury. A CT scan will localize depressed skull fractures[71] and will detect focal brain damage that can be treated surgically.

There is no consensus on the clinical indications for an immediate CT scan in blunt head trauma. All patients with either a Glasgow Coma Scale (GCS) less than 15, an ab-

normal mental status, or a persistent or focal neurologic deficit should be considered for an immediate CT head scan[67] (Table 3-1). Patients with a GCS of 15, a normal mental status, and a normal neurologic examination in the emergency department have an exceedingly small chance of developing serious complications from minor head trauma, and these patients can easily be observed.[67] Table 3-1 lists GCS criteria for patients who are at high risk for intracranial injury and who should undergo an immediate CT scan.[56,59,71] Another study[72] also recommends emergent CT scans on all patients with a history of loss of consciousness or amnesia following head trauma. Patients with a normal CT scan, a GCS of 15, and a mild head injury can be safely observed at home by family members.[72]

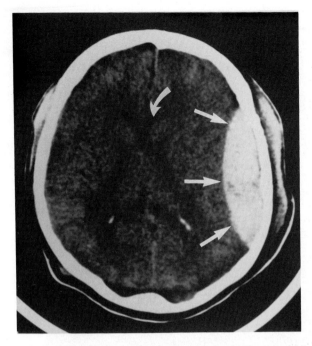

Fig. 3-22. Nonenhanced CT scan shows a classic biconvex high-density extracerebral collection as a result of an epidural hematoma *(arrows)*. Also note the midline shift *(curved arrow)*.

Different types of intracranial injury can be demonstrated on the CT scan. Epidural hematomas develop between the dura and the inner table of the skull. They are produced by arterial bleeding and are often associated with temporal bone fractures, which result in trauma to the middle meningeal artery. Epidural hematomas appear as biconvex extra-axial abnormalities on the CT scan (Fig. 3-22). This configuration is caused by the intimate attachment of the dura to the inner table of the skull, which inhibits diffuse spread of the blood as seen in subdural hematomas.[73] Adherence of the dura to the skull is greatest in infancy and old age so that epidural hematomas are seen less commonly at the extremes of life.[73] Secondary mass effect from the hematoma may produce displacement of the midline structures. Epidural hematomas are best visualized on a nonenhanced CT scan. Fresh blood on the CT scan appears as a white area of increased density. Epidural hematomas are a true neurosurgical emergency and must be treated expeditiously.

Subdural hematomas are the most common extra-cerebral intracranial lesion.[71] In comparison to epidural hematomas, subdural hematomas occur under the dura, are usually diffuse, and involve venous bleeding. Subdural hematomas appear on a CT scan as a convex configuration along the inner table with a concave inner margin as it

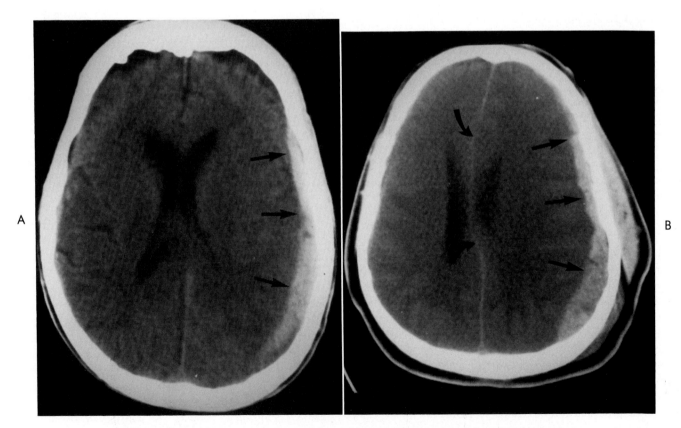

Fig. 3-23. A and **B,** Nonenhanced CT scans in two different patients reveal high-density extracerebral collections *(arrows)* conforming to the contour of the cerebral cortex, representative of acute subdural hematomas. Note also midline shift *(curved arrows)* in **B** and marked soft tissue swelling. (Courtesy Elizabeth Eelkema, MD.)

conforms to the contours of the brain (Fig. 3-23). Occasionally, localized subdural hematomas may be convex and resemble epidural hematomas[71,74] (Fig. 3-24).

Subdural hematomas may be classified as acute (high density) if less than 24 hours old, subacute (high density to isodense) if 2 to 10 days old, and chronic (low density) if greater than 10 days old.[75] Acute subdural hematomas are high-density lesions on the CT scan and appear white. Chronic subdural hematomas appear as low-density lesions. The subdural collection of blood tends to become isodense with the adjacent brain usually in 15 to 90 days. During this time, the high absorption index of the blood dependent on the protein concentrations in hemoglobin decreases with time.[71,75] Thus chronic subdural hematomas may sometimes be difficult to detect since they become isodense with the surrounding brain tissue. High-dose intravenous contrast material infusion may enhance the surrounding brain to make an isodense subdural hematoma more apparent[73] (Fig. 3-25). Similarly, the contrast material may collect in the subdural hematoma to make it more visible.[73] Midline shift present on a CT scan may help in the diagnosis of an isodense subdural hematoma (Fig. 3-26). A false negative CT scan sometimes occurs with bilateral isodense subdural hematomas and no midline shift[73] (Fig. 3-27). Prompt neurosurgical evaluation with surgical intracranial decompression, if necessary, improves outcome, reduces mortality, and improves functional recovery.[76,77]

An acute intracerebral hematoma (Fig. 3-28) appears on a CT scan as a circumscribed area of high density sur-

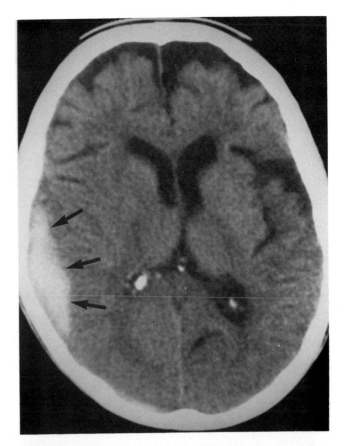

Fig. 3-24. Nonenhanced CT scan demonstrates acute subdural hematoma resembling an epidural hematoma *(arrows)*. This can occasionally be seen when atrophy is present. (Courtesy Elizabeth Eelkema, MD.)

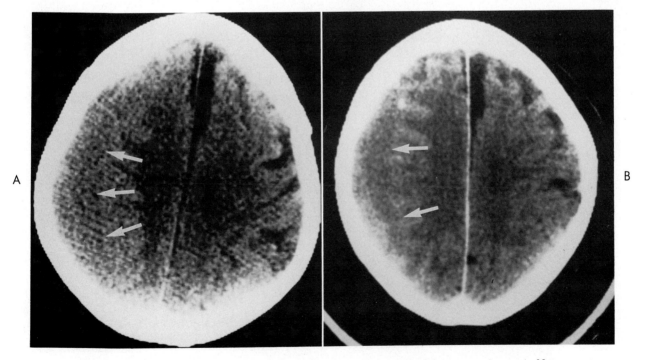

Fig. 3-25. A, Nonenhanced CT scan shows an isodense subdural hematoma *(arrows)*. Note asymmetry of sulci from right to left as a clue to diagnosis. **B,** Enhanced CT scan better differentiates underlying parenchyma from overlying isodense subdural hematoma *(arrows)*. These scans were taken on a first generation CT scanner. Note the poor definition.

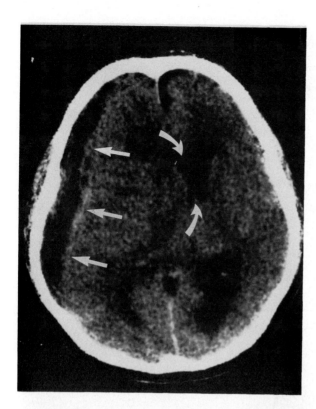

Fig. 3-26. Enhanced CT scan showing chronic (low-density) subdural hematoma with enhancement of a membrane *(arrows)* and marked midline shift *(curved arrows).*

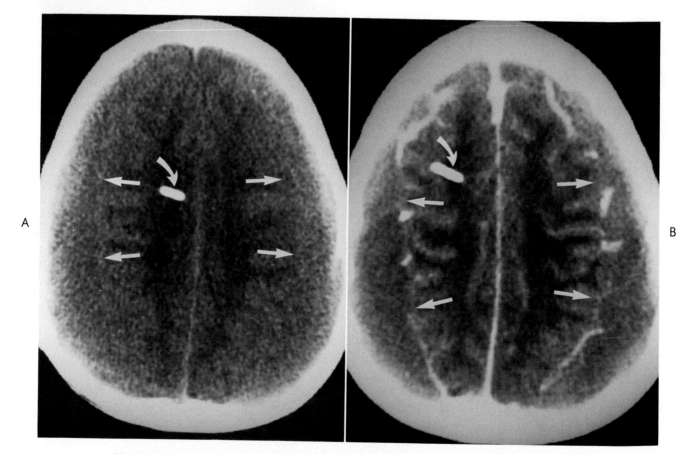

Fig. 3-27. A, Nonenhanced CT scan showing bilateral isodense subdural hematomas *(arrows).* The absence of sulci suggests the diagnosis. **B,** Enhanced CT scan demonstrates the findings much more clearly *(arrows).* These subdural hematomas developed following the insertion of a ventricular shunt *(curved arrows)* for treatment of hydrocephalus. (Courtesy Elizabeth Eelkema, MD.)

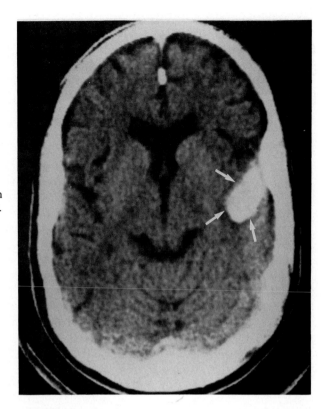

Fig. 3-28. Nonenhanced CT scan showing a high-density collection in the left temporal lobe *(arrows)* representing an intracerebral hematoma.

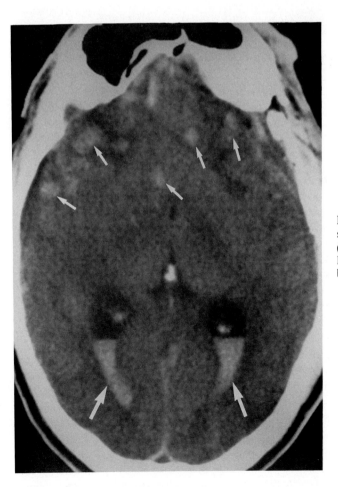

Fig. 3-29. Nonenhanced CT scan showing multiple small high-density areas in the frontal lobes bilaterally, representing contusions *(short arrows)*. Also note the presence of intraventricular blood, which layers out due to the supine position *(long arrows)*. (Courtesy Elizabeth Eelkema, MD.)

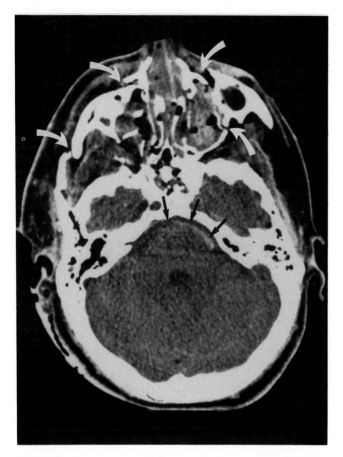

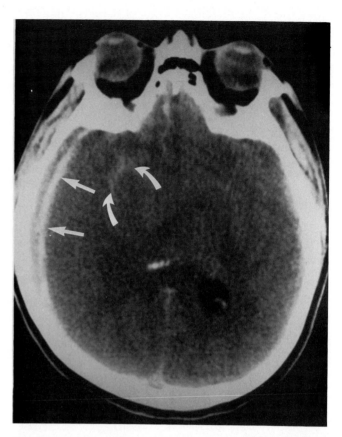

Fig. 3-30. Nonenhanced CT scan demonstrating a high-density collection *(dark arrows)* in the prepontine cistern due to subarachnoid hemorrhage. This resulted from severe craniofacial trauma as shown by multiple complex facial fractures *(curved arrows)*. (Courtesy Elizabeth Eelkema, MD.)

Fig. 3-31. Nonenhanced CT scan demonstrating both subarachnoid blood *(curved arrows)* in the sylvian fissure and also an acute subdural hematoma *(arrows)*. (Courtesy Elizabeth Eelkema, MD.)

rounded by a rim of low density due to associated edema that exerts a mass effect.[70,75] Several days after injury, the hematoma becomes less dense and the area of surrounding edema enlarges.[74]

Cerebral contusion (Fig. 3-29) is a very common posttraumatic injury. A contusion appears on a CT scan as a nonhomogenous area of high and low densities[71,74] caused by the presence of extravasated blood in swollen, edematous brain. A mass effect may be present due to swelling.

Ninety percent of subarachnoid hemorrhages can be visualized on a CT scan if the scans are performed within 5 days of the event.[71] A subarachnoid hemorrhage (Figs. 3-30 and 3-31) appears as an area of increased density in the region of the falx and basal cisterns on a nonenhanced CT scan. This may be followed by an enhanced CT scan to help identify arteriovenous (AV) malformations and aneurysms[71] or to help better quantify the parenchymal involvement. A CT scan may be normal in about 10% of patients with a subarachnoid hemorrhage. A lumbar puncture should be performed in a patient with suspected subarach-

noid hemorrhage with a normal neurologic examination and after a normal CT scan in order to detect the 10% of subarachnoid hemorrhages that are not visible on the scan.

Magnetic resonance imaging for blunt head injury. At the current time, magnetic resonance imaging (MRI) is not recommended for the evaluation of acute head trauma since computed tomography is superior to MRI in managing patients with acute moderate-to-severe head injury.[78] Both CT scans and MRI detect acute hemorrhagic lesions equally well,[79,80] but the CT scan is faster, more readily available, and easier to perform in patients requiring life-support equipment. A CT scan detects cerebral trauma amenable to surgical intervention.[78,80] In addition, CT scans depict skull fractures[81] while lack of signal-generating protons in bone renders bone invisible on MRI. CT scans are equal to or better than MRI in detecting subarachnoid hemorrhages.[78,79,81]

MRI is superior to CT scans in detecting intracranial injuries in the subacute or chronic stage[78] and in patients

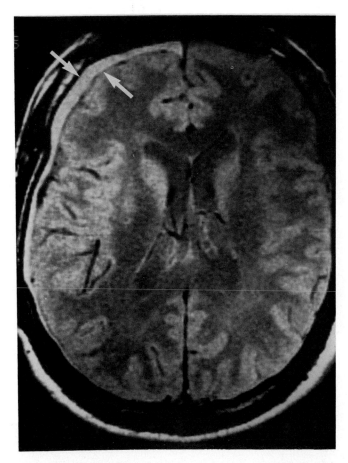

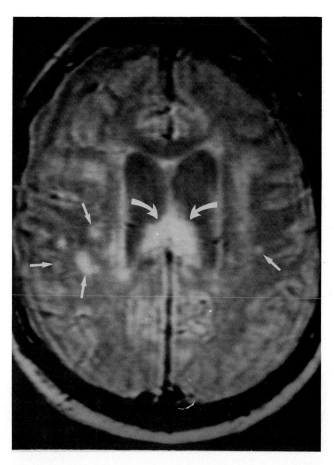

Fig. 3-32. Axial MRI proton-density image demonstrating an area of increased signal intensity conforming to the cerebral cortex *(arrows)* representing a subdural hematoma. The patient had previously undergone a CT scan that was normal. (Courtesy Elizabeth Eelkema, MD.)

Fig. 3-33. Comatose male with no apparent abnormality on CT scan following a motor vehicle accident. Axial proton-density MRI image shows multiple areas of high-signal intensity in the white matter bilaterally *(arrows)*. This is seen in shearing injuries. Also note high-signal intensity in the corpus callosum *(curved arrows)*, which may be due to a contusion. (Courtesy Elizabeth Eelkema, MD.)

with minor head trauma. Both isodense subdural hematomas[80,82] and small acute subdural hematomas that are insufficient to cause any mass effect[78,81,83] are better visualized on MRI than on a CT scan. In 100 patients[78] evaluated by both MRI and computed tomography, a CT scan missed 58% of small subdural hematomas and 80% of transversely oriented subdural hematomas. MRI was equal to or superior to the CT scan in 94 of 95 patients in the subacute or chronic phases of their injury (Fig. 3-32).

MRI also identifies shearing brain injuries and nonhemorrhagic contusions that are not visible on CT scans[78,80,84,85] (Fig. 3-33). These are the brain injuries that often result from NAT and that may lead to seizure disorders.[81] Thus MRI may detect milder forms of NAT than the CT scan.

In summary, MRI is not recommended for detecting surgically correctable lesions in the acutely traumatized patient with moderate-to-severe head injury. MRI is superior to the CT scan, however, in detecting small subdural hematomas, subdural hematomas in the subacute or chronic phase, nonhemorrhagic contusions, or shearing injuries. In these clinical situations, MRI, when available, will probably replace the CT scan as the procedure of choice.

Penetrating cranial trauma

The initial management and resuscitation of patients with penetrating injuries to the skull is similar to the management of those with blunt trauma.

AP and lateral skull radiographs must be obtained early in the evaluation of the patient to determine the location and extent of skull penetration (Figs. 3-34 and 3-35). Bihemispheric involvement secondary to the missile crossing the midline carries a very poor prognosis[86] and is considered lethal by some.[87] Tangential radiographs to the site of penetration may be helpful in determining skull penetration in low-velocity missile wounds and stab wounds or if a foreign body is imbedded in the skull.

A CT scan should be obtained expeditiously on all patients with skull penetration. The scan can reveal the bullet or knife track with any accompanying intracranial injuries[88] (Fig. 3-36). A CT scan with a knife blade in place can yield

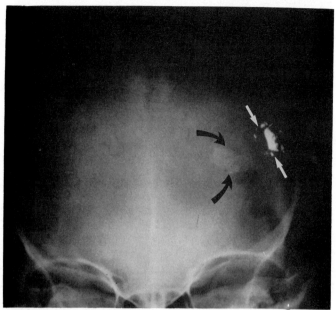

Fig. 3-34. AP skull radiograph showing multiple bullet fragments *(arrows)* and also a bony fragment *(curved arrows)* in the left cerebral hemisphere.

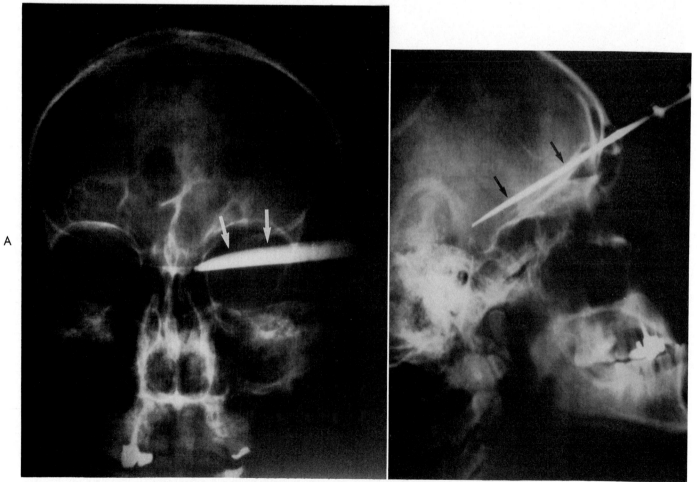

A

B

Fig. 3-35. AP **(A)** and left lateral **(B)** radiographs of a patient showing a large knife that has penetrated the cranial vault *(arrows).* (Courtesy John A Marx, MD.)

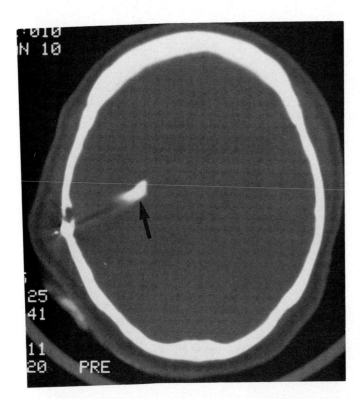

Fig. 3-36. CT scan showing an intracranial bony fragment *(arrow)* secondary to a gunshot wound.

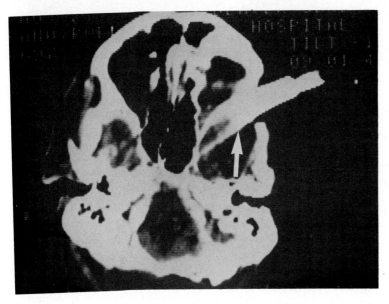

Fig. 3-37. CT scan of the same patient in Fig. 3-35 showing location of knife blade in the middle cranial fossa *(arrow)*. (Courtesy John A Marx, MD.)

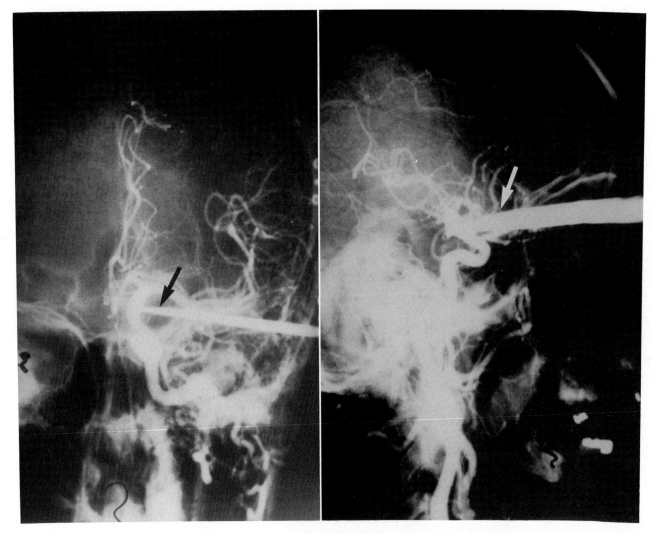

Fig. 3-38. AP (**A**) and left lateral (**B**) carotid angiograms of the same patient as in Figs. 3-35 and 3-37, showing relationship of knife tip to be within a few millimeters of the supra-clinoid carotid artery. (Courtesy John A Marx, MD.)

useful information despite the metal artifact[88] (Fig. 3-37).

Following the CT scan, angiography is indicated for patients with a stab wound to the cranium with the knife in place, unless precluded by rapid clinical deterioration.[88] The angiogram guides the removal of the knife blade and alerts the surgeon to the potential for massive intraoperative hemorrhage (Fig. 3-38).

SUMMARY

Injuries to the head and neck are among the most complicated and difficult to manage. Emergent intervention may be life-saving. Early and appropriate use of radiographic imaging will lead to more accurate diagnosis of the injury and will expedite appropriate treatment.

REFERENCES

1. Narrod JA, Moore EE: Initial management of penetrating neck wounds—a selective approach, *J Emerg Med* 2:14, 1984.
2. Jurkovich GJ, Zingarelli W, Wallace J et al: Penetrating neck trauma: diagnostic studies in the asymptomatic patient, *J Trauma* 25:819, 1985.
3. Shama DM, Odell J: Penetrating neck trauma with tracheal and oesophageal injuries, *Br J Surg* 71:534, 1984.
4. Orgog GJ, Albin D et al: 110 bullet wounds to the neck, *J Trauma* 25:238, 1985.
5. Belinkie SA, Russell JC, DaDilva J et al: Management of penetrating neck injuries, *J Trauma* 23:235, 1983.
6. Dunbar LL, Adkins RB, and Waterhouse G: Penetrating injuries to the neck—selective management, *Am Surg* 50:198, 1984.
7. Obeid FN, Haddad GS, Horst HM et al: A critical reappraisal of a mandatory exploration policy for penetrating wounds of the neck, *Surg Gynecol Obstet* 160:517, 1985.
8. Fitchett VH, Pomerantz M, Butsch AW et al: Penetrating wounds of the neck, *Arch Surg* 119:574, 1984.
9. Fogelman MS, Stewart RD: Penetrating wounds of the neck, *Am J Surg* 91:581, 1956.
10. Knightly JJ, Swaminathan AP, and Rush BP: Management of penetrating wounds of the neck, *Am J Surg* 126:575, 1973.

11. McInnis WA, Cnz AB, and Aust JB: Penetrating injuries to the neck, *Am J Surg* 130:416, 1975.

12. Roon AJ, Christensen N: Evaluation and treatment of penetrating cervical injuries, *J Trauma* 19:391, 1979.

13. Weaver Aw, Fromm SH, and Wah AJ: The management of penetrating wounds of the neck, *Surg Gynecol Obstet* 133:49, 1971.

14. Meyer JP, Barrett JA et al: Mandatory vs. selective exploration for penetrating neck trauma, *Arch Surg* 122:592, 1987.

15. Golueke PJ, Goldstein AS, Sclafani SJA et al: Routine versus selective exploration of penetrating neck injuries: a randomized prospective study, *J Trauma* 24:1010, 1984.

16. Metzdorff MT, Lowe DK: Operation or observation for penetrating neck wounds? *Am J Surg* 147:646, 1984.

17. Massac E, Siram SM, and Leffall LD: Penetrating neck wounds, *Am J Surg* 145:263, 1983.

18. Ayuyao AM, Kaledzi YL et al: Penetrating neck wounds: mandatory versus selective exploration, *Ann Surg* 202:563, 1985.

19. Rao PM, Bhatti MF, Gaudino J et al: Penetrating injuries of the neck: criteria for exploration, *J Trauma* 23:47, 1983.

20. Wood J, Fabian T, and Mangiante EC: Penetrating neck injuries: recommendations for selective management, *J Trauma* 29:5 602-605, 1989.

21. Saletta JD, Folk FA, and Freeark RJ: Trauma to the neck region, *Symp Head Neck Surg* 53:73, 1973.

22. Narrod JA, Moore EE: Selective management of penetrating neck injuries, *Arch Surg* 119:574, 1984.

23. Rivers SP, Yashwant P et al: Limited role of arteriography in penetrating neck trauma, *J Vasc Surg* 8:112, 1988.

24. Sclafani SJA, Panetta T, Goldstein AS et al: The management of arterial injuries caused by penetration of zone III of the neck, *J Trauma* 25:871, 1985.

25. Calcateria TC, Holt GP: Carotid artery injuries, *Laryngoscope* 82:321, 1972.

26. Spenler CW, Benfield JR: Esophageal disruption from blunt and penetrating external trauma, *Arch Surg* 111:663, 1976.

27. Symbas PN, Hatcher CR et al: Esophageal gunshot injuries, *Ann Surg* 191:703, 1980.

28. Glatterer MS, Toon RS et al: Management of blunt and penetrating external esophageal trauma, *J Trauma* 25:784, 1985.

29. Sheely CH, Mattox KL, Beall AC et al: Penetrating wounds of the cervical esophagus, *Am J Surg* 130:707, 1975.

30. Thompson JN, Strausbaugh PL et al: Penetrating injuries of the larynx, *South Med J* 77:41, 1984.

31. Fakhry SM, Jaques PF, and Proctor HJ: Cervical vessel injury after blunt trauma, *J Vasc Surg* 8:501, 1988.

32. Bessen HA, Mooney RP: Delayed hemiparesis following nonpenetrating carotid artery trauma, *Am J Emerg Med* 6:341, 1988.

33. Jernigan WR, Gardner WC: Carotid artery injuries due to closed cervical trauma, *J Trauma* 11:429, 1971.

34. Yamada S, Kindt GW, and Youmans JR: Carotid artery occlusion due to nonpenetrating injury, *J Trauma* 7:333, 1967.

35. Perry MO, Snyder WH, and Thal ER: Carotid artery injuries caused by blunt trauma, *Ann Surg* 192:74, 1980.

36. Mooney RP, Bessen HA: Delayed hemiparesis following nonpenetrating carotid artery trauma, *Am J Emerg Med* 6:341, 1988.

37. McNab AA, Fabinyl, and Milne PY: Blunt trauma to the carotid artery, *Aust NZ J Surg* 58:651, 1988.

38. Crissey MM, Bernstein EF: Delayed presentation of carotid initial tear following blunt craniocervical trauma, *Surgery* 75:574, 1974.

39. Richardson JD, Simpson C, and Miller FB: Management of carotid artery trauma, *Surgery* 104:673, 1988.

40. Chedid M, Deeb Z et al: Major cerebral vessel injury caused by a seatbelt shoulder strap: case report, *J Trauma* 29:1601, 1989.

41. Beal S, Pottmeyer EW, and Spisso JM: Esophageal perforation following external blunt trauma, *J Trauma* 28:1425, 1988.

42. Foley JR, Gahremoni EG, and Rogers JA: Reapprasial of contrast material used to detect upper gastrointestinal perforations, *Diagn Radiol* 144:231, 1982.

43. Camnitz PA, Shepherd SM, and Henderson RA: Acute blunt laryngeal and tracheal trauma, *Am J Emerg Med* 5:157, 1987.

44. Butler RM, Moser FH: The padded dash syndrome: blunt trauma to the larynx and trachea, *Laryngoscope* 78:1172, 1968.

45. Reece GP, Shatney CH: Blunt injuries of the cervical trachea: review of 51 patients, *South Med J* 81:1542, 1988.

46. Spira R, Bolanos R: Perforation of the hypopharynx: demonstration by computerized tomography, *South Med J* 5:658, 1988.

47. Schaefer SD: Primary management of laryngeal trauma, *Ann Otol Rhinol Laryngol* 91: 1982.

48. Gussack GS, Jurkovich GJ: Treatment dilemmas in laryngotracheal trauma, *J Trauma* 10:1439, 1988.

49. Schild JA, Denneny EC: Evaluation and treatment of acute laryngeal fractures, *Head Neck Surg* 11:491-6, 1989.

50. Fuhrman GM, Stieg FH, and Buerk CA: Blunt laryngeal trauma: classification and management protocol, 1:87, 1990.

51. Guertler AT: Blunt laryngeal trauma associated with shoulder harness use, *Ann Emerg Med* 17:838, 1988.

52. Line WS: Strangulation: a full spectrum of blunt neck trauma, *Ann Otol Rhinol Laryngol* 94:542, 1985.

53. Iverson KV: Strangulation: a review of ligature, manual, and postural neck compression injuries, *Ann Emerg Med* 13:179, 1984.

54. McHugh T, Stout M: Near-hanging injury, *Ann Emerg Med* 12:774, 1983.

55. Harwood-Nash DC, Hendrick EB, and Hudson AR: The significance of skull fractures in children, *Pediatr Radiol* 101:151, 1971.

56. Masters, SJ: Evaluation of head trauma: efficacy of skull films, *AJR* 135:539, 1980.

57. Eyes B, Evans AF: Post-traumatic skull radiographs, *Lancet* 2(8080):85, 1978.

58. Zimmerman RA, Bilaniok LT: Computerized tomography in pediatric head trauma, *J Neuroradiol* 8:257, 1981.

59. Masters SJ, McClean PM, Arcarese JS et al: Skull x-ray examinations after head trauma, *N Engl J Med* 316:84, 1987.

60. North S, Pollak EW: Skull roentgenography in the evaluation of head injury, *South Med J* 76:468, 1983.

61. Fisher RP, Carlson J, and Perry JF: Post-concussive hospital observation of alert patients in a primary trauma center, *J Trauma* 21:920, 1981.

62. Dacey RG, Alves WM, Rimel RW et al: Neurosurgical complications after apparently minor head injury, *J Neurosurg* 65:203, 1986.

63. Young HA, Schmidek HH: Complications accompanying occipital skull fracture, *J Trauma* 22:914, 1982.

64. Bell RS, Loop JW: The utility and futility of radiographic skull examination for trauma, *N Engl J Med* 284:236, 1971.

65. DeSmet AA, Fryback DG, and Thornbury JR: A second look at the utility of radiographic skull examination for trauma, *AJR* 132:95, 1979.

66. Bligh AS, Davies ER, Ennis WP et al: Cost and benefits of skull radiography for head injury, *Lancet* 2(8250):791, 1981.

67. Feuerman T, Wackym PA, Gade GF et al: Value of skull radiography, head computed tomographic scanning, and admission for observation in cases of minor head injury, *Neurosurgery* 22:449, 1988.

68. Stevenson BE: Initial management of the acute head injury, *Otolaryngol Clin North Am* 12:279, 1979.

69. Roberts E, Shopener CE: Plain skull roentgenograms in children with head trauma, 114:230, 1970.

70. Servadei F, Ciucci G et al: Skull fractures as a factor of increased risk in minor head injuries—indication for a broader use of cerebral computed tomography scanning, *Surg Neurol* 30:364, 1988.

71. McMicken DB: Emergency CT head scans in traumatic and atraumatic conditions, *Ann Emerg Med* 15:274, 1986.

72. Stein SC, Ross SE: The value of computed tomographic scans in patients with low-risk head injuries, *Neurosurgery* 26:638, 1990.

73. Davis KR, Taveras JM, Roberson GH et al: Computed tomography in head trauma, *Semin Roentgenol* 12:53, 1977.

74. Bruce DA, Schut L: The value of CAT scanning following pediatric head injury, *Clin Pediatr* 11:719, 1980.

75. Danziger A, Price H: The evaluation of head trauma by computed tomography, *J Trauma* 19:1, 1979.

76. Seelig JM, Becker DP, Miller D et al: Traumatic acute subdural hematoma, *N Engl J Med* 304:1511, 1981.

77. Haselsberger K, Pucher R, and Auer LM: Prognosis after acute subdural or epidural haemorrhage, *Acta Neurochir Wien* 90:111, 1988.

78. Kelly AB, Zimmerman RD, Snow RB et al: Head trauma: comparison of MRI and CT experience in 100 patients, *AJNR* 9:699, 1988.

79. Gentry LR, Godersky JC, Thompson B et al: Prospective comparative study of intermediate-field MR and CT in the evaluation of closed head trauma, *AJNR* 150:673, 1988.

80. Zimmerman RA, Bilaniuk LT, Hackney DB et al: Head injury: early results of comparing CT and high-field MR, *AJNR* 147:1215, 1986.

81. Alexander RC, Schor DP, and Smith WL: Magnetic resonance imaging of intracranial injuries from child abuse, *J Pediatr* 109:975, 1986.

82. Sipponen JT, Sepponen KE, and Sivula A: Chronic subdural hematoma: demonstration by magnetic resonance, *Radiology* 150:79, 1984.

83. Gandy SE, Snow RB, Zimmerman RD et al: Cranial nuclear magnetic resonance imaging in head trauma, *Ann Neurol* 16:254, 1984.

84. Hesselink JR, Dowd CF: MR imaging of brain contusions: a comparative study with CT, *AJR* 150:1133, 1988.

85. Gentry LR, Godersky JC, and Thompson BH: Traumatic brain stem injury: MR imaging, *Radiology* 171:177, 1989.

86. Nagib MG, Rockswold GL, Sherman RS et al: Civilian gunshot wounds to the brain: prognosis and management, *Neurosurgery* 18:553, 1986.

87. Selden BS, Goodman JM, Cordell WC et al: Outcome of self-inflicted gunshot wounds of the brain, *Ann Emerg Med* 17:247, 1988.

88. Haworth CS, deVilliers JC: Stab wounds to the temporal fossa, *Neurosurgery* 23:431, 1988.

Facial Trauma

John McGill
Louis J. Ling
Saul Taylor

The emergency radiographic evaluation of facial trauma should be limited to moderately injured patients. Physical examination will suffice for patients with minimal injury whereas patients with severe injury require evaluation and stabilization of life-threatening injuries before facial trauma is addressed. Airway obstruction may result from severe facial injuries, and the decision to stabilize the airway is always based on clinical assessment and should never wait for radiographic evaluation. Other major injuries associated with facial trauma include intracranial and cervical spine injuries and injuries to the globe and optic nerve. These injuries must be excluded before proceeding with the assessment of facial trauma. Even major Le Fort and central smash fractures can be radiographically ignored in the emergency department. The first radiographic evaluation of these injuries is frequently obtained in conjunction with a CT scan of the head.

Radiographic evaluation of facial injuries is especially challenging because the complex facial structure results in a confusing overlapping of densities on the radiograph.[1] The use of multiple facial views from differing angles is helpful in optimally illustrating these facial structures. It is important for the clinician to know what views are best for the suspected fractures and how patient position may affect the appearance of the radiograph.[2]

The PA Waters view (Fig. 4-1) is the single most valuable view in evaluating facial injuries. In this projection, the maxillary sinuses are projected above the petrous ridges. The resulting image displays the maxillary sinus, the malar portion of the zygoma, the arch of the nasal bone, and the nasal septum. In the cooperative patient, an upright Waters view (Fig. 4-2) may demonstrate an air-fluid level in the maxillary sinus representing blood after acute injury. When the patient is uncooperative or has a potential cervical spine injury, an AP (reverse) Waters

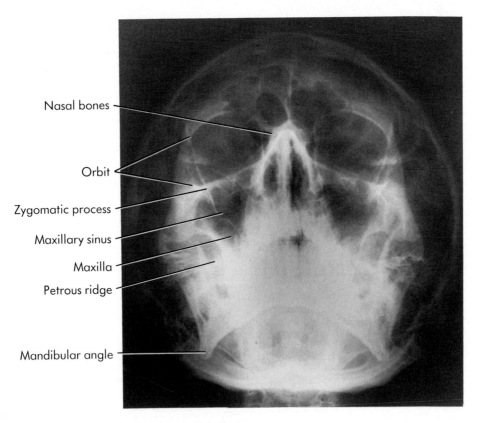

Nasal bones

Orbit

Zygomatic process

Maxillary sinus

Maxilla

Petrous ridge

Mandibular angle

Fig. 4-1. Waters view showing normal facial anatomic landmarks and structures. (Ballinger PW: *Merrill's atlas of radiographic positions and radiologic procedures,* ed 7, vol 2, St Louis, 1991, Mosby–Year Book.)

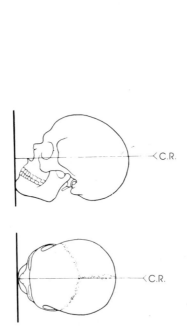

Fig. 4-2. Position of skull during normal PA upright Waters view. (Ballinger PW: *Merrill's atlas of radiographic positions and radiologic procedures,* ed 7, vol 2, St Louis, 1991, Mosby–Year Book.)

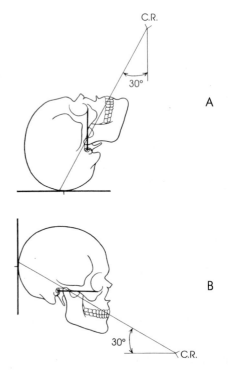

Fig. 4-3. Position of skull during normal AP supine Waters view. **A,** Table radiography. **B,** Upright radiography. (Ballinger PW: *Merrill's atlas of radiographic positions and radiologic procedures,* ed 7, vol 2, St Louis, 1991, Mosby–Year Book.)

view (Fig. 4-3) can be taken of the supine patient. However, in this view, an air-fluid level is not visible and blood will appear as a diffuse haziness in the sinus. Also, because facial bones are further from the cassette in the reverse Waters, there is loss of bony detail as a result of scatter of the x-ray beam. If there is inadequate head tilt when positioning the patient, the petrous bones will be superimposed over the inferior portion of the maxillary sinus and will obscure pathology in this area.

In the Caldwell view (Fig. 4-4), the orbital floor is pro-

jected above the petrous ridges. The frontal and ethmoid sinuses and superior orbits are easily seen as is the outline of the mandible. However, the maxillary sinus is not well visualized. This view differs from a true PA skull view in which the petrous bones are superimposed over the orbit. If the patient is upright, air-fluid levels may be seen. In patients who are uncooperative or on a backboard, the AP view can be substituted, but will provide less resolution of bony detail.

The lateral facial view (Fig. 4-5) is particularly difficult

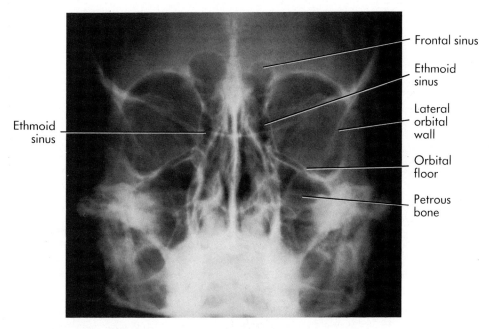

Fig. 4-4. Caldwell view showing normal facial anatomic landmarks and structures.

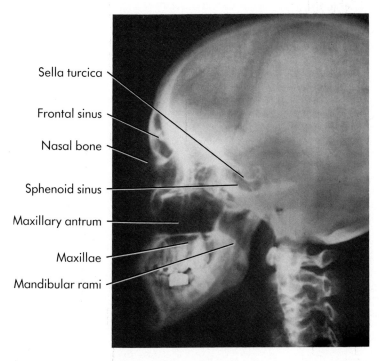

Fig. 4-5. Lateral view showing normal facial anatomic landmarks and structures. (Ballinger PW: *Merrill's atlas of radiographic positions and radiologic procedures,* ed 7, vol 2, St Louis, 1991, Mosby–Year Book.)

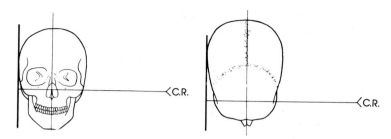

Fig. 4-6. Position of patient during upright lateral views. (Ballinger PW: *Merrill's atlas of radiographic positions and radiologic procedures,* ed 7, vol 2, St Louis, 1991, Mosby–Year Book.)

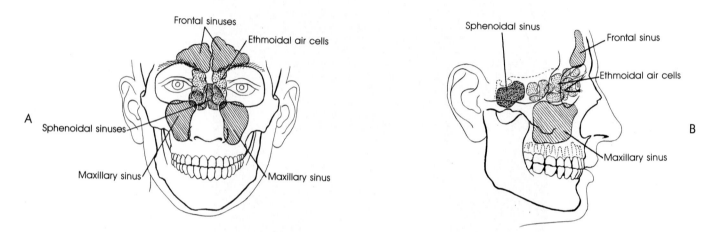

Fig. 4-7. A, Anterior aspect of paranasal sinuses, showing lateral relation to each other and to surrounding parts. **B,** Anteroposterior relation of paranasal sinuses to each other and surrounding parts. (Ballinger PW: *Merrill's atlas of radiographic positions and radiologic procedures,* ed 7, vol 2, St Louis, 1991, Mosby–Year Book.)

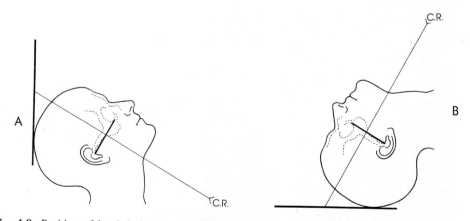

Fig. 4-8. Position of head during a submental vertex view. **A,** Upright radiography. **B,** Table radiography. (Ballinger PW: *Merrill's atlas of radiographic positions and radiologic procedures,* ed 7, vol 2, St Louis, 1991, Mosby–Year Book.)

to interpret because of the superimposition of bilateral structures. Air-fluid levels may be present in the sinuses, but their appearance will depend on whether the patient is upright (Fig. 4-6) or supine. This is the only view in which the sphenoid sinus, the posterior frontal and maxillary sinus walls, and the pterygoids are visualized (Fig. 4-7). A lateral skull view cannot substitute for the lateral view of the facial bones because the increased exposure required to penetrate the cranium results in loss of facial bony detail. Fractures of the upper cervical spine and cranium occasionally can be seen on this view.

The submental vertex view (Fig. 4-8) is obtained primarily when a zygomatic arch fracture is suspected. Because it is necessary to underexpose this view to visualize the zygomatic arch, evaluation of other structures is difficult. If the patient is not correctly centered, one of the arches may be hidden by the skull. In addition to visualizing the zygomatic arches, the submental vertex view may provide information about the mandible, the lateral wall of the maxillary sinus, and both walls of the frontal sinus.

The mandible is best evaluated with a panoramic view

(Fig. 4-9, *A*). This view requires the patient to stand or sit erect motionless for 30 seconds. Other mandibular views may be obtained with the patient in the recumbent position if necessary (Fig. 4-9, *B*). Insufficient tilting of the head may result in superimposition of the bodies of the mandible. The Towne projection can be performed in the sitting or supine position (Fig. 4-10) and outlines the condyles and ascending rami of the mandible. Suboptimal imaging can result from an insufficient angle, incomplete mouth opening, rotation, and overexposure.

A lateral nasal view (Fig. 4-11) is coned down to examine the fine bony structure. While the nose can be seen on the lateral view of the sinuses, the overexposure necessary to penetrate the skull results in a loss of detail of the nasal bones.

In summary, the physician has a variety of plain film radiographic views that can be used for the evaluation of facial injury. The appropriate selection is based firmly on a careful history and physical examination. Most facial trauma has associated signs and symptoms suggesting the presence of a fracture. Repeated radiographic examina-

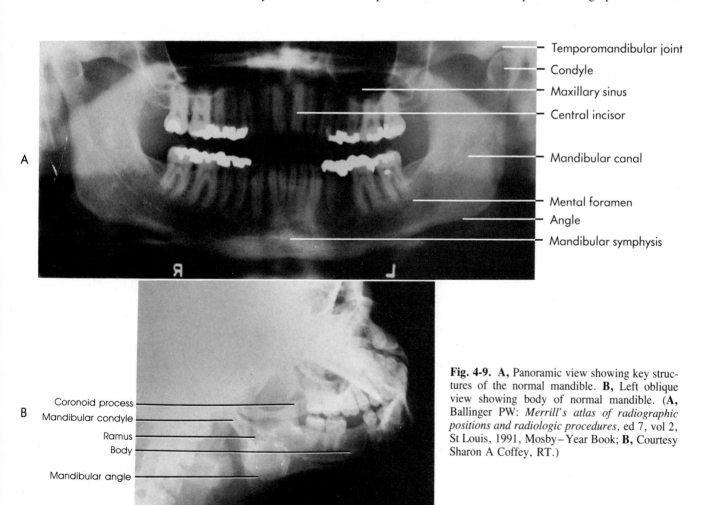

A

Temporomandibular joint
Condyle
Maxillary sinus
Central incisor

Mandibular canal

Mental foramen
Angle
Mandibular symphysis

B

Coronoid process
Mandibular condyle
Ramus
Body

Mandibular angle

Fig. 4-9. A, Panoramic view showing key structures of the normal mandible. **B,** Left oblique view showing body of normal mandible. (**A,** Ballinger PW: *Merrill's atlas of radiographic positions and radiologic procedures,* ed 7, vol 2, St Louis, 1991, Mosby–Year Book; **B,** Courtesy Sharon A Coffey, RT.)

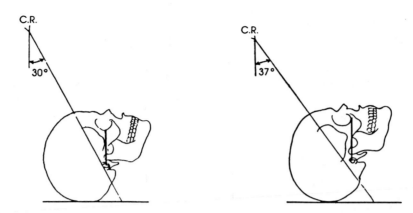

Fig. 4-10. Towne projection of mandible in a supine patient.(Ballinger PW: *Merrill's atlas of radiographic positions and radiologic procedures,* ed 7, vol 2, St Louis, 1991, Mosby–Year Book.)

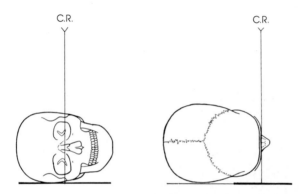

Fig. 4-11. Position of head during lateral nasal views. (Ballinger PW: *Merrill's atlas of radiographic positions and radiologic procedures,* ed 7, vol 2, St Louis, 1991, Mosby–Year Book.)

tions may be necessary in the uncooperative intoxicated patient.

MANDIBULAR FRACTURE

Even though it is the strongest of the facial bones, because of its isolated position and prominence, two thirds of all facial trauma occurs at the mandible[3] (Figs. 4-12 to 4-17). Mandibular fractures with their associated swelling, bleeding, and loss of support for the tongue may threaten the airway, which is the first priority in patient management.

Fracture of the body of the mandible often occurs at the canine tooth since the curvature is the greatest at that point.[4] Other common fracture sites are through the mental foramen, the angle, and the neck.[3] The absence of teeth in adults results in bone resorption and weakening, which predispose to fractures (Fig. 4-12). Fractures in children occur in the same areas but are complicated because of unerupted permanent teeth, which also weaken the body of the mandible[3,5] (see Fig. 4-17). Fracture of the condyles often occurs when the chin is struck and the force is trans-

mitted posteriorly. In children, this is frequently a greenstick fracture.[5] Fracture of the symphysis is usually associated with an additional fracture.[4]

The most frequent bilateral fracture combinations are bilateral condyles, bilateral angles, and the body of the mandible and contralateral angles.[4] A blow to one side of the jaw can fracture the body of the mandible and contralateral subcondylar region.[3] Fractures to the symphysis can occur with fractures at any other site.[6] Alveolar fractures often occur at the incisors since that area tends to receive a high proportion of direct blows. These fractures are often associated with avulsed teeth.

Clinical findings

The sensation of malocclusion perceived by the patient is a very sensitive indicator of fracture. However, this sensation can also be caused by swelling and paresthesia from a soft tissue injury. Fracture of the subcondylar region can result in inability to completely close the mouth at the incisors. Bleeding from around a tooth or loss of the normal relationship between teeth can indicate an underlying alveolar or mandibular fracture. Palpation around the mandibular body externally, inside the mouth, and under the tongue can detect tenderness, step-off, or a hematoma from a fracture. Palpation for tenderness of the subcondylar areas and condyles via the anterior aspect of the external ear canal is a requisite part of this examination. Anesthesia of the lower lip may be present if the fracture has disrupted the inferior alveolar nerve as it courses through the mandibular body. Tenderness with palpation, ecchymosis, and mobility of teeth on either side of the fracture may help localize the site. Because pain with movement is prominent, patients will minimize movement when speaking, swallowing, or eating, resulting in drooling and salivation from stimulation of the salivary glands. Patients may also notice a grinding sound as fragments shift with movement. This is painful and should not be purposefully

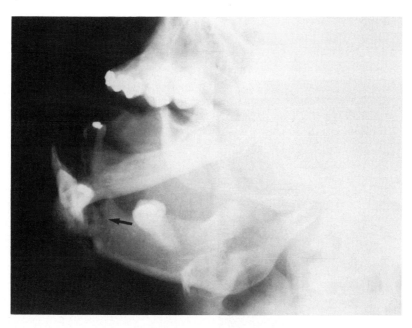

Fig. 4-12. Right oblique view of mandible demonstrating a right body fracture *(arrow)*. Because this patient had very few teeth, the mandible resorbed to a great extent, causing increased weakness.

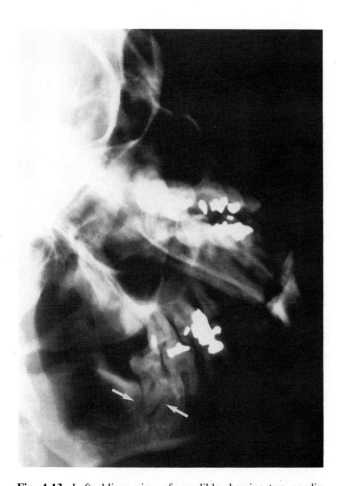

Fig. 4-13. Left oblique view of mandible showing two nondisplaced fractures of the body just anterior to the angle *(arrows)*. Fractures extend to the root of the teeth, which frequently are relatively weak areas.

elicited. When the mouth is opened, there may be an abnormal shift toward the site of the fracture.

Radiographic evaluation

Indications for radiographs are crepitus, malocclusion sensed by the patient, localized tenderness by palpation, hematoma, avulsed teeth, and inability to open or fully close the mouth.

A standard series includes the two lateral oblique views (see Figs. 4-12 and 4-13) where each side of the mandible is projected without overlapping the opposite side. The condyles are best seen on a Towne projection (see Figs. 4-14 and 4-15) and can also be seen on a PA view. The symphysis is the most difficult area to examine on plain radiographs. A panoramic view (see Figs. 4-16 and 4-17) may replace the other views but requires a special unit and cooperation from the patient, and the symphysis may not be seen well on this view.

Displacement of the segments depends on the force of the blow, the location of the fracture, the direction of the fracture line, and the direction of forces of the muscles at the fracture site. The geniohyoid and digastric muscles pull the anterior mandible downward and backward while the masseter, temporal, and medial pterygoid muscles pull the angle upward and forward. The result is that fractures running downward and forward from the molars will be nondisplaced because the muscles pull the segments together. However, fractures of the mandibular body coursing downward and posterior are often displaced, requiring open reduction. Fractures of the subcondylar area frequently show lateral angulation at the fracture and loss of the smooth straight line from the mandibular angle to the

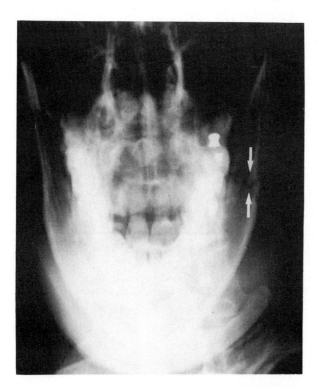

Fig. 4-14. Towne projection showing fracture of the left ramus of the mandible *(arrows)* without angulation. Notice the elongated view of the mandibular body.

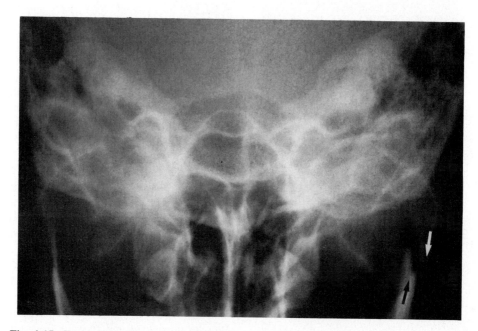

Fig. 4-15. Towne projection demonstrating disruption and loss of continuity in the left subcondylar area of the mandible *(arrows)*. This should be compared to the smooth, continuous line noted on the contralateral side.

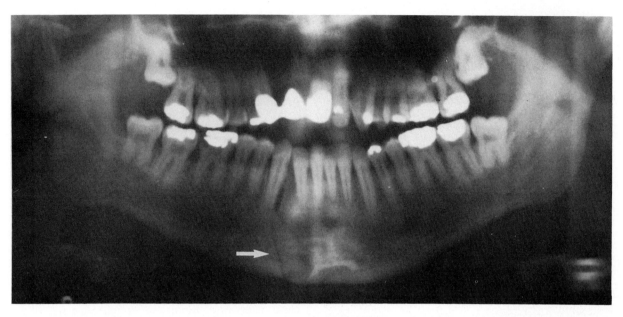

Fig. 4-16. Panoramic view demonstrating a nondisplaced fracture into the root of a tooth on the right symphysis of the mandible *(arrow)*.

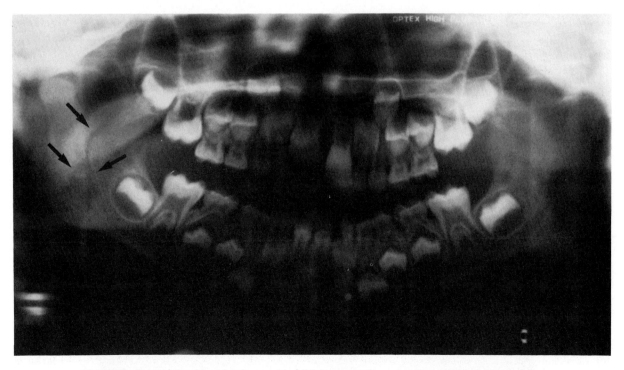

Fig. 4-17. Panoramic view of a 6-year-old child demonstrating a nondisplaced right subcondylar fracture of the mandible *(arrows)*. Note the unerupted underlying permanent teeth, which cause areas of bone weakness.

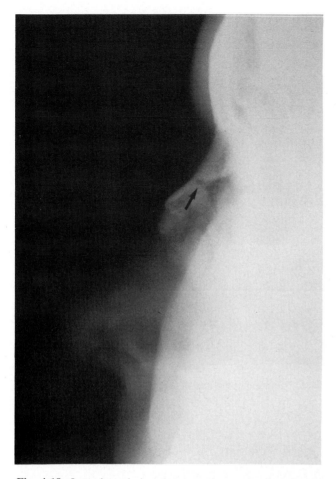

Fig. 4-18. Lateral nasal view demonstrating a comminuted nasal fracture with fracture lines perpendicular to the bridge of the nose *(arrow)*. These lines should not be confused with the nasal frontal suture, which is more superior. This suture runs parallel to the bridge of the nose and is normally seen on all lateral views. Note that the frontal sinus and other facial structures are not seen because of underexposure.

condylar head. This indicates disruption of the joint capsule and ligament. Less commonly, these are intact and the fracture has no angulation.

Special studies

Because of the detail of panoramic views, there usually is no need for conventional tomography or CT scans. When there is a need to view the symphysis, an occlusal view can be done where the patient holds the film with the incisors and the beam is directed upward from below the chin.

Treatment and disposition

If there is upper airway obstruction from an unstable mandibular fracture, from foreign bodies such as broken dentures or teeth, or from vomitus or an ongoing hemorrhage, then immediate active airway intervention with suction and endotracheal intubation or cricothyrotomy must be performed. All patients with mandibular fractures should be referred to a consultant since most will require operative stabilization. Those patients who have significant limitation of jaw excursion or potential for increased swelling or recurrent hemorrhage should be admitted for close observation in order to minimize the risk of aspiration and to treat any airway compromise. The vast majority may also need to be admitted for occlusal fixation with dental wire or internal plating, depending on the condition of the teeth and the displacement and alignment of the fracture. Open fractures should be treated with intravenous antibiotics. All missing teeth or dentures should be accounted for and, if necessary, a plain chest radiograph should be obtained to rule out radio-opaque foreign bodies.

NASAL BONES FRACTURE

Direct trauma to the midface frequently causes a nasal fracture (Figs. 4-18 and 4-19) with or without other frac-

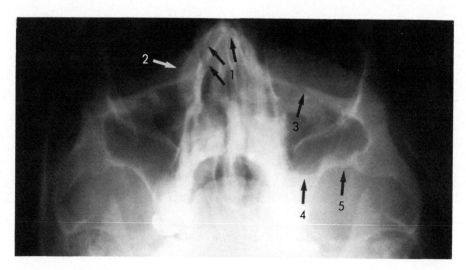

Fig. 4-19. Exaggerated Waters view of a comminuted fracture of the nose with lateral displacement and multiple bony fragments of the arch of the nose *(arrow 1)*. There is soft tissue swelling to the right side of the nose *(arrow 2)*. Also note the fracture of the infraorbital floor *(arrow 3)* and the air-fluid level in the left maxillary sinus *(arrow 4)*. The lateral maxillary wall is also fractured *(arrow 5)*.

tures. Because of the prominence of the nose, it is one of the most frequent fracture sites seen.[3] Cartilage supports the lower two thirds of the nose and the paired nasal bones support the upper third.[3] The nasal bones join the face at the frontal and maxillary bones where they are relatively thick and articulate with each other at the midline. They become thin distally as they articulate with the cartilage and are supported by the bony nasal septum.

Clinical findings

Direction and severity of the force, previous nasal injury, and appearance of the nose before injury are all helpful historic factors.

Most nasal fractures are easily recognizable clinically by deformity and displacement. Evaluation should be done as soon as possible, however, since once swelling ensues the injuries may be more difficult to see. Since many people have slightly displaced nasal bones, it is important to have the patient look in a mirror or have a friend help determine if the deformity is new. This is especially true if a patient has had previous fractures. Edema of the lids, periorbital ecchymosis, and subconjunctival hemorrhage may be associated findings.[3] The presence of movement or bony crepitus makes the diagnosis easy; however, these signs may be absent if the nose is impacted or telescoped. Epistaxis, mucosal tears in the nasal cavity, and hematoma are sometimes seen with fractures.[3] A septal hematoma should be specifically excluded on examination since increasing pressure will cause ischemia of the septum.

The diagnosis of a fracture in children is very difficult and should be suspected after trauma-induced epistaxis.[3,5] Examination may need to be done under anesthesia in order to make the diagnosis.[3]

If the clinical examination demonstrates a fracture, radiographic studies add little and do not alter management since they are of no aid in subsequent reduction. Although some single nasal bone fractures are undetectable by examination and may only be diagnosed by radiographs, they usually do not require manipulation.[7] Radiographic studies may be helpful in supplying concrete documentation of the fracture for legal reasons.

Radiographic evaluation

The typical nasal plain series includes a lateral view (Fig. 4-18) coning down on the nose and a Waters view. The normal Waters view should show an intact arch and septum. Fragmentation or loss of clarity of the arch are signs of a fracture (Fig. 4-19). Unfortunately, normal patients and cadaver skulls have a high incidence of deformities that mimic acute fractures.[8] Severely comminuted fractures may be indicative of more severe maxillary and orbital injuries, and soft tissue swelling may be seen overlapping the orbits. The lateral nasal view shows sutures parallel to the bridge of the nose. Any perpendicular line reaching the anterior wall of the nasal bone indicates a fracture. The lateral facial or skull radiograph can also show these fractures but will require a bright light for ex-

amination since the nasal bones will be relatively overexposed. In children, there is a suture along the bridge of the nose so that fractures often have over-riding of one nasal bone on the other.[5]

Special studies

There is no need for computed tomography, conventional tomography, or other more advanced imaging for simple nasal fractures. Examination under anesthesia may be helpful when the diagnosis is uncertain.

Treatment and disposition

Once a septal hematoma is ruled out or drained and epistaxis is controlled, the patient can be followed as an outpatient in 5 days. At that time, the swelling should have subsided and manipulation of the fracture can be done if there is a cosmetic or functional deformity.

BLOW-OUT FRACTURE

Blow-out fractures (Figs. 4-20 to 4-23) are common fractures of the midface. They result from blunt trauma directly to the globe in which the force is transmitted through the relatively incompressible soft tissues of the orbit and causes the orbital floor or medial wall to fracture. Blow-out fractures occur most commonly in the orbital floor because of the large cross-sectional area and thinness (0.5 to 1 mm) of the orbital plate of the maxilla. The orbital plate of the ethmoid sinus, the lamina papyracea, forms the medial wall of the orbit and is actually thinner (0.2 to 0.4 mm) than the orbital floor but is strengthened and buttressed by the bony septa of the ethmoidal cells. Medial wall fracture is infrequently diagnosed in isolation but has been reported to occur in greater than 50% of all orbital floor fractures.[9] Medial wall fractures, however, are rarely of clinical significance.[10] The exception is a large defect fracture with prolapse or entrapment of soft tissue into the ethmoid sinus.

Up to 30% of patients with blow-out fractures have associated serious eye injury.[11] Ocular injuries include globe rupture, vitreous hemorrhage, hyphema, lens dislocation, choroidal rupture, and retinal detachment.

Clinical findings

The most important part of the evaluation of a patient with isolated orbital trauma is an eye examination. Due to the rapidly increasing swelling often seen with blunt injuries to the orbit, it is imperative that this examination be performed early. The examination includes testing of visual acuity, pupillary reactivity, and extraocular motion. Funduscopic examination should also be performed when possible. Lid retractors are sometimes necessary to complete the examination.

Most of the signs and symptoms of blow-out fracture result from the involvement of extraocular soft tissue, with edema, extraocular muscle entrapment, or actual prolapse of the periorbital contents through the fracture site into the surrounding sinuses. The most common symptom associ-

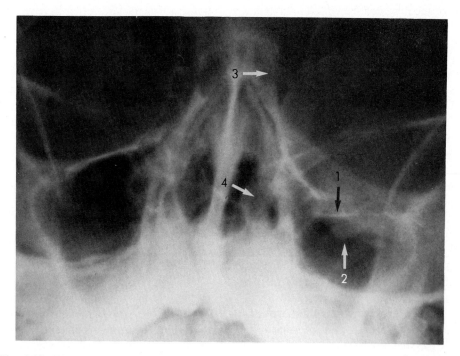

Fig. 4-20. Waters view of left blow-out fracture with linear density high in the maxillary antrum representing displaced fragment of the orbital floor *(arrow 1)*. A soft tissue density, "tear-drop" sign, represents soft tissue prolapse into the maxillary sinus *(arrow 2)*. Also noted is opacification of the left ethmoid sinus *(arrow 3)* and disappearance of the lamina papyracea, indicating medial wall fracture *(arrow 4)*.

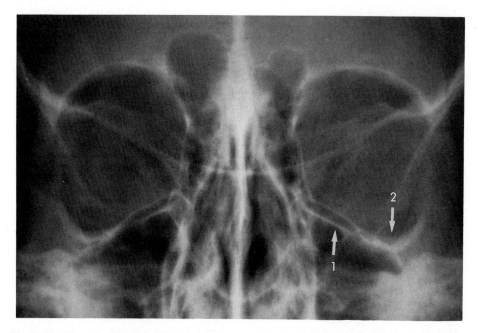

Fig. 4-21. Normal radiograph (Caldwell view, central portion) of posteromedial orbital floor *(arrow 1)* seen clearly above and running parallel with the orbital rim *(arrow 2)*. The posteromedial cortex is normally symmetric; a marked asymmetry or discontinuity represents orbital floor fracture.

A

B

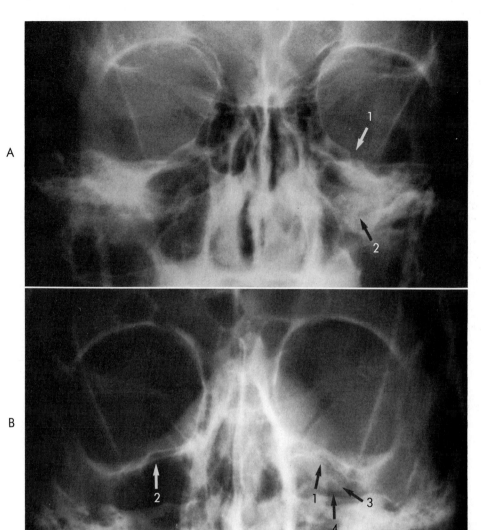

Fig. 4-22. A, Caldwell view of left blow-out fracture of orbital floor demonstrating discontinuity of the medial floor of the orbit *(arrow 1)*. There is also increased haziness of the left maxillary sinus *(arrow 2)*, suggesting fluid in the sinus. B, Caldwell view demonstrating an absent left posterior floor cortex *(arrow 1)* that can be clearly seen on the right for comparison *(arrow 2)*. An abnormal linear density *(arrow 3)* represents the displaced fragment. A "tear-drop" sign in the roof of the maxillary antrum represents a prolapse of periorbital soft tissue *(arrow 4)*. Note the left maxillary sinus opacification often seen on a supine film.

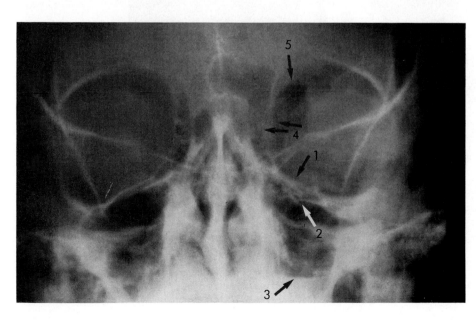

Fig. 4-23. Caldwell view of left blowout fracture of the orbital floor and medial wall. Left posterior floor cortex is missing *(arrow 1)* and is seen as several linear opacities displaced into the maxillary antrum in this view *(arrow 2)*. There is an air-fluid level *(arrow 3)*, the lamina papyracea is also absent, and the left ethmoid sinus is opacified *(arrow 4)*. There is also superomedial orbital emphysema *(arrow 5)*.

ated with blow-out fractures is diplopia, occurring in up to 80% of cases.[12] Examination may reveal limitation of extraocular movement, especially upward gaze, suggesting at least transient entrapment of infraorbital soft tissue. Less common is limitation of lateral gaze, indicating medial wall fracture with entrapment of the medial rectus muscle. Hypesthesia in the distribution of the infraorbital nerve is frequently observed. Enophthalmos is rare immediately following trauma and indicates a large bony defect with prolapse of orbital contents into the adjacent sinuses. An apparent ptosis may signal an underlying enophthalmos. A history of sudden puffing of the eye with noseblowing is most commonly associated with fracture of the medial wall into the ethmoid sinus. Careful palpation of the periorbital soft tissues, particularly in the superior and medial quadrants, may identify subcutaneous emphysema.

Radiographic evaluation

Patients sustaining blunt trauma to the orbit who present with marked periorbital swelling and ecchymosis should undergo plain film radiographic evaluation of the orbits. Patients with signs of orbital injury, including diplopia, limitation in extraocular movement, or infraorbital hypesthesia, should also be evaluated radiographically.[13] Patients with moderate periorbital swelling without other signs of orbital trauma do not need radiographic evaluation. The standard radiographs for evaluating the orbit are the Waters and Caldwell views. The Waters view (see Fig. 4-2) is the most informative, with its excellent display of the inferior orbital rims, the nasoethmoid complex, and the maxillary sinus. The Caldwell view (see Fig. 4-4) is better for evaluating the lateral orbital rim and ethmoid bones. The lateral view (see Fig. 4-5), plagued by superimposition of multiple bones, is the least useful in detecting fracture but may be of use in confirming an air-fluid level.

Definitive radiographic diagnosis of blow-out fracture is bone discontinuity or displacement (Fig. 4-20). In orbital floor fractures, this usually occurs in the posterior aspect of the orbital plate of the maxilla just medial to the infraorbital groove. The remarkable symmetry between the orbital plates of the maxilla (Fig. 4-21) allows for detection of subtle orbital floor fracture (Fig. 4-22, A).

The most common radiographic finding associated with orbital floor fracture is an air-fluid level in the maxillary sinus.[14] Other presumptive evidence includes a soft tissue density in the roof of the maxillary sinus (i.e., the "teardrop" sign) (Fig. 4-22, B), opacification of the maxillary sinus, and orbital emphysema. These associated findings correlate closely with fracture and should alert one to the presence of orbital floor fracture. Fracture of the medial orbital wall is rarely seen on plain radiographs. This diagnosis is usually made presumptively on the basis of unilateral clouding of the ethmoid sinus or by the presence of orbital emphysema[9] (Fig. 4-23).

Special studies

Emergency acquisition of special studies in patients with blow-out fractures is rarely indicated. An important exception is the patient with unexplained visual loss or suspected injury to the globe. In this setting, computed tomography has largely replaced conventional tomography.[15] Conventional tomography requires repositioning of the patient

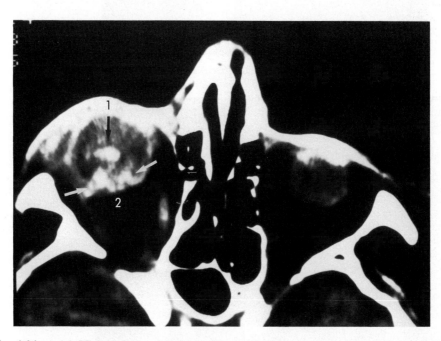

Fig. 4-24. Axial CT scan demonstrating significant soft tissue swelling of the right eyelid and, most significantly, an oval radiodensity in the middle of the globe, representing a dislocated lens *(arrow 1)*. Also noted is increased radiodensity located posteriorly in the globe, representing blood *(arrow 2)*.

for coronal and sagittal planes; a CT scan requires only that the patient be in the neutral supine position. A CT scan readily identifies injuries involving the globe, the optic nerve, the extraocular muscles, and intraorbital vascular structures, while exposing the patient to less radiation than conventional tomography (Fig. 4-24).

Treatment and disposition

All patients with blow-out fracture and unexplained visual loss require emergency ophthalmologic consultation and admission. Blow-out fractures with entrapment and enophthalmos previously were considered indications for early surgery. It is now realized that the majority of these symptoms resolve spontaneously and most surgeons delay the decision to operate for 10 to 14 days, at which point the amount of residual diplopia and enophthalmos can be determined. If there are clinical indications for surgery, elective CT scans or, if unavailable, conventional tomograms may be obtained at this time. Other patients with isolated blow-out fractures require early subspecialty follow-up.

TRIPOD FRACTURE

Zygomaticomaxillary (tripod) fracture (Figs. 4-25 to 4-30) is the most common fracture involving the orbit and paranasal sinuses.[16] The classic tripod fracture results from a blunt high-energy force to the body of the zygoma, or malar eminence, resulting in three fractures. These fractures include (1) the zygomaticomaxillary suture, and (2) the zygomaticofrontal suture diastasis, (3) the zygomatic arch. Tripod fractures may also involve the orbital processes of the frontal bone or zygoma rather than the suture lines. The most devastating injury associated with an isolated tripod fracture is injury to the eye and optic nerve.[17]

Clinical findings

The patient with tripod fracture usually presents with a significant degree of periorbital swelling and ecchymosis. Visual acuity is usually normal and should be documented on all patients. If abnormal, it suggests possible injury to the globe or optic nerve. Other physical findings largely depend on the degree of displacement of the zygoma. Nondisplaced fractures should produce no cosmetic defect other than soft tissue swelling. Displacement of the zygoma will result in malar flattening if seen early. This finding becomes obscured in the presence of marked soft tissue swelling. When there is inferior displacement of the zygoma, the lateral canthal angle may be displaced inferiorly because of its ligamentous attachment to the zygoma. Because tripod fractures involve the orbital floor, they share some of the signs and symptoms associated with blow-out fractures. Hypesthesia in the distribution of the infraorbital nerve is usually present. Diplopia, entrapment, and enophthalmos are less common. Simultaneous palpation of both orbital rims in patients without marked soft tissue swelling may reveal step-off deformities in the regions of the zygomaticomaxillary and zygomaticofrontal sutures. When pain and associated soft tissue swelling prevents adequate examination by palpation, intraoral palpation of the malar eminence in the compliant patient is suggested; an upwardly directed force to the undersurface of the malar eminence should elicit pain in the presence of tripod fracture. If there is no pain, tripod fracture is unlikely; the presence of pain, however, does not accurately predict tripod fracture.[18] An inferiorly displaced tripod fracture may limit the motion of the mandible by impingement of either the zygomatic arch or the body of the zygoma on the temporalis muscle or coronoid process of the mandible.

Radiographic evaluation

Patients who have sustained blunt trauma to the lateral midface and have clinical findings suggestive of possible tripod fracture should undergo radiographic evaluation. Additionally, patients who have marked periorbital soft tissue swelling that precludes adequate examination should also undergo plain film radiographic evaluation. The standard series for tripod fractures commonly employs three views: Waters, Caldwell, and underexposed submental vertex. The Waters view is best suited for illustrating the inferior orbital rim and maxillary extension of the zygoma as well as the maxillary sinus. The Caldwell projection well illustrates the zygomaticofrontal suture and the frontal process of the zygoma. The underexposed submental vertex is the preferred view for evaluating the zygomatic arch.

Tripod fracture most commonly involves fracture sites through the zygomaticomaxillary suture, the zygomaticofrontal suture, and the zygomatic arch (Figs. 4-25 and 4-26, A). The orbital floor is also involved as the fracture line extends laterally from the area of the infraorbital fora-

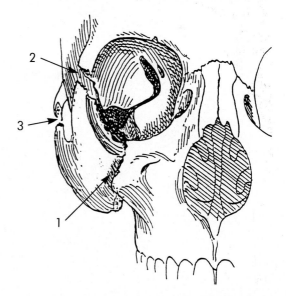

Fig. 4-25. Schematic drawing demonstrating the classic lines of tripod fracture. *1,* zygomaticomaxillary suture; *2,* zygomaticofrontal suture; *3,* zygomatic arch. (Zizmor J, Noyek AM: Orbital trauma. In Newton TH, Potts DG, eds: *Radiology of the skull and brain,* vol 1, St Louis, 1971, CV Mosby.)

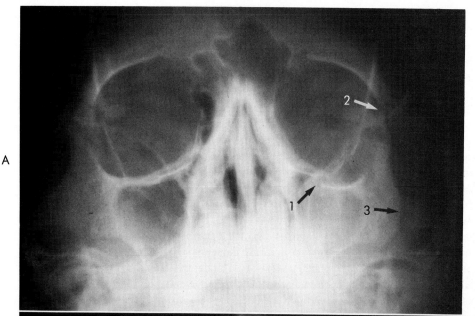

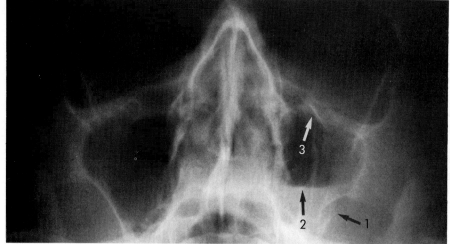

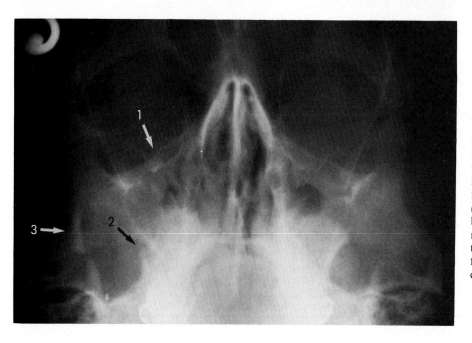

Fig. 4-26. A, Waters view of left tripod fracture illustrating classic lines of zygomaticomaxillary complex fracture involving zygomaticomaxillary suture *(arrow 1),* and zygomaticofrontal suture *(arrow 2),* and zygomaticotemporal suture *(arrow 3).* There is also opacification of the left maxillary sinus. **B,** Waters view demonstrating several of the findings suggestive of tripod fracture. There is a fracture of the lateral wall of the maxillary sinus *(arrow 1)* with associated air-fluid level *(arrow 2).* There is also evidence of orbital floor disruption with a linear opacity extending into the maxillary antrum *(arrow 3).* In the absence of the lateral maxillary sinus wall fracture, this radiograph would be interpreted as a blow-out fracture.

Fig. 4-27. Waters view of right tripod fracture demonstrating a step-off of the inferior rim with slight inferior displacement of the zygomaticomaxillary complex *(arrow 1).* There is a fracture in the lateral wall of the maxillary sinus *(arrow 2)* and increased density at the temporal process takeoff from the zygoma, indicating overlying bone fragments of zygomatic arch fracture *(arrow 3).* There is opacification of both maxillary sinuses although the right seems slightly more involved than the left. There is no evidence of fracture on the left. This may represent chronic inflammation.

men up the lateral orbital wall to the zygomaticofrontal suture. Another component of tripod fracture that is invariably present is a fracture of the lateral wall of the maxillary sinus. This fracture and its associated maxillary sinus opacification or air-fluid level is readily apparent on the Waters view (Fig. 4-26, *B*). Variations of the classic tripod fracture result from fractures through the relatively thin orbital processes of the frontal bone or zygoma rather than through the sutures. Regardless, the body of the zygoma becomes a free fragment that may either be nondisplaced, partially displaced with a degree of rotation, or completely displaced with or without rotation. The clinical significance of these fractures is a function of the degree of displacement and rotation.

The zygomaticomaxillary component of the tripod frac-

ture is often visualized by a step-off at the inferior orbital rim and buckling or displacement of the lateral maxillary wall. The Waters view is optimal for illustrating these findings (Fig. 4-27). Tripod fractures involving the infraorbital rim and the lateral wall of the maxillary sinus may simulate the lateral extension of a Le Fort II fracture. A distinguishing feature is that the Le Fort II fracture tends to involve the medial orbital rim and floor as opposed to the more common lateral rim involvement with tripod fractures.[19] The Caldwell view is best for demonstrating diastasis at the zygomaticofrontal suture (Fig. 4-28). Significant medial displacement of the zygoma may be recognized by the presence of a unilateral small maxillary antrum (Fig. 4-29). This is clinically significant because such medial displacements are more likely to impinge on the in-

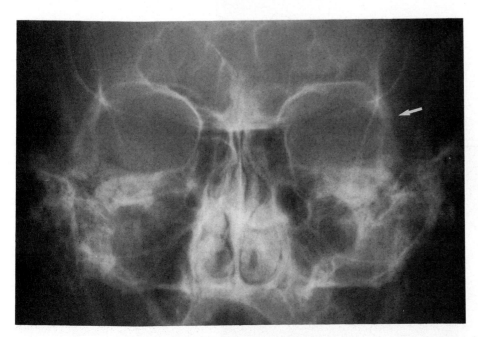

Fig. 4-28. Caldwell view of left zygomaticofrontal suture diastasis clearly demonstrating zygomaticofrontal disruption associated with tripod fracture *(arrow)*.

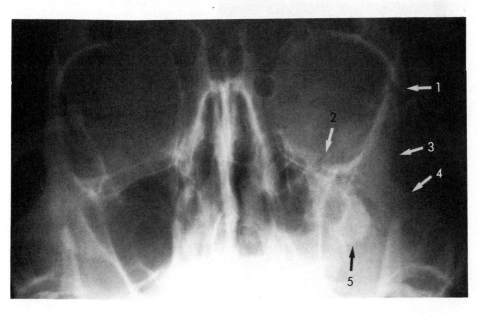

Fig. 4-29. Waters view of left tripod fracture with comminuted body of zygoma demonstrating diastasis at the zygomaticofrontal suture *(arrow 1)* and zygomaticomaxillary suture *(arrow 2)*. A lateral orbit fragment is displaced inferomedially *(arrow 3)*, and there is severe comminution of the body of the zygoma *(arrow 4)*. A rotated fragment of zygoma appears as an increased radiodensity *(arrow 5)*.

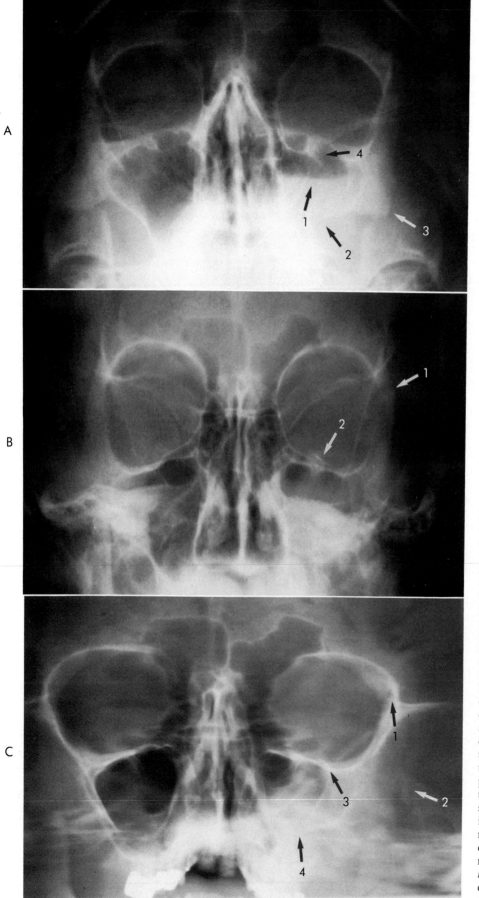

Fig. 4-30. Left tripod fracture demonstrated on plain radiographs (**A** and **B**) and pantomography (**C**). **A,** Waters view shows an obvious air-fluid level *(arrow 1)* as well as buckling of the lateral wall of the maxillary sinus *(arrow 2).* There is also a zygomaticotemporal suture diastasis *(arrow 3)* and, consistent with orbital floor fracture, punctate radiodensities in the superior aspect of the maxillary antrum and a vague linear radiodensity extending into the maxillary sinus from the orbital floor *(arrow 4).* **B,** Caldwell view demonstrates as well a zygomaticofrontal suture diastasis *(arrow 1)* and a vague linear radiodensity in the area of the orbital floor *(arrow 2),* consistent with orbital floor fracture. **C,** Pantomogram shows two classic sites of tripod fracture, the zygomaticofrontal suture *(arrow 1)* and zygomaticotemporal suture diastases *(arrow 2).* In addition, it demonstrates irregularity of the inferior orbit in the region of the zygomaticomaxillary suture, which most likely represents a fracture of this suture *(arrow 3).* There is also a fracture of the lateral wall of the maxillary sinus *(arrow 4)* with opacification of the sinus.

fraorbital foramen with greater potential for optic nerve injury.[19] The Caldwell view also demonstrates a comminuted fracture of the body of the zygoma, a relatively uncommon injury indicating an unusually large amount of force applied directly to the zygoma.

Special studies

In the absence of an eye injury, plain film radiography is sufficient for the emergency evaluation of an isolated tripod fracture without associated complications. Another modality, pantomography, may supplement information obtained from standard radiographs. The basic technology—initially used to image teeth, alveolar processes, and the mandible—has been advanced to include programs that study various zones of the head and neck. The pantomogram is a thick-slice tomogram that produces maxillozygomatic imaging with excellent details of the inferior orbital rim and zygomatic arch and thus may provide clarification if these regions are in question. Because this study is taken with the patient in a sitting position, there should be no suspicion of cervical spine injury. Patient compliance is also necessary for this study. The midface pantomogram may clarify suspicions arising from the standard radiographs but rarely identifies previously unsuspected fractures and thus has minimal impact on patient management (Fig. 4-30).

Treatment and disposition

Patients rarely require hospitalization for isolated zygomaticomaxillary complex fracture. The exception is a tripod fracture complicated by visual loss or severe limitation of mouth opening that might threaten the patient's airway if vomiting were to occur. Both of these conditions require admission. The use of antibiotics and antihistamines in tripod fracture is controversial and should be prescribed based on the preference of the consultant.

ZYGOMATIC ARCH FRACTURE
Clinical findings

An isolated zygomatic arch fracture is an infrequent injury, usually resulting from well-localized blunt trauma as seen in baseball injuries or blows from a pool cue. When seen early, a depressed zygomatic arch should be obvious from observation and palpation. If seen later, overlying soft tissue swelling may obscure the depression, and tenderness may prevent adequate examination by palpation. If there has been marked displacement, the patient may have difficulty opening the mouth because of impingement of the fracture fragments on the temporalis muscle or coronoid process of the mandible.

Given the proximity of the zygomatic arch to the squamous portion of the temporal bone and its underlying middle meningeal artery, consideration should be given to the possibility of an epidural hematoma in patients with isolated zygomatic arch fracture.

Radiographic evaluation

The optimal view for visualizing fractures of the zygomatic arch is the underexposed submental vertex. The zygomatic arch fracture is also frequently visualized on the Waters view or on an underexposed Towne projection.

Depressed zygomatic arch fractures generally involve three fracture sites and have a V-shaped configuration. The depressed apex of the V represents the point of impact, and there are usually nondisplaced fractures at the two other points of the V (Fig. 4-31). The previous section on tripod fractures includes illustrations of zygomatic arch fracture associated with zygomaticomaxillary complex fractures.

Special studies

Plain film radiographs are sufficient for the emergency evaluation of all isolated zygomatic arch fractures. In pa-

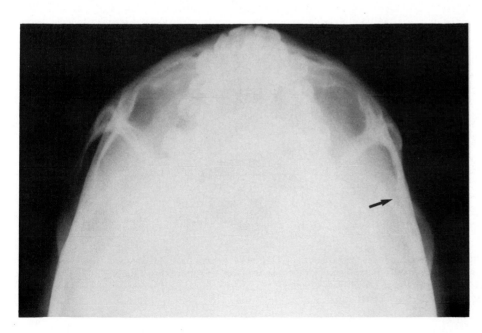

Fig. 4-31. Submental vertex view demonstrating a markedly depressed left zygomatic arch with the maximum point of depression indicated *(arrow)*.

tients with limitation of jaw mobility after zygomatic arch fracture, conventional tomography or more commonly CT scans may be used to evaluate the cause of this disability. These special studies, however, are normally performed on an elective basis.

Treatment and disposition

Patients with uncomplicated zygomatic arch fractures do not require hospitalization. Most patients with mild trismus and limitation of jaw motion also may be discharged home. The exception to this is the patient whose fracture severely limits the ability to open the mouth, which results in an increased risk of aspiration with vomiting. All patients should receive follow-up consultation to determine the need for surgery.

LE FORT FRACTURE

Fractures of the midface are due to direct trauma. Major fractures in this region are classified according to the system devised by Rene Le Fort (Fig. 4-32). A Le Fort I is a horizontal fracture of the maxilla at the level of the nasal floor. A Le Fort II fracture (Fig. 4-33) includes fractures through the maxilla, antrum, nasal bones, and infraorbital rim, resulting in a mobile maxillary segment. A Le Fort III fracture or craniofacial separation includes fracture or separation of the zygomaticofrontal suture, or the zygoma, and the frontal bone above the nose. Often, the fractures are asymmetric so that there may be combinations of one Le Fort fracture (Fig. 4-34) with another type of Le Fort fracture, a tripod, or another incomplete fracture on the opposite side. A Le Fort I and III are rarely present to-

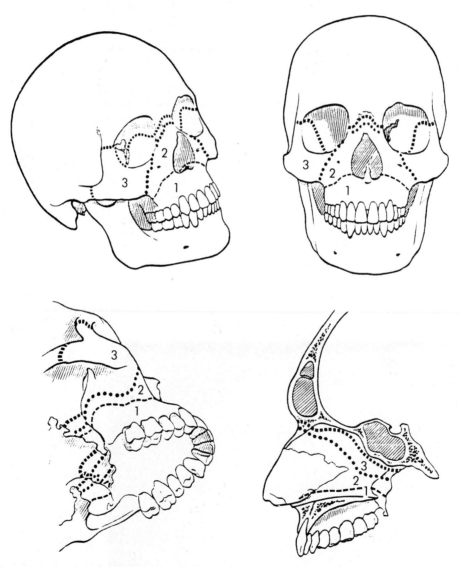

Fig. 4-32. Le Fort I fracture on the level of the nasal floor *(1)*; Le Fort II through the nasal bones, infraorbital rims, and maxilla *(2)*; and Le Fort III through the frontozygomatic suture, orbits, and the zygomatic arch *(3)*. (Used with permission from Dingman RO, Natvig P: *Surgery of facial fractures,* Philadelphia, 1964, WB Saunders.)

gether. These patterns are the same in children. Cases where many of the facial bones are fractured into small fragments may not be amenable to classification and have been termed "central facial smash"[20] (Fig. 4-35).

Clinical findings

Le Fort fractures usually occur after motor vehicle accidents and are the result of massive forces spread diffusely across the face. Physical examination for Le Fort I fractures includes testing for mobility of the palate while stabilizing the forehead. Le Fort II fractures exhibit mobility of the maxilla. Le Fort III fractures are associated with facial and periorbital edema and complete movement of the face compared to the cranial vault. The clinical examination is more accurate than initial radiographs, which are usually taken with the patient in the supine position using portable equipment.

Radiographic evaluation

In Le Fort fractures, there should be air-fluid levels in the sinuses (Figs. 4-33 and 4-34). Pterygoid fractures are also present and are best visualized on the lateral view (Fig. 4-34, *A*). Pterygoid fractures can also be seen on lateral cervical spine radiographs. The second most helpful view is the Waters projection (Fig. 4-34, *B*). If the patient is unable to lie prone, then a reverse Waters view with the patient supine should be performed. The detail in this will be less than in the true Waters because of increased magnification.

In a Le Fort I, the fracture is horizontal across the inferior maxilla. Fracture of the lateral wall of the maxillary sinus may be visible. The Le Fort II fracture is most easily seen as disruption of the inferior rim of the orbit lateral to the infraorbital canal with associated medial orbital wall and nasofrontal fracture. Because a Le Fort III causes the midface to be free floating, the orbits may be elongated and the ethmoid sinuses opacified. There are fractures through the zygomaticofrontal suture and the zygomatic arch. Both Le Fort II and III fractures are associated with blood seen as air-fluid levels in or opacification of the maxillary sinus. Not all of these radiographic findings may be present, and a clinical examination suggesting a fracture warrants further study.

Special studies

Most Le Fort fractures can be evaluated by a CT scan at 4 mm to 5 mm slice thicknesses (Fig. 4-35, *A*). A Le Fort I fracture may be difficult to identify on CT scan because of its transverse location, but the pterygoid fracture and extension into the palate may be seen.[19] A Le Fort II fracture is recognized on CT scan by involvement of the ethmoid sinuses and medial orbital wall and floor and can be differentiated from a Le Fort III by lack of disruption above the zygoma[19] (Fig. 4-36). Le Fort III fractures also have more lateral involvement of the orbital floor and disruption of the maxillary sinus only at the roof. A central facial smash will have multiple bony fragments smaller than the typical Le Fort segments (Fig. 4-35, *B*).

Treatment and disposition

All patients with suspected Le Fort fractures should be admitted to the hospital for CT scan and eventual fixation. Nasal packing may be necessary to control persistent epistaxis.

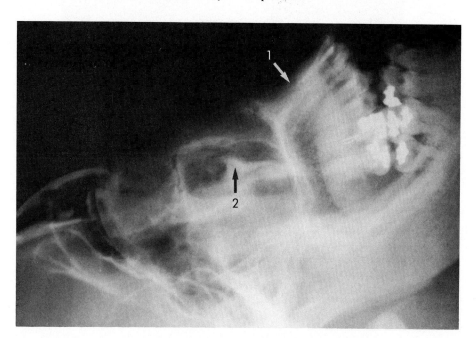

Fig. 4-33. Supine lateral view showing a Le Fort II fracture, noted by disruption of the anterior maxillary wall *(arrow 1)* and an air-fluid level in the maxillary sinus *(arrow 2)*.

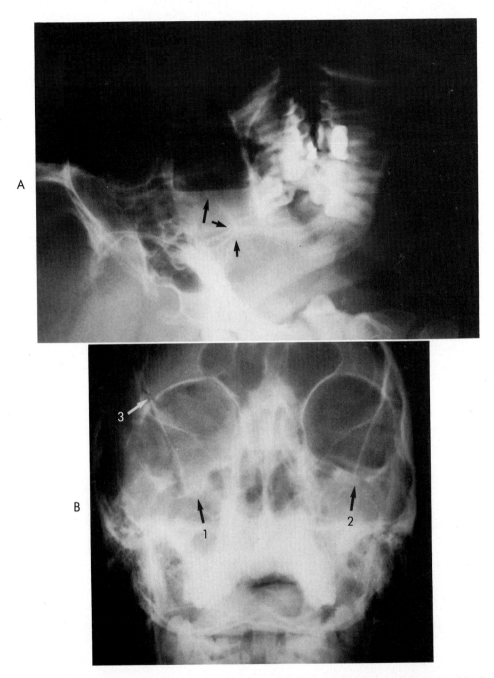

Fig. 4-34. A, Supine lateral view of a bilateral Le Fort fracture showing an air-fluid level in the maxillary sinus *(long arrow)* and fracture of both pterygoid plates *(small arrows)*. The Le Fort classification cannot be defined from this particular radiograph. **B,** Waters view showing clouding indicative of blood in both maxillary sinuses and ethmoid sinuses as well as disruption of both infraorbital floors *(arrows 1 and 2)*. There is considerable clouding of the right orbit indicative of soft tissue swelling and widening of the right frontozygomatic suture *(arrow 3)*.

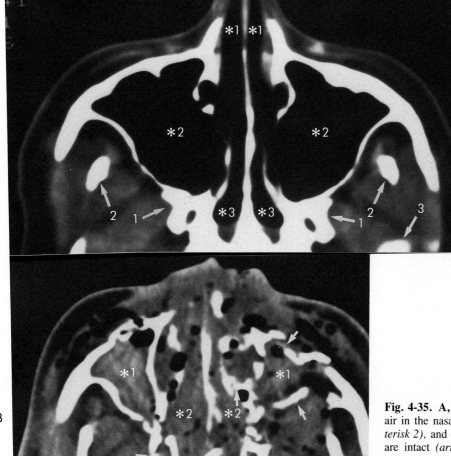

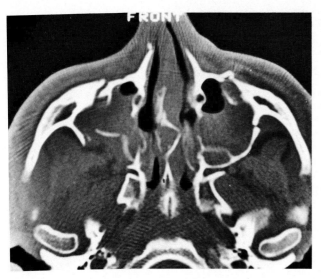

Fig. 4-35. **A,** CT scan of normal maxillary sinus showing air in the nasal cavity *(asterisk 1),* maxillary sinuses *(asterisk 2),* and ethmoid sinuses *(asterisk 3).* The pterygoids are intact *(arrow 1),* and the mandibular coronoid processes *(arrow 2)* and the condyle *(arrow 3)* can be seen. **B,** CT scan of central facial smash showing multiple fractures and fragmentation of the facial bones. Note blood in both maxillary sinuses *(asterisk 1)* and complete disruption of the anterior, posterior, and medial walls of the left maxillary sinus *(small arrows).* There is also obliteration of the ethmoid sinuses *(asterisk 2)* and fractures of the pterygoid *(long arrow)* as well as soft tissue swelling of the face and in the nasal cavity.

Fig. 4-36. Axial CT scan showing Le Fort II fracture. On more caudal scans, the pterygoid plates were visualized as fractured, while on more cranial scans the ethmoid sinuses and orbital floors were fractured. (Som PM, Bergeron RT: *Head and neck imaging,* ed 2, St Louis, 1991, Mosby–Year Book.)

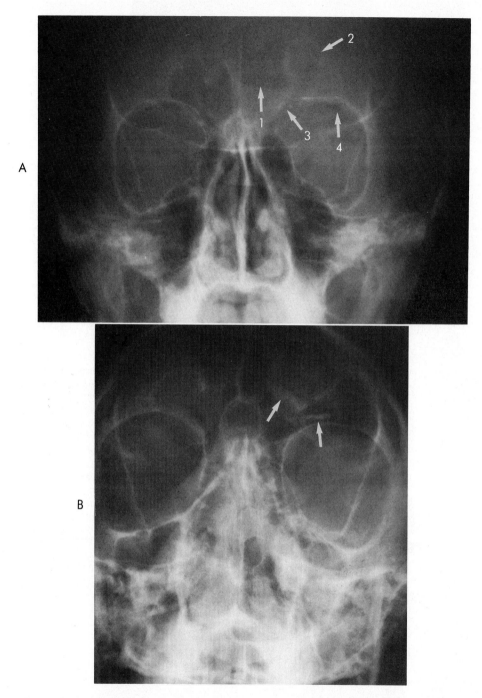

Fig. 4-37. A, Caldwell view of frontal sinus fracture demonstrating an air-fluid level in the frontal sinus *(arrow 1)* and opacification of the left aspect of the sinus *(arrow 2)*. In addition, there is loss of definition of the medial supraorbital rim *(arrow 3)* and a radiolucency in the superior orbit indicating orbital emphysema *(arrow 4)*. These findings indicate a complex frontal sinus fracture with orbital rim and roof involvement. **B,** Caldwell view demonstrating several depressed fragments overlying the frontal sinus *(arrows)*.

The presence of a central facial smash or Le Fort II or III fracture may cause airway compromise and complicate active airway management. If orotracheal intubation is contraindicated or unsuccessful, then emergency cricothyrotomy should be performed. After control of the airway and other life-threatening problems have been treated or ruled out, consultation should be obtained and definitive treatment of these fractures may be delayed until the patient's overall condition permits elective surgical reduction and stabilization.

FRONTAL SINUS FRACTURE

Up to 8% of all facial fractures involve the frontal sinus[21] (Fig. 4-37). The mechanism of injury is usually high-impact blunt or penetrating trauma. A high proportion of frontal sinus fractures are open.[22] The force necessary to fracture the frontal sinus is significantly greater than that associated with fractures of the maxillary or ethmoid sinuses. Therefore the incidence of intracranial complications associated with these fractures is greater than those seen in mid or lower facial injuries.[23]

Fractures of the frontal sinus may involve the anterior wall, the posterior wall, or both. They may be seen in isolation or with associated supraorbital rim or nasoethmoidal complex fractures. Anterior wall fractures are classified as displaced or nondisplaced. In one series of isolated anterior wall fractures, 60% were nondisplaced.[24] The most common frontal sinus fracture, resulting from high-veloc-

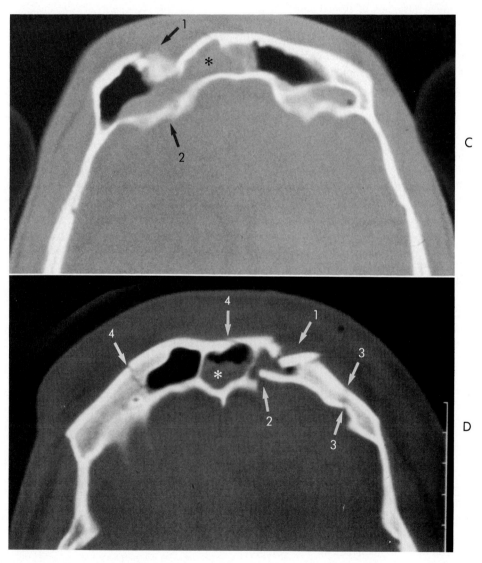

Fig. 4-37, cont'd. C, Axial CT scan demonstrating a depressed, comminuted fracture of the anterior wall of the right frontal sinus *(arrow 1)*. There is also homogeneous radiodensity in the right frontal sinus, representing fluid *(asterisk)*. The posterior wall is intact *(arrow 2)*. **D,** Axial CT scan demonstrating a depressed comminuted fracture of the anterior wall of the left frontal sinus *(arrow 1)* with accompanying displaced posterior wall fracture *(arrow 2)*. There are also *(arrow 3)* linear nondisplaced fractures involving both walls of the left frontal sinus as well as nondisplaced fractures involving the anterior wall of the right frontal sinus *(arrow 4)*. Fluid is noted in the left frontal sinus as well *(asterisk)*.

ity blunt injury to the forehead, is a comminuted anterior wall fracture (eggshell deformity).[19]

The emergency diagnosis of frontal sinus fracture is of particular importance because it is one of the few facial injuries that frequently requires early surgical exploration. A delayed catastrophic complication of unrecognized frontal sinus fracture is CNS infection resulting from posterior wall fracture with disruption of the dura. Post-traumatic frontal sinusitis is another complication seen following this fracture. In children under age 15, the frontoethmoidal sutures are not closed; even minor fractures, when associated with infected nasal sinus secretions, can lead to the rapid development of periorbital abscess.[25]

Clinical findings

The basis for clinical suspicion of frontal sinus fracture should be the mechanism of injury resulting in trauma to the low-to-mid central forehead. The degree of soft tissue swelling is not a reliable predictor of this fracture. Open wounds overlying the frontal sinus should be carefully inspected and palpated for evidence of fracture since some fractures that are not detectable on plain radiographs can be identified during wound examination.[26]

Clinical diagnosis of closed frontal sinus fracture is difficult because of overlying soft tissue swelling that frequently accompanies this fracture. Anesthesia of the supraorbital nerve may be present, and cerebral spinal fluid rhinorrhea may result from posterior wall fracture.

Radiographic evaluation

Routine facial views employing the Waters, Caldwell, and lateral projections are used in the detection of frontal sinus fracture. The Caldwell projection provides the best detail of fractures involving the anterior table of the frontal sinus. The lateral projection may demonstrate displacement of the anterior frontal wall but rarely demonstrates posterior wall fractures (Fig. 4-37, A and B).

Special studies

Frontal sinus fractures usually require a CT scan to determine if there is posterior wall frontal sinus involvement (Fig. 4-37, C and D).

Treatment and disposition

Patients with fractures involving the frontal sinus require hospitalization. A CT scan is generally performed. Fractures found to involve the posterior wall sinus are usually surgically explored. Frontal sinus fracture associated with supraorbital rim or nasoethmoidal fractures has a high incidence of nasofrontal duct involvement; the compromised or obstructed duct prevents frontal sinus drainage and is often an indication for exploration. In the stable patient, open displaced anterior wall fractures are usually repaired immediately while the decision to repair closed anterior wall fractures can be delayed until the soft tissue swelling has subsided. The use of prophylactic antibiotics is controversial.

SUMMARY

In summary, the diagnosis and treatment of facial bone fractures may be safely delayed for hours or days after the patient's airway has been secured and hemorrhage controlled. Plain film radiographs should be followed by special diagnostic imaging such as a CT scan when better definition is necessary to plan definitive surgical care.

REFERENCES

1. Dolan KD, Jacoby CG, and Smoker W: The radiology of facial fractures, *Radiographics* 4(4):599, 1984.
2. Ballinger PW: *Merrill's atlas of radiographic positions and radiologic procedures,* ed 7, St Louis, 1991, Mosby–Year Book.
3. Dingman RO, Natvig P: *Surgery of facial fractures,* Philadelphia, 1964, WB Saunders.
4. Keats T, ed: *Emergency radiology,* Chicago, 1988, Year Book Publishers.
5. Spicer TE: Facial and soft tissue trauma in childhood. In Mayer TA, ed: *Emergency management of pediatric trauma,* Philadelphia, 1985, WB Saunders.
6. James RB, Frederickson C, and Kent JN: Prospective study of mandible fractures, *J Oral Surg* 39:275, 1981.
7. Clayton ML, Lesser THJ: The role of radiography in the management of nasal fractures, *J Laryngol Otol* 100:797, 1986.
8. deLacey GJ, Wignall BK, Hussain S et al: The radiology of nasal injuries: problems of interpretation and clinical relevance, *Radiology* 50:412, 1977.
9. Zilka A: Computed tomography of blow-out fracture of the medial orbital wall, *AJR,* 137:963, 1981.
10. Hammerschlag SB, Hughes S, and O'Reilly GV: Another look at blow-out fractures of the orbit, *AJR* 139:133, 1982.
11. Kersten RC: Blow-out fracture of the orbital floor with entrapment caused by isolated trauma to the orbital rim, *Am J Ophthalmol* 103(2):219, 1987.
12. Hammerschlag SB, Hugher, and O'Reilly GV: Blow-out fractures of the orbit: a comparison of computed tomography and conventional radiography with anatomical correlation, *Radiology* 143(2):489, 1982.
13. Berardo N, Leban SG, and Williams FA: A comparison of radiographic treatment methods for evaluation of the orbit, *J Oral Maxillofac Surg* 46:845, 1988.
14. Putterman AM, Smith BC, and Lismen RD: Blowout fractures. In Smith BC, Rocca RC, Nesi FA, eds: *Ophthalmic, plastic and reconstructive surgery,* vol 1, St Louis, 1987, CV Mosby.
15. Unger M: Orbital apex fractures: the contribution of computed tomography, *Radiology* 150:713, 1984.
16. Noyek AM, Kassel EK, and Wortzman G: Contemporary radiologic evaluation in maxillofacial trauma, *Otolaryngol Clin North Am* 16(3)480, 1983.
17. Godtfredsen E: Unilateral optic atrophy following head injury, *Acta Ophthalmol* 41:693, 1963.
18. Banovetz JD, Duvay AJ: Zygomatic fractures, *Otolaryngol Clin North Am* 9(2):499, 1976.
19. Kassel EE: Traumatic injuries of the paranasal sinuses, *Otolaryngol Clin North Am* 21(3):455, 1988.
20. Dolan KD, Jacoby CG: Facial fractures, seminars in roentgenology, *Radiographics* 13(1):37, 1978.
21. Luce EA: Frontal sinus fractures: guidelines to management, *Plast Reconstr Surg* 80:500, 1987.
22. Calvert: *Fractures of facial skeleton,* Baltimore, 1955, Rowe, Williams & Wilkins.
23. Toombs BD, Sandler CM, eds: *Computed tomography in trauma,* Philadelphia, 1987, WB Saunders.
24. Whited RE: Anterior table frontal sinus fractures, *Laryngoscope* 89:1951, 1979.
25. Pollak K, Payne EE: Fractures of the frontal sinus, *Otolaryngol Clin North Am* 9(2):517, 1976.
26. Newman MH: Frontal sinus fractures, *Laryngoscope* 83:1281, 1973.

C H A P T E R **5**

Chest Trauma

D. Michael Hunt
Frederick J. Schwab

Thoracic trauma is second only to head injury as a leading cause of traumatic death and accounts for approximately one fourth of the 100,000 annual civilian trauma deaths in the United States.[1] Radiographically, the spectrum of definable injury involves the soft tissue and bony structures of the thoracic cage: the ribs, pulmonary parenchyma and pleura, diaphragm, esophagus, heart, and great vessels. The imaging modalities presently available for the examination of damage to these structures in the emergency department setting are somewhat limited, given time constraints for diagnosis before initiating therapy. They generally involve three tools: plain radiography, computed tomography, and angiography. When available, echocardiography, radionuclide scanning, and esophagography may contribute vital information to patient management.

IMAGING MODALITIES
Plain radiography

Perhaps no other radiograph depends more on technical features of production for accurate interpretation than the chest radiograph.[2] Ideally, the chest radiograph should be obtained with the patient in the upright position using a posteroanterior (PA) projection. With proper positioning, accurate exposure, and a cooperative patient, the technically correct, normal-appearing chest should demonstrate several features. These include a midline trachea, a central and symmetric location of the medial borders of the clavicles over the superior mediastinum, and equally dense lung fields and pulmonary hila with symmetric vascular markings. Additionally, the thoracic spine outline should be visible through the mediastinum, the ribs behind the heart, and vascular markings identifiable behind the ribs. The borders of the hemidiaphragms should be well defined, the costophrenic and cardiophrenic angles sharp, and the dome of the right hemidiaphragm between 0.5 and 2.5 cm above the left.[3]

Ironically, it is the trauma patient who may most benefit from a technically precise radiograph, but for whom it frequently cannot be obtained. Because of the nature and severity of patient injuries, the initial radiograph is often done using an anteroposterior (AP) projection with the patient supine and with the potential for numerous objects (in the form of clothing, jewelry, backboards, neck-immobilizing devices, tubing, and monitor wires) to lie in the path of the x-ray beam. Variable patient cooperation, suboptimal positioning, and attention to other diagnostic and therapeutic maneuvers can also diminish the yield of the initial chest radiograph. When such an inadequate radiograph is obtained, the astute clinician appropriately relies on clinical confirmation for decision-making until a study of reasonable quality is available. It can be as important to interpret correctly what is revealed as it is to recognize what is obscured or distorted.

The AP projection is notorious for producing "abnormal" radiographs on the basis of technique alone. A large hemothorax, which is apparent on the PA projection, may be missed or misinterpreted as resulting from patient rotation on the supine AP view.[3] The cardiac silhouette can appear enlarged and the mediastinum, widened, in the AP projection because of magnification differences and normal increases in mediastinal venous dilatation (Fig. 5-1). Such

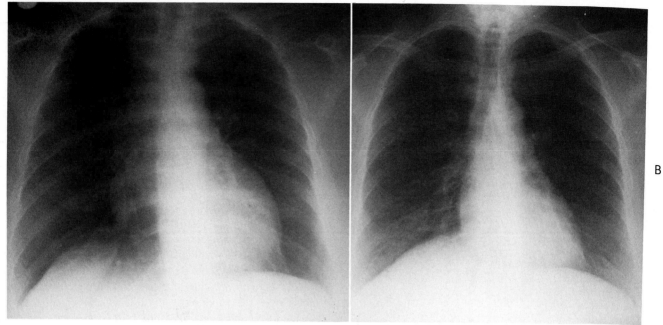

Fig. 5-1. These radiographs demonstrate the difference projection and patient posture can make. **A,** AP projection with the patient supine. There is a suggestion of mediastinal widening and an enlarged heart. **B,** Normal appearance of such structures in the PA upright radiograph.

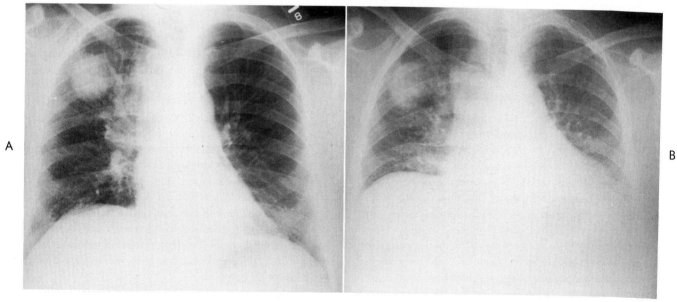

Fig. 5-2. These radiographs demonstrate changes in radiographic appearance as affected by respiratory phase alone. **A,** Normal inspiratory view. **B,** Apparent findings of cardiac enlargement, mediastinal widening, and pulmonary vascular engorgement during expiratory view. (Carcinoma in the right upper lobe is an incidental finding.)

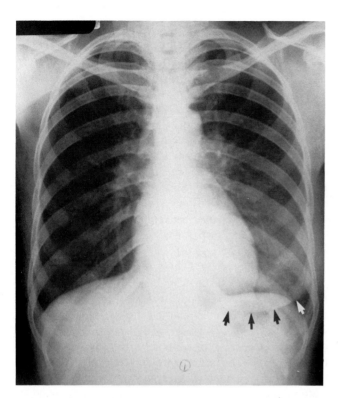

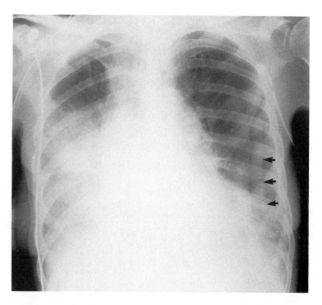

Fig. 5-4. Superimposed skinfold mimicking a left-sided pneumothorax *(arrows)*.

Fig. 5-3. Superimposed soft tissue structures may simulate pathologic conditions unless the radiograph is examined carefully. What may be interpreted as a left-sided infiltrate or pulmonary contusion is merely an increase in density from breast tissue compared to the right side where a mastectomy was performed. The key finding is the inferior breast border *(arrows)* seen on the left side only.

findings may require confirmation with other views if intervention in the form of pericardiocentesis or angiography is considered. The patient who cannot or will not cooperate with a deep inspiration may provide a radiograph that shows small, abnormally dense lungs, an enlarged heart, and engorged pulmonary vascular markings (Fig. 5-2). Unless the incomplete expansion is recognized, fluid overload or underlying congestive heart failure may be diagnosed.[4] Conversely, a radiograph of a patient performing a valsalva maneuver (forced expiration against a closed glottis) will demonstrate a smaller than expected heart and hilar blood vessels due to the reduced venous return and cardiac output.[3]

Certain normal anatomic structures may also be misinterpreted if their presence is not recognized or anticipated.[5] Breasts, nipples, scapulae, muscles, or skinfolds are all potential sources for diagnostic error. Breast shadows are most likely to cause confusion when they are asymmetric in size or position, or the patient has undergone a mastectomy (Fig. 5-3). Muscle shadows can be identified by tracing their course beyond the chest wall. "Companion shadows" are superimposed folds of skin and subcutaneous tissue that may be misinterpreted as the abnormal pleural position associated with a pneumothorax (Fig. 5-4). The three most common places to see such

shadows are parallel to the superior clavicular border, near the inferomedial border of the second rib, and extending cephalad from the costophrenic angle for 1 to 2 cm.[5] Although the shadows can be confused with pneumothorax, pleural thickening, and effusion, they are usually differentiated by their symmetric, bilateral appearance and extension beyond the lung margins.

There are some basic principles common to all radiographic interpretation that warrant reiteration to ensure that complete and accurate information is obtained from a particular study. After confirming the patient's identity on the radiograph and being satisfied that the study is adequate, the most important principle is to evaluate the radiograph systematically. The method employed does not matter as much as does the habitual application of the same process to each AP or PA projection. While it is natural for the physician to look first to the areas of obvious or expected abnormalities (and critical if immediate intervention is required), the entire radiograph must be examined so that important information is not overlooked. One routine for evaluation is to proceed peripherally from the central chest region.[3]

The trachea should be examined for midline location and to differentiate pathology from positioning if it does not lie centrally. The mediastinum should be inspected for widening, displacement, or free air, and the heart size and shape should be assessed. The lung fields should be free of local or asymmetric fluid accumulations or densities that cannot be accounted for by extraparenchymal structures. Vascular markings should be traceable to the periphery throughout the lungs. Bronchioles should be inspected for the abnormal finding of air on both sides of the wall. The costophrenic angles should be sharp. (A supine AP projection may conceal several 100 ml of blood in a hemithorax.) The hemidiaphragms should be distinct, appropriately curved, and the right higher in position than the left. The ribs and sternum should be inspected for any irregularity in their course, indicating fracture or displacement.

Finally, and frequently overlooked, the structures on the radiograph lying outside the boundaries of the thoracic cage should be thoroughly scrutinized. Fractures, soft tissue air suggestive of a pneumothorax, or a foreign body

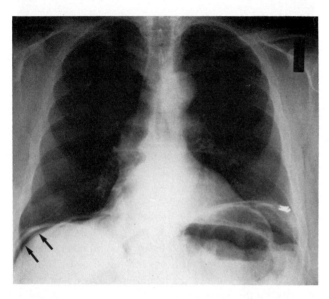

Fig. 5-5. Free abdominal air. A gunshot wound to the lower chest shows that the peritoneal cavity was also violated, mandating laparotomy. Free air is noted under right hemidiaphram *(arrows)*.

can be identified on the periphery of the study. Free intraperitoneal air from abdominal viscus disruption may be seen on an upright radiograph (Fig. 5-5). Tubes and catheters should be traced for continuity and proper location.

Computed tomography

While plain radiography is more readily available and provides sufficient information for the majority of chest trauma studies, the CT scan can add details that may alter patient management. Of course, the benefit of acquiring additional data must be weighed against the practical considerations of the added time required and difficulties inherent in monitoring and managing the trauma patient outside the emergency department. Unstable patients do not belong in the gantry of a CT scanner.

Advantages of the CT scan imaging[3] include the increased ability to distinguish between soft tissue structures, identify fluid accumulations, demonstrate axial relationships, delineate individual mediastinal structures, recognize pulmonary contusions[6] and diaphragmatic injuries, and trace the course of pulmonary vessels and bronchi (Fig. 5-6). The CT scan can greatly increase diagnostic yield, identifying up to three or four times as many abnormalities due to thoracic trauma as can plain radiographs[7,8] (Fig. 5-7). Contrast-enhanced studies offer even greater advantage in providing diagnostic accuracy.[9] Oral contrast agents can increase the yield of esophageal studies, and the dynamic CT scan with intravenous contrast material can demonstrate vascular abnormalities that may not otherwise be appreciated.

The major disadvantages in obtaining a CT scan lie in removing the patient from the observation of the emergency department as well as the extra time necessary to

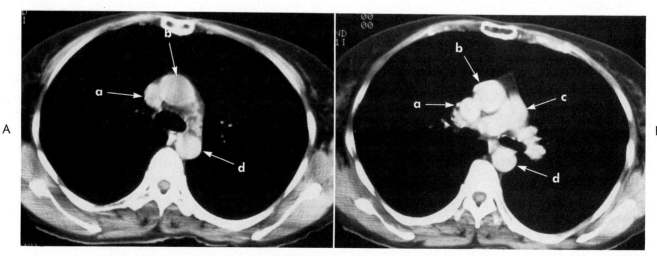

A   B

Fig. 5-6. Normal contrast-enhanced CT scans of thorax. **A,** Below the carina. **B,** Caudal to aortic arch. Visualized structures include the superior vena cava *(a)*, ascending thoracic aorta *(b)*, pulmonary artery *(c)*, and descending thoracic aorta *(d)*. Mediastinal fat pads are well defined, without fluid collection.

obtain the scan. Also longer scanning times (especially in older equipment) and patient movement can result in blurred images and even falsified information.

Angiography

Angiography remains the primary imaging technique for the diagnosis of aortic disruption following blunt chest trauma and arterial occlusion or dissection following penetrating or avulsive injury.[2] Angiography can demonstrate subtle injury to the vessel wall and provides a surgical "road map" to plan and organize appropriate surgical intervention. The study can be performed safely and rapidly with small diameter catheters and rapid imaging equipment. The major imaging limitation of angiography is that only the arterial wall and lumen are studied. Compared to a CT scan, for example, little additional information is obtained regarding injury to other organ systems. The major logistic drawback to angiography is the investment of time and technical support required to accomplish the procedure. Again, it also requires physically removing the potentially unstable patient from the confines of the emergency department.

Magnetic resonance imaging

One of the newest and most exciting imaging modalities, magnetic resonance imaging (MRI), is not readily available to most emergency trauma patients and its true utility in this setting remains undefined. Although MRI can provide a wealth of information, the long scanning times previously required (up to 1 hour per patient) and the need for complete patient cooperation made this study impractical for most trauma victims. Presently, however, advances in the area of rapid scanning times and of vascular imaging may allow MRI to become a noninvasive alternative to the CT scan and angiography.

Echocardiography

The use of two-dimensional echocardiography to document cardiac injury from blunt trauma is gaining popularity and respect as a diagnostic tool in the emergency department. It can be used in the chest trauma patient to demonstrate pericardial effusion, dyskinetic heart motion, papillary disruption, valve incompetence, and the presence of thrombi. While it is portable, noninvasive, and can be applied to the chest wall of the trauma patient without disrupting resuscitative efforts, it requires the availability of someone proficient in the operation of the equipment and in interpretation of the echocardiograms if the information is to be of value.[10,11]

SPECIFIC INJURIES
Extrathoracic findings

The emergency physician should make use of all information available on the plain radiograph and avoid focusing exclusively on the area in question. Specific attention should be placed on the extrathoracic bony structures such as the clavicles and humerus, looking for the otherwise unexpected fracture, separation, subluxation, or dislocation (Fig. 5-8). Soft tissue injuries and especially the presence

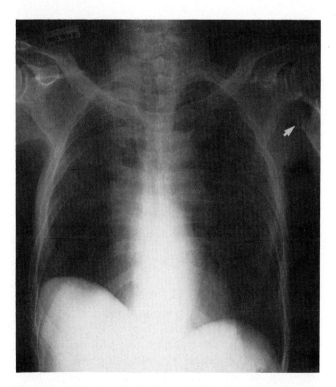

Fig. 5-8. While attention is frequently drawn to the center of a film, the entire radiograph should be examined for additional information about patient injuries. This study has the incidental finding of a fractured left humerus *(arrow)* that may not be appreciated initially in the comatose patient yet has clear implications for increased morbidity.

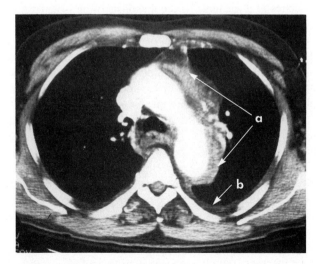

Fig. 5-7. Contrast-enhanced CT scan of patient who sustained blunt chest trauma. Initial chest radiograph was normal, and CT scan shows moderate mediastinal hemorrhage *(a)*. Small pleural effusion is also identified *(b)*. Aortogram was normal, and patient was managed conservatively.

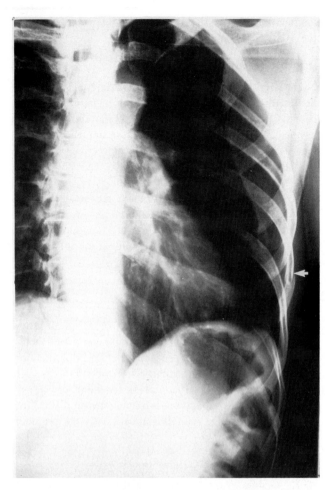

Fig. 5-9. Fractured left sixth rib. This oblique radiograph shows an isolated fracture. Its location and appearance suggest a compressive force as the mechanism of trauma.

of foreign bodies may be detected when they might otherwise be missed. The identification of air in the soft tissue of the chest wall of the blunt trauma victim should prompt a careful search for a pneumothorax and associated rib fracture(s). In the patient sustaining penetrating trauma to the chest, soft tissue air may be visible as the result of dermal penetration by a knife, a bullet, or other projectile, and residual foreign bodies should be recognized.

Chest wall

Rib fracture. Isolated rib fractures are the most frequently encountered manifestation of nonpenetrating thoracic trauma.[12-14] Since bone elasticity is greatest in the younger age group, rib fractures are relatively uncommon in the pediatric population. Fractures occur with increasing frequency and with decreasing amounts of requisite force in older patients.[12,15] Fractures result from either compression of the chest wall or from a direct blow.[2] The former mechanism most typically produces fractures at the posterior angle (the structurally weakest segment), involving the fourth through ninth ribs[12,14] (Fig. 5-9). The radiographic

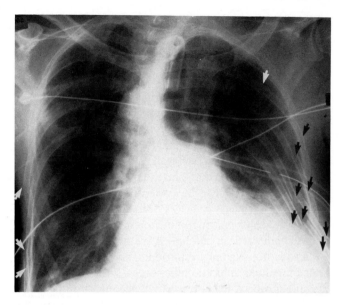

Fig. 5-10. Flail chest. This patient sustained fractures in two places along each of the left fourth through eighth ribs, creating a flail segment *(dark arrows)*. Note also the right rib fractures *(white arrows)*. A central flail may be created when multiple ribs at the same level are fractured on both sides of the sternum.

appearance is of outward buckling or a "spring fracture" and is infrequently associated with underlying injuries to the lung and pleura.[12] Direct trauma is more likely to produce an inwardly directed fracture and pneumothorax and parenchymal lacerations.[2] Incomplete or nondisplaced rib fractures may not be identified on the initial radiograph in 10% to 50% of the cases.[14,16] Signs of fracture include linear or irregular lucency and cortical disruption or displacement. Occasionally, an extrapleural hematoma at the site of injury or pain and tenderness at the site may be the only evidence of a fracture.[4] If the diagnosis of an isolated fracture is important, it may be obtained using the oblique views of a rib series or a set of delayed studies.[2,12] More importantly, a radiograph should be obtained to determine the possibility of associated underlying pleural, pulmonary, and visceral injuries or to predict the potential complications of atelectasis and pneumonia.[12,14]

First through third ribs are less frequently fractured, ostensibly because of the additional protection afforded by the clavicles, scapulae, and large muscle groups of the upper chest and back.[2] When fractures in this region are identified, it must be assumed that a tremendous amount of force has been imparted to the upper chest. The possibility of tracheobronchial and great vessel injury should be given full consideration.[13] It is has been reported that fractures of the first rib may be associated with aortic avulsions in 50% of cases,[17] with a patient mortality of up to 36%.[18] However, these figures are misleading. When *isolated* first rib fracture cases are examined, these patients were found to have a mortality of only 1.5%.[19] Nevertheless, identification of first rib fractures has implication for further

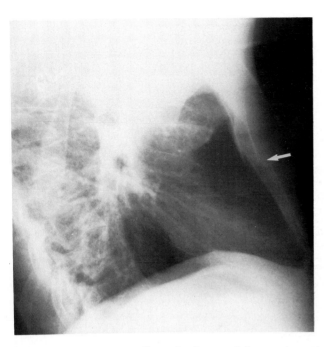

Fig. 5-11. Lateral chest radiograph of a sternal fracture *(arrow)*.

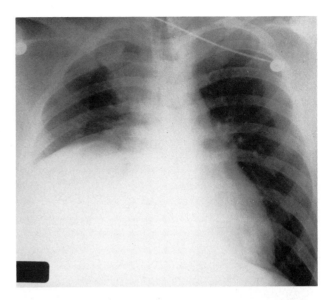

Fig. 5-12. Diaphragmatic herniation. The apparent elevation of the right hemidiaphragm is caused by the liver herniating into the pleural cavity through a large right diaphragmatic rent.

study, specifically angiography to rule out vascular injury. Such further studies should be considered when the fracture is displaced or the patient has a pulse deficit or brachial plexus injury.[20]

Fractures of the tenth, eleventh, and twelfth ribs are also infrequent because of the increased flexibility afforded by their less secure anterior attachments. Rib fractures at these levels should raise the question of accompanying splenic, hepatic, or renal injury.[2,15]

Multiple rib fractures are also indicators of severe trauma, with the chance for associated intrathoracic trauma increasing approximately 10% for every rib fractured.[21] A flail chest exists when three or more consecutive ribs are fractured at two or more points (Fig. 5-10). The radiographic significance of a flail segment is that it mandates the need to search for subtle hemopneumothorax and cardiac and pulmonary contusion. Even if the radiographic studies cannot identify these, the patient needs to be carefully observed for respiratory insufficiency and may require prophylactic thoracostomy if active mechanical ventilation is to be used for surgery or respiratory assistance.

Sternal fracture. Sternal fractures are the result of severe blunt trauma, most often caused by striking the steering wheel in motor vehicle accidents.[14] These fractures rarely involve the manubrium[16] but can contribute to the creation of a central flail chest. They have tremendous potential for associated serious injuries, including myocardial and pulmonary contusion, vascular disruption, and cardiac rupture. Electrocardiographic abnormalities have been observed in up to 62% of patients with such fractures.[22] The mortality rate of over 40% is usually attributed to the asso-

ciated injuries.[12,14] The best view to identify these fractures is the lateral chest radiograph (Fig. 5-11). Although the diagnosis can frequently be made clinically on the basis of exquisite tenderness, oblique views may also be helpful. Surgical correction is rarely required, and treatment is appropriately directed toward management of the concomitant injuries.[12,14,22]

Diaphragm

The diagnosis of traumatic diaphragmatic rupture can be quite challenging and the pursuit of substantial findings elusive. Blunt trauma tends to produce predominantly left-sided injuries given the protective and supporting location of the liver under the right hemidiaphragm. Stab wounds of the diaphragm are also more often discovered on the left side (presumably due to a higher proportion of right-handed assailants) although gunshot wounds are more evenly distributed between either side.[23,24]

Imaging studies most likely to contribute to the diagnosis of diaphragmatic rupture are plain chest radiographs, upper gastrointestinal tract contrast studies, and computed tomography.[25] The initial upright chest radiograph may demonstrate several direct and indirect features of a diaphragmatic tear[23]: an indistinct or elevated hemidiaphragm, pleural effusion, mediastinal shift, pneumothorax, or the presence of viscera in the chest (Fig. 5-12). The diagnosis can be made in up to 40% of patients based on the chest radiograph alone,[26] but, when the findings are not conclusive, additional procedures should be employed. The passage of a nasogastric tube into an obscure, ill-defined shadow in the thorax may be a sign of a herniated stomach. An upper gastrointestinal series or a barium en-

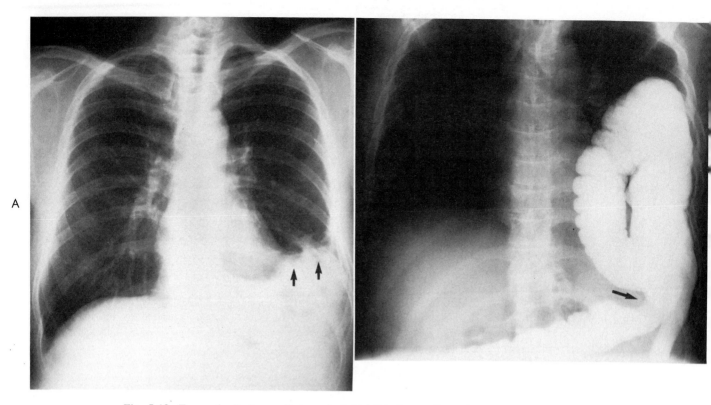

A

Fig. 5-13. Traumatic diaphragmatic tear. **A,** Initial PA chest radiograph demonstrates elevation of the left hemidiaphragm with a "cystic" mass suggested at the left base *(small arrows).* **B,** Barium enema demonstrates entrapment of the colonic splenic flexure *(arrow)* in the tear.

ema can demonstrate a contrast-filled viscus above the diaphragm or point to the location of a small rent when visualization of the bowel is abruptly cut off (Fig. 5-13). The ancillary use of the CT scan in demonstrating diaphragmatic herniation has proved useful when planned for the diagnosis of other injuries, when the administration of oral or rectal contrast material is impractical, and when the patient's stability permits (Fig. 5-14). Finally, the use of radionuclide scanning to assist in making the diagnosis of traumatic diaphragmatic rupture has been attempted with limited success. Liver-spleen scans tend to be nondiagnostic unless these particular organs have, in fact, herniated through the diaphragm. Transdiaphragmatic migration of technetium-labelled colloid has been demonstrated convincingly in animal models but has yet to be proved an effective diagnostic tool in humans.[27] The most sensitive test of diaphragmatic injury secondary to penetrating trauma is diagnostic peritoneal lavage (DPL) with a positive red blood cell threshold of 5000 RBCs/ mm^3.

Pleura and mediastinum

Pneumothorax. Pneumothorax occurs as a result of blunt trauma in 15% to 50% of patients. It occurs almost exclusively from pleural violation by associated rib fractures but may also result from a ruptured bleb, alveoli, or

bronchus.[15] Penetrating trauma may introduce air through the wound track or through a parenchymal laceration.[13]

Pneumothorax is typically categorized as simple, communicating, or tension. A simple pneumothorax is one that neither connects with the external chest nor demonstrates a progressive accumulation of air in the pleural space (Fig. 5-15). The radiographic diagnosis of this entity is usually based on the appearance of increased lung field lucency and the loss of peripheral lung markings that are otherwise expected to extend all the way out to the chest wall. Loss of lung markings is frequently accompanied by a line of visceral pleura. The diagnosis may be difficult if the pneumothorax is obscured by ribs. The diagnosis may be mistakenly made if there are pleural blebs or superimposed skinfolds and clothing.

Techniques to delineate the presence of a small or otherwise undetectable pneumothorax should include upright expiratory views or a lateral decubitus view with the side of interest up (Fig. 5-16). The presence of subcutaneous emphysema should prompt the clinician to conclude a pneumothorax is present when penetrating injury is involved and as an absolute indication of pleural disruption in the blunt trauma victim. Yet the emergency physician need not be overly concerned over radiographic proof of pneumothorax since it is unwise to conclude that air was

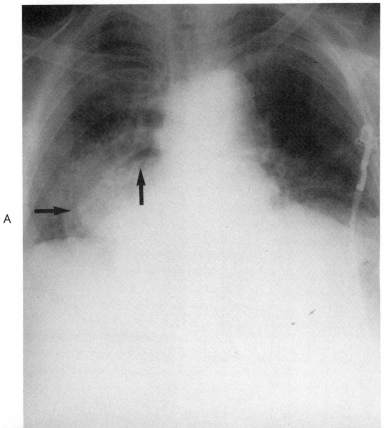

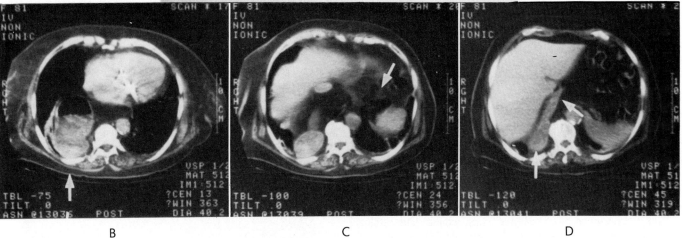

Fig. 5-14. Diaphragmatic herniation. **A,** Initial portable AP chest radiograph demonstrates large mass *(horizontal arrow)* with air-fluid level *(vertical arrow)* suggested within the right lower lobe. **B,** CT scan confirms mass with an air-fluid level *(arrow)* within the gastric fundus. **C** and **D,** CT scans further define mass as representing stomach herniated into the right chest. CT scan **(C)** demonstrates the absence of the stomach within the left upper abdomen *(arrow)*, while CT scan **(D)** demonstrates gastric body and antrum *(arrows)* herniated through the lesser sac. (Courtesy Neal H Rosner, MD.)

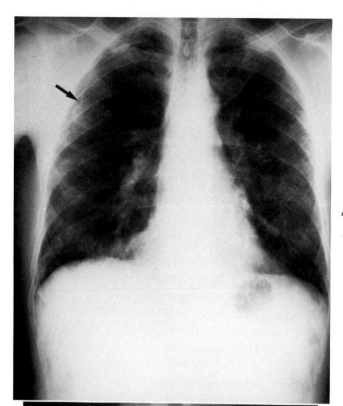

Fig. 5-15. Simple pneumothorax. Distinct pleural line in the right apex indicates the presence of a small pneumothorax *(arrows)* (less than 15%). This finding could result from any penetrating injury.

introduced by the penetrating instrument. It is more prudent to perform a thoracostomy and use further radiographic studies to assess tube placement. Attempts to accurately estimate the volume of a pneumothorax on the basis of a two-dimensional study can be difficult, and assessment of size is easiest to grade in general terms. A small pneumothorax is considered to be anything under 15%, a moderate pneumothorax is a collapse of about 15% to 60%, and anything over this figure is large.[15]

A communicating pneumothorax involves free air passage between the pleural cavity and the external environment. This is usually a clinical diagnosis made by observing the presence of a "sucking" chest wound. The clinical identification of this type of pneumothorax is easy although the only radiographic documentation may come from sequential respiratory phase views. Compared to the closed pneumothorax, these views demonstrate paradoxical collapse and expansion with inspiration and expiration, respectively.

A tension pneumothorax is a potentially life-threatening condition created by progressive collection of air in the pleural space because of unidirectional air flow from a visceral pleura defect (Fig. 5-17). This leads to an incremental shift in the mediastinal structures toward the unaffected

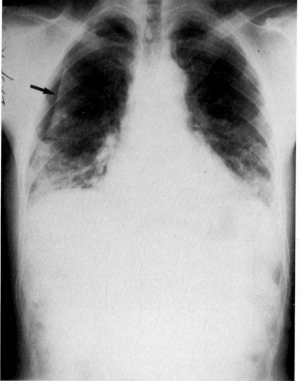

Fig. 5-16. Upright inspiratory (**A**) and expiratory (**B**) chest radiographs demonstrate accentuation of right pneumothorax *(arrows)*.

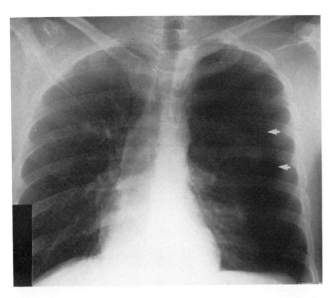

Fig. 5-17. Tension pneumothorax. The progressive accumulation of air in the left pleural cavity has induced a mediastinal shift to the right. Note left pleural margin *(arrows)*.

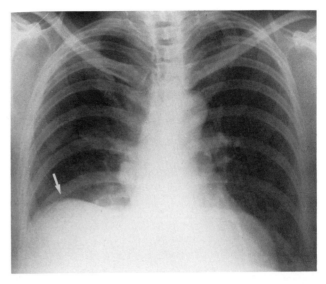

Fig. 5-19. Right-sided subpulmonic effusion. Note the elevation of the hemidiaphragm as well as the lateral displacement of the dome *(arrow)*, findings characteristic of this condition.

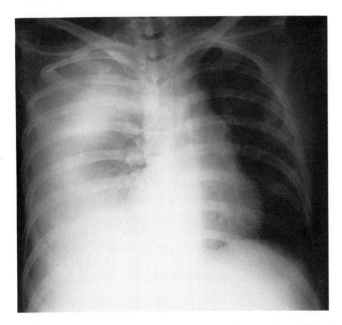

Fig. 5-18. Massive right hemothorax. PA chest radiograph reveals near total opacification of the right hemithorax.

side with a gradual reduction in venous return to the heart. Unremedied, this can rapidly progress to decreased cardiac output, precipitous hemodynamic collapse, and death. Although it has been remarked that the presentation is usually so dramatic that treatment should be rendered on the basis of clinical suspicion alone (absent breath sounds, respiratory distress, hypotension, and tachycardia) before confirmatory radiographs are obtained, plain radiographic findings reveal the diagnosis in up to three fourths of the cases.[28] As the pressure around the collapsed lung takes

time to rise, a chest radiograph may reveal mediastinal shift before the patient exhibits any clinical signs of a tension pneumothorax. Although it is always prudent to compare radiographic with clinical findings, this is one instance where the radiographic finding of shift should mandate rapid thoracostomy rather than waiting for the clinical signs of a tension pneumothorax. The discovery of a massive pneumothorax with contralateral mediastinal shift, a hyperinflated hemithorax, or depression of the ipsilateral hemidiaphragm in a patient with cardiovascular compromise should prompt immediate decompression of the affected side.

Hemothorax. Radiographic documentation of free blood in the thoracic cavity depends on the view obtained (supine vs. upright) and the volume of fluid present (Fig. 5-18). Because many studies are initially done with the patient supine, the only findings may be that of diffuse unilateral haziness although the dependent fluid can also be manifested indirectly as a thickened pleural or paraspinal stripe. An upright radiograph will demonstrate a hemothorax of greater than 250 ml[16] by costophrenic angle blunting or diaphragmatic obscuration. A volume of blood less than this may go undetected in the posterior sulcus in the upright position but can be readily demonstrated by a lateral decubitus view. As the amount of free fluid in the chest increases, the ipsilateral lung undergoes progressive parenchymal compression and atelectasis. Subpulmonic effusions are manifested by the apparent elevation of the hemidiaphragm and lateral displacement of the dome from its normal position (Fig. 5-19). A horizontal line in the chest should be taken as prima facie evidence of a hemopneumothorax and indicates urgent decompression by tube thoracostomy (Fig. 5-20).

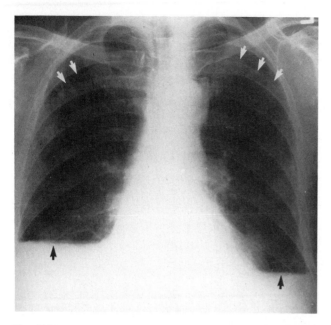

Fig. 5-20. Bilateral hemopneumothorax. A straight line *(black arrows)* in the chest on an upright view is indicative of an air-fluid interface, and, when it extends across the pleural space in trauma patients, a hemopneumothorax is present. The pleural margins *(white arrows)* are obscured by ribs on the left side.

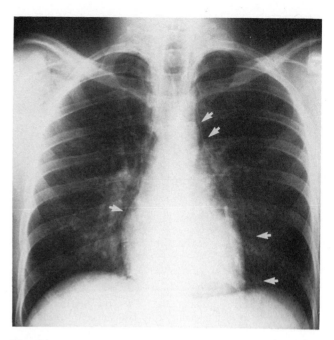

Fig. 5-21. Pneumomediastinum. Notice the bilateral paramediastinal linear densities extending inferiorly from the level of the clavicles *(arrows)*.

Pneumomediastium. Introduction of air into the mediastinal region can occur through traumatic communication with the pleura, upper airways, esophagus, or abdomen (Fig. 5-21). It can result as a consequence of extrathoracic chest wall compression, increased intraluminal pressure, or penetrating trauma. The radiographic sign pathognomonic for this condition is a thin, vertically oriented paramediastinal lucency and increased adjacent lateral density representing outwardly compressed pleural structures. Occasionally, the pneumomediastinum may dissect inferiorly and be confused with a pneumopericardium or may be associated with subcutaneous emphysema (Fig. 5-22). A pneumomediastinum can be differentiated radiographically from a medial pneumothorax using views in the lateral decubitus position or in different phases of respiration. Using the latter technique will demonstrate the pneumomediastinum to be static while the pneumothorax size will fluctuate with lung volume.

Lung parenchyma

Pulmonary contusion. Pulmonary contusion is the most common lung injury in nonpenetrating chest trauma.[7] It is characterized by edema and blood in the interstitial and alveolar compartments without tissue laceration (Fig. 5-23). Typically a deceleration injury from a motor vehicle accident, pulmonary contusion has also been described in association with falls and nonpenetrating missile and concussive injuries.[29] Although severe contusions occur in the absence of rib fractures (particularly in young people),

pulmonary contusion should be considered whenever a rib or sternal fracture is identified and should be assumed present in any case of flail chest.[30] Appearing as an irregular region of alveolar infiltrates, a contusion may not be seen on the plain radiograph until several hours after the initial injury. The infiltrates may be either discrete or confluent and are distinguished from the type of opacities seen after aspiration in the multiple trauma patient by their lack of anatomic confinement to particular lobes or segments.[7] Occasionally, the contusion will become consolidated although most contusions begin to clear radiographically within a few days.[15] When the patient demonstrates physiologic signs of contusion (progressively increasing hypoxemia, increasing respiratory rate, and carbon dioxide retention) that are unconfirmed by a plain radiograph, a CT scan of the chest should be considered (Fig. 5-24).

Pulmonary laceration. The radiographic picture of pulmonary laceration is generally similar to that of pulmonary contusion. The clinical difference is that this entity involves a tear, avulsion, or laceration of the parenchyma (Fig. 5-25). These injuries result from lung penetration by fractured ribs or foreign bodies or, rarely, a torn pleural adhesion.[14,15] The use of computed tomography has suggested that many presumed pulmonary contusions are, in fact, lacerations, and the primary mechanism of injury is compression of the chest wall.[7] While a CT scan can demonstrate lacerations of the lung tissue directly (Fig. 5-26), the plain radiograph may only present evidence of a localized, cystic air-fluid interface within the lung parenchyma.

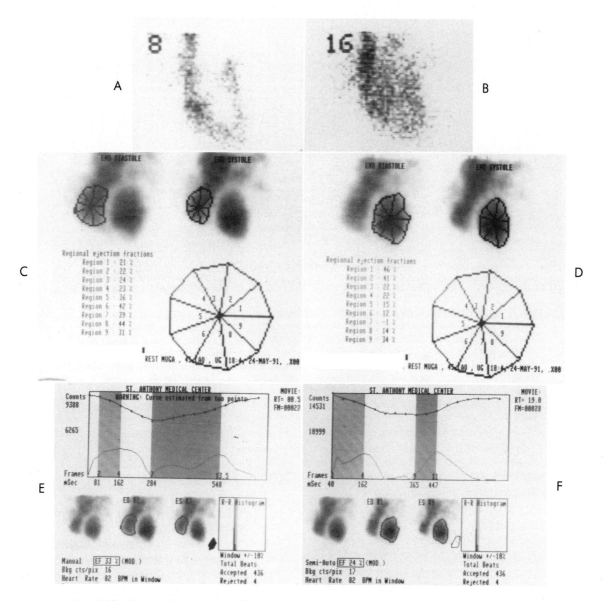

Fig. 5-28. Myocardial contusion. First-pass radionuclide angiograms localize the right ventricle (**A**) and left ventricle (**B**). Multi-gated acquisition analysis (MUGA) images in equilibrium and computer analyses graphs demonstrate mildly diminished ejection fraction of the right ventricle (**C** and **E**) and markedly diminished ejection fraction of the left ventricle (**D** and **F**). (Courtesy Jung Kuo, MD.)

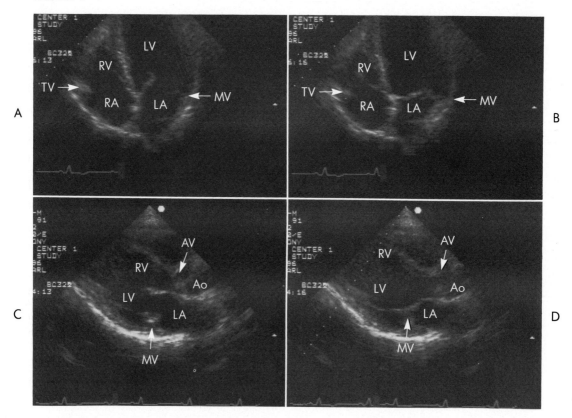

Fig. 5-29. Two-dimensional echocardiogram demonstrating myocardial contusion. Apical four-chamber view in diastole (**A**) and systole (**B**) and parasternal long axis views in diastole (**C**) and systole (**D**). These views demonstrate normal contractility of the right ventricle and minimal contractility of the left ventricle in systole in a patient with a diminished ejection fraction. Note the open and closed positions of the tricuspid and mitral valves corresponding to diastole and systole, respectively; also the open and closed position of the aortic valve corresponding to systole and diastole, respectively. *RA*, right atrium; *LA*, left atrium; *TV*, tricuspid valve; *LV*, left ventricle; *RV*, right ventricle; *MV*, mitral valve; *Ao*, aorta; *AV*, aortic valve. (Courtesy Yoshio Takamiya, MS.)

and predictive value (97%, 86%, and 88%, respectively), this modality has the promise of providing rapid, accurate, and relatively inexpensive diagnostic information in the emergency department setting.[36]

Myocardial puncture and tamponade. Acute pericardial tamponade should be suspected in any patient who presents with a penetrating wound to the thorax or upper abdomen and manifests an elevated CVP, hypotension, and tachycardia after tension pneumothorax has been ruled out.

When myocardial injury occurs in the context of an intact or resealed pericardium, tamponade from immediate bleeding or effusion in the form of delayed serous or serosanguinous fluid accumulation may develop. If acute pericardial tamponade is suspected, then emergency echocardiography is the diagnostic procedure of choice since plain film radiography is often normal. Plain films can be helpful in detecting large pericardial effusions (Fig. 5-30). Such films should be followed by echocardiography since it is the definitive tool to identify the presence of pericardial fluid (Fig. 5-31).

Vascular trauma

Thoracic vascular trauma may result from rapid deceleration in an automobile accident, a fall resulting in an avulsion of the aorta, or from a direct penetrating wound. Both arterial and venous injuries are possible but are managed differently. Patients with major arterial injuries often deteriorate rapidly, so efficient diagnostic assessment is essential.

Aortic injury. Aortic transection or tear is usually the result of a rapid deceleration injury. While the descending aorta is anatomically fixed, the aortic arch and ascending aorta are relatively mobile. Severe shearing forces can be produced at specific points of attachment: immediately distal to the origin of the left subclavian artery, at the aortic root, and at the diaphragm.

Chest radiographic evidence of an aortic transection is a function of the degree of bleeding into the mediastinum and pleural spaces from accompanying organ injuries. However, severe injuries can be present with only subtle changes on a chest radiograph. A large tear in the aortic wall can be temporarily contained by the adventitia, with

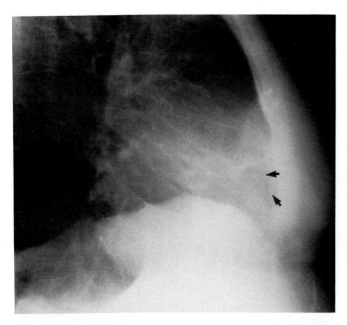

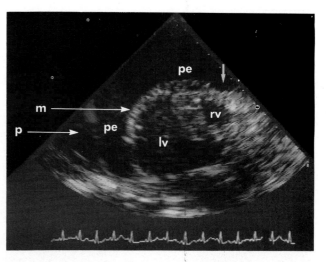

Fig. 5-31. Two-dimensional echocardiogram of patient with cardiac tamponade. Pericardium *(p)*, large pericardial effusion *(pe)*, myocardium *(m)*, left ventricle *(lv)*, right ventricle *(rv)*. Note compression of right ventricle due to tamponade effect *(arrow)*.

Fig. 5-30. Pericardial effusion on lateral chest radiograph. There is an anterior radiolucency indicative of pericardial effusion caused by separation of the normal radiolucent bands of pericardial and epicardial fat *(arrows)*.

minimal leakage into the mediastinum. However, a less severe venous injury can produce signs of substantial bleeding that will mandate angiography.

Widening of the mediastinum is the most common radiographic finding in aortic tear but is neither sensitive nor specific for the diagnosis. As most severely traumatized patients undergo an AP supine chest radiograph initially, it is important to differentiate the normal mediastinal widening produced as a result of this projection, from the widening due to a pathologic condition. Mediastinal widening on a supine radiograph may disappear when a standard upright PA chest radiograph is performed; therefore, if the patient's condition permits, this study should be performed before making the decision to order a CT scan or angiography to rule out the presence of mediastinal hemorrhage or great vessel injury. In addition to mediastinal widening, there are other radiographic findings indicative of transection, which include loss of definition of the aortic knob or mediastinal borders, deviation of a nasogastric tube or trachea to the right, depression of the left mainstem bronchus, left hemithorax, or apical cap, and associated displaced fractures of the first through third ribs (Fig. 5-32, *A* to *C*).

Additional evaluation will depend on the status of the patient. Thoracic angiography is most sensitive and is the "gold standard" for defining the site of transection (Fig. 5-32, *D*). However, thoracic angiography will not delineate the size of a mediastinal hematoma or define the site of venous bleeding. While a CT scan is very sensitive for detecting the presence of hemorrhage into the mediastinum, it has poor specificity and must be followed by an-

giography immediately in order to determine if an aortic or great vessel injury is present and its location.

Patients with clinical findings and chest radiography suggestive of transection generally should undergo emergent angiography before surgical exploration if their clinical condition is stable. A CT scan should be limited to patients who have unimpressive mechanisms of injury but who have radiographic chest abnormalities as discussed previously. In these situations, a normal CT scan of the mediastinum probably obviates the need for angiography. However, angiography is required if mediastinal hemorrhage is present[37] (Fig. 5-33).

Penetrating injuries. Knife or gunshot wounds can produce injuries to the great vessels or their branches at the shoulder. Vascular injuries can range from complete transection or occlusion to subtle intimal dissection or pseudo-aneurysm. Severe injuries to vessels such as the subclavian artery are usually found clinically because of difference in pulse pressure between affected and unaffected arms. Angiography is then used as a pre-operative "road map" to guide vascular bypass or repair (Fig. 5-34). Occasionally, proximal vascular injuries will initially produce little or no pulse deficit. Angiography, therefore, is useful in excluding any significant injury and should be employed if the potential for vascular compromise exists.

Esophagus

Whether injury occurs as a result of esophageal instrumentation, an external penetrating force, or because of the effects of high luminal pressure on an anatomically weakened region of the esophagus, violation of the wall integrity has implications for high morbidity and mortality. Because the esophagus lacks a serosal barrier to contain spill-

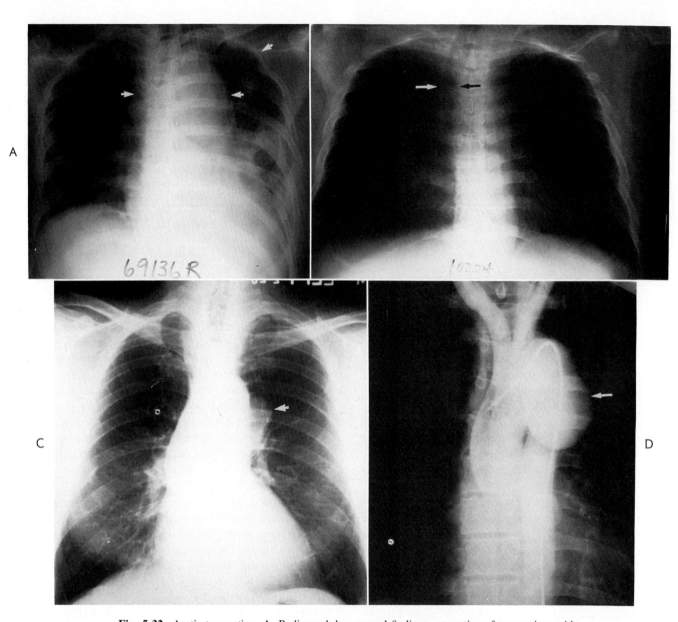

Fig. 5-32. Aortic transection. **A,** Radiograph has several findings suggestive of transection: widened mediastinum *(opposed arrows),* obscured aortic knob, and a left second rib fracture *(top arrow).* **B,** In addition to an obscured aortic knob and widened mediastinum, the trachea is markedly deviated to the right *(arrows).* **C,** Density adjacent to the aortic knob in the left lung field is a pseudo-aneurysm *(arrow)* found after a delayed presentation for blunt chest trauma. **D,** Large post-traumatic pseudo-aneurysm *(arrow).* This angiogram is the companion study for the plain radiograph in **C.**

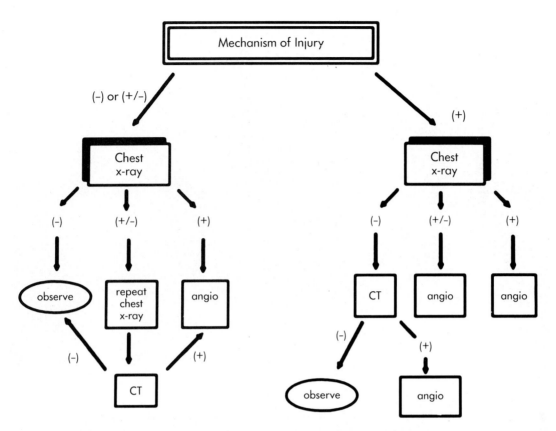

Fig. 5-33. Algorithm to guide the use of diagnostic modalities for possible aortic transection in blunt chest trauma. If the mechanism of injury supports the possibility of transection and the chest radiograph has suggestive findings, angiography is the indicated procedure. For an equivocal or unremarkable mechanism, the chest radiographic results should guide further diagnostic procedures. Any positive CT scan should be followed by angiography.

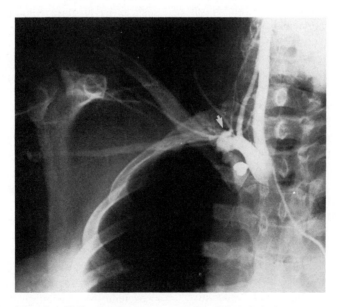

Fig. 5-34. Angiography. Bullet in chest transected the right subclavian artery *(arrow)*. Angiogram provides crucial information for anticipated surgical intervention.

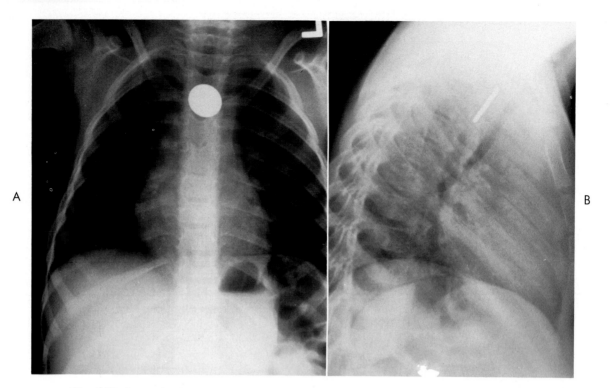

Fig. 5-35. Ingested coin in the esophagus. This en face appearance on the PA chest radiograph (**A**) is typical for coins lodged in the esophagus as is the impacted location at the level of the aortic arch. On the lateral chest radiograph (**B**) the coin is seen on end.

age from a rent or perforation of the wall, material usually confined to the lumen then has direct access to the retropharyngeal space of the cervical esophagus and to the mediastinum over the lower two thirds of its course.[23] The resulting mediastinitis and attendant complications of pneumothorax, pleural effusion, respiratory failure, and sepsis are responsible for a mortality approaching 30%,[38] thus supporting the need for rapid diagnosis and treatment.

Over two thirds of esophageal perforations are the result of endoscopy, dilatation, or the placement of tubes or devices for the purpose of airway protection or gastric access to facilitate decompression or feeding.[39] Although the vast majority of these procedures are accomplished without complication, the fact that most occur in patients with some predisposing condition (congenital malformation, prior surgery, previous injury, or chemical burn) should prompt the physician to elicit such a history when time permits.[40] A foreign body may cause perforation directly or secondarily through induced pressure necrosis of the esophagus. More frequently, a foreign body will result in a complete or partial obstruction. Children tend to have foreign body obstruction due to the relative narrowing of the cricopharyngeal region and their propensity to explore their world orally. Adults, on the other hand, frequently ingest bone or large food boluses. Recurrence of obstruction in any age group is an indication to rule out a structural abnormality.

Radiographic diagnosis of a foreign body is relatively straightforward. PA and lateral projections of the chest will identify and localize most radio-opaque objects (see Chapter 24). Occasionally, the foreign body is radiolucent or relatively obscured by chest structures. In these instances, obtaining oblique views or using indirect clues such as an air-fluid column may confirm the diagnosis. The most likely areas for a foreign body to become impacted include the regions of the cricopharyngeous muscle, the aortic arch, and at the esophagogastric junction.[15] Impacted food in the esophagus of adults is usually not apparent on a plain radiograph and a contrast examination is usually necessary to confirm and locate the offending bolus. Coins tend to be a commonly swallowed object in the pediatric population. Their presence in the esophagus can be differentiated from an airway location by their typical en face appearance in the AP projection and their side view position on a lateral radiograph (Fig. 5-35).

Less frequent sources of esophageal injury include spontaneous rupture (Boerhaave syndrome) or penetration by an external source such as a knife. The latter cases typically involve damage to other regional structures and, unless the possibility of esophageal damage is considered when dealing with mediastinal trauma and efforts are made to exclude the possibility, the effects can be devastating. Although rare, Boerhaave syndrome should be considered in extremely ill patients with severe abdominal, back, or chest pain after vomiting. Perforation in these patients tends to occur in the distal left posterior region of the

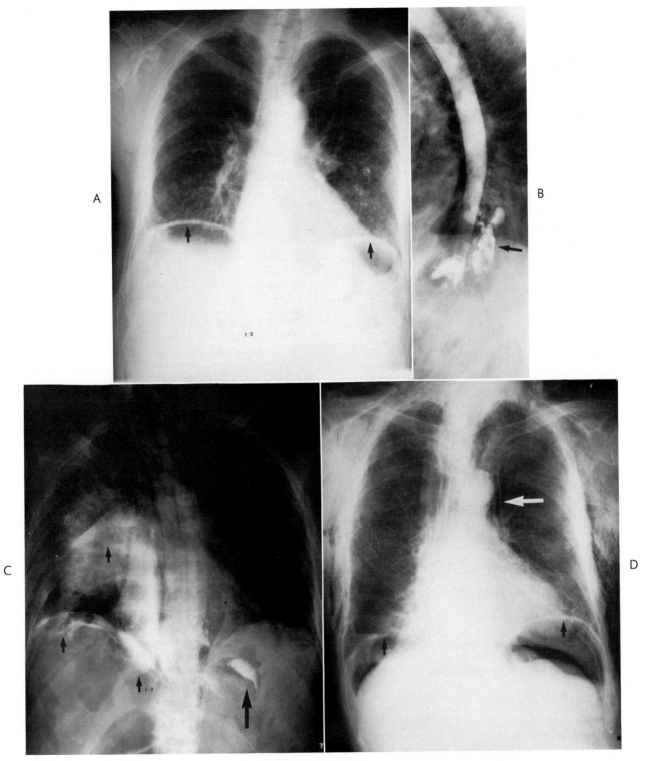

Fig. 5-36. Esophageal perforation secondary to endoscopic dilatation. **A,** Upright chest radiograph demonstrates free air underlying hemidiaphragms *(small arrows).* **B,** Lateral view of barium swallow demonstrates site of perforation *(horizontal arrow).* **C,** Supine view shows extent of extrapleural and peritoneal extravasation *(small arrows).* Note barium in gastric fundus *(large vertical arrow).* **D,** Upright chest radiograph of esophageal perforation secondary to Heimlich maneuver demonstrates more typical appearance of pneumoperitoneum *(small arrows),* pneumomediastinum *(horizontal arrow),* and extensive subcutaneous emphysema within cervical and thoracic regions.

esophagus and may occur without an emetic history.[41]

When the diagnosis of possible esophageal perforation is entertained, several indirect signs should be considered in the examination of the plain radiograph.[23] Mediastinal air, pneumothorax, a left pleural effusion, a widened mediastinum, and the presence of subcutaneous air should suggest this problem (Fig. 5-36, *A* and *D*). An esophagogram can be performed to confirm the diagnosis and should be done initially with a water-soluble contrast agent. A negative examination should be followed with a barium swallow for the added detail provided by this denser medium (Fig. 5-36, *B* and *C*).

SUMMARY

In summary, traumatic injuries to the thorax can result in several life-threatening conditions and can present the clinician with many challenges. The proper selection and sequencing of diagnostic imaging studies is very important. However, emergency treatment and stabilization of life threats such as tension pneumothorax should never be delayed in order to obtain diagnostic studies. Communication with consulting radiologists and surgeons should occur in a timely fashion in order to facilitate diagnostic studies and therapeutic intervention in these patients.

We are indebted to S. David Rockoff, M.D., and Peter E. Doris, M.D., for providing the radiographs reproduced in this chapter.

REFERENCES

1. National Safety Council: Accident facts: preliminary condensed edition, March, 1983.
2. Harris JH, Harris HW: *The radiology of emergency medicine,* ed 2, Baltimore, 1981, Williams & Wilkins.
3. Watkins PR: *A practical guide to chest imaging,* Edinburgh, 1984, Churchill-Livingstone.
4. Landay MJ: *Interpretation of the chest roentgenogram,* Boston, 1987, Little, Brown.
5. Simon G: *Principles of chest x-ray diagnosis,* ed 4, London, 1978, Butterworths.
6. Schild HH et al: Pulmonary contusion: CT vs. plain radiograms, *J Comput Assist Tomogr* 13(3):417, 1989.
7. Wagner RB et al: Classification of parenchymal injuries of the lung, *Radiology* 167(1):77, 1988.
8. Toombs BD et al: Computed tomography of chest trauma, *Radiology* 140:733, 1981.
9. Moss AA, Goldberg HI, eds: *Computed tomography, ultrasound and x-ray: an integrated approach,* New York, 1980, Academic Press.
10. Mayfield W, Hurley EJ: Blunt cardiac trauma, *Am J Surg* 148:162, 1984.
11. Miller FA et al: Two-dimensional echocardiography findings in cardiac trauma, *Am J Cardiol* 50:1022, 1982.
12. Dronen SC: Disorders of the chest wall and diaphragm, *Emerg Clin North Am* 1(2):449, 1983.
13. Van Moore A et al: Radiologic evaluation of acute chest trauma, *CRC Crit Rev Diagn Imaging* 19(2):89, 1983.
14. Vukich DJ, Markovchick VJ: Pulmonary and chest wall injuries. In Rosen P, Baker FJ II, Barkin R et al: *Emergency medicine: concepts and clinical practice,* ed 2, vol 1, St Louis, 1988, CV Mosby.
15. Levy RC et al: *Radiology in emergency medicine,* St Louis, 1986, CV Mosby.
16. Kirsh MM, Sloan H, eds: *Blunt chest trauma,* Boston, 1977, Little, Brown.
17. Corso PJ: Chest trauma, *Primary Care* 5:543, 1978.
18. Harrison WH et al: Severe non-penetrating injuries to the chest: clinical results in the management of 216 patients, *Am J Surg* 100:715, 1960.
19. Yee ES et al: Isolated first rib fracture: clinical significance after blunt chest trauma, *Ann Thorac Surg* 32:278, 1981.
20. Phillips EH et al: First rib fractures: incidence of vascular injury and indications for angiography, *Surgery* 89(1):42, 1981.
21. Bassett JS et al: Blunt injuries to the chest, *J Trauma* 8:418, 1968.
22. Buckman R et al: The significance of stable patients with sternal fractures, *Surg Gynecol Obstet* 164:261, 1987.
23. Hurst JG, Markovchick VJ: Esophageal and diaphragmatic injuries. In Rosen P, Baker FJ II, Barkin R et al: *Emergency medicine: concepts and clinical practice,* ed 2, vol 1, St Louis, 1988, CV Mosby.
24. Wise L et al: Traumatic injury to the diaphragm, *J Trauma* 13:946, 1973.
25. Morgan AS et al: Blunt injury to the diaphragm: an analysis of 44 patients, *J Trauma* 26(6):565, 1986.
26. Rodriguez-Morales G et al: Acute rupture of the diaphragm: analysis of 60 patients, *J Trauma* 26(5):438, 1986.
27. Pecoraro JP et al: Radioisotope assisted diagnosis of traumatic rupture of the diaphragm, *Am Surg* 51(12):687, 1985.
28. Blair E et al: Delayed or missed diagnosis in blunt chest trauma, *J Trauma* 11:129, 1971.
29. Wilson RE et al: Nonpenetrating thoracic injuries, *Surg Clin North Am* 57:17, 1977.
30. Trinkle JK et al: Management of flail chest without mechanical ventilation, *Ann Thorac Surg* 19:355, 1975.
31. Bodai BI et al: The role of emergency thoracotomy in blunt trauma, *J Trauma* 22(6):487, 1982.
32. Shorr RM et al: Blunt thoracic trauma: analysis of 515 patients, *Ann Surg* 206(2):200, 1987.
33. Rodriguez A, Shatney C: The value of technetium pyrophosphate scanning in the diagnosis of myocardial contusions, *Am Surg* 48:472, 1982.
34. Fenner JE et al: The use of gated radionuclide angiography in the diagnosis of cardiac contusion, *Ann Emerg Med* 13(9):688, 1984.
35. Rothstein RJ: Myocardial contusion diagnosed by first-pass radionuclide angiography, *Am J Emerg Med* 4(3):210, 1986.
36. Pandian NG et al: Immediate diagnosis of acute myocardial contusion by two-dimensional echocardiography: studies in a canine model of blunt chest trauma, *Am Coll Cardiol* 2:488, 1983.
37. Richardson P, Mirvis SE, Scorpio R et al: Value of CT in determining need for angiography when findings of mediastinal hemorrhage on chest radiographs are equivocal, *AJR* 156:273, 1991.
38. Loop FD, Graves LK: Esophageal perforations: collective review, *Ann Thorac Surg* 10:571, 1970.
39. Triggiani E, Belsey R: Oesophageal trauma: incidence, diagnosis and management, *Thorax* 32:241, 1977.
40. Berry BE, Ochsner JL: Perforation of the esophagus: a 30 year review, *J Thorac Cardiovasc Surg* 65:1, 1973.
41. Schwartz JA et al: Boerhaave's syndrome: an elusive diagnosis, *Am J Emerg Med* 4(6):532, 1986.

Abdominal Trauma

Edward J. Newton
Yuri R. Parisky

Abdominal injury represents one of the most common and challenging problems in emergency care since potentially serious abdominal trauma is seen on an almost daily basis in most emergency departments. Of the thousands of yearly fatalities caused by trauma, approximately 10% are the direct result of abdominal injuries.[1] In addition, abdominal trauma contributes significantly to survivor morbidity. The role of the emergency physician, in concert with other members of the trauma team, is to accurately detect all significant traumatic injuries within a limited time frame, while minimizing the risk to the patient from invasive procedures, radiation exposure, and financial cost.

Abdominal trauma is classically divided into two categories: blunt and penetrating. Historically, considerable experience has been acquired in the penetrating category, largely as a result of the treatment of military casualties. Blunt trauma, however, has become epidemic in the 20th century, with the advent of high-speed transportation.[2]

Overall, blunt trauma accounts for approximately two thirds of the abdominal injury patients who come to the emergency departments[3] although, in certain urban locations, the incidence of penetrating trauma may predominate. Motor vehicle accidents account for up to 80% of blunt trauma injuries, with the remainder being caused by falls, assault, and industrial accidents.[4]

There are substantial differences between penetrating and blunt abdominal trauma in terms of the mechanism of injury, incidence of particular organ injury, and, consequently, diagnostic approach. Table 6-1 lists the incidence of organ injury in both categories.[5] The incidence of organ injury in penetrating trauma is approximately proportional to the cross-sectional area of the organ in question. However, in blunt trauma, injury to solid viscera is more common and results from direct compression, from sudden deceleration forces that tend to avulse vascular and mesenteric attachments, or from laceration by adjacent skeletal fractures. Hollow viscus injuries may also result from sudden compressive increases in intraluminal pressure, causing either bursting of the intestinal wall or vascular disruption.

As in all forms of emergency care, diagnosis of intra-abdominal injury must take place within the context of a systematic and orderly resuscitation of the patient. Up to two thirds of blunt abdominal trauma patients have significant injuries to other systems as well,[3] and these injuries may take precedence in terms of diagnosis and treatment.

Twelve percent to 16% of patients with abdominal trauma present to the emergency department in a state of profound shock.[4,6] Failure of these patients to respond to initial resuscitative measures mandates immediate surgical intervention to identify and correct the source of bleeding, whether in the chest, abdomen, or pelvis. It is a potentially lethal error to delay surgery in these patients in order to obtain radiographic clarification of their injuries. If the patient's condition permits, plain radiographs of the chest, cervical spine, and pelvis should be obtained while the patient is in the emergency department. However, unstable patients should not be sent to the radiology suite for definitive studies. Foley et al.,[7] in a review of preventable

Table 6-1. Incidence of organ injury in blunt and penetrating trauma

Blunt		Penetrating	
Spleen	25.0%	Liver	37.0%
Kidney	12.0%	Small bowel	26.0%
Intestine	15.0%	Stomach	19.0%
Liver	15.0%	Colon	16.5%
Retroperitoneum	13.0%	Vascular retroperitoneum	11.0%
Mesentery	5.0%	Mesentery	9.5%
Pancreas	3.0%	Spleen	7.0%
Diaphragm	2.0%	Diaphragm	5.5%
Urinary bladder	6.0%	Kidney	5.0%
Urethra	2.0%	Pancreas	3.5%
Vascular	2.0%	Duodenum	2.5%
		Biliary system	1.0%
		Other	1.0%

From Anderson CB, Ballinger WF: Abdominal injuries. In Zuidema GD, Rutherford RB, and Ballinger WF, eds: *The management of trauma*, ed 4, Philadelphia, 1985, WB Saunders.

deaths of trauma patients occurring in the emergency department noted that four of six patients died in the radiology suite secondary to intra-abdominal hemorrhage from splenic injury.

There remains, then, a large group of trauma patients who are either hemodynamically stable on initial presentation or who respond quickly to initial fluid resuscitation. These patients fall into one of three categories. First, there are patients who, although hemodynamically stable, demonstrate a clear need for laparotomy. Indications for laparotomy in this group include unequivocal signs of peritoneal irritation, evisceration of abdominal contents, impalement injuries, gross blood detected on rectal or vaginal examination, blood in the nasogastric tube, and all but the most clearly tangential gunshot wounds.[8]

A second group of patients includes those who are alert, free from the influence of drugs or alcohol, and who have no other distracting, painful injuries. A normal physical examination in these patients is generally reliable[9] although they should be observed over a period of hours and cautioned to return for re-evaluation should abdominal pain occur. Patients with a history of a serious mechanism for potential injury—for example, a fall from a height of more than 20 feet—should be observed for up to 24 hours.

The final category of patients who need to be evaluated are those in whom physical examination is unreliable or who demonstrate equivocal findings. The reliability of physical examination is often compromised by head or spinal cord injury, intoxication due to drugs or alcohol, advanced pregnancy, or general anesthesia. In addition, very young patients and those with previous mental debilitation may not be able to reliably report pain. Finally, the physical examination may be confusing in patients with painful injuries adjacent to the abdomen, such as lower rib or pel-

vic fractures or abdominal wall contusions. Up to 80% or more of patients presenting to the emergency department with multiple trauma may fall within this group.[4] Clearly, it is this category of patients who present the greatest diagnostic difficulty.

DIAGNOSTIC MODALITIES

The emergency physician has an ever-increasing diagnostic armamentarium that will permit highly accurate detection of otherwise occult intra-abdominal injuries. This armamentarium includes history and physical examination, plain radiographs with and without contrast, ultrasonography, radionuclide scanning, angiography, diagnostic peritoneal lavage, and enhanced/nonenhanced computed tomography. The specific imaging technique chosen depends not only on the condition of the patient but also on the availability of the test, the experience of the radiologist, the preference of the consulting surgeon, and the usual practice in a particular institution. The use of each diagnostic modality should be viewed as complementary rather than mutually exclusive, and the role of the trauma physician is to employ the optimal technique at the proper time in a given clinical circumstance.

Physical examination

Physical examination, although limited in accuracy in certain cases, remains the mainstay of diagnosis. In addition to the obvious indications for laparotomy listed previously, certain findings will indicate the need for further diagnostic tests in stable patients. For example, the combination of left upper quadrant tenderness and pain radiating to the left shoulder in association with left lower rib fracture is strong presumptive evidence of splenic injury and mandates further investigation. The value of repeated abdominal examination cannot be stressed enough. Certain injuries that may initially cause few symptoms, such as bowel perforations and pancreatic contusions, become progressively symptomatic within a brief period and may be detected by serial abdominal examinations.

Despite this caution, the accuracy of physical examination is clearly limited, particularly in patients with abnormal mental status. Various series have demonstrated a diagnostic error in physical examination of blunt abdominal trauma ranging from 16% to 45%[10,11] with an overall accuracy of 66% in one large study.[12] Certain physical findings are more reliable than others. Diffuse abdominal rigidity, rebound tenderness, progressive abdominal distention, and shock unexplained by thoracic or pelvic injury are highly suggestive of intra-abdominal injury. On the other hand, presence or absence of bowel sounds is an unreliable indicator in the immediate post-injury assessment. Whereas positive findings on abdominal examination will prompt further diagnostic evaluation, the main danger in reliance on physical examination alone is its lack of sensitivity to certain abdominal injuries. Retroperitoneal injuries are notoriously silent on initial examination since the peritoneum is not irritated, and these injuries have significantly higher morbidity and mortality if treatment is delayed.[13]

Laboratory tests

Reliance on laboratory tests is similarily fraught with error. Serial determination of the patient's hematocrit is useful in detecting significant hemorrhage and should be performed in all patients sustaining significant trauma. However, a common occurrence is that a lesser amount of blood loss will produce only a slight decrease in hematocrit, which may be ascribed to the dilutional effect of intravenous fluid administration. In addition, injury to the pancreas, hollow viscera, and diaphragm will often result in minimal blood loss. Certain injuries causing "third space" loss of extracellular fluid, such as traumatic pancreatitis, may in fact produce hemoconcentration and may confuse the clinical picture provided by reliance on a falling hemoglobin concentration to detect hemorrhage. Rather than being falsely reassured by a single normal value, the trend of changes in hemoglobin concentration is much more important in detecting hemorrhage.

Other blood assays have been used to identify injury to particular organs but without much success. Determination of serum amylase is often made in cases of abdominal trauma. However, this test has been shown to be both insensitive[14] and nonspecific[15] in the detection of pancreatic injury. Urinalysis, on the other hand, is a useful initial screening test and should be performed in all cases of abdominal trauma (see Chapter 7).

Diagnostic laparotomy

Based on military experience of improved outcome with a more aggressive approach to treating penetrating abdominal trauma, it became standard practice to perform a diagnostic laparotomy in virtually all patients with symptomatic abdominal injuries.[9,16] Quite apart from the enormous cost of this policy, concerns were raised regarding the morbidity and mortality of negative laparotomies for abdominal trauma. Several studies have noted mortality of up to 1.6% and morbidity ranging from 5% to 29% for laparotomies based on clinical findings alone, which can result in a negative laparotomy rate greater than 30%.[9,16,17]

Diagnostic peritoneal lavage

In an effort to improve on the diagnostic accuracy of physical examination and laboratory testing, a multitude of investigational tests, both radiographic and surgical, have been introduced. Abdominal paracentesis and the "four-quadrant tap" have been used with some success in the diagnosis of abdominal injury, achieving up to 86% accuracy.[18,19] More recently, however, these techniques have been supplanted by diagnostic peritoneal lavage.[20]

Diagnostic peritoneal lavage (DPL) is based on the detection of free intraperitoneal blood, bile, urine, food, or fecal material in the effluent lavage fluid. Elevation of

---

> ### Criteria for positivity of peritoneal lavage[4]
>
> - Aspiration of more than 10 ml gross blood on initial tap.
> - RBC count in lavage fluid:
>   Blunt trauma: >100,000 RBC/ml lavage fluid.
>   Penetrating trauma: >10,000 RBC/ml lavage fluid.
> - WBC count in lavage fluid greater than 500/ml.
> - Amylase concentration in lavage fluid >175 μg/100 ml.
> - Return of food particles, bile, urine, or stool.
> - Efflux of lavage fluid through Foley catheter or chest tube.

WBCs and amylase also constitute a positive lavage although, in the acute setting, detection of RBCs is of prime importance. The box above summarizes the criteria for positivity of peritoneal lavage.[4]

The sensitivity of DPL in detecting intraperitoneal blood exceeds 95% with a specificity greater than 90% and an overall accuracy consistently approaching 98% in multiple series.[21,22] This approach has greatly enhanced the ability of the trauma physician to identify virtually all patients with significant intra-abdominal injuries since as little as 5 ml of free intraperitoneal blood can be detected by this method.[23]

There are, however, several injuries that are poorly detected by DPL and others that give false positive results. In addition, DPL does not provide organ-specific information, and relatively insignificant injuries, such as minor liver lacerations that have ceased bleeding, will give positive DPL results often prompting an unnecessary laparotomy.

DPL is a relatively insensitive technique for detecting injury to retroperitoneal structures such as the pancreas and some duodenal injuries, traumatic diaphragmatic herniations, and fully contained subcapsular hematomas of the liver or spleen.[12,24] There is also a relatively high incidence of false positivity in association with pelvic fractures.[25]

Despite these shortcomings, DPL has contributed enormously to accurate and early detection of otherwise occult intra-abdominal injury. Where question as to the source of blood loss is pertinent in a marginally stable patient, DPL may be extremely useful in distinguishing intraperitoneal from other sources of blood loss. Patients with less than optimal response to fluid resuscitation should not be transported from the emergency department for specialized radiographic testing as their condition may deteriorate precipitously. In these cases, peritoneal lavage is the preferred diagnostic technique.

Because of its high sensitivity to intraperitoneal blood, exclusive reliance on DPL has resulted in a continued high incidence of negative laparotomy, particularly of concern in this era of nonoperative treatment of certain stable splenic and hepatic injuries.[9,16,26-31] In many centers, nonoperative treatment of pediatric splenic trauma has become the rule rather than the exception, and Powell et al.[12] suggest that a positive DPL in hemodynamically stable pediatric patients is an indication for further investigation rather than automatic laparotomy. Other authors[32] advise caution with this approach in adults, however, since the risk of post-splenectomy sepsis appears to be much less in this group and because there is greater risk of concomitant bowel injury. The nonoperative approach in adults has proven relatively less successful, thus far, in comparison to the pediatric splenic trauma population.[32,33]

Diagnostic imaging

Plain radiography. Radiographs in the emergency department or trauma unit should be performed in an expeditious manner following resuscitation and stabilization of the injured patient. Optimally, the resuscitation area should have fixed radiographic equipment that facilitates radiographic examination and allows simultaneous intense observation, monitoring, and treatment of the patient. Less optimally, the use of portable radiographic equipment may accomplish a similar task. However, portable equipment is bulky and limits access to the patient during the course of the radiographic examination. Transfer of the patient to the radiology department for initial radiographs is discouraged. The time wasted and the reduction of emergency personnel to accompany the patient may result in an unfavorable outcome. Appropriate shielding should be employed by all personnel when exposed to radiation.

Initial radiographs. It cannot be stressed often enough that the radiographic approach to the multiple trauma patient must be dictated by the patient's clinical condition. All stable patients and those who respond to initial fluid therapy should undergo radiographic studies of the cervical spine, chest, and pelvis because of the relatively high incidence and potentially devastating results of injury to these areas.

In severely injured patients, considerable clinical judgment must be exercised regarding radiographic investigation. Patients presenting in profound shock with clear evidence of thoracic or intra-abdominal injury do not tolerate any immediate radiographic confirmation of their injuries before surgical intervention. Where time and the patient's condition permit, the most important radiograph to obtain is the chest radiograph. As clinical circumstances dictate, the patient should be placed in as upright a position as possible and the direction of the radiographic beam should be as perpendicular as possible to the long axis of the patient. In hypotensive patients and in those in whom radiographic or clinical clearance of the spine have not yet been obtained, it is inadvisable to sit the patient upright for the chest radiograph. Consequently, supine chest radiographs are more commonly obtained on initial survey. The AP chest radiograph offers evaluation of the mediastinum and pulmonary parenchyma. Integrity of the bony skeleton and hemidiaphragms should be ascertained as radiographic abnormalities of these structures are frequently accompanied by intra-abdominal injury. The principal use of the chest radiograph in the severely injured trauma patient is to identify major thoracic injury. However, it also serves to distinguish between intrathoracic and intra-abdominal sources of bleeding in situations in which the source of bleeding is unclear. A normal chest radiograph in a patient in shock usually points to an infradiaphragmatic source, whether intraperitoneal or retroperitoneal.

The upright chest radiograph is a relatively sensitive means of detecting pneumoperitoneum. However, the upright chest radiograph must be obtained before peritoneal lavage to be useful since the lavage will automatically introduce air into the peritoneal cavity. Gross pneumoperitoneum can be identified as lucent, semilunar air collections beneath the hemidiaphragms, more likely to be located on the left than the right. Small collections of air from minor bowel perforations may not be initially apparent on the upright or semi-upright AP chest radiograph as it may take up to 10 minutes for free air to rise to the highest point in the peritoneal cavity.[34] Nevertheless, it is possible, with optimal radiographic technique, to demonstrate as little as 1 cc of free air on the upright chest radiograph.[35]

The next most crucial radiographic examination is the cervical spine lateral view that must include all cervical vertebrae and the C7/T1 interspace to be complete. A swimmer's view of the cervical spine may be necessary to confirm alignment of the vertebrae although much anatomic detail is lost in this view compared to the cross-table lateral view. Attempts to visualize the entire cervical spine should not interfere with aggressive resuscitation and assessment of potentially life-threatening injuries. If necessary, the patient's spine may remain immobilized prophylactically while other essential treatment, including laparotomy, is carried out.

In the appropriate clinical setting, a supine AP pelvic radiograph should be obtained. Evaluation of the pelvic bony skeleton may indicate the potential for severe vascular injury and hemorrhage. Pelvic fractures are identified in 5% of multiple trauma victims in some series.[36] Evaluation of the soft tissues of the pelvis may demonstrate free intraperitoneal fluid or blood. In hemodynamically stable patients, more definitive radiographic examinations may be performed as necessary.

Some controversy exists as to whether supine radiographs of the abdomen (Fig. 6-1) should be obtained as part of the initial series.[18] In general, plain abdominal radiographs should not be obtained in a patient with blunt trauma since the patient will likely undergo more sophisticated examinations such as peritoneal lavage or CT scan to adequately assess abdominal injury. In the setting of penetrating trauma, plain radiographs in two dimensions may be necessary for localization and documentation of bullets

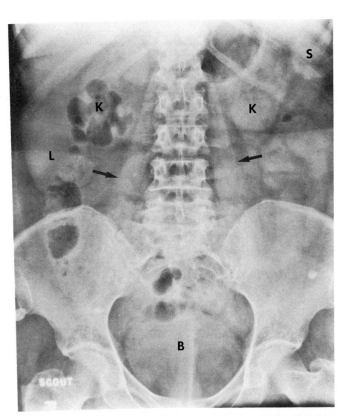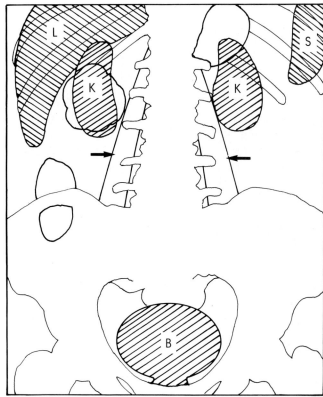

Fig. 6-1. Normal radiograph of the abdomen (KUB). Note the sharp inferior border of the liver *(L)* and the psoas shadows *(arrows)*. The kidney *(K)*, bladder *(B)*, and spleen *(S)* outlines are readily apparent.

or other projectiles. Marking entrance and exit wounds with small radio-opaque skin clips is helpful in determining the trajectory of the projectile and in detecting cases where the projectile may have embolized to other parts of the body.

Every attempt should be made by the radiologist or the resuscitation team to remove unnecessary opaque devices either on the patient or between the patient and the film cassette. Small pieces of metal may simulate bullets or other fragmented projectiles. Debris may obscure or simulate fractures. Unnecessary clothing, sheets, or blankets can cause creases that may mimic free air within the thorax or abdomen.

The trauma physician and radiologist should familiarize themselves with the radiographic appearance of equipment commonly used in resuscitation such as cervical collars, nasogastric tubes, monitor wires and electrodes, and intravenous catheters. Careful attention should be paid to the appearance and course of catheters inserted during resuscitation.

There is benefit to the placement of a nasogastric tube. Displacement of the tube by a mediastinal hematoma resulting from intrathoracic rupture of the aorta is well documented.[37] Likewise, the abnormal position of the nasogastric tube within the stomach may suggest an adjacent hematoma, diaphragmatic rupture and herniation of the stomach, or gastric rupture. A nasogastric tube decreases

the likelihood of aspiration, decompresses gastric dilatation, and allows for the administration of dilute contrast material before the CT scan.

With the advent of more advanced diagnostic imaging techniques such as high-resolution CT scan, the roles of upper and lower GI contrast studies are somewhat limited. Upper GI examination still plays an important role in the diagnosis of suspected duodenal hematoma and of diaphragmatic hernia. The barium enema may have some utility in the diagnosis of diaphragmatic hernia by demonstrating herniation of the contrast-filled colon through a rent in the diaphragm during fluorscopy.

SPECIFIC RADIOGRAPHIC FINDINGS

Pneumoperitoneum. Pneumoperitoneum is commonly seen in the context of penetrating abdominal or pelvic trauma. Gross pneumoperitoneum appears as lucent collections of gas conforming to the inferior surfaces of the diaphragm (Fig. 6-2). Gastric dilatation, which is often seen in the setting of abdominal trauma or cardiopulmonary resuscitation, may obscure gas beneath the left hemidiaphragm. Air seen within a dilated stomach will demonstrate the thickness of the stomach wall and hemidiaphragm underlying the lung base. The diaphragms are structures that should not exceed 2 mm in thickness. This finding is often obscured by the presence of associated

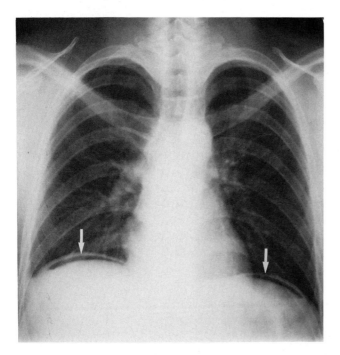

Fig. 6-2. Pneumoperitoneum on an upright chest radiograph. Semilunar collections of air *(arrows)* outline the inferior surfaces of the diaphragm in a 27-year-old male with a stab wound to the colon.

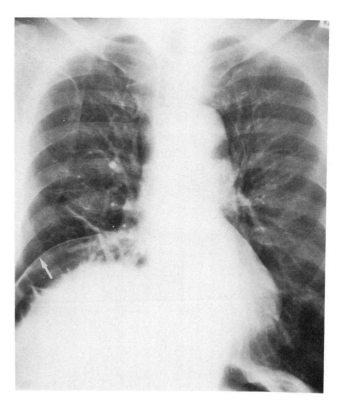

Fig. 6-3. Normal variant mimicking free intraperitoneal air. Occasionally, the colon becomes interposed between the liver and the right diaphragm *(arrow)*.

pleural reaction or pleural effusion, especially in the setting of a partially upright chest radiograph. Consequently, gastric decompression by means of nasogastric tube suction may be helpful. Occasionally, dilated loops of colon or small bowel may radiographically mimic free air (Fig. 6-3) or even obscure it entirely. A lateral decubitus radiograph of the abdomen, preferably with the left side down, will demonstrate air against the right edge of the liver or right abdominal wall.

There are several subtle signs of pneumoperitoneum on the supine abdominal view. Visualization of the falciform ligament is demonstrated when free air is present on both sides of this ligament in the right upper quadrant (Fig. 6-4). It is demonstrated as a curvilinear density projected adjacent to the right paravertebral space underlying the liver. Similarly, when free intraperitoneal air outlines the serosal surface of bowel, in the presence of intraluminal gas, the characteristic full thickness of the bowel wall is demonstrated by Rigler's sign (Fig. 6-5). A lucent oval appearance to the central abdomen is termed the "football" sign. Free air rises in the central abdomen and is responsible for this sign that mimics the shape of a football.[38]

A CT scan is not very accurate in detecting bowel perforation since significant numbers of false negative examinations occur. It is capable of detecting minute amounts of free intraperitoneal and retroperitoneal gas. While pneumoperitoneum suggests the presence of bowel perforation, caution must be taken to exclude other causes before sur-

gery is performed for presumptive ruptured bowel. A retrospective review of 547 pediatric abdominal CT scans performed for blunt trauma revealed an alarming incidence of false positive pneumoperitoneum.[39] Of nine patients with pneumoperitoneum, only four (44%) had ruptured bowel at laparotomy. Other sources of pneumoperitoneum included pneumomediastinum, prior peritoneal lavage, and bladder perforation. Equally alarming was the fact that of six patients who were found to have a ruptured bowel at laparotomy, only four (67%) were identified pre-operatively by CT scan.

Hemoperitoneum. Hemoperitoneum is the most common finding in patients with abdominal injury. Blood may initially localize adjacent to the injured tissue, be contained by the capsule of an injured organ, or be distributed throughout the abdominal cavity.

Plain radiographs of the abdomen are relatively insensitive for the detection of hemoperitoneum. Intraperitoneal volumes of greater than 800 ml are usually necessary for the demonstration of classic plain radiographic signs.[40] Free intraperitoneal fluid gravitates to the most dependent portions of the abdomen. Thus, in the supine patient, the intraperitoneal portion of the pelvis collects free fluid. Because of this and the frequent occurrence of pelvic fracture in blunt abdominal trauma, the supine abdominal radiograph should include the pelvic contents.

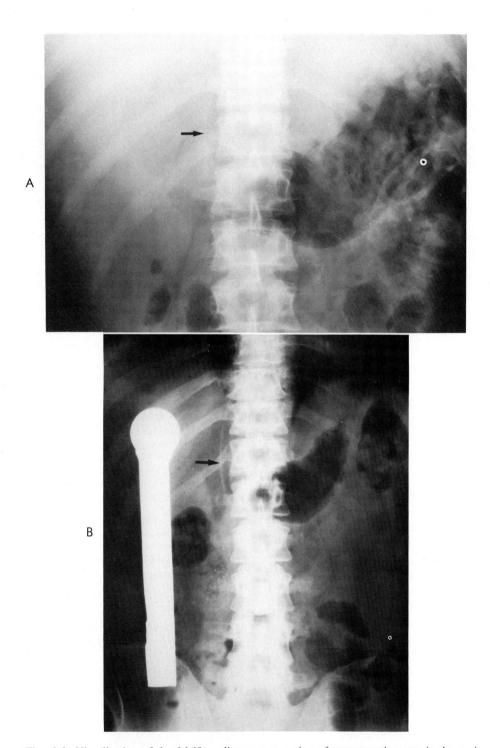

Fig. 6-4. Visualization of the falciform ligament as a sign of pneumoperitoneum in the supine radiograph of the abdomen. **A,** A thin curvilinear ligament projects adjacent to the paravertebral border *(arrow)*. Free air on both sides of the ligament allows its visualization. **B,** A 36-year-old male truck driver impaled on a metallic gear shift with subtle pneumoperitoneum *(arrow)* and a less subtle foreign body in the abdomen.

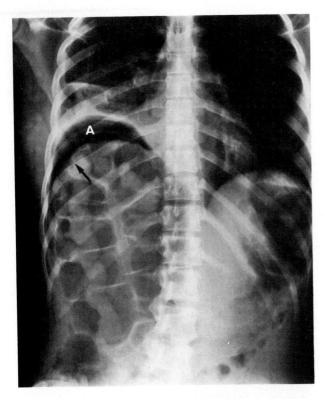

Fig. 6-5. Pneumoperitoneum. Massive free air *(A)* outlining the serosal surface *(arrow)* of the colonic hepatic flexure in the right upper quadrant. Bowel wall thickness can only be demonstrated by apposing collections of gas. In this case of colonic perforation by a stab wound, intraluminal and free intraperitoneal gas outline the bowel wall.

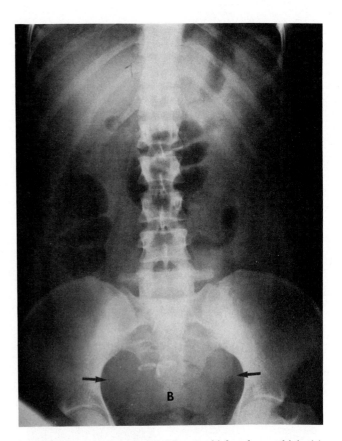

Fig. 6-6. Hemoperitoneum. A 37-year-old female was kicked in the abdomen by a horse and sustained a splenic laceration. At surgery, 1 L of blood was found in the pelvis, in addition to a large splenic hematoma. The soft tissue densities projecting superior to the bladder *(B)* and lateral to the uterus *(note the intrauterine device)* are commonly referred to as "bladder ears" or "dog ears" *(arrows)*, which represent collections of blood in the intraperitoneal lateral vesicle recesses.

Accumulation of intraperitoneal blood within the dependent portion of the pelvis, the pouch of Douglas, presents as the classic radiographic finding known as "dog ears" or "bladder ears" (Fig. 6-6). This finding results from the accumulation of blood within the lateral recesses of the bladder, producing soft tissue densities that project superolaterally to the bladder. Accompanying this finding is a thin lucent line following the contour of the dome of the bladder. This lucent line is produced when extraperitoneal fat is interposed between the blood-distended pelvic peritoneum and the urinary bladder. Fig. 6-7 demonstrates the appearance of hemoperitoneum on a CT scan in the same patient as does the radiograph in Fig. 6-6.

Hemoperitoneum resulting from either splenic or hepatic injury may obscure the relatively sharply outlined margins of the injured organ. Normal spleen surrounded by fat or bowel commonly gives a distinct inferior outline. Subcapsular hematoma will expand the outline, while adjacent hematoma will obliterate the distinct margin. The same observation applies to the readily visible inferior aspect of the right hepatic lobe (see Fig. 6-1).

Within the true abdomen, the most dependent intraperitoneal areas are within the paracolic gutters. Blood tracking from injured liver or spleen will gather in the respec-

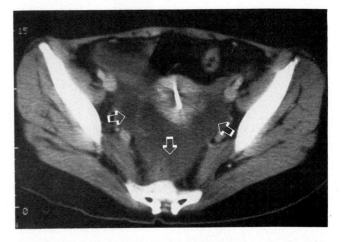

Fig. 6-7. Hemoperitoneum. CT scan demonstrates blood *(open arrows)* outlining the uterus posteriorly and laterally. (Note the intrauterine device.) Intraperitoneal blood in the lateral vesicle recesses corresponds to the finding of "dog ears" on plain radiographs (see Fig. 6-6).

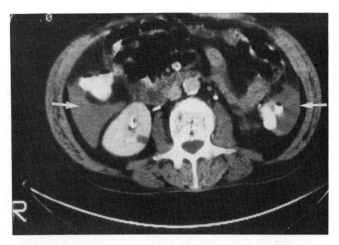

Fig. 6-10. Hemoperitoneum. CT scan demonstrates blood of a splenic injury in a 62-year-old male tracking along both paracolic gutters *(arrows)*. Note that the contrast-opacified right and left colon are somewhat displaced medially. Blood increases the distance between the colon and the abdominal wall and obscures the normally present fat, producing the "flank stripe" finding on plain radiographs (see Fig. 6-8).

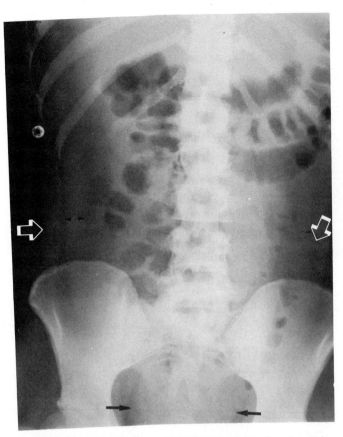

Fig. 6-8. Hemoperitoneum. Plain radiograph of a liver laceration in a 19-year-old male victim of a motor vehicle accident. The patient presented in shock and at exploratory laparotomy was found to have 1 L of blood in the peritoneal cavity. Note the bilateral "flank stripe" *(open arrows)* in which blood obscures the normal fat margin between the lateral colonic wall and the abdominal wall. Blood is also seen distending the lateral vesicle recesses *(solid arrows)*.

tive gutter, appearing as a soft tissue mass. This collection of blood will displace the right or left colon medially, widening the space between the lateral wall of the colon and the radiolucent vertical flank stripe. The gasless fluid-filled colon will blend imperceptibly into the soft tissues. Hematoma or inflammation within the lateral abdominal wall will obscure the radiolucent fat of the flank stripe. On occasion, a fluid-filled small bowel may interpose between the lateral colonic wall and the abdominal wall, mimicking fluid within the gutter (Figs. 6-8 to 6-10).

Diagnostic peritoneal lavage is an extremely sensitive tool in detecting hemoperitoneum and has become the "gold standard" in this respect over the past 20 years. Defining the source of bleeding and the degree of organ injury lies beyond the scope of peritoneal lavage but falls favorably within the capability of modern cross-sectional imaging.

Ultrasonography

Ultrasonography is rarely used, except as a complementary imaging modality, in the initial evaluation of abdominal trauma in adults although there are many reports of its successful use in pediatric trauma. It is often used as a primary screening device in Europe and Japan, but its use in the United States has been largely superceded by the use of DPL and the abdominal CT scan. Despite its accurate anatomic delineation and relatively high sensitivity for both hemoperitoneum and solid organ injury, the limitations of ultrasonography outweigh its immediate benefits.

Successful and accurate ultrasonographic examination depends on the skills of the radiologist and ultrasonographer and the sophistication of the equipment. A cooperative patient, capable of suspending respirations and able to

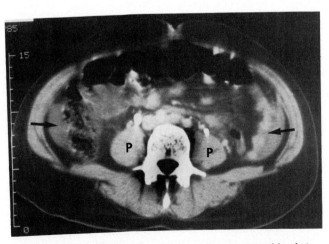

Fig. 6-9. Hemoperitoneum. CT scan demonstrates blood *(arrows)* tracking along the paracolic gutter the entire length of the ascending and descending colon. Note that the blood has a greater density than fat and is of similar density as muscle (*P*, psoas muscle).

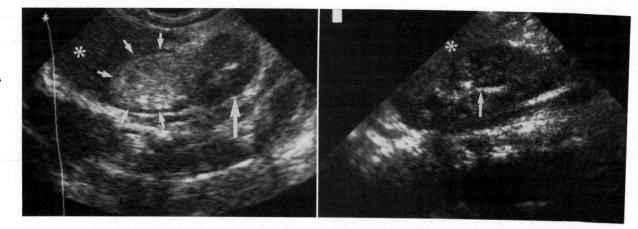

Fig. 6-11. Resolution of an adrenal hematoma confirmed by ultrasonography. **A,** Ultrasonogram demonstrates right kidney *(large arrow)* and overlying adrenal hematoma *(small arrows)* and adjacent liver *(asterisk).* **B,** Ultrasonogram performed 3 months later clearly demonstrates resolution of the hematoma. The right kidney *(arrow)* and liver *(asterisk)* are well visualized. (Courtesy Marian P Demus, MD.)

alter position, is required. Performance of a thorough ultrasonographic examination may require up to 30 minutes.

Unsuitable patients include those who are critically ill, uncooperative, or who have superficial abdominal injuries. Stable patients can be evaluated on an initial screening basis for hemoperitoneum and solid organ injury. Ultrasonography may serve an adjunctive role in patients with equivocal findings. Currently, the usefulness of ultrasonography in trauma is in the determination of the resolution or progression of lesions in patients with established diagnoses (Fig. 6-11).[41]

There exists a small group of patients in whom peritoneal lavage is relatively contraindicated and in whom ultrasonography may be considered an alternative—those who have conditions such as coagulopathy, obesity, or previous abdominal surgery.[31]

Hemoperitoneum can be accurately diagnosed by ultrasonography in technically successful examinations. The localization of relatively echo-free fluid depends on the volume of blood present and on visualization of the dependent portions of the abdomen or pelvis. Free peritoneal fluid conforms to the anatomic space that it occupies. Consequently, this fluid can be visualized as a lenticular collection in the subphrenic space, triangular in Morrison's pouch, and ovoid in the pelvis.[41] Residual peritoneal lavage fluid is indistinguishable from hemoperitoneum, and the diagnosis of hemoperitoneum by ultrasonography under these circumstances should be made with caution.

Solid organ injury can be recognized by subcapsular or intraparenchymal hematomas. The ultrasonographic appearance of a hematoma varies depending on multiple factors, most notably the age of the hematoma. The initial hematoma is echogenic but gradually progresses to sonolucency over 96 hours. This is related to formation and subsequent resolution of clot, initial hematocrit, and presence of fibrinogen.[42-44]

A recent prospective study by Gruessner et al.[45] comparing ultrasonography to peritoneal lavage failed to establish ultrasonography as an acceptable alternative for the initial evaluation of abdominal trauma.

Radionuclide scanning

Before the general acceptance of the CT scan as the standard for imaging the abdomen of the injured patient, radionuclide scanning shared this role with angiography. The two most commonly injured organs in the abdomen, the liver and the spleen, are well suited for study by radionuclide scanning. The liver/spleen scan uses technetium (Tc 99m) sulfur colloid, a readily available radiopharmaceutical. Uptake of this labelled colloid by reticuloendothelial cells in the liver and spleen results in an image permitting excellent evaluation of the blood supply, displacement of normal parenchyma by hematoma, or disruption of the organ contour by laceration or rupture (see Fig. 6-19). Initially, however, use of the planar gamma camera required multiple projections to accurately map the topography of the organ, and planar images were less sensitive in detecting small intraparenchymal hematomas. Recently, single photon emission computed tomography (SPECT) imaging offers cross-sectional imaging similar to computed tomography.

Following intravenous injection of Tc 99m sulfur colloid, images are obtained within several minutes. Accuracy in the detection of splenic injury has ranged from 90% to 98.5% in a review of multiple series.[46,47] False positive findings most often are the result of anatomic variants that are misread as lacerations. True positive findings, filling defects, disruption of the normal contour, or loss of activity in devitalized tissue correspond well with surgical findings.[48,49]

. Even though cross-sectional imaging with SPECT enhances the sensitivity of radionuclide scanning, there are several drawbacks to the use of radionuclide scanning.[50] The patient must be sufficiently stable to be transported to the nuclear medicine department. Overlying resuscitation equipment such as chest tubes and backboards may interfere with image acquisition. Finally, the primary reasons for decreased use of radionuclide scanning in the initial assessment of trauma are its limitation to the evaluation of liver and spleen and its failure to provide information regarding adjacent or remote injury to other structures.

Therefore limited application of radionuclide scanning in evaluating trauma patients presently includes follow-up of liver or spleen injuries to determine the resolution of hematoma or to document organ function.[49,51,52] In the setting of hepatic injury involving the biliary tree, the use of a biliary scanning agent such as Tc 99m–HIDA can demonstrate a biloma or bilious fluid leakage and fistula.[49] In certain circumstances, radionuclide angiography can demonstrate small vascular injuries that may exceed the sensitivity of conventional angiography. This technique uses either Tc 99m sulfur colloid for single pass determination or the more sensitive Tc 99m–labelled RBC study that may demonstrate bleeding as minimal as 1 ml/minute.[53]

Computed tomography

Just as peritoneal lavage has dramatically enhanced clinical diagnostic accuracy, the introduction of the CT scan has revolutionized abdominal imaging. Although the exact role of the CT scan in evaluation of abdominal trauma has yet to be determined, increasing availability and experience with the technique has provided a non-invasive alternative to peritoneal lavage in detecting otherwise occult injuries to both intra-abdominal and retroperitoneal structures and in grading the severity of specific parenchymal injuries. Although no single technique is ideal in every situation, a large number of trauma patients who attain relative hemodynamic stability and present diagnostic dilemmas because of equivocal physical findings or alterations in consciousness are suitable candidates for a CT scan. In addition, patients in whom peritoneal lavage is relatively contraindicated, such as those with multiple previous surgeries, massive obesity, or bleeding diathesis, are better evaluated by a CT scan.

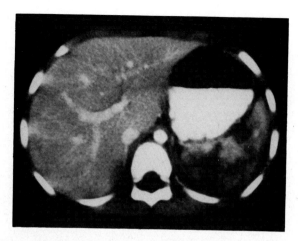

Fig. 6-12. CT scan of 5-year-old girl involved in a motor vehicle accident. New technology allows scanning of the entire abdomen and pelvis in 32 seconds, which virtually eliminates motion artifact and expedites patient triage. This contrast-enhanced scan demonstrates a splenic laceration. (Courtesy Picker International.)

No other technique offers a simultaneous anatomic view of the entire abdomen and retroperitoneum with such resolution. There is an obvious advantage to the use of a CT scan over other modalities in that patients with relatively stable injuries can be easily identified and undergo a period of nonoperative observation rather than an unnecessary laparotomy. In addition, unsuspected pathology, such as spinal and pelvic fractures,[54] unsuspected malignancy, or congenital anomalies, may be demonstrated by a CT scan.

The CT scan technology has rapidly evolved through "generations" of scanners to the point now where technical quality, resolution, rapidity of examination, and availability of scanners have made a significant impact in the management of trauma. The newest generation of scanners are capable of generating a complete abdominal examination in less than a minute, virtually eliminating motion artifact, particularly in pediatric and minimally cooperative patients (Fig. 6-12). As radiologists gain further experience with the use of the CT scan in abdominal trauma, accuracy will continue to improve.

Although a head CT scan can readily detect fresh intracranial hemorrhage without the use of contrast material, an abdominal CT scan requires administration of both intravenous and oral contrast material in order to maximize resolution and to accurately assess parenchymal structures. The box on p. 113 describes the technique of abdominal CT scan for blunt injuries. Figs. 6-13 to 6-15 demonstrate normal anatomy on abdominal CT scans with and without contrast material.

There have been a multitude of studies comparing the accuracy of the CT scan with peritoneal lavage,[55-61] radionuclide scanning,[62] ultrasonography,[151] and magnetic resonance imaging [63] in selected patients with abdominal

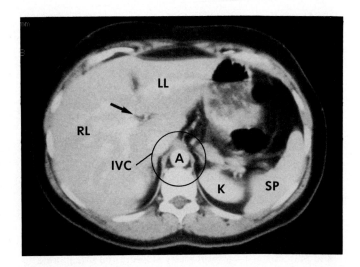

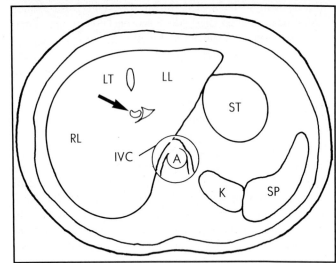

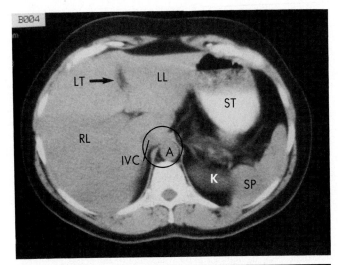

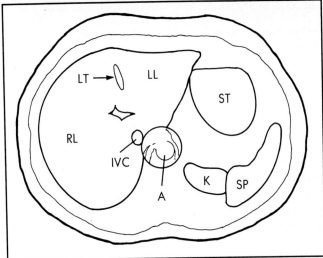

Fig. 6-13. Nonenhanced CT scan of the upper abdomen demonstrating normal anatomy. Oral contrast material opacifies the stomach *(ST)*. The liver occupies the upper right abdomen *(RL, right lobe, LL, left lobe)* and extends across the midline. The sagittally oriented low-density area is fat within the intersegmental fissure, which contains the ligamentum teres *(LT)*. The spleen *(SP)* occupies the posterior lateral portion of the left upper abdomen. The tissue density of the spleen is normally slightly less than the liver density in the nonenhanced CT scan. The relatively low-density structure medial to the spleen is the "volume-averaged" superior pole of the left kidney *(K)*. In the liver, note that the unopacified blood-filled inferior vena cava *(IVC)* and the adjacent aorta *(A)* have a somewhat lower density than the liver *(circle)*.

Fig. 6-14. Enhanced CT scan of the upper abdomen demonstrating normal anatomy. Following rapid bolus administration of intravenous contrast material, there is opacification of the parenchymal organs of the upper abdomen *(RL, right lobe of the liver; LL, left lobe of liver; ST, stomach; SP, spleen; K, kidney)*. The density of the opacified blood in the aorta *(A)* and inferior vena cava *(IVC)* equals or exceeds the density of the normally opacified liver parenchyma. Liver and spleen parenchymal density are now similar. The coronally oriented low-density area posterior to the intersegmental fissure, which contains the ligamentum teres *(LT)*, is the fat-filled intrahepatic portal space *(arrow)*. The density within the portal space is a branch of the hepatic artery.

trauma. The results have varied greatly, resulting in considerable controversy concerning the use of the CT scan as the primary diagnostic imaging modality in the initial evaluation of trauma. The discrepancy in the reported results to some extent reflects differences in patient selection, available technology, and in level of expertise in the performance and interpretation of abdominal CT scans from center to center. Sensitivity of the CT scan has been reported from as low as 25%[59] to as high as 96.5%[60]; however, accuracy of the scan is consistently reported as greater than 90%.[55,57-60] In addition, many of the injuries missed by the CT scan are, in fact, of minor significance and would not alter the course of the patient's management had they been demonstrated. The fact that these minor injuries are detected by peritoneal lavage and often result in unnecessary laparotomy is precisely the reason why the CT scan may be the better technique. In other words, the lower sensitivity of the CT scan compared to peritoneal lavage may allow for

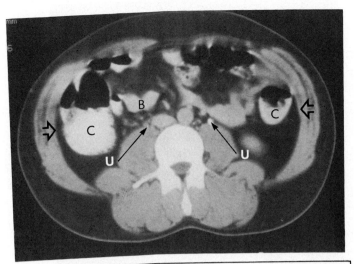

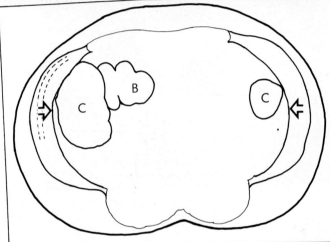

Fig. 6-15. Enhanced CT scan of the normal midabdomen demonstrating paracolic gutters. Oral contrast material opacifies the ascending and descending colon *(C)* and small bowel *(B)*. Ureters *(U)* opacified by excretion of intravenous contrast material overlie the psoas muscles. The paracolic gutters and adjacent fat outline the "flank stripe" bilaterally *(open arrows)*.

greater accuracy in detecting significant injuries and, thus, result in a lower unnecessary laparotomy rate. The CT scan has been reported to be highly accurate in the detection of solid viscus and retroperitoneal injuries. The principal source of false negative examinations has been in the detection of hollow viscus and pancreatic injuries. Coincidentally, these two injuries are also poorly detected by peritoneal lavage although the sensitivity of peritoneal lavage in detecting bowel injury is greater than the CT scan.[60]

Another controversy lies in the ability of the CT scan to predict which patients might be suitable for nonoperative management. Some findings to date have been contradictory (see later discussions of splenic and hepatic injury).

There has been debate regarding the timing of peritoneal lavage and the CT scan when both tests are used (Fig. 6-16). Centers using the CT scan as the initial diagnostic

---

CT scan technique in blunt abdominal trauma

1. Patients should be continually observed. Monitoring devices should be positioned to avoid causing artifact. A physician or nurse should always accompany the patient.
2. Dilute (0.5% to 1.0%) water-soluble gastrograffin (400 to 500 ml) is administered orally or through a nasogastric tube 45 minutes before scanning. While the patient is being placed in the scanner, an additional 200 ml of oral contrast material should be administered. The nasogastric tube should be partially withdrawn into the distal esophagus to minimize artifact.
3. Intravenous contrast material is administered via rapid drip or bolus technique. In adults, 40 g of iodine delivered in 150 to 300 ml of saline will provide satisfactory opacification of visceral parenchyma.
4. Patients are scanned supine without angulation of the gantry.
5. Scanning should coincide with the initial arterial phase of opacification and should proceed rapidly in order to image the upper abdomen within the first 2 to 3 minutes.
6. The scan is performed at 1-cm intervals from the level of the hemidiaphragms through the kidneys. The remainder of the scan is performed at intervals of 1.5 or 2.0 cm to the level of the pubic symphysis.

mode tend to reserve peritoneal lavage to detect occult hollow viscus injuries that may be missed by the CT scan. In addition, angiography may be performed following a CT scan to assess the rate of bleeding in hepatic and splenic injuries that are being considered for nonoperative observation although the use of contrast material during the CT scan may interfere with subsequent angiography.

When peritoneal lavage is used as the initial assessment, its greater sensitivity detects virtually all intraperitoneal injuries. A positive lavage in a stable patient is an indication for a CT scan or angiography to more clearly delineate the anatomic detail of the injuries and to assist in the decision regarding operative treatment vs. nonoperative observation. However, prior installation and incomplete removal of peritoneal lavage fluid confuses the assessment of hemoperitoneum by the CT scan since residual lavage fluid may mimic hemoperitoneum. Because assessment of the extent of hemoperitoneum may have prognostic significance in scoring the severity of injury, some authors[64] argue that peritoneal lavage should follow the CT scan. However, performing lavage before the CT scan offers the advantage of using a highly sensitive nonanatomic diagnostic assessment before an organ-specific imaging modality. Patients with a negative lavage then need not undergo the relatively more expensive CT scan unless the lavage is equivocal or complicated (i.e., positive return of

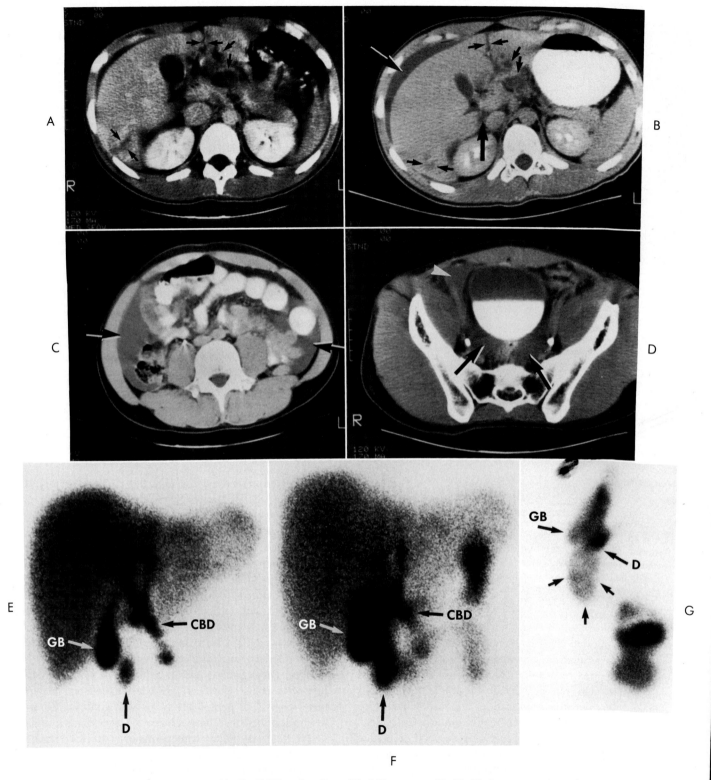

Fig. 6-16. CT scans **(A, B, C, D)** and radionuclide biliary scans **(E, F, G)** demonstrate hemoperitoneum secondary to a lacerated liver and common bile duct in a patient with true positive diagnostic peritoneal lavage (DPL). **A,** Initial CT scan demonstrates hepatic lacerations *(opposing paired small arrows)* and hepatic hematomas *(small arrows)*. CT scans **(B, C, D)** filmed at a different window settings and 4 days later clearly demonstrate an increasing hemoperitoneum *(large arrows),* stable hepatic lacerations *(opposing paired small arrows),* hepatic hematomas *(small arrows),* and an evolving biloma *(large arrowhead).* Biliary scans **(E, F, G)** obtained at 20 min, 60 min, and 16 hours, respectively, confirm extravasation of radionuclide *(small arrows)* from common bile duct *(CBD)* adjacent to gallbladder *(GB)* and duodenum *(D).* (Courtesy Paul J Petrozzo, MD, and Marylyn Rosencranz, DO.)

lavage fluid) since the incidence of serious injury is low with a negative lavage. It should be noted that there is a significant incidence of underlying serious injury in patients with indeterminate lavage results, and these patients are ideally suited for a CT scan.[4]

There are methods of determining the density of various fluids by the CT scan, thereby differentiating hemoperitoneum from residual lavage fluid.[64,65] Collections of fluid with low Hounsfield units (HU) (density measurement) are compatible with residual lavage fluid; those with high HU suggest hematoma. However, this distinction is imprecise because of the variability in the density of intraperitoneal blood as it lyses.

Magnetic resonance imaging

Currently, magnetic resonance imaging (MRI) because of its technical limitations does not play a role in the initial evaluation of the acutely injured patient. The principle of MRI is based on the induction and subsequent release of a high-strength, large-field magnetic polarization around the patient being examined. The image is produced by the recording of a radiofrequency generated by the release of hydrogen proton signals within the patient as a result of this alternating magnetic pulse (see Appendix). Presently, MRI is restricted to cooperative patients who do not require continuous monitoring and who can remain immobile during the course of the lengthy examination.

There is a role for MRI following the stabilization of the trauma patient. The multiplanar imaging capability offered by MRI is clearly advantageous when specific anatomic information is sought. Because of this and the superior visualization of soft tissues compared to the CT scan, MRI is well suited to serial follow-up examination of central nervous system trauma. Certain anatomic areas such as the brachial plexus and the large peripheral joints are studied with excellent anatomic definition using MRI. In addition, with the advent of MRI spectroscopy, physiologic function will be ascertained and tissue viability, hematoma resolution, edema, and blood flow parameters will become commonplace evaluations.

The case demonstrated in Fig. 6-17 illustrates the exquisite capability of MRI multiplanar imaging. Subdiaphragmatic, subcapsular, and intraparenchymal hematomas are well delineated.

ABDOMINAL TRAUMA EVALUATION
Spleen

Splenic injury is common in both blunt and penetrating trauma. Although it may occur as an isolated injury, the majority of patients with splenic trauma have associated intra-abdominal injuries.[47,61,66,67] The location of the spleen appears relatively well protected in adults, but its high-density, limited stromal infrastructure, and thin capsule make it susceptible to fracture. The proximity of the spleen to the left lower ribs also makes it vulnerable to puncture or laceration by fractures. Splenic injuries can be

---

CT scan classification of splenic injuries[67]

Grade I: Capsular avulsion; superficial laceration(s); or subcapsular hematoma <1 cm.
Grade II: Parenchymal laceration(s) 1 to 3 cm deep; central/subcapsular hematoma(s) <3 cm.
Grade III: Laceration(s) >3 cm deep; central/subcapsular hematoma(s) >3 cm.
Grade IV: Fragmentation of three or more sections or devascularized nonenhanced spleen.

---

classified according to severity, ranging from simple contusion to intraparenchymal and subcapsular hematomas, lacerations, fractures, and complete pulverization or avulsion of the spleen from the vascular pedicle (see the box above).

Clinical findings. The clinical presentation of splenic injury depends on the rate of blood loss and the nature of associated injuries. A significant number of patients present with signs of hemorrhagic shock, a progressively distending abdomen, or diffuse peritoneal irritation with falling hemoglobin levels. Specific signs of splenic injury may be elicited in a minority of cases. Pain radiating from the left subcostal area to the left shoulder, left upper quadrant tenderness, left lower rib or thoracic transverse process fractures, and dullness to percussion over the stomach area have all been described as indicative of a splenic injury, but the absence of these signs does not preclude severe trauma.

Delayed rupture of subcapsular splenic hematomas is well documented anecdotally, but the exact incidence is not known.[28,46,68] It may be that the majority of "delayed ruptures" are in fact caused by continual blood loss from an initially undetected splenic injury.[69-71]

In addition to performing serial hematocrits to detect blood loss, the finding of unexplained leukocytosis to levels of 30,000/ml should suggest the possibility of splenic injury.[5] However, there are no specific laboratory tests that detect splenic injury.

Diagnostic peritoneal lavage. Diagnostic peritoneal lavage (DPL) is a technique for detecting splenic injury with a 98% sensitivity rate.[66] False negative results may rarely be obtained if the spleen has herniated through the diaphragm and thus bleeds into the chest rather than the abdomen, or if there is a completely contained subcapsular hematoma. The principal disadvantage to DPL in detecting splenic injuries is that it fails to differentiate relatively insignificant superficial lacerations from severe injuries requiring operative intervention. In addition, DPL does not differentiate between a lesion that has ceased bleeding and one in which active bleeding is occurring. Consequently, many laparotomies are performed for relatively stable splenic injuries. While it is certainly better to perform an unnecessary operation than to miss a potentially fatal

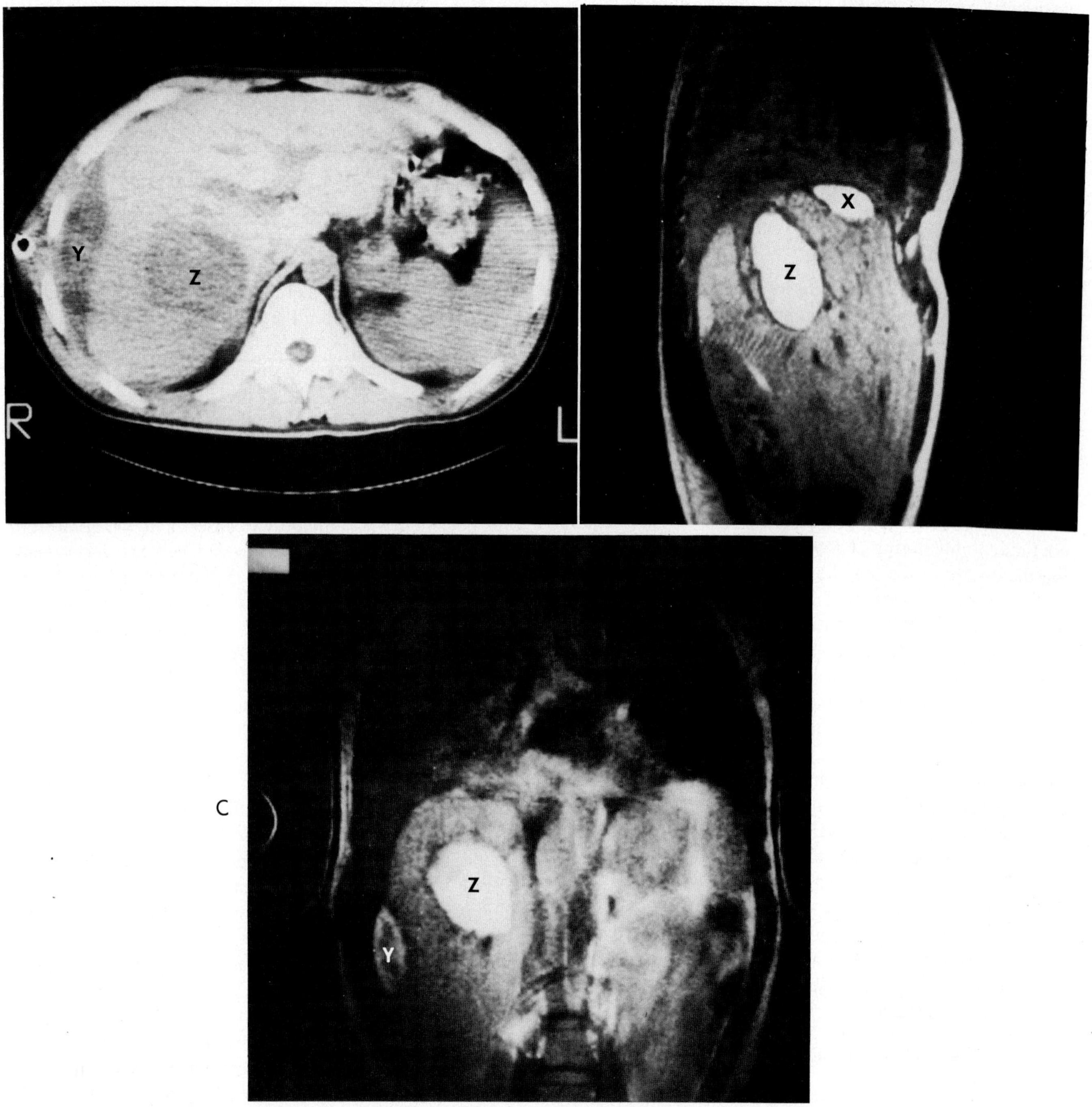

Fig. 6-17. Hepatic trauma. Correlation of the CT scan and MRI findings in a patient with blunt abdominal trauma. **A,** Standard CT scan with oral and intravenous contrast shows subcapsular *(Y)* and intraparenchymal *(Z)* hematomas. **B,** Sagittal MRI image demonstrates subdiaphragmatic *(X)* and intraparenchymal *(Z)* hematomas. **C,** Coronal MRI image demonstrates hepatic intraparenchymal hematoma *(Z)* and another view of subcapsular hematoma *(Y)*.

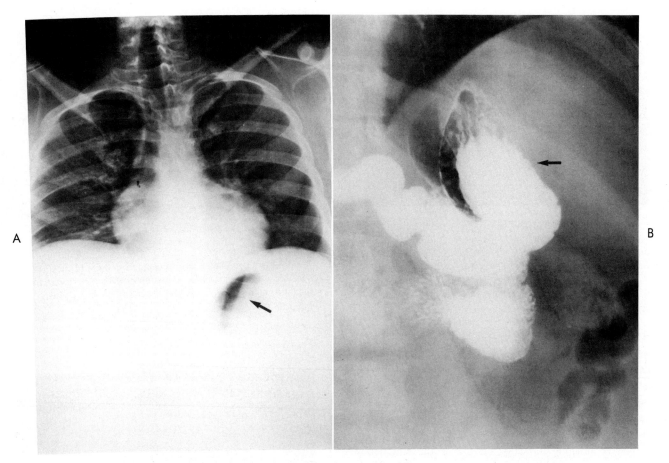

Fig. 6-18. Medial displacement of the stomach by a splenic hematoma. **A,** Semi-upright AP chest radiograph shows a mass in the left upper quadrant and a medially displaced stomach gas bubble (*arrow*) in a patient with a splenic laceration from blunt abdominal trauma. **B,** The contrast-filled stomach more clearly demonstrates displacement by the splenic hemorrhage (*arrow*).

splenic injury, the current emphasis on nonoperative treatment of splenic injuries, especially in the pediatric population, has dictated a need for more precise definition of the splenic injury before surgery is undertaken.

Diagnostic imaging. Because of the high frequency of injuries to the spleen, particularly in blunt trauma, the usefulness of various imaging modalities in abdominal trauma depends largely on their reliability in detection of splenic injury. Methods for initial screening must have a high sensitivity for splenic injury to be of any value.

Plain radiographs of the abdomen have limited usefulness. The findings on the plain radiographs are usually nonspecific and relate to the finding of hemoperitoneum. More specific findings may occasionally include medial displacement of the stomach (Fig. 6-18), evidence of a mass in the left upper quadrant, elevation of the left hemidiaphragm, downward displacement of the splenic flexure of the colon, and overlying left lower rib fractures. These findings are often subtle and, therefore, frequently missed. Significant splenic injury may occur without any abnormalities on these plain radiographs. The addition of oral contrast material may demonstrate these findings more clearly.

Radionuclide scanning of the spleen has been used extensively in the past with relatively good results although the availability of this test on short notice remains a problem in many centers. Positive findings include nonvisualization of the spleen, focal areas of decreased uptake, "cold" bands across the organ representing fracture, displacement of the spleen by adjacent hematoma, fragmentation of the organ, loss of normal splenic contour, reduced size of the spleen due to failure to perfuse an avulsed distal fragment, and subcapsular hematoma[48,49] (Fig. 6-19).

The principal role of radionuclide scanning in abdominal trauma in the past has been the detection of occult splenic injuries. This modality has largely been replaced by the CT scan, which has the advantage of providing greater sensitivity and specificity, better anatomic detail, and much more information regarding injury to adjacent abdominal structures. In addition accessory spleens and congenital clefts occasionally result in false positive findings.[72] The radionuclide scan of the spleen is useful in documenting healing of established splenic injuries treated nonoperatively although the CT scan is increasingly used for this purpose as well.

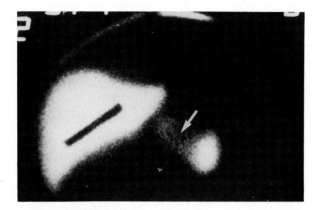

Fig. 6-19. Radionuclide scan of the spleen demonstrating a subcapsular hematoma (*arrow*) in a patient with blunt abdominal trauma. The liver/spleen scan demonstrates loss of vitalized splenic tissue due to the compressive effect of the hematoma.

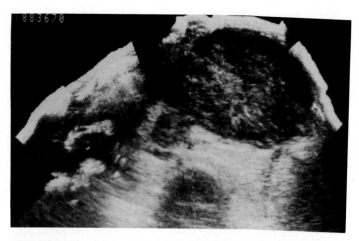

Fig. 6-20. Ultrasonography demonstrating a splenic hematoma in a young soccer player who presented 2 days after suffering a severe blow to his left flank. (Hagen-Ansert S: *Textbook of diagnostic ultrasonography,* ed 3, St Louis, 1989, Mosby–Year Book.)

Ultrasonography is a relatively sensitive technique for assessing splenic injury in a well prepared patient. The sensitivity and specificity of ultrasonography in this respect is similar to that of the CT scan, and, in fact, ultrasonography is used as the primary screening device in patients with abdominal trauma in some pediatric centers.[73] Although it is a relatively inexpensive, accessible, and noninvasive imaging modality, its use in the emergency department is limited by the frequent presence of overlying abdominal wall injuries and excessive bowel gas due to paralytic ileus that makes the examination technically difficult to perform. Gruessner et al.[45] performed a prospective study comparing ultrasonography with peritoneal lavage in the evaluation of patients with blunt trauma. The results confirmed an overall accuracy of 86% and a predictive value of 89% for ultrasonography compared to 99% and 96% for lavage. They concluded that ultrasonography cannot replace lavage as the primary screen of patients with abdominal trauma.[45] Positive ultrasonographic findings include the detection of hematoma either within or contiguous to the spleen, deformation of the spleen and displacement of upper abdominal organs by adjacent hematoma, and perisplenic fluid collections[41] (Fig. 6-20). The echogenicity of a splenic hematoma varies with the age of the blood since as the blood elements are lysed the hematoma becomes more highly echogenic. In addition, valuable information can be simultaneously obtained regarding the integrity of the liver, pancreas, and kidneys.[74]

Arteriography was the gold standard in the past for diagnosing splenic injuries and remains a relatively sensitive and specific technique although false negative studies do occur. In addition to showing extravasation either freely into the peritoneum or into the perisplenic area, positive findings include alteration of the normal arterial architecture caused by compressing subcapsular hematomas, col-

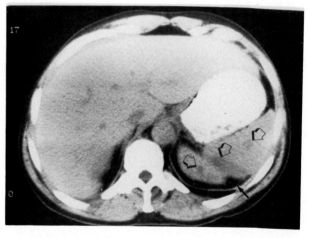

Fig. 6-21. Splenic contusion. CT scan of a 39-year-old male with blunt abdominal trauma and multiple splenic contusions (*open arrows*), which appear as low-density rounded areas within the spleen. Note the congenital cleft in the spleen (*closed arrow*), which may be misconstrued as a laceration on a radionuclide spleen scan.

lections of contrast material within the pulp of the spleen indicative of subcapsular and intraparenchymal hematomas, and early filling of the splenic vein and arterial spasm.[75] Angiographic embolization of actively bleeding splenic vessels is a controversial area with an unacceptable complication rate in some series.[76]

The CT scan using oral and intravenous contrast material has proved to be highly accurate in detecting splenic injuries and has become the radiographic procedure of choice for both detecting and following the resolution of splenic injuries treated conservatively. The reported 96%

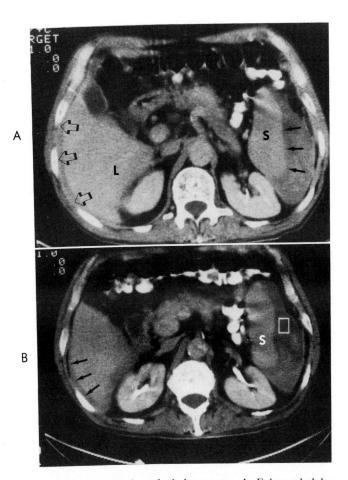

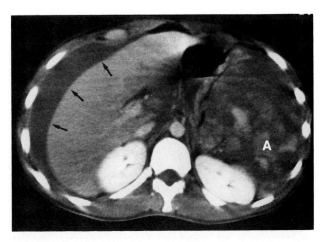

Fig. 6-23. CT scan demonstrating pulverization or complete disruption of the splenic integrity *(A)* in a 20-year-old male skier with blunt abdominal trauma. The patient had a recent viral illness that may have predisposed him to splenic injury because of splenic enlargement. Areas of high density within the splenic bed may represent leaking contrast material due to active bleeding or perfusion of splenic remnants. Note the large hemoperitoneum *(arrows)* adjacent to the liver.

Fig. 6-22. Subcapsular splenic hematoma. **A,** Enhanced abdominal CT scan demonstrates a low-density hematoma *(solid arrows)* compressing adjacent perfused splenic tissue *(S)*. The low-density rim surrounding the liver *(L) (open arrows)* represents hemoperitoneum. **B,** Enhanced abdominal CT scan, in another patient, was performed using standard window/level parameters *(L,* 40; *W,* 320). The cursor demonstrates that the subcapsular splenic hematoma has a density of 30 Hounsfield units (HU), which suggests hematoma rather than normally opacified splenic parenchyma. Note that the higher density *(S)* in the opacified residual splenic parenchyma may be due in part to compression of splenic tissue by the hematoma. Note also the thin rim of blood adjacent to the posterior edge of the liver *(solid arrows)*.

to 98% sensitivity of the CT scan in detecting splenic injury is comparable to that reported for peritoneal lavage, but the CT scan provides the advantage of visualizing the anatomic detail of the splenic injury and also of detecting many concurrent abdominal injuries that might make nonoperative treatment imprudent.[77,78] Despite this theoretic advantage, the ultimate decision on the feasibility of nonoperative treatment depends on the clinical status of the patient. Efforts to predict the clinical course of the patient with CT scans have met with mixed results. Buntain et al.[79] report a 97% accuracy in predicting the need for splenectomy using the CT scan to assess the degree of splenic injury and presence of associated injuries. Resciniti et al.[80] had similarly excellent results in cases of pediatric splenic

trauma but significantly less success in adult patients, which underscores the hazards of the nonoperative approach in adults. Brick et al.[81] found no correlation between the extent of hemoperitoneum and the need for surgery and emphasize that the clinical status of the patient must dictate the decision to operate or observe.

Fig. 6-21 shows multiple splenic contusions and a small intrasplenic hematoma in a 39-year-old male who presented with blunt trauma of the head and abdomen and a progressively falling hematocrit. Fig. 6-22 demonstrates more extensive subcapsular splenic hematomas using varied "windows" to enhance differences between injured and normal splenic tissue. On a nonenhanced CT scan, a perisplenic clot is isodense or of high density in comparison to intact splenic parenchyma. After administration of intravenous contrast material, intact splenic parenchyma exhibits density greater than an adjacent hematoma or splenic laceration[82] (Fig. 6-23). However, inadequate administration of intravenous contast material may result in a situation in which the hematoma is isodense with normal splenic parenchyma.[72,79,83] In general, the finding of heterogenous splenic tissue density suggests splenic hematoma juxtaposed with undamaged parenchyma. However, false positive findings may occur because of differences in regional blood flow within the spleen.[84,85]

Liver

Because of its abundant blood supply and frequent involvement in both penetrating and blunt trauma, injuries to the liver account for a large share of the morbidity and mortality associated with abdominal trauma. Due to its large cross-sectional area, the liver is involved in 37% of

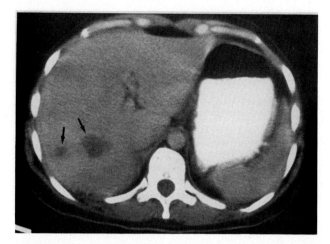

Fig. 6-24. Intraparenchymal hematoma of the liver. Low-density hematomas (*arrows*) are demonstrated within the liver in a patient who received both oral and intravenous contrast material.

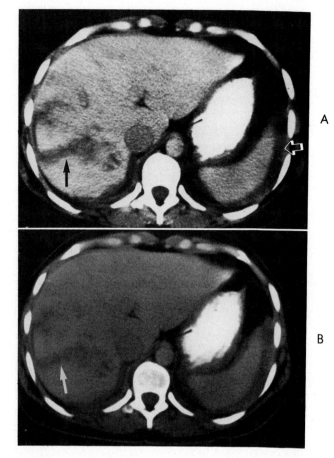

Fig. 6-25. Differing windows on the CT scan. A 27-year-old female victim of a motor vehicle accident remained stable despite the liver injury seen in these scans. She was successfully treated nonoperatively. **A,** CT scan shows an intrahepatic hematoma (*solid arrow*) and low-density blood adjacent to the spleen. **B,** Narrower window more clearly demonstrates the liver fracture (*arrow*) but the perisplenic hematoma is less well seen (*open arrow*).

penetrating wounds to the abdomen (see Table 6-1). In blunt trauma the incidence of liver injury ranges from 35% to 45% in patients treated in trauma centers.[4] The density, ligamentous attachments, location, and intrinsic architecture predispose the liver to fracture, internal disruption, laceration by overlying rib fragments, and "tethering" injuries at ligamentous points of fixation. The box on p. 121 grades liver injuries on the CT scan.[86]

As with splenic injuries, considerable interest has been generated recently by nonoperative management of a subset of relatively stable patients with liver injuries.[87] Patients considered suitable for nonoperative management include those who are hemodynamically stable, have no other injuries requiring surgical repair, have either simple laceration of the liver or intrahepatic hematoma, and have less than 250 ml of hemoperitoneum.[87,88] Clearly, in these cases it is necessary to use a diagnostic technique that will provide anatomic detail of the extent of the liver injury, detect other abdominal injuries, and quantify the amount of hemoperitoneum.

The majority of patients who can be managed expectantly undergo abdominal CT scan as the initial diagnostic imaging study and, then, subsequent scans to follow the progress of liver lesions. As with splenic trauma, there is controversy regarding the ability of the CT scan to predict the clinical course of liver injuries based on the morphology of the lesion[89] although nonoperative management of liver injuries, even in adults, is much more successful than nonoperative management of splenic injuries.

The diagnostic approach to liver injuries must be tailored to the clinical situation. Patients presenting in shock should be resuscitated with volume infusions and directed to surgery as quickly as possible. If time permits, a chest radiograph may provide useful information regarding coexistent hemothorax, pneumothorax, or thoracic vascular injury, but laparotomy should not be delayed in unstable patients in order to obtain diagnostic tests. Patients who achieve and maintain hemodynamic stability should undergo more thorough evaluation to precisely define their injuries and to identify those in whom expectant management is feasible.

Clinical findings. The history and physical findings in liver injury are nonspecific and consist of signs and symptoms of blood loss and peritoneal irritation. Tenderness confined to the right upper quadrant with or without right shoulder or periscapular pain is suggestive of an isolated liver injury. Rarely, a palpable mass is discovered in the right upper quadrant, consistent with an expanding liver hematoma. In the subacute phase, persistent presence of blood in the GI tract suggests possible disruption of the biliary tree. Development of jaundice is rare following trauma but suggests disruption of the bile ducts.

Diagnostic peritoneal lavage. Diagnostic peritoneal lavage (DPL) is an extremely sensitive technique for detecting liver injury with a diagnostic accuracy upward of

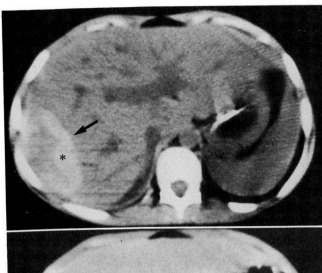

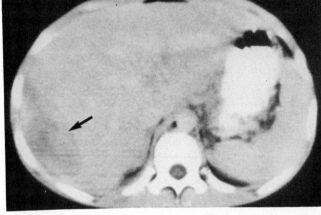

Fig. 6-26. Subcapsular hematoma of the liver in an 8-year-old male. **A,** Before administration of oral and intravenous contrast material, the hematoma (*arrow*) appears to be of high density in relation to the normal liver parenchyma. **B,** Following administration of oral and intravenous contrast material, the same hematoma (*arrow*) appears to be of low density since it is not perfused with contrast-laden blood.

CT scan classification of liver injuries[86]

Grade I: Capsular avulsion; superficial laceration(s) <1 cm deep; subcapsular hematoma <1 cm maximal thickness; periportal blood tracking only.

Grade II: Laceration(s) 1 to 3 cm deep; central/subcapsular hematoma(s) 1 to 3 cm diameter.

Grade III: Laceration(s) >3 cm deep; central/subcapsular hematoma(s) >3 cm diameter.

Grade IV: Massive central/subcapsular hematoma >10 cm; lobar tissue destruction (maceration) or devascularization.

Grade V: Bilobar tissue destruction (maceration) or devascularization.

97% in some series.[22] DPL has detected many significant liver injuries in which surgical repair would otherwise have been delayed. Concern has been raised, however, and discussed previously that exclusive reliance on peritoneal lavage has resulted in an excessive number of unnecessary laparotomies. Peritoneal lavage cannot distinguish trivial from severe injuries nor differentiate lesions that continue to bleed from those that have ceased bleeding. Because of the recent trend towards nonoperative management, more organ-specific diagnostic techniques have been sought.

Diagnostic imaging. Plain radiographs of the chest and abdomen are highly unreliable in detecting liver injury, but certain radiographic findings are useful when detected. An increase in opacification of the right upper quadrant, representing perihepatic hematoma with a resultant shift of intestine away from that area, is suggestive of liver injury[90] and is occasionally seen as an incidental finding. In general, when liver injury is suspected, more sensitive techniques than plain radiographs such as the CT scan should be employed in diagnosis.

Considerable experience has now been gained with the use of the CT scan in the diagnosis of liver injuries. This modality has sensitivity and specificity comparable to peritoneal lavage and provides specific anatomic delineation of liver injury as well.[88] All grades of liver injury are readily detectable by CT scan, including contusions, subcapsular and intraparenchymal hematomas (Fig. 6-24), lacerations and fractures (Fig. 6-25), and major crush or avulsion injuries. Hematomas and fractures of the liver appear as lucent areas surrounded by normal opaque parenchyma when intravenous contrast is used. Fig. 6-26 shows abdominal CT scans of the same patient taken before and after oral and intravenous contrast administration, demonstrating that the subcapsular hematoma of the right lobe of the liver changes from high density on the initial radiograph (Fig. 6-26, *A*) to low density after the administration of contrast material (Fig. 6-26, *B*). A CT scan classification of liver injury is outlined in the box above.[86]

Ultrasonographic examination of the liver is limited by the same conditions as outlined for splenic injury and is similarly accurate in detecting significant injury (Fig. 6-27). With more rapid availability and portable equipment, ultrasonography may yet prove to be an excellent screening device in liver as well as splenic and pancreatic injuries.

Angiography is accurate in detecting liver injury and offers the added advantage of arterial embolization as a therapeutic measure, if indicated. Fig. 6-28 demonstrates angiographic embolization with subsequent resolution of an intrahepatic hemorrhage in a patient who sustained a gunshot wound to the liver with pseudo-aneurysm formation of the left hepatic artery. The positive angiographic findings in liver angiography are classified in the same manner as in splenic injury.

Radionuclide scanning of the liver is largely obsolete in the acute setting as other modalities are more accurate,

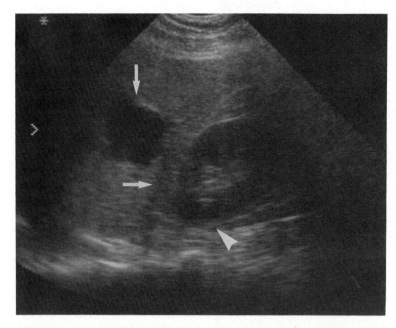

Fig. 6-27. Ultrasonogram of traumatic liver injury demonstrates hepatic hematoma *(vertical arrow)* and hepatic laceration *(horizontal arrow)* overlying superior pole of right kidney *(large arrowhead)*. (Courtesy Tony KY Chan, MD.)

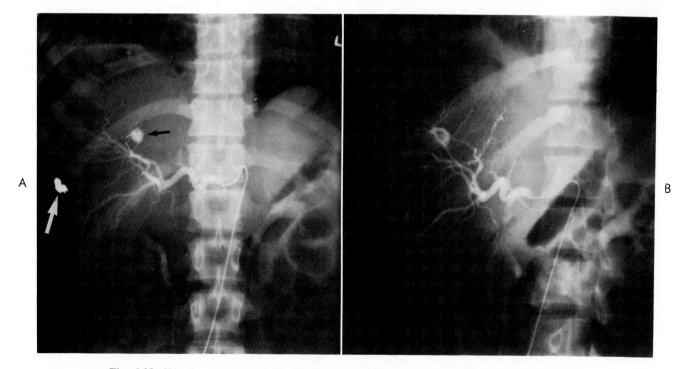

Fig. 6-28. Hepatic angiography and embolization. A 23-year-old male with a gunshot wound to the liver exhibited persistent hemobilia following surgery. **A,** Pseudo-aneurysm of the left hepatic artery *(small arrow)* is revealed adjacent to surgical clips. Note deformed bullet *(large arrow)*. **B,** Following embolization, repeat angiography reveals obliteration of the pseudo-aneurysm.

faster, and accessible. Positive findings are identical to those discussed under splenic injury.

Pancreas

The pancreas is the least commonly injured solid viscus yet contributes disproportionately to overall mortality and morbidity in abdominal trauma. Injury to the pancreas occurs in approximately 2% to 12% of all abdominal trauma cases.[91] Unlike other solid viscus injuries, penetrating wounds (particularly gunshot wounds) to the pancreas account for up to 80% of the cases of pancreatic trauma.[92,93] Gunshot wounds involve the head, body, and tail of the pancreas with uniform frequency depending on the course of the projectile. In blunt pancreatic trauma, injuries to the neck of the gland are more common as this area of the pancreas is directly compressed between the vertebral column and the external force, usually a steering wheel in motor vehicle accidents. In children the most common mechanism is direct compression by the wheels of a vehicle or by a "handlebar" injury in cycling accidents.

Overall mortality in pancreatic injuries in a collected series ranged from 17% to 32%[94] although the majority of deaths were due directly to associated injuries. Mortality is greatly increased when there is co-existent rupture of either the duodenum or colon.[94] When the pancreas alone is injured, mortality as low as 3% has been reported.[95] However, because of its relatively well protected location in the abdomen, the pancreas is rarely the only abdominal injury present. Virtually all cases of penetrating pancreatic trauma and the vast majority of blunt trauma cases have associated injuries. In one large retrospective series, over 98% of patients with pancreatic injury had an average of 3.5 associated injuries/patient.[93]

Penetrating injuries to the upper abdomen tend to be explored at laparotomy without much prior investigation, and many pancreatic injuries are found fortuitously. Similarly, in blunt abdominal trauma the high frequency of associated injuries often results in laparotomy based either on physical findings or a positive peritoneal lavage. Diagnostic difficulty arises in cases of blunt abdominal trauma where the pancreas is the only organ injured.

Clinical findings. Because of its retroperitoneal location, severe pancreatic injuries may be clinically silent on initial presentation. Over a period of hours to days symptoms suggestive of pancreatic injury may appear but these symptoms are relatively nonspecific. Patients complain of moderate-to-severe constant epigastric pain radiating to the midback, with associated symptoms of nausea, vomiting, anorexia, and occasionally, diarrhea.[91] In the early phase, abdominal findings may be minimal or absent. Once the peritoneum becomes irritated by pancreatic juice, abdominal findings may range from epigastric and left upper quadrant tenderness to frank generalized peritonitis and shock.

Diagnostic peritoneal lavage. Ancillary studies to detect the relatively silent pancreatic injury have included mea-

surement of serum amylase and diagnostic peritoneal lavage (DPL). Although one would expect serum amylase to be significantly elevated in pancreatic trauma, it is a suprisingly unreliable measurement.[14] Olsen[96] reported that of all trauma patients with hyperamylasemia in a series, only 8% proved to have pancreatic injury. Conversely, in a small series, Moretz et al.[15] noted that only three of five patients with pancreatic injury had elevated serum amylase. In recent large series, serum amylase was reported to be elevated in 56%[93] and 80%[95] of pancreatic injuries. Persistent or rising serum amylase levels are thought to be more specific indicators of pancreatic injury, but this is of limited usefulness during the initial phase of evaluation.

Initial criteria for positivity of DPL include elevation of lavage fluid amylase; however, subsequent questions as to the usefulness of this measurement have rendered it largely obsolete.[97] Nevertheless, Smego et al.[95] reported a success rate of 97% in detecting pancreatic injury using a combination of physical findings and peritoneal lavage, despite a false negative rate of 23.5% in patients undergoing peritoneal lavage. The high rate of success of peritoneal lavage in this context is somewhat misleading since the majority of positive results were due to associated intraperitoneal injuries. Isolated pancreatic injury is poorly detected because of its retroperitoneal location and late involvement of the peritoneum.

Diagnostic imaging. Despite greater awareness of the possibility of pancreatic injury in the modern era, the complication rate for pancreatic injuries has remained a high 33%.[94] Complications include pancreatic fistula, intra-abdominal abscess, and pseudocyst formation. Pseudocyst formation occurs in 12% of cases and may be the initial presentation of pancreatic trauma.[5] The radiographic approach to pancreatic injury is limited. Plain radiographs of the abdomen may demonstrate nonspecific findings, including the "sentinel loops" of bowel representing localized ileus overlying the epigastric area (Fig. 6-29), widening of the sweep of the duodenum due to intervening pancreatic hematoma, and displacement of the stomach and hollow viscera laterally, anteriorly, and inferiorly. The generalized haziness of the abdomen associated with ascites may be a late finding and is nonspecific.

Ultrasonography is a useful tool in the acute evaluation of the injured pancreas but is subject to the same limitations in its use as it is for other areas of the abdomen (Fig. 6-30). It is particularly useful in the detection and observation of pancreatic pseudocysts and abscesses. Positive findings include the detection of peripancreatic hematomas, retroperitoneal fluid, and direct visualization of pancreatic fracture or focal edema.

The role of the CT scan in detecting pancreatic trauma is controversial. Critics point out a relatively high incidence of false positive and negative results, whereas proponents note a considerable degree of accuracy, considering that no other commonly used technique can provide more precise diagnostic information. A 91% accuracy has

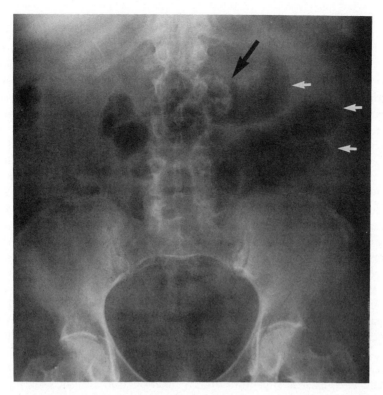

Fig. 6-29. Plain radiograph of the abdomen demonstrates "sentinel loops" *(small arrows)* secondary to acute pancreatitis. Pancreatic calcifications *(large arrow)* confirm underlying chronic pancreatitis.

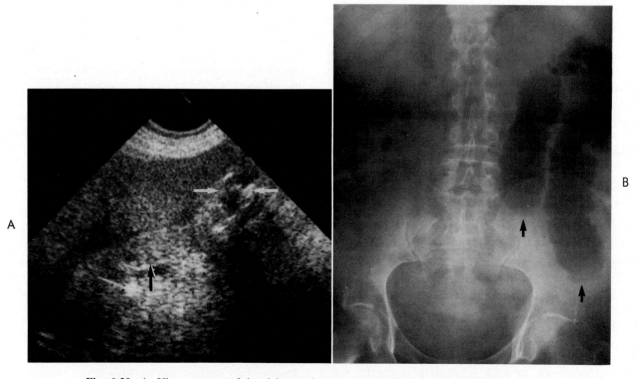

Fig. 6-30. A, Ultrasonogram of the abdomen demonstrates "sentinel loops" *(horizontal arrows)* resulting in acoustic shadowing that obscures the tail of the inflamed pancreas. The head of the pancreas *(vertical arrow)* is not involved. **B,** Corresponding plain radiograph of the abdomen also demonstrates "sentinel loops" *(small arrows)*. (Courtesy Neal H Rosner, MD.)

been reported by experienced examiners.[61,98] Positive findings may be subtle and must be actively sought. These include parenchymal disruption, focal or diffuse enlargement of the gland, peripancreatic fluid collections, and areas of diminished attenuation, representing fracture.[61] In addition, thickening of the anterior prerenal fascia, particularly on the left, may represent inflammation caused by autodigestion from spillage of extrapancreatic enzyme[94] (Fig. 6-31). False positive studies may be due to faulty technique, motion artifact, adjacent nonopacified bowel loops appearing as a peripancreatic hematoma, intraperitoneal fluid in the lesser sac, and peripancreatic hematoma from injury to other upper abdominal organs including the liver, spleen, and kidney.[61] There is also a substantial delay in the development of traumatic pancreatitis in many cases. Performance of the CT scan before the development of ultrastructural changes in the gland may result in a false negative result. Also, a significant fracture of the pancreas may be present with no abnormalities on the CT scan.[98]

Endoscopic retrograde cholangiopancreatography (ERCP) is the only technique available that can appraise the integrity of the pancreatic ductal system, which is a prime determinant of the clinical course of traumatic pancreatitis (Fig. 6-32). There is little reported experience with ERCP in the context of acute trauma evaluation, and its use would seem more appropriate for investigation of subacute and questionable cases in stable patients. ERCP may be indicated in cases in which primary diagnostic studies are equivocal.[99]

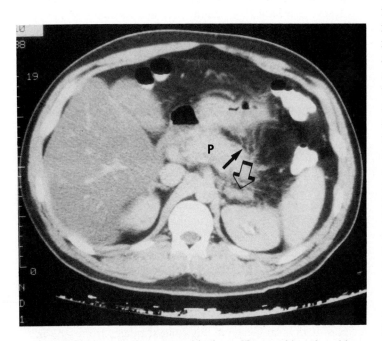

Fig. 6-31. Traumatic pancreatitis in a 29-year-old male with blunt trauma to the abdomen from a motor vehicle accident. The pancreas *(P)* is edematous. There is stranding of the parapancreatic fat indicative of inflammation *(closed arrow)* and thickening of the left anterior renal fascial plane *(open arrow)*. Both serum and urinary amylase were elevated.

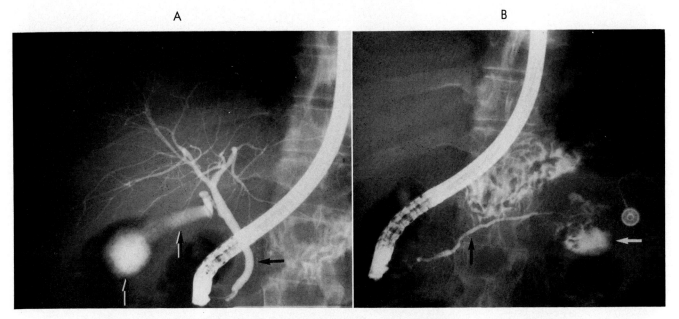

Fig. 6-32. Endoscopic retrograde cholangiopancreatography (ERCP). **A,** Radiograph demonstrates contrast-filled cystic duct and gallbladder *(vertical arrows)*, common bile duct *(horizontal arrow)*, and normal biliary tree. **B,** Radiograph demonstrates contrast-filled pancreatic duct *(vertical arrow)* and pancreatic pseudocyst *(horizontal arrow)*. The proximal two thirds of the pancreatic duct is normal; the distal third is narrowed and irregular as it connects with a pseudocyst in a patient with acute pancreatitis. (Courtesy Tony KY Chan, MD.)

Hollow viscus

Hollow visceral injury occurs much more commonly with penetrating wounds than with blunt trauma. In some series, 80% to 90% of the hollow viscus injuries reported result from penetrating wounds.[100,101] There is a suggestion that the incidence of blunt intestinal injury is increasing as a result of increased seat belt use[102] although this may be an acceptable price to pay for the overall increased survival rate associated with such use.

Intestinal injuries may be intraperitoneal, retroperitoneal, or both, depending on the site of injury. Multiple intestinal injuries occur in a majority of patients with a penetrating mechanism and in 25% of patients with blunt traumatic hollow visceral injury.[100,103] Significant intestinal injuries include perforation of the viscus with spillage of its contents, mesenteric avulsions with consequent ischemic bowel necrosis, severe contusion of the bowel wall with ultimate potential for necrosis, and luminal obstruction by intramural hematoma. Potentially significant injuries include serosal tears, "blast injuries" from high-velocity gunshot wounds, and prolonged ileus.

Clinical findings. The diagnosis of intestinal injury is one of the most difficult and controversial aspects of trauma care. Depending on the organ involved, symptoms related to an isolated bowel injury may be delayed for many hours. In small bowel injury, the frequent absence of severe bleeding, a neutral pH, and absence of heavy bacterial and enzyme concentrations make intraperitoneal spillage relatively nonirritating and signs of peritonitis may be delayed.[104] The acid pH of the stomach and high bacterial concentration in colonic contents will produce symptoms earlier, but, in the immediate post-injury assessment, symptoms of peritonitis may also be absent. Consequently, these injuries are often overlooked, and substantial delays may occur in detection and treatment. Several studies have shown a dramatic increase in mortality from 0% to 5% with early repair compared to 47% to 65% when repair is delayed beyond 24 hours.[13,105]

Diagnostic peritoneal lavage. Although diagnostic peritoneal lavage (DPL) is highly sensitive in detecting intraperitoneal blood, it is much less sensitive in detecting isolated bowel injury since it may take between 3 to 6 hours for the lavage WBC count to become significantly elevated in cases of hollow viscus rupture.[106] In addition, retroperitoneal injury of the duodenum and rectum are not easily detected by peritoneal lavage. The reported sensitivity of peritoneal lavage in this context ranges from 50% in a series of duodenal injuries[100] to 85% overall.[106] Engrav et al.[107] also reported a 16% false negative rate for peritoneal lavage in intestinal trauma. Furthermore, peritoneal

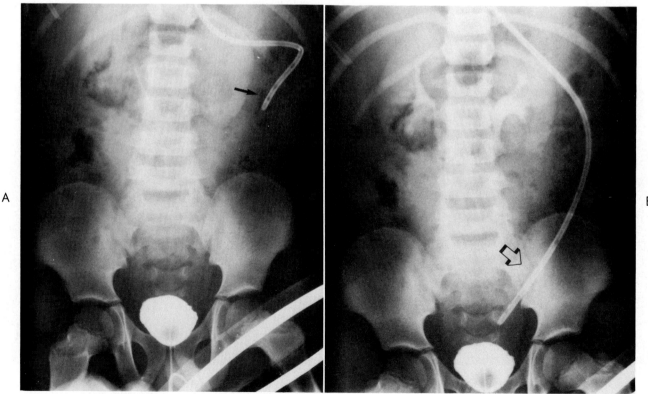

Fig. 6-33. Gastric rupture. Intravenous pyelogram of a 6-year-old male blunt trauma victim with free intraperitoneal rupture of the stomach and laceration of the spleen. **A,** Initial abdominal radiograph shows suspicious course of the nasogastric tube. **B,** Further displacement of the nasogastric tube into the pelvis confirms gastric rupture.

lavage does not differentiate relatively minor serosal tears and mesenteric or intraluminal hematomas from significant injuries requiring laparotomy. Consequently, there is a substantial rate of unnecessary laparotomies with bowel injuries. Although the measurement of lavage fluid amylase is controversial, significant elevations are considered reason for further investigation. Serum amylase is relatively insensitive in detecting bowel injuries since elevations occur in as few as 25% of cases of blunt intestinal trauma.[106]

Diagnostic imaging. Plain radiographs of the abdomen are also relatively insensitive in detecting bowel injury. Rupture of a hollow viscus may produce free air either intraperitoneally or retroperitoneally, but this finding is rare in the early phase of assessment. Whereas stomach and colon may contain substantial amounts of bowel gas, the normal small intestine contains very little. Robbs et al.[105] detected free air in only 43% of patients with intestinal perforation from trauma. Additional findings suggesting bowel injury on plain radiographs are nonspecific and include scoliosis and free intraperitoneal fluid. Rigler's "double wall" sign (see Fig. 6-5), in which both sides of

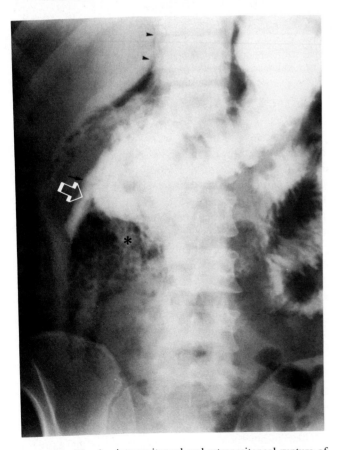

Fig. 6-34. Massive intraperitoneal and retroperitoneal rupture of the duodenum. Generalized "stippling" of upper abdominal gas adjacent to the duodenum *(asterisk)* represents retroperitoneal free air. Extravasation of contrast material is seen on the right side of the duodenum *(open arrow).* The inferior edge of the liver and the falciform ligament are outlined by gas *(small arrowheads).*

the bowel wall are clearly visualized because free intraperitoneal and intraluminal gas outline the bowel wall, is highly specific but rarely observed in traumatic bowel rupture. Retroperitoneal rupture is suggested by the presence of stippled air bubbles outlining the margins of the psoas muscles or retroperitoneal structures such as the kidney or pancreas and by obliteration of the psoas shadow by associated leakage of fluid. Detection of retroperitoneal air is difficult, and the findings are often very subtle. These findings have been reported to occur in 20% to 40% of patients with duodenal rupture.[108,109]

Fig. 6-33, *A,* shows the suspicious course of a nasogastric tube in a 6-year-old male with blunt abdominal trauma and free intraperitoneal rupture of the stomach. The patient also had a splenic injury. Fig. 6-33, *B,* confirms the diagnosis of stomach rupture as the nasogastric tube is advanced into the pelvis. Fig. 6-34 shows massive free intraperitoneal and retroperitoneal air in a patient who presented after being kicked in the abdomen during an altercation. He was subsequently found to have a duodenal rupture.

Contrast studies employing water-soluble contrast material are extremely useful in detecting perforation and intraluminal obstruction in stable patients. However, the delays involved in obtaining these tests preclude their initial use in the emergency department or in unstable patients. Positive findings include extravasation of contrast, obstruction to the flow of contrast material past an obstructing hematoma, the "coiled spring" or "stacked coin" sign associated with a small bowel hematoma (Fig. 6-35), and displacement of the bowel by a compressing extraneous mass such as a splenic or hepatic hematoma. Fig. 6-36, *A,* demonstrates the typical radiographic appearance of a duodenal hematoma on an upper GI contrast examination, in this case involving a lap seat belt injury in a 27-year-old male. The flow of contrast is obstructed by the intramural hematoma with a characteristic convex "cap" of contrast material. Fig. 6-36, *B,* is the abdominal CT scan of the same patient in which the full extent of the massive duodenal hematoma is seen. Duodenal hematoma may also be detected by ultrasonography as demonstrated in Fig. 6-36, *C,* although upper GI contrast examination is the "gold standard" for diagnosing these injuries.

The use of the CT scan as the primary screening device in abdominal trauma has been resisted in part because of a fear that it is insensitive in detecting bowel injuries.[32,110,111] Furthermore, injury to the bowel or mesentery is responsible for the greatest disparity between the diagnostic accuracy of the CT scan and peritoneal lavage. In a series of 301 hemodynamically stable blunt abdominal trauma patients who underwent both the CT scan and peritoneal lavage, 19 patients had a negative CT scan, a positive peritoneal lavage, and bowel injury confirmed at laparotomy.[112] A retrospective study comparing the diagnostic accuracy of the CT scan and peritoneal lavage found the overall ac-

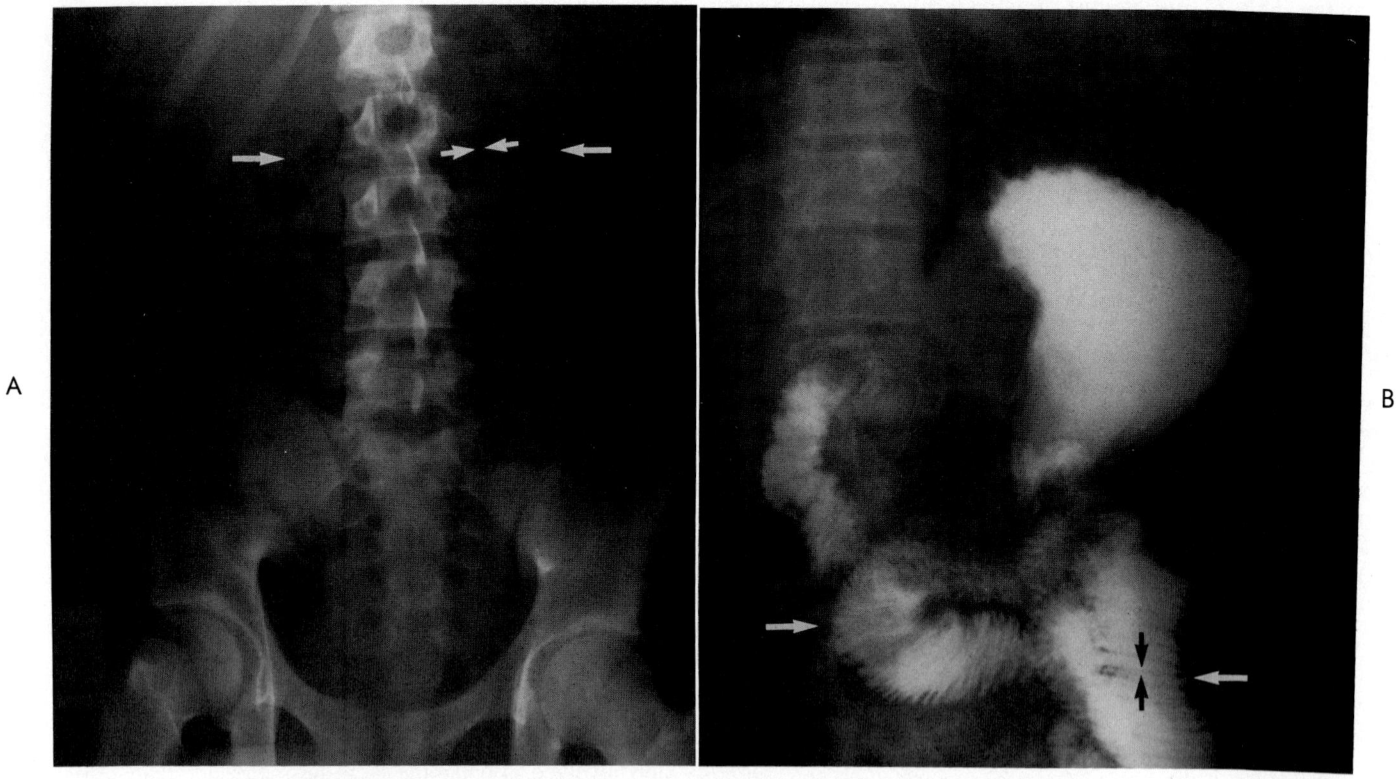

Fig. 6-35. Hollow viscus injury. **A,** Supine radiograph of the abdomen demonstrates mildly dilated loops of jejunum *(horizontal arrows)* with prominent valvulae conniventes *(paired small arrows)*. **B,** Small bowel series with barium confirms these findings and demonstrates the "coiled spring" sign associated with a small bowel hematoma.

curacy of the CT scan to be excellent, but it was unreliable in detecting bowel injury.[113]

Another study,[114] demonstrating increased sensitivity of the CT scan, was reasonably successful in differentiating surgical from nonsurgical candidates. In this study of 51 patients with suspected bowel or mesentery injury, the CT scan identified 89% of bowel hematomas or mesenteric injuries in 19 nonsurgical patients. In another subgroup, a preoperative CT scan identified surgically confirmed bowel injuries in 26 of 28 patients.[114] Clearly, the role of the CT scan in this context is evolving and, with further experience, proficiency in detecting bowel injury may improve.

Some CT scan findings that correlate well with surgical findings include the detection of free intraperitoneal fluid, mesenteric infiltration, and thickened bowel wall (Fig. 6-37). Free intraperitoneal fluid is a nonspecific finding that may be caused by injury to solid viscera and blood vessels in addition to the bowel. In the absence of obvious hepatic or splenic injury on the CT scan, the appearance of free intraperitoneal fluid should be considered strongly suggestive of bowel injury since this may be the only positive CT scan finding. A more specific finding is the "sentinel clot" that represents the focal accumulation of high-density clotted blood adjacent to the injured bowel. In a retrospective review of 116 patients with abdominal trauma, the sentinel clot was the only positive finding in 32% of the cases with bowel or mesenteric injury.[115]

Appropriate CT imaging technique is essential for detection of the often subtle signs of bowel and mesenteric injury. Patient preparation requires oral administration of a dilute water-soluble contrast material in a 400-ml dose up to 1 hour before scanning and a second identical dose immediately preceding the scan. Bolus intravenous administration of contrast material is helpful for evaluating solid parenchyma but is less likely to contribute in the evaluation of bowel and mesenteric trauma. Standard imaging protocols and slice/interval thicknesses suffice. Manipulation of CT window settings requires the addition of wide windows (1000 to 1500 HU) to optimize visualization of free intraperitoneal gas.[114]

The duodenum is the most frequently injured portion of the small bowel in blunt trauma. Not uncommonly, the injury involves both the intra- and retroperitoneal portions of the duodenum, resulting in both free subdiaphragmatic gas and more localized retroperitoneal "stippling."

Positive findings on the CT scan include the detection of either intraperitoneal or retroperitoneal free air, extravasation of contrast material, bowel wall thickness greater than 3 mm or narrowing of the lumen (representing intramural hematoma), thickening or infiltration of the mesentery, and hemoperitoneum. Retroperitoneal gas tends to localize near the site of injury, often accompanied by fluid, either blood or intestinal contents. However, because of the great sensitivity of the CT scan in detect-

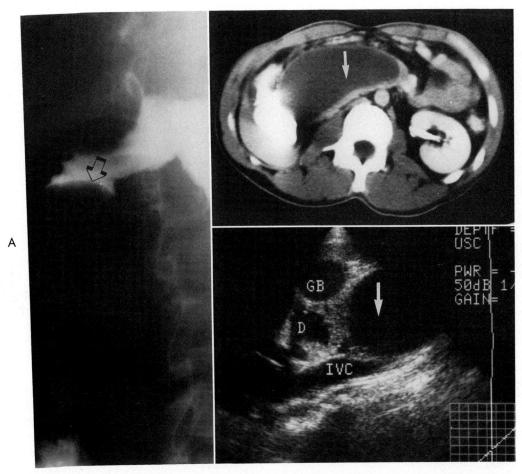

Fig. 6-36. Duodenal hematoma in a 27-year old male with blunt abdominal trauma from a motor vehicle accident. **A,** Upper GI series with oral contrast material. The submucosal duodenal hematoma effaces the duodenal lumen, resulting in obstruction. Oral contrast material outlines the superior aspect of the hematoma *(open arrow).* **B,** CT scan clearly demonstrates the full extent of the duodenal hematoma *(arrow)* in the same patient. **C,** Ultrasonogram demonstrates the hematoma *(white arrow)* on the left of the duodenal lumen *(D).* The gallbladder *(GB)* and inferior vena cava *(IVC)* are also well seen.

ing free air, it is not unusual to find small focal collections of retroperitoneal gas that are remote from the injury site.

Rupture of the duodenum is less common than nonperforating injury. Duodenal hematoma has a characteristic appearance on CT scan (see Fig. 6-36, *B*). With opacification of the bowel by oral contrast material, the hematoma is of lower density. Without oral contrast material, the density of the hematoma depends on its age, and it may become isodense with the surrounding bowel wall.

Injuries to the mesenteric vessels are often immediately fatal and patients who survive to reach the emergency department are often critically unstable. Consequently, the majority of these cases are taken directly to surgery without further diagnostic procedures. For those who achieve relative hemodynamic stability, angiography is useful in precisely locating the injury.

Diaphragm

Diaphragmatic injuries occur in up to 8% of patients with blunt abdominal trauma[116] and in 15% of cases of stab wounds and 46% of gunshot wounds to the lower thorax and upper abdomen.[117] Penetrating wounds directly lacerate the diaphragm causing relatively small defects that can remain asymptomatic for long periods of time until abdominal contents herniate through the diaphragmatic tear. Sudden application of blunt force to the abdomen causes dramatic increases in intra-abdominal pressure that can result in large explosive diaphragmatic tears. In both cases, the frequency and severity of associated injuries, 100% in one series,[118] tended to overshadow the often asymptomatic diaphragmatic tears.

Although it is traditionally taught that 95% of diaphragmatic tears occur on the left,[116,119,120] recent findings indicate only a slight preponderance of left-sided tears.[116,120-122] Herniation, on the other hand, is more

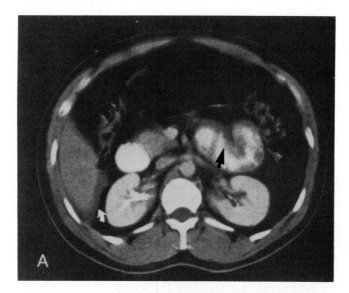

Fig. 6-37. CT scan of jejunal hematoma and laceration *(arrow)*. Proximal jejunum has a thick wall, representing intramural hematoma.

commonly observed on the left since the liver tends to prevent the egress of viscera into right-sided defects. Although the most commonly involved organs are the stomach, colon, liver, small bowel, and spleen,[122] virtually every abdominal organ has been reported within a diaphragmatic hernia.

Clinical findings. Diaphragmatic injuries are frequently missed in the initial evaluation phase because acute herniation occurs in only 32% of cases,[120] and the tear itself is relatively asymptomatic until herniation occurs. Saber et al.[123] in a review of delayed presentation of diaphragmatic rupture note that 33% to 47% of these injuries are missed in the immediate post-traumatic phase.[123] The pull from negative intrathoracic pressure eventually draws abdominal contents into the chest, producing symptoms of respiratory compromise and bowel obstruction or strangulation. Once strangulation occurs, mortality may be as high as 80%.[123] The use of positive pressure ventilation may prevent herniation in the acute phase by negating the thoraco-abdominal pressure gradient.

Diagnosis of diaphragmatic injury is difficult because none of the imaging modalities can reliably detect a tear before herniation has occurred. Many diaphragmatic tears are discovered fortuitously at laparotomy done for associated injuries although even laparotomy may fail to detect a substantial number of these injuries.[124]

Diagnostic peritoneal lavage. Because a diaphragmatic rupture may not bleed severely or may bleed into the chest rather than the abdomen, diagnostic peritoneal lavage (DPL) may be falsely negative in 36% of cases[24,125] although some authors[120,126] report a higher success rate by lowering the RBC threshold of positivity to 5000-10,000 ml. Occasionally, recovery of lavage fluid through a chest tube will be diagnostic of diaphragmatic tears.

Diagnostic imaging. The role of the plain chest radiograph in diagnosing diaphragmatic tears is similarily controversial. A majority of chest radiographs are abnormal although most of the findings are nonspecific. One third of the chest radiographs are entirely normal in some series.[127] Payne and Yellin[122] noted an abnormal chest radiograph in 94% of their series, with findings diagnostic of diaphragmatic hernia in only 43% of cases. Nonspecific findings include an indistinct or elevated hemidiaphragm, pleural effusion, atelectasis with shift of the mediastinum to the contralateral side, hemothorax or pneumothorax, and lower rib fractures. Specific findings are visualization of bowel loops or solid masses above the diaphragm and loss of the normal diaphragmatic contour. Insertion of a nasogastric tube before performing the chest radiograph will increase the accuracy of plain film diagnosis in cases involving herniation of the stomach since the tube will be visualized in the thorax.[128] Whenever vague infiltrates of the lower lung fields are seen in a trauma patient, the possibility of diaphragmatic injury should be considered and further diagnostic studies should be pursued. Fig. 6-38, illustrates this point. Although no clearly visible loops of bowel or solid masses are seen in the thorax, the presence of an unexplained infiltrate on the chest radiograph in a trauma victim raises the suspicion of diaphragmatic herniation. The unusual course of the chest tube in Fig. 6-39 is caused by herniation of the stomach into the chest in a 37-year-old male victim of blunt trauma. The herniated stomach in this case mimicked a pneumothorax, prompting insertion of the chest tube. There are reports of "tension gastrothorax," in which needle or tube thoracostomy was performed to relieve a suspected tension pneumothorax.[129]

When the patient's condition permits and particularly when chronic herniation is suspected, contrast studies should be used to clearly delineate the hernia. Both an upper GI series and barium enema examinations are useful, depending on the viscus involved in the hernia. Positive findings include visualization of contrast-filled loops of bowel above the diaphragm, bowel obstruction at the level of the diaphragm, and failure of contrast material to advance into distal bowel segments on repeated examinations.[122] Because of the risk of bowel necrosis, water-soluble contrast material should be used. The barium enema shown in Fig. 6-40 demonstrates colonic obstruction at the level of the diaphragm in a patient with a previously missed diaphragmatic rupture due to a penetrating injury, resulting in strangulation of the colon.

Other radiographic investigations such as radionuclide scanning might incidentally be able to detect a diaphragmatic tear if either the liver, spleen, or kidney are involved within the hernia. Chest CT scan will readily show herniated abdominal contents but is unreliable in diagnosing diaphragmatic tears before herniation. Fluoroscopic examination of the motion of the diaphragm is accurate and useful in detecting chronic diaphragmatic hernias but is not commonly used in the acute setting.

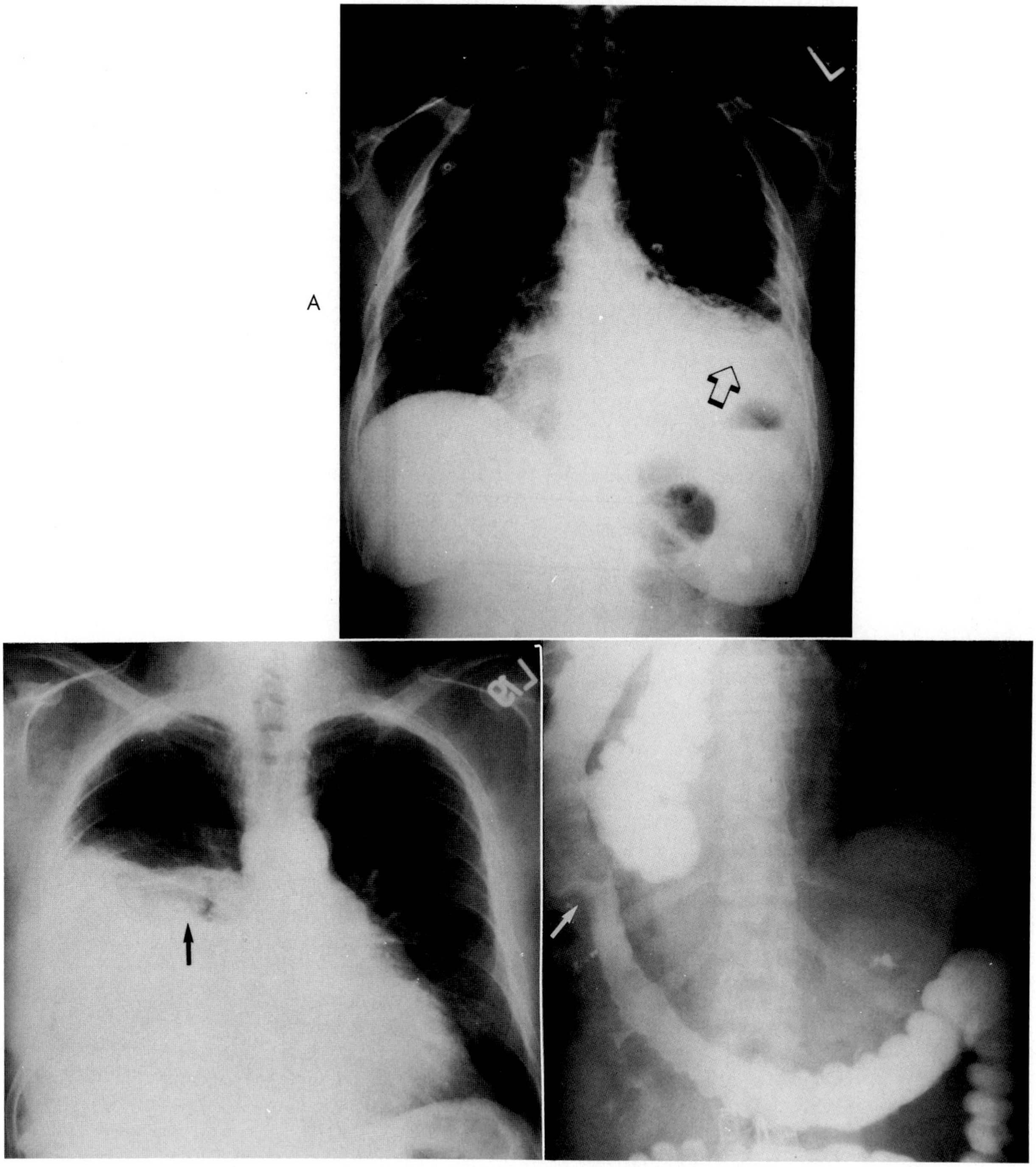

Fig. 6-38. Diaphragmatic hernia. **A,** Subtle changes in the left lung base in a trauma patient suggest the possibility of diaphragmatic herniation. In this case, the air-fluid level lies higher in relation to the diaphragm than usual. The margins of the left hemidiaphragm are obscured, and there is a pulmonary infiltrate in the left lung base. **B,** Portable AP chest radiograph demonstrates entrapment of the hepatic flexure in a traumatic diaphragmatic tear. There is opacification of the lower two thirds of the right hemithorax with a questionable cavitary mass *(arrow).* **C,** Barium enema confirms entrapment of hepatic flexure *(arrow).*

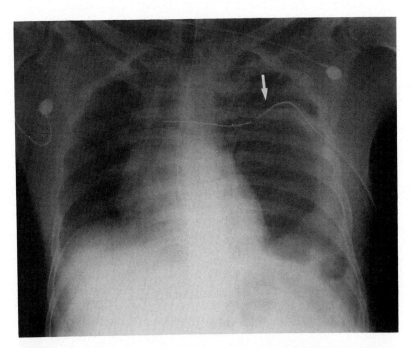

Fig. 6-39. Diaphragmatic hernia. A 37-year-old male victim of blunt abdominal trauma presented with respiratory distress and diminished breath sounds in the left chest, which prompted insertion of a chest tube for suspected pneumothorax. In fact, the patient had sustained a massive rupture of the left hemidiaphragm with herniation of the stomach into the thorax. Note the unusual course of the chest tube (*arrow*) as it courses over the stomach.

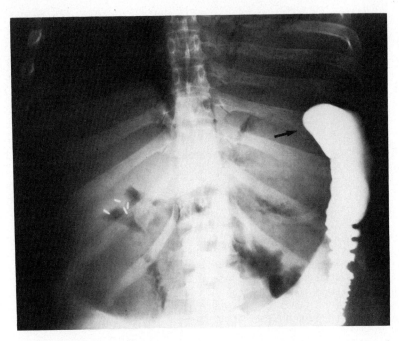

Fig. 6-40. Diaphragmatic hernia. A barium enema demonstrates entrapment of the colonic splenic flexure in a traumatic diaphragmatic tear (*arrow*).

Other abdominal injuries

Retroperitoneal injury. The most frequently injured retroperitoneal structures are the great vessels (31%), GI tract (26%), GU tract (21%), and musculoskeletal system (19%).[130] Pelvic fractures are frequently associated with extensive retroperitoneal hematoma and account for a disproportionate number of deaths.[131] The vast majority of these cases are due to blunt injury. Retroperitoneal hematomas are approached differently depending on their location. Multiple or distracted pelvic fractures should suggest the possibility of significant vascular injury. Inability to account for blood loss in either the chest or abdomen in a patient with ongoing transfusion requirements should dictate angiographic investigation. The potential for simultaneous angiographic embolization of actively bleeding pelvic vessels is well documented[133,134] and may be lifesaving since opening the retroperitoneum to control bleeding is associated with high mortality.[130] Other treatment modalities that may be useful are external fixation of pelvic fractures and application of the MAST suit to assist in the tamponade of bleeding vessels.[135] Fig. 6-41, *A* and *B*, correlates angiographic and CT findings in a patient with a penetrating wound of the pelvis that resulted in a traumatic pseudo-aneurysm; Fig. 6-41, *C* demonstrates the angiographic resolution of the pseudo-aneurysm following embolization.

Upper abdominal retroperitoneal hematomas are associated with injury to major vessels, including the aorta and inferior vena cava. Aortic rupture may be relatively well contained in only a minority of patients, and urgent aortography should be performed. If the patient deteriorates before repair can be undertaken, emergency thoracotomy with cross-clamping of the descending aorta may be lifesaving.

Penetrating abdominal trauma. Penetrating abdominal trauma is epidemic in inner city areas. Penetrating wounds of the abdomen, both accidental and intentional, are increasingly common presentations in the emergency department. The use of high-velocity automatic weapons has also increased not only the incidence but also the lethality and complexity of resultant injuries.

Gunshot wounds. Gunshot wounds may range from the trivial, superficial wound inflicted by a low-caliber, low-velocity weapon to devastating, lethal injuries with massive tissue loss and vascular disruption from high-velocity weapons and close-range shotguns.

The high incidence of peritoneal penetration and visceral injury seen with gunshot wounds has mandated a much more aggressive surgical approach. Consequently, the radiographic approach to penetrating abdominal trauma differs from blunt trauma in several respects. Many centers advocate mandatory exploration of all gunshot wounds to the abdomen and lower thorax. In these centers, the contribution of diagnostic radiology is usually confined to the detection of thoracic injury by chest radiography. In stable patients, plain radiographs of the abdomen can occasionally demonstrate evidence of free intraperitoneal air and blood, as with blunt trauma. In addition, plain radiographs taken at 90° to each other can assess the location and approximate course of a bullet and document bullet embolization (Fig. 6-42). As a general rule, the number of holes in the patient plus the number of bullets should add up to an even number. If not, bullet embolization or a previous gunshot wound should be suspected. Contrast studies are of limited usefulness but may demonstrate bowel injuries and diaphragmatic herniation.

Stab wounds. The incidence of peritoneal penetration and visceral injury is much lower for stab wounds, and a more conservative approach to treatment is common. Selective local exploration and observation of abdominal stab wounds has greatly reduced the incidence of unnecessary laparotomies in large series of patients.[136-141] The use of "sinograms" in which contrast material is injected along the suspected course of the stab wound to determine the presence of peritoneal penetration is an insensitive technique because the track of the wound may seal very quickly producing false negative results.[142] Local wound exploration may be valuable when the track can be clearly identified as penetrating the anterior fascia mandating DPL. Nevertheless, false negative results may occur (Fig. 6-43).

Adoption of more stringent criteria for positivity of diagnostic peritoneal lavage, in penetrating trauma has improved the sensitivity of this test in this context[4] (see box on p. 103) although specificity for serious injury remains a problem.

The CT scan has been effective in the evaluation of abdominal stab wounds, with a high degree of accuracy in predicting the need for surgical exploration although it is relatively insensitive in detecting bowel injuries and diaphragmatic tears. Consequently, it should not be used as the only diagnostic technique in penetrating abdominal wounds because of the high incidence of associated bowel injury.[143]

Positive findings on the CT scan include those previously described for blunt trauma. In addition, the CT scan can often show the exact course of a stab wound by detecting air along the track of the knife (Fig. 6-44).

Flank and back wounds. Both serial physical examinations and diagnostic peritoneal lavage (DPL) are relatively insensitive in detecting retroperitoneal injuries and diaphragmatic tears resulting from penetrating back and flank wounds. These injuries must be aggressively evaluated in stable patients with penetrating trauma to avoid the morbidity and mortality that results from delayed diagnosis.

Nevertheless, Peck et al.[140] have shown sequential physical examination to be relatively safe in this group of patients although patients developing signs of peritoneal penetration and visceral injury will do so at a later stage of their injury using this clinical approach. The accuracy of the CT scan in evaluating the retroperitoneum makes these patients candidates for screening so as to detect significant injury at an earlier stage.

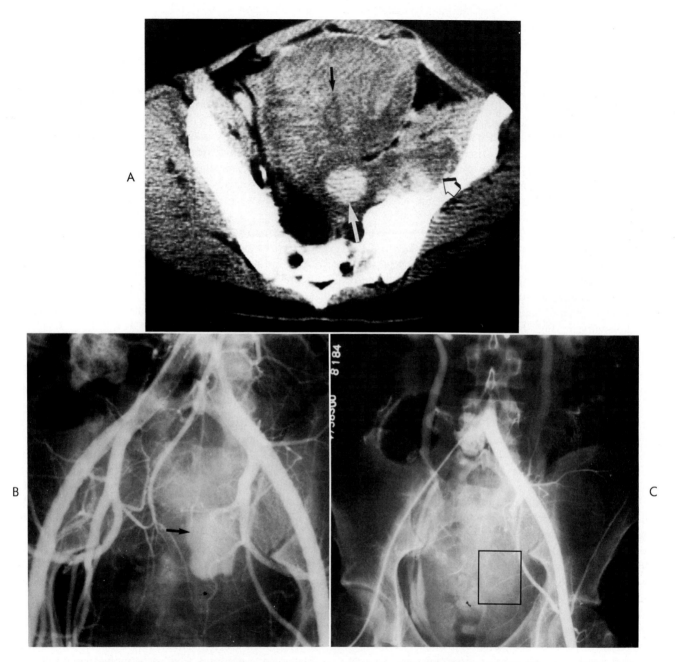

Fig. 6-41. A, Young male who sustained a stab wound to the pelvis. Contrast-enhanced CT scan of the pelvis reveals a large soft tissue density area *(small dark arrow)*, which is a hematoma. A smaller hematoma extends along the left iliac fossa *(open arrow)*. The round dense mass posterior to the pelvic hematoma is a contrast-opacified pseudo-aneurysm from a branch of the left internal iliac artery *(large white arrow)*. **B,** A pelvic angiogram via a right femoral artery approach shows the same large pseudo-aneurysm containing extravasated contrast material *(dark arrow)*. **C,** Post-embolization angiogram of the left iliac artery, which was embolized with coils *(inside box)*. No evidence of extravasation or pseudo-aneurysm is seen. The patient required no subsequent surgery or intervention.

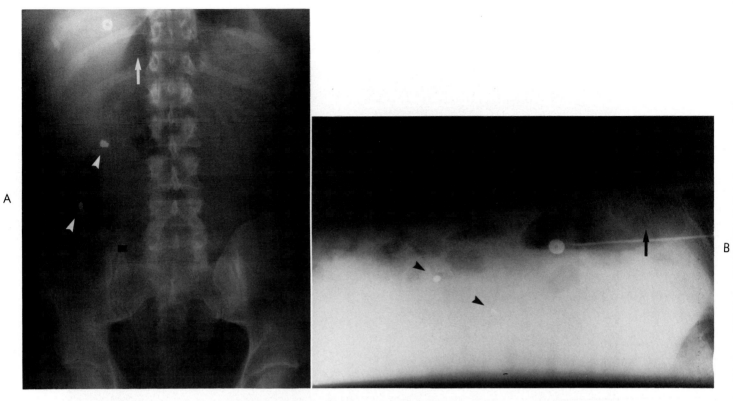

Fig. 6-42. Plain radiographs of abdomen demonstrating trajectory of bullet following gunshot wound. **A,** Supine radiograph demonstrates trajectory of major and minor bullet fragments *(arrowheads)*. Note free air within lesser sac *(vertical arrow)*. **B,** Cross-table radiograph permits localization of bullet fragments *(arrowheads)* in the AP plane. Note free air underlying anterior abdominal wall *(vertical arrow)*. No comment can be made regarding associated organ injury. (See also Fig. 6-44). (Courtesy Walter S Tan, MD.)

The role of the CT scan in penetrating trauma has been questioned because of its relative insensitivity to small perforations of hollow viscera although addition of oral and intravenous contrast material does improve this sensitivity. The CT scan is an excellent imaging modality for assessing penetrating wounds of the flank and back since retroperitoneal structures are well visualized. Meyer et al.[144] in a study of 205 patients with stab wounds to the back found the CT scan an excellent means of evaluating these injuries with a sensitivity of 89% and overall accuracy of 98%. Kelly et al.[145] suggest the initial use of the nonenhanced CT scan to detect bowel wall injuries followed by the addition of oral and intravenous contrast to detect other injuries; however, this has not become standard practice at this point. The "triple contrast" scan using oral, intravenous, and barium contrast enhances the accuracy of a CT scan in the detection of penetrating injuries by demonstrating extravasation of contrast material from a perforated colon.[146,147]

Shotgun wounds. Shotgun wounds can vary in severity from devastating at short range to relatively benign at long range. Clearly, the former group require surgical repair of the extensive injuries produced. The diagnostic difficulty arises in the latter group in trying to determine whether the

peritoneum has been penetrated and whether visceral injury, primarily bowel perforation, has occurred. Attempts to localize pellets intraperitoneally with plain radiographs of the abdomen can be a frustrating experience since the abdominal surface is rounded and technical variations on successive radiographs may produce confusion (Fig. 6-45). Reliance on clinical examination entails a substantial delay before signs of peritoneal irritation occur. Diagnostic peritoneal lavage, using the stringent criteria for penetrating wounds, will detect the vast majority of cases of peritoneal penetration, but not all of these patients will have visceral injury or require surgical treatment. In addition, the lavage should be performed at least 3 hours after injury in order for the lavage fluid WBC count to be reliable. The CT scan can anatomically localize intra-abdominal pellets with great precision and in many cases reveals the presence and extent of both intraperitoneal and retroperitoneal injuries although the presence of metallic fragments producing streak artifacts tends to limit the technical quality of the scan.

PEDIATRIC TRAUMA

While the mechanisms of abdominal injury in children are essentially the same as in adults, there are several im-

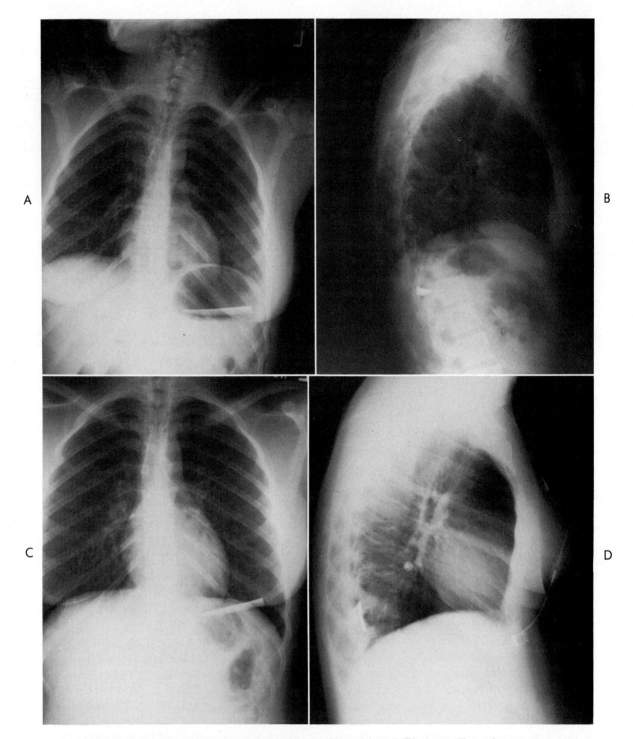

Fig. 6-43. Localization of stab wound. Initial PA **(A)** and lateral **(B)** chest radiographs suggest a stab wound localized to the left upper quadrant of the abdomen, despite the absence of a pneumoperitoneum. Repeat PA **(C)** and lateral **(D)** chest radiographs confirm and localize a stab wound to the left lower hemithorax, despite the absence of a pneumothorax. (See Fig. 6-44 regarding the role of the CT scan.) (Courtesy A Melinda Liller, MD.)

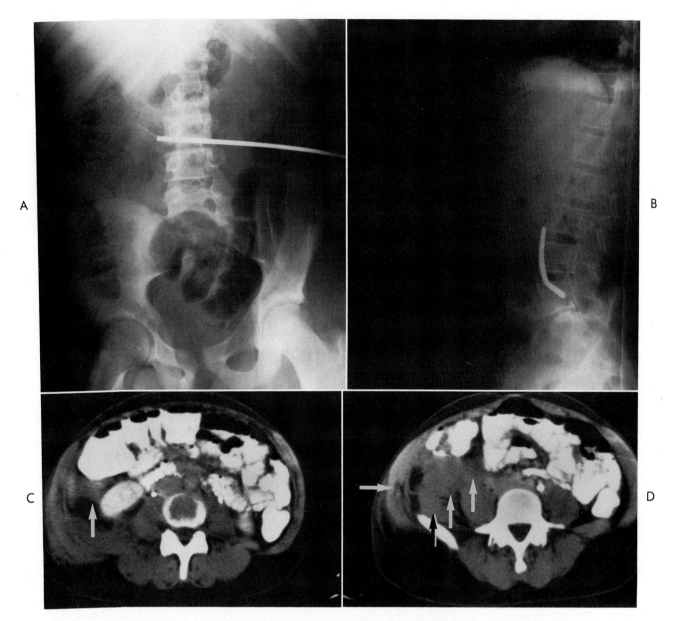

Fig. 6-44. Role of the CT scan in evaluating penetrating abdominal trauma. **A,** Initial supine radiograph of abdomen demonstrates stab wound in the left flank below the left renal shadow. **B,** Cross-table lateral radiograph raises questions of vascular and ureteral injury. IVP, aortogram, and inferior vena cavogram were negative. In another patient, CT scan **(C)** at level of inferior pole of right kidney and CT scan **(D)** below inferior pole of right kidney demonstrate track of penetrating injury *(horizontal arrow)* and a hematoma in the pararenal space *(vertical arrows)* and confirm integrity of the right kidney and inferior vena cava. The CT scan provides more information regarding the extent of injury than plain radiographs and often obviates the necessity for other interventional studies to exclude the presence of organ injury. (Courtesy Joseph J Porada, MD.)

portant differences that should be noted. First, the vast majority of traumatic abdominal injuries in children are due to blunt trauma, and co-existent neurologic and orthopedic injury is very common. Furthermore, the treating physician must always consider the possibility of nonaccidental trauma (NAT) or neglect in every case of pediatric trauma, and a careful assessment of the family situation should be made before releasing children to their families. When suspicion of NAT is high, a skeletal survey should be part of the diagnostic workup.

Certain anatomic variables in children result in greater exposure of upper abdominal organs to trauma. Both the liver and spleen lie relatively lower in the abdomen than in adults and the greater compliance of the rib cage results in

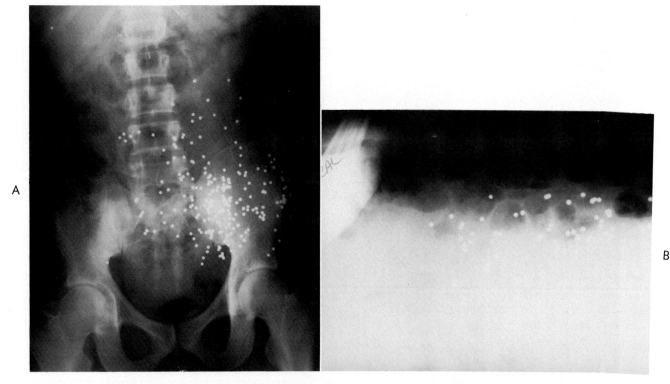

Fig. 6-45. Localization of shotgun pellets. **A,** Supine radiograph of abdomen demonstrates multiple shotgun pellets in a single plane. **B,** Cross-table radiograph of abdomen permits limited pellet localization in the AP plane. No comment can be made regarding associated organ injury. (See also Fig. 6-44.) (Courtesy A Melinda Liller, MD.)

frequent injury to these organs without overlying rib fractures. Conversely, organ injury due to puncture by rib fragments is less common than in adults.

Because of limited verbal skills and the frequent co-existence of head injury in injured children, physical examination is often less reliable in this group than in adults. Consequently, diagnostic peritoneal lavage (DPL) has been commonly employed in some centers to detect intraperitoneal injury in children. Several series report considerable success with DPL in children, demonstrating a diagnostic accuracy of 98.6% with only 0.4% false negativity.[148] However, Powell et al[73] note that the high incidence of unnecessary laparotomy (42% in the series) and its attendant cost and complications in a pediatric trauma population makes exclusive reliance on peritoneal lavage in children unwise.

Several studies have assessed the role of the CT scan in pediatric trauma and found it to be a highly sensitive technique for detecting injuries but less useful in terms of determining which specific injuries required surgery as opposed to observation.[39,81,149-151] Because motion artifact is common in children undergoing a CT scan, sedation must often be used, and there is an inherent risk of respiratory depression and hypotension in patients who may be hypovolemic or head injured. Children who are sedated and

who leave the emergency department for diagnostic tests must be carefully monitored at all times. The latest generation CT scanners, with extremely rapid scan times, should faciltate obtaining an abdominal CT scan in pediatric patients.

Filiatrault et al.[73] have reported excellent success in using ultrasonography in conjunction with intravenous pyelography, when indicated, as the initial imaging modality in pediatric trauma. However, they did not compare the accuracy of ultrasonography with the other imaging modalities. Ultrasonography has the advantage of portability, with the ability to detect hemoperitoneum and injury involving most solid viscera with considerable accuracy and can usually be performed without the sedation requirements needed for either a CT scan or peritoneal lavage. However, ultrasonography is subject to technical limitations discussed previously. Babcock and Kaufman[151] reported higher accuracy with the CT scan in children compared to ultrasonography. However, because of cost differential, portability of the ultrasonographic equipment, and ease of the examination, they prefered ultrasonography as the initial examination, reserving the CT scan for cases in which greater anatomic detail was desired or in which ultrasonographic examination was technically difficult.[151] However, despite the advantages of ultrasonography, the

CT scan is emerging as the procedure of choice for diagnosing intra-abdominal injury in stable pediatric patients.

SUMMARY

Both blunt and penetrating abdominal injuries are common in our society. Emergency physicians are often the first to encounter patients with such injuries, and they must be thoroughly familiar with all diagnostic modalities applicable in treating abdominal trauma. Any experienced trauma physician has learned to treat abdominal trauma with respect, as the physical signs of injury may be misleading and apparently stable patients may deteriorate precipitously.

Over the past 20 years, tremendous strides have been made in improving our ability to accurately distinguish patients with serious injury from those without. While diagnostic peritoneal lavage (DPL) continues to be an excellent method for detecting abdominal injury, a more precise definition of the extent of injury is possible by the use of the CT scan, provided careful attention is paid to correct technique and patient preparation and stability. This is particularly relevant in an era in which nonoperative management of certain intra-abdominal injuries has become more commonplace. As CT technology advances and further experience with its use in abdominal trauma occurs, the "occult" abdominal injury may well become more obsolete.

Clinicians must not only be familiar with the imaging modalities available but must also carefully consider the clinical status of the patient before undertaking any investigation. Patients leaving the emergency department for diagnostic tests must be accompanied by qualified personnel and must be continually monitored and re-evaluated to avoid unnecessary adverse outcomes.

ACKNOWLEDGEMENT

We are indebted to Dr. Peter E. Doris, M.D., for providing some of the radiographs in this chapter.

REFERENCES

1. Budnick LD, Chaiken BP: The probability of dying of injuries by the year 2000, *JAMA* 254:3350, 1985.
2. Ward RE: Study and management of blunt trauma in the immediate post-impact period, *Radiol Clin North Am* 19:3, 1981.
3. Strauch DO: Clinical findings in abdominal trauma, *Radiol Clin North Am* 11:555, 1973.
4. McClellan BA, Hanna SS, Montoya DR et al: Analysis of peritoneal lavage parameters in blunt abdominal trauma, *J Trauma* 25:393, 1985.
5. Anderson CB, Ballinger WF: In Zuidema GD, Rutherford RB, and Ballinger WF, eds: *The management of trauma*, ed 4, Philadelphia, 1985, WB Saunders.
6. Federle MP, Crass RA, Jeffrey RB et al: Computed tomography in blunt abdominal trauma, *Arch Surg* 117:645, 1982.
7. Foley RW, Harris LS, and Pilcher DB: Abdominal injuries in automobile accidents: review of care of fatally injured patients, *J Trauma* 17:611, 1977.
8. American College of Surgeons: *Advanced Trauma Life Support Manual*, 1981, Committee on Trauma.
9. Shah R, Max MH, and Flint LM: Negative laparotomy: mortality and morbidity among 100 patients, *Am Surg* 188:150, 1978.
10. Parvin S, Smith DE, Asher M et al: Effectiveness of peritoneal lavage in blunt abdominal trauma, *Ann Surg* 181:255, 1975.
11. Olsen WR, Redman HC, and Hildreth DH: Quantitative peritoneal lavage in blunt abdominal trauma, *Arch Surg* 104:536, 1972.
12. Powell DC, Bivins BA, and Bell RM: Diagnostic peritoneal lavage, *Surg Gynecol Obstet* 155:257-64, 1982.
13. Rizzo MJ, Federle MP, and Griffiths BG: Bowel and mesenteric injury following blunt abdominal trauma: evaluation with CT, *Radiology* 173:143, 1989.
14. Takahashi M, Maemura K, Sawada Y et al: Hyperamylasemia in critically injured patients, *J Trauma* 20:951, 1980.
15. Moretz JA, Campbell DP, Parker DE et al: Significance of serum amylase level in evaluating pancreatic trauma, *Am J Surg* 130:739, 1975.
16. Peterson SR, Sheldon GF: Morbidity of a negative finding at laparotomy in abdominal trauma, *Surg Gynecol Obstet* 149:23, 1979.
17. Lowe RJ, Boyd DR, Folk FA, et al: The negative laparotomy for abdominal trauma, *J Trauma* 12:853, 1972.
18. Davis JJ, Cohn I, and Nance FC: Diagnosis and management of blunt abdominal trauma, *Ann Surg* 183:672, 1976.
19. Olsen WR, Hildreth DH: Abdominal paracentesis and peritoneal lavage in blunt abdominal trauma, *J Trauma* 11:824, 1971.
20. Root HD, Hauser CW, McKinley CR et al: Diagnostic peritoneal lavage, *Surgery* 57:633, 1965.
21. Strum JT, Cicero JJ, and Perry JF: Peritoneal lavage for the diagnosis of abdominal visceral injury, *Am J Emerg Med* 2:246, 1984.
22. Fischer RP, Beverlin BC, Engrav LH et al: Diagnostic peritoneal lavage: fourteen years and 2,586 patients later, *Am J Surg* 136:701, 1978.
23. Gumbert JL, Froderman SE, and Marcho JP: Diagnostic peritoneal lavage in blunt abdominal trauma, *Ann Surg* 165:70, 1967.
24. Freeman T, Fisher RP: The inadequacy of peritoneal lavage in diagnosing acute diaphragmatic rupture, *J Trauma* 16:538, 1976.
25. Hubbard SG, Bivins BA, Sachatello CR et al: Diagnostic errors with peritoneal lavage in patients with pelvic fractures, *Arch Surg* 114:844, 1979.
26. Ein SE, Shandling B, Simpson JS et al: The morbidity and mortality of splenectomy in childhood, *Ann Surg* 185:307, 1976.
27. Oakes DD, Charters AC: Changing concepts in the management of splenic trauma, *Surg Gynecol Obstet* 153:181, 1981.
28. Gruenberg JC, Horan DP: Delayed splenic rupture: the phoenix, *J Trauma* 23:150, 1983.
29. Pearl RH, Wesson DE, Spence LJ et al: Splenic injury: a 5-year update with improved results and changing criteria for conservative management, *J Pediatr Surg* 24:121, 1989.
30. Kakasseril JS, Stewart D, Cox JA et al: Changing treatment of pediatric splenic trauma, *Arch Surg* 117:758, 1982.
31. Soderstrom CA, DuPriest RW, and Cowley RA: Pitfalls of peritoneal lavage in blunt abdominal trauma, *Surg Gynecol Obstet* 151:513, 1980.
32. Mahon PA, Sutton JE: Nonoperative management of adult splenic injury due to blunt trauma: a warning, *Am J Surg* 149:718, 1985.
33. Malangoni MA, Levine AW, Droege EA et al: Management of injury to the spleen in adults: results of early operation and observation, *Ann Surg* 200:702, 1984.
34. Bryant LR, Wiot JF, and Kloecker RJ: A study of the factors affecting the incidence and duration of postoperative pneumoperitoneum, *Surg Gynecol Obstet* 117:145, 1963.
35. Miller RE, Nelson SW: The roentgenologic demonstration of tiny amounts of free intraperitoneal gas: experimental and clinical studies, *AJR* 112:574, 1971.
36. Mucha P, Farnell MB: Analysis of pelvic fracture management, *J Trauma* 24:379, 1984.
37. Fisher RG, Hadlock F, and Ben-Menachem Y: Laceration of the thoracic aorta and brachiocephalic arteries by blunt trauma: report of 54 cases and review of the literature, *Radiol Clin North Am* 19:91, 1981.
38. Burrell M, Toffler R, Lowman R: Blunt trauma to the abdomen and

gastrointestinal tract: plain films and contrast study, *Radiol Clin North Am* 11:561, 1973.

39. Bulas DI, Taylor GA, and Eichelberger MR: The value of CT in detecting bowel perforation in children after blunt abdominal trauma, *AJR* 153:561, 1989.

40. Blaisdell FW, Trunkey DD: Abdominal trauma, In Blaisdell FW, Trunkey DD, eds: *Trauma management,* vol 1, New York, 1982, Thieme Stratton.

41. Kuligowska E, Mueller PR, Simeone JF et al: Ultrasound in upper abdominal trauma, *Semin Roentgenol* 19:281, 1984.

42. Sigel B, Coehlo JCU, Spigos DG et al: Ultrasonography of blood during stasis and coagulation, *Invest Radiol* 16:71, 1981.

43. Coehlo JCU, Sigel B, Ryva JC et al: B-mode sonography of blood clots, *J Clin Ultrasound* 10:323, 1982.

44. Sigel B, Coehlo JCU, Schade SG et al: Effect of plasma proteins and temperature on echogenicity of blood, *Invest Radiol* 17:29, 1982.

45. Gruessner R, Mentges B, Duber C et al: Sonography vs. peritoneal lavage in blunt abdominal trauma, *J Trauma* 29:242, 1989.

46. Hertzanu Y, Mendelsohn D: Delayed splenic rupture,: a true entity, *Clin Radiol* 35:393, 1984.

47. Gilday DL, Alderson PO: Scintigraphic evaluation of liver and spleen injury, *Semin Nucl Med* 4:357, 1974.

48. Solheim K, Nerdrum HJ: Radionuclide imaging of splenic laceration and trauma, *Clin Nucl Med* 4:528, 1979.

49. McConnell BJ, McConnell RW, and Guiberteau MJ: Radionuclide imaging in blunt trauma, *Radiol Clin North Am* 19:37, 1981.

50. Rosenberger A, Adler OB, and Troupin RH: *Trauma imaging in the thorax and abdomen,* Chicago, 1987, Year Book Medical Publishers.

51. Fischer KC, Eralkis A, Rossello P et al: Scintigraphy in the followup of pediatric splenic trauma treated without surgery, *J Nucl Med* 19:3, 1978.

52. Mishalany HG, Miller JH, and Wooley MM: Radioisotope spleen scan in patients with splenic injury, *Arch Surg* 117:1147, 1982.

53. Alavi A: Detection of gastrointestinal bleeding with 99mTc sulfur colloid, *Semin Nucl Med* 12:126-38, 1982.

54. Ang JGP, Hanslits ML, Clark RA et al: Computed tomography of abdominal and pelvic trauma, *J Emerg Med* 3:311, 1985.

55. Pertzman AB, Makaroun MS, Slasky BS et al: Prospective study of computed tomography in initial management of blunt abdominal trauma, *J Trauma* 26:585, 1986.

56. Goldstein AS, Sclafani SJA, Kupferstein NH et al: The diagnostic superiority of computerized tomography, *J Trauma* 25:938, 1985.

57. Meyer DM, Thal ER, Weigelt JA et al: Evaluation of computed tomography and diagnostic peritoneal lavage in blunt abdominal trauma, *J Trauma* 29:1168, 1989.

58. Fabian TC, Mangiante EC, White TJ et al: A prospective study of 91 patients undergoing both computed tomography and peritoneal lavage following blunt abdominal trauma, *J Trauma* 26:602, 1986.

59. Marx JA, Moore EE, Jorden RC et al: Limitations of computed tomography in the evaluation of acute abdominal trauma: a prospective comparison with diagnostic peritoneal lavage, *J Trauma* 25:933, 1985.

60. Kearney PA, Vahey T, Burney RE et al: Computed tomography and diagnostic peritoneal lavage in blunt abdominal trauma: their combined role, *Arch Surg* 124:344, 1989.

61. Cook DE, Walsh JW, Vick CW et al: Upper abdominal trauma: pitfalls in CT diagnosis, *Radiology* 159:65, 1986.

62. Berg BC: Complementary roles of radionuclide and computed tomographic imaging in evaluating trauma, *Semin Nucl Med* 13:86, 1983.

63. Cohen JM, Weinreb JC, and Maravilla KR: Fluid collections in the intraperitoneal and retroperitoneal spaces: comparison of MR and CT, *Radiology* 155:705, 1985.

64. Federle MP, Jeffrey RB: Hemoperitoneum studied by computed tomography, *Radiology* 148:187, 1983.

65. Kane NM, Dorfman GS, and Cronan JJ: Efficacy of CT following peritoneal lavage in abdominal trauma, *J Cat* 11:998, 1987.

66. Livingston CD, Sirinek KR, Levine BA et al: Traumatic splenic injury: its management in a patient population with a high incidence of associated injury, *Arch Surg* 117:670, 1982.

67. Mirvis SE, Whitley NO, and Gens DR: Blunt splenic trauma in adults: CT classification and correlation with prognosis and treatment, *Radiology* 171:33, 1989.

68. Sziklas JJ, Spencer RP, and Rosenberg RJ: Delayed splenic rupture: a suggestion for predictive monitoring, *J Nucl Med* 26:609, 1985.

69. Olsen WR, Polley TZ: A second look at delayed splenic rupture, *Arch Surg* 112:422, 1977.

70. Taylor CR, Rosenfield AT: Limitations of computed tomography in the recognition of delayed splenic rupture, *J Cat* 8:1205, 1984.

71. Fagleman D, Hertz MA, and Ross AS: Delayed development of splenic subcapsular hematoma: CT evaluation, *J Cat* 9:815, 1985.

72. Mall JC, Kaiser JA: CT diagnosis of splenic laceration, *AJR* 134:265, 1980.

73. Filiatrault D, Longpre D, Patriquin H et al: Investigation of childhood blunt abdominal trauma: a practical approach using ultrasound as the initial diagnostic modality, *Pediatr Radiol* 17:373, 1987.

74. Foley LC, Teele RL: Ultrasound of epigastric injuries after blunt trauma, *AJR* 132:593, 1979.

75. Osborne DJ, Glickman MG, Grnja V et al: The role of angiography in abdominal non-renal trauma, *Radiol Clin North Am* 11:579, 1973.

76. Castaneda-Zuniga WR, Hammerschmidt DE, Snachez R et al: Non-surgical splenectomy, *AJR* 129:805, 1977.

77. Korobkin M, Moss AA, Callen PW et al: Computed tomography of subcapsular splenic hematoma, *Radiology* 129:441, 1978.

78. Jeffrey RB, Laing FC et al: Computed tomography of splenic trauma, *Radiology* 141:729, 1981.

79. Buntain WL, Gould HR, and Maull KI: Predictability of splenic salvage by computed tomography, *J Trauma* 28:24, 1988.

80. Resciniti A, Fink MP, Raptopoulos V et al: Nonoperative treatment of adult splenic trauma: development of a computed tomographic scoring system that detects appropriate candidates for expectant management, *J Trauma* 28:828, 1988.

81. Brick SH, Taylor GA, Potter BM et al: Hepatic and splenic injury in children: the role for CT in the decision for laparotomy, *Radiology* 165:643, 1987.

82. Federle MP, Griffiths B, Minagi H et al: Splenic trauma: evaluation with CT, *Radiology* 162:69, 1987.

83. Federle MP: Computed tomography of blunt abdominal trauma, *Radiol Clin North Am* 21:461, 1983.

84. Kaufman RA, Towbin R, Babcock DS et al: Upper abdominal trauma in children: imaging evaluation, *AJR* 142:449, 1984.

85. Glazer GM, Axel L, Goldberg HI et al: Dynamic CT of the normal spleen, *AJR* 137:343, 1981.

86. Mirvis SE, Whitley NO, Vainwright JR et al: Blunt hepatic trauma in adults: CT-based classification and correlation with prognosis and treatment, *Radiology* 171:27, 1989.

87. Meyer AA, Crass RA, and Lim RC Jr: Selective non-operative management of blunt liver injury using computed tomography, *Arch Surg* 120:550, 1985.

88. Moon KL, Federle MP: Computed tomography in hepatic trauma, *AJR* 141:309, 1983.

89. Jeffrey RB Jr: CT diagnosis of blunt hepatic and splenic injuries: a look to the future, *Radiology* 171:17, 1989.

90. Feliciano DV, Pachter HL: Hepatic trauma revisited, *Curr Probl Surg* 26:49, 1989.

91. Northrup WF, Simmons RI: Pancreatic trauma: a review, *Surgery* 71:27, 1972.

92. Feliciano DV, Martin TD, Cruise PA et al: Management of combined pancreatoduodenal injuries, *Ann Surg* 205:673, 1987.

93. Stone HH, Fabian TC, Satiani B et al: Experiences in the management of pancreatic trauma, *J Trauma* 21:257, 1981.

94. Sims EH, Mandal AK, Schlater T et al: Factors affecting outcome in pancreatic trauma, *J Trauma* 24:125, 1984.

95. Smego DR, Richardson D, and Flint LM: Determinants of outcome in pancreatic trauma, *J Trauma* 25:771, 1985.

96. Olsen WR: The serum amylase in blunt abdominal trauma, *J Trauma* 13:200, 1973.

97. Alyono D, Perry F: The value of quantitative cell count and amylase activity of peritoneal lavage fluid, *J Trauma* 21:345, 1981.

98. Jeffrey RB Jr, Federle MP, and Crass RA: Computed tomography of pancreatic trauma, *Radiology* 147:491, 1983.

99. Bozymski EM, Orlando RC, and Holt JW III: Traumatic disruption of the pancreatic duct demonstrated by endoscopic retrograde pancreatography, *J Trauma* 21:244, 1981.

100. Levison MA, Petersen SR, Sheldon GF et al: Duodenal trauma: experience of a trauma center, *J Trauma* 24:475, 1984.

101. Shorr RM, Greaney GC, and Donovan AJ: Injuries of the duodenum, *Am J Surg* 154:8, 1987.

102. Schenck WG, Lonchya V, and Moylan JA: Perforation of the jejunum from blunt abdominal trauma, *J Trauma* 23:54, 1983.

103. Kelly G, Norton L, Moore G et al: The continuing challenge of duodenal injuries, *J Trauma* 18:160, 1978.

104. Harris CR: Blunt abdominal trauma causing jejunal rupture, *Ann Emerg Med* 14:916, 1985.

105. Robbs JV, Moore SW, and Pillay SP: Blunt abdominal trauma with jejunal injury: a review, *J Trauma* 20:308, 1980.

106. Burney RE, Mueller GL, Coon WW et al: Diagnosis of isolated small bowel injury following blunt abdominal trauma, *Ann Emerg Med* 12:71, 1983.

107. Engrav LM, Benjamin CI, Strate RG et al: Diagnostic peritoneal lavage in blunt abdominal trauma, *J Trauma* 15:854, 1975.

108. Corley RD, Norcross WJ, Shoemaker WC et al: Injuries to the duodenum: a report of 98 cases, *Ann Surg* 181:92, 1975.

109. Snyder WH III, Weigelt JA, Watkins WL et al: The surgical management of duodenal trauma, *Arch Surg* 115:422, 1980.

110. Fischer RP, Miller-Crotchett P, and Reed RL: Gastrointestinal disruption: the hazard of nonoperative management in adults with blunt abdominal injury, *J Trauma* 28:1445, 1988.

111. Buckman RF, Piano G, Dunham CM et al: Major bowel and diaphragmatic injuries associated with blunt spleen or liver rupture, *J Trauma* 28:1317, 1988.

112. Meyer DM, Thal ER, Weigelt JA et al: Evaluation of computed tomography and diagnostic peritoneal lavage in blunt abdominal trauma, *J Trauma* 29:1168, 1989.

113. Kearney PA, Vahey T, Burney RE et al: Computed tomography and diagnostic peritoneal lavage in blunt abdominal trauma, *Arch Surg* 124:344, 1989.

114. Rizzo MJ, Federle MP, and Griffiths BG: Bowel and mesenteric injury following abdominal trauma: evaluation with CT, *Radiology* 173:143, 1989.

115. Orwig D, Federle MP: Localized clotted blood as evidence of visceral trauma on CT: the sentinel clot sign, *AJR* 153:747, 1989.

116. Waldschmidt ML, Laws HL: Injuries of the diaphragm, *J Trauma* 20:587, 1980.

117. Jarrett F, Bernhardt LC: Right-sided diaphragmatic injury: rarity or overlooked diagnosis, *Arch Surg* 113:737, 1978.

118. Ward RE, Flynn TC, and Clark WF: Diaphragmatic disruption secondary to blunt abdominal trauma, *J Trauma* 21:35, 1981.

119. Leaman P: Rupture of the right hemidiaphragm due to blunt trauma, *Ann Emerg Med* 12:351, 1983.

120. Rodriguez-Morales G, Rodriguez A, and Shatney CH: Acute rupture of the diaphragm in blunt trauma: analysis of 60 patients, *J Trauma* 26:438, 1986.

121. Shea L, Graham AD, Fletcher JC et al: Diaphragmatic injury: a method for early diagnosis, *J Trauma* 22:539, 1982.

122. Payne JH, Yellin AE: Traumatic diaphragmatic hernia, *Arch Surg* 117:18, 1982.

123. Saber WL, Moore EE, Hopeman AR et al: Delayed presentation of traumatic diaphragmatic hernia, *J Emerg Med* 4:1, 1986.

124. Feliciano DV, Cruse PA, Mattox KL et al: Delayed diagnosis of injuries to the diaphragm after penetrating wounds, *J Trauma* 28:1135, 1988.

125. Miller L, Bennett EV Jr, Root D et al: Management of penetrating and blunt diaphragmatic injury, *J Trauma* 24:403, 1984.

127. Freeman T, Fisher RP: The inadequacy of peritoneal lavage in diagnosing acute diaphragmatic rupture, *J Trauma* 16:358, 1976.

128. Perlman SJ, Rogers LF, Mintzer RA et al: Abnormal course of nasogastric tube in traumatic rupture of left hemidiaphragm, *AJR* 142:85, 1984.

129. Ordog GJ, Wassenberger J, and Balasubramaniam S: Tension gastrothorax complicating post-traumatic rupture of the diaphragm, *Am J Emerg Med* 2:219, 1984.

130. Weil PH: Management of retroperitoneal trauma, *Curr Prob Surg* 20:545, 1983.

131. Grieco JG, Perry JF: Retroperitoneal hematoma following trauma: its clinical importance, *J Trauma* 20:733, 1980.

133. Maull KI, Sachatello CR: Current management of pelvic fractures: a combined surgical-angiographic approach to hemorrhage, *South Med J* 69:1285, 1976.

134. Evers BM, Cryer HM, Miller FB: Pelvic fracture hemorrhage: priorities in management, *Arch Surg* 124:422, 1989.

135. Flint LM, Brown A, Richardson JD et al: Definitive control of bleeding from severe pelvic fractures, *Am Surg* 189:709, 1979.

136. Nance FC, Wennar MH, Johnson LW et al: Surgical judgement in the management of penetrating wounds of the abdomen: experience with 2212 patients, *Ann Surg* 179:639, 1974.

137. Zubkowski R, Nallathambi M, Ivatury R et al: Selective conservatism in abdominal stab wounds: the efficacy of serial abdominal examination, *J Trauma* 28:1665, 1988.

138. Lee WC, Uddo JF, and Nance FC: Surgical judgement in the management of abdominal stab wounds, *Ann Surg* 199:549, 1984.

139. Demetriades D, Rabinowitz B, Sofianos C et al: The management of penetrating injuries of the back: a prospective study of 230 patients, *Ann Surg* 207:72, 1987.

140. Peck JJ, Berne TV: Posterior abdominal stab wounds, *J Trauma* 21:298, 1981.

141. McAlvanah MJ, Shaftan GW: Selective conservativism in penetrating abdominal wounds: a continuing reappraisal, *J Trauma* 18:206, 1978.

142. Aragon GE, Eiseman B: Abdominal stab wounds: evaluation of sinography, *J Trauma* 16:792, 1976.

143. Rehm CG, Sherman R, and Hinz TW: The role of CT scan in evaluation for laparotomy in patients with stab wounds of the abdomen, *J Trauma* 29:446, 1989.

144. Meyer DM, Thal ER, Weigelt JA et al: The role of abdominal CT in the evaluation of stab wounds to the back, *J Trauma* 29:1226, 1989.

145. Kelly J, Rastopoulos V, Davidoff A et al: The value of non-contrast-enhanced CT in blunt abdominal trauma, *AJR* 152:41, 1989.

146. Hauser CJ, Huprich JE, Bosco P et al: Triple-contrast computed tomography in the evaluation of penetrating posterior abdominal injuries, *Arch Surg* 122:1112, 1987.

147. Phillips T, Sclafani SJA, Goldstein A et al: Use of the contrast-enhanced CT-enema in the management of penetrating trauma to the flank and back, *J Trauma* 26:601, 1986.

148. Drew R, Perry JF, and Fischer RP: The expediency of peritoneal lavage for blunt trauma in children, *Surg Gynecol Obstet* 145:885, 1977.

149. Karp MP, Cooney DR, Berger PE et al: The role of computed to-mography in the evaluation of blunt abdominal trauma in children, *J Pediatr Surg* 16:316, 1981.

150. Taylor GA, Fallat ME, Potter BM et al: The role of computed to-mography in blunt abdominal trauma in children, *J Trauma* 28:1660-4, 1988.

151. Babcock DS, Kaufman RA: Ultrasonography and computed tomography in the evaluation of the acutely ill pediatric patient, *Radiol Clin North Am* 21:527, 1983.

C H A P T E R 7

Genitourinary Trauma

Ann L. Harwood-Nuss
Carl M. Sandler

Approximately 10% of all traumatic injuries involve the genitourinary tract, most often the kidney. The majority of renal injuries occur in association with blunt multisystem trauma in males younger than 40 years, are limited in extent, and do not require surgical intervention. Although genitourinary trauma is seldom the cause of death, there is potential for serious morbidity if such injuries are missed. Accurate radiographic staging defines the presence and extent of injury and permits selective management. The emergency evaluation of genitourinary trauma must be integrated into the overall management of the trauma patient.

In subsequent sections of this chapter, specific organ injuries (kidney, ureter, bladder, and urethra) will be distinguished. But it must be emphasized that the urinary tract is continuous, with significant overlap of signs and symptoms of injury to both the upper and lower portions. Significant injuries usually have a common denominator—vi-

olent blunt or penetrating trauma. Multiple radiographic studies may be necessary to fully evaluate and stage genitourinary system injuries. Recommendations for the order and timing of imaging studies are based principally on the patient's clinical status—stable vs. unstable. In the critically injured patient, complex and time-consuming radiographic studies are usually contraindicated unless therapy is incorporated into the study (e.g., embolization). The evaluation of the genitourinary tract is a lower priority than the abdomen, chest, or head in such patients.[1] Even when the luxury of an orderly evaluation is available, what does not exist is a universal set of recommendations that are based on scientific study. Our recommendations on the order of studies are based on experience and currently available literature. It is also clear that there is no universal imaging policy that works in all cases or even in all institutions.[2] We have attempted to provide recommendations based on acceptable preferences.

RENAL TRAUMA
Anatomy

The kidney is located high in the retroperitoneum, bounded by the diaphragm superiorly, abdominal muscles laterally, abdominal viscera anteriorly, lumbar quadrate muscle and the twelfth rib posteriorly, and the psoas muscle and second lumbar vertebra medially. The kidney is also in close approximation to the lung and pleura. The anterior surface of the kidney is crossed by the sixth to the tenth ribs, and the posterior surface is crossed by the eleventh and twelfth ribs. Both kidneys are highly mobile. The kidneys are invested in the perinephric fascia that may act as effective wall to tamponade hemorrhage. Trauma to the right side of the abdomen may injure the second portion of the duodenum, the right lobe of the liver, and the hepatic flexure of the right colon. On the left side of the abdomen, the stomach, pancreas, spleen, and splenic flexure of the left side of the colon may be injured.[3] As result of these anatomic relations, associated injuries to these organs are common and should be anticipated, especially with penetrating trauma.

Mechanism of injury

Blunt trauma causes 94% of all renal injuries, with motor vehicle, motorcycle, and auto-pedestrian accidents (75%); falls (9% to 20%); blows (5% to 15%); and sports injuries (5%) accounting for the majority of cases.[4] Penetrating wounds cause the remaining 6% of renal injuries, with gunshot wounds (4.5%) and stab wounds (1.5%) being the most common. Blunt trauma results in major renal injury in only 5% to 15% of cases. In contrast, penetrating trauma is associated with a 50% to 60% incidence of major renal injury.[2,5]

Associated injuries

Renal trauma is often accompanied by serious injury to other important structures. The incidence of associated injuries is significantly higher with penetrating trauma (80% to 90%) than with blunt renal trauma (14% to 34%).[2,5,6] Blunt trauma typically injures solid organs; spleen and liver injuries are seen in 20% of cases of blunt renal trauma.[2,5,7,8] To a lesser extent, injuries to the pancreas, bowel, chest, and central nervous system are seen. Penetrating renal trauma is associated with concomitant abdominal injury to the liver, small and large intestine, stomach, diaphragm, and chest.[2,5]

Classification of renal injuries

There is no universally accepted classification system for renal trauma. A functional classification in which the injuries are grouped according to severity and therapeutic implications is used in this discussion. One should be aware that one or more types of injury may occur in the same kidney.

Minor injuries constitute 85% of blunt renal trauma injuries. Included in this category are renal contusions (70%) and minor lacerations, including cortical disruption not involving the collecting system or deep medulla (15%). In penetrating renal trauma, about 50% of injuries are considered minor, consisting of 34% renal contusions and 17% minor lacerations.

Intermediate injuries from blunt trauma (10%) consist of deep lacerations of the renal parenchyma and segmental vascular infarcts. The majority are lacerations with parenchymal disruption involving the collecting system or deep renal medulla. A renal parenchymal laceration from blunt trauma typically transects the kidney transversely, beginning at the border of the cortex and moving into the medulla and collecting system as it increases in severity. The deeper the laceration, the greater the likelihood of major renal bleeding because the major arteries and veins are located in the central portion of the kidney. Extensive perirenal hematoma is usually present. If the collecting system is involved, extravasation is present. Surgery may be required because other serious associated injuries are common.

Major injuries compose only 5% of cases of blunt renal trauma and include the shattered or fractured kidney, renal rupture (multiple renal lacerations), renal pedicle injury,

and laceration or avulsion of the renal pelvis. Conversely, almost 50% of renal injuries from penetrating trauma are major. These injuries virtually always require surgical exploration because of either a threat to the viability of the kidney or extensive hemorrhage.

Although grouped in the major injury category of most classification systems, vascular pedicle injury and ureteropelvic junction disruption warrant separate discussions. They both are unusual injuries, may occur in the context of blunt or penetrating renal trauma, and may be particularly difficult to diagnose initially.

Vascular pedicle injury

A vascular pedicle injury involves a complete or partial tear of the renal artery or renal vein. The majority (75%) of vascular injuries are caused by blunt, multisystem trauma (deceleration falls, auto-pedestrian accidents, and direct blows to the abdomen). The remainder (25%) are due to penetrating trauma.[2]

The kidney is mobile in the retroperitoneum, and the main renal artery is anchored to the aorta. With rapid deceleration, the artery undergoes excessive stretching. The intimal layer of the artery ruptures, initiating thrombus formation, resulting in total arterial occlusion and renal ischemia. Many authorities have emphasized that hematuria may be absent with a renal vascular injury. Cass and Luxenberg[9] reported a 25% incidence of documented pedicle injury in the absence of hematuria. Conversely, Mee and McAninch[4] reported that no vascular injuries occurred without either gross hematuria or microhematuria and shock.

The initial imaging study is usually an intravenous pyelogram (IVP). Unilateral nonvisualization (absence of contrast excretion) on the IVP suggests renal artery occlusion and is an indication for either computed tomography (CT scan) or angiography. Although there are advocates for both studies, most authorities seem to favor the CT scan.[10-14] Advocates of CT scan maintain that it is faster, noninvasive, identifies other causes of nonvisualization that may not require an angiogram, and provides important information about other associated injuries.[3,9,11,13-16] Bretan et al.[3] recommends angiography only for indeterminate CT scans (most often associated with large perirenal hematoma) and suspected venous laceration. Lang et al.[12] recommends augiography for suspected arterial injuries not clarified with a CT scan, for preoperative evaluation, and for persistent bleeding where angiography may be combined with embolization. The choice of the study is often ultimately dictated by the fact that the majority (98%) of patients with renal pedicle injuries have severe multisystem trauma and are critically ill, with mortality rates of 12% to 44%.* Although pre-operative radiographic assessment is necessary because surgical exploration may miss a thrombosed artery, other more life-threatening injuries may take precedence. If the patient is unstable, prolonged

---

*References 2, 5, 9, 14, 17, 18.

imaging is contraindicated. If the patient can tolerate a brief radiographic study and revascularization is anticipated, an angiogram is recommended. Success of revascularization is reduced with time. Although the precise warm ischemia time is not known, if ischemia lasts more than 6 to 8 hours, severe tubular necrosis and dysfunction occur and long-term function is poor. Even early intervention may not result in a salvage rate of greater than 33% (with such patients experiencing a relatively poor late outcome).[17,19]

Ureteropelvic junction avulsion

Isolated avulsion of the ureteropelvic junction is rare, occurring primarily in children. The ureter is relatively fixed in the retroperitoneum and may be torn from its attachment to the renal pelvis during rapid deceleration.[20] The injury occurs primarily in children who lack retroperitoneal fat to cushion the kidney during sudden deceleration.[20] An IVP will demonstrate extravasation of contrast material. Massive extravasation, especially if the renal outline appears intact and the ureter does not fill, is strongly suggestive of a ureteropelvic junction disruption.[2,20] Gross extravasation of urine may be seen with a deep medullary laceration, but it may also reflect a collecting system disruption or a ureteropelvic junction avulsion. A CT scan will further clarify the extent of the injury. Avulsion of the ureteropelvic junction may occur in association with renal vascular pedicle injury.

Blunt renal trauma

Blunt renal trauma constitutes 94% of all renal injuries in most study series. Associated injuries are the principal determinants of morbidity and mortality.[8] Although most patients with renal trauma have abdominal (69%) or flank tenderness (91%), these symptoms do not identify those most likely to have sustained major renal trauma.[4] A flank mass is suggestive of severe renal hemorrhage or extravasation. However, pre-existing renal disease should also be considered because it is present in up to 25% of children with renal trauma.[21]

Hematuria. Hematuria is the single best indicator of renal injury and is present in about 95% of all cases of blunt renal trauma. Hematuria may be reliably detected with either microscopic analysis or dipstick test method.[22,23] Goldner et al.[24] compared both methods and found a wide range of microscopic hematuria for each dipstick test value. Despite this apparent discrepancy, both methods have a high degree of sensitivity and specificity for the detection of hematuria. The identification of more than 5 to 10 red blood cells (RBC)/high-power field (HPF) or a positive dipstick test result are indicative of hematuria.[22,23] Because both hemolysis and rhabdomyolysis may result in positive results for the urine dipstick test for blood, a positive dipstick result must be followed by a microscopic analysis. The presence of RBCs confirms the diagnosis of hematuria. It is generally agreed that, although the presence of hematuria is suggestive of renal injury, the degree

of hematuria does not correlate well with the severity of blunt renal trauma.[25,26] Thus, as a staging criterion, hematuria is unreliable.[4,25-27]

Indications and recommendations for imaging. A recent study by Mee and McAninch[4] found that the only clinical signs that correlated with significant blunt renal injury were (1) gross hematuria and (2) microscopic hematuria and shock (systolic blood pressure <90 mm Hg). These criteria were shown to accurately define patients for radiographic staging of blunt renal trauma. In patients who sustained blunt trauma with microhematuria and no shock, the incidence of significant renal injuries was low, with greater than 90% demonstrating renal contusions on IVP.[4,28,29] A recent study by Stalker[30] suggests that similar criteria may be safely applied to children.

Stable patient. The stable multisystem trauma patient customarily undergoes routine radiographs of the neck, chest, and pelvis. Fifty percent of patients with renal trauma have associated fractures (32%, rib fractures; 10%, pelvic fractures; and 7%, vertebral fractures). A plain abdominal scout radiograph should be obtained before any subsequent studies with contrast material are done. It may demonstrate a retroperitoneal hematoma or urinoma with obliteration of the psoas margin. In patients with a normal pulse rate and blood pressure and no history of hypotension in the prehospital phase of care, renal imaging should be obtained only for those individuals who exhibit gross hematuria. The IVP remains the screening examination of choice. Those patients with normal IVP results are not likely to have clinically significant renal injury and do not need further evaluation.[31] The IVP documents the presence of both kidneys, defines the renal parenchyma, and delineates the collecting system. It also provides a general assessment of both renal perfusion and renal function. If the IVP results are abnormal or indeterminate, a CT scan is indicated. The CT scan is the imaging technique of choice for those renal injuries thought to be extensive or incompletely assessed with an IVP.[2,14,32,33] The CT scan is the most accurate staging examination (98% to 100%) for renal trauma.[2-4,10,13-16,32,33] It is noninvasive and rapid and provides both physiologic and anatomic information. A CT scan delineates nonviable tissue, parenchymal lacerations, contusions, intrarenal and extrarenal hematomas, and extravasation.[2] It should be done with both oral and intravenous contrast materials.

In the context of blunt multisystem trauma, there appears to be wide variation between institutions regarding the next stage of evaluation. There is no doubt that, in the evaluation of an isolated renal injury resulting from blunt trauma, the CT scan is the "gold standard". However, there is debate concerning the optimal evaluation of nonrenal injuries secondary to blunt abdominal trauma. The two diagnostic tools most widely available are the abdominal CT scan and diagnostic peritoneal lavage (DPL). In the medical literature, there is some evidence that the two may be comparable in sensitivity and specificity for detecting intra-abdominal injury (97% to 98%).[34,35] Proponents of the abdominal CT scan contend that it provides more specific information about intra-abdominal and retroperitoneal injury. It allows for accurate staging and permits nonoperative management.[36]

Conversely, Marx et al.[37] maintain that the CT scan has a high incidence of false-negative results for significant abdominal injuries in both blunt and penetrating trauma. Therefore local preferences must dictate the next phase of evaluation. Either DPL or an abdominal CT scan is indicated to evaluate potential abdominal injury in the "stable" patient with head injury, altered mental status (i.e., from drugs or alcohol), neurologic injury, or in other situations in which serial abdominal radiographic examinations cannot be accurately interpreted or monitored. However, the urgency to determine the presence of intraperitoneal injury may make DPL the priority study because it can be rapidly performed in the emergency department. DPL accurately detects intraperitoneal blood, but it provides no information about the status of the kidneys. If further evaluation of the kidneys is indicated because of an abnormal IVP, a contrast-enhanced CT scan will be necessary. A prior DPL may obscure CT scan findings, but valuable information may still be obtained. If a CT scan is preferred to evaluate intra-abdominal injuries, the initial IVP is not necessary because the kidneys will be adequately evaluated at the time of the abdominal CT scan.[35,36]

Selective renal angiography is invasive and time consuming. It is indicated in the stable patient with indeterminate CT scan results if there is suspicion of a renal artery injury and anticipation for revascularization. Clinical evidence of this injury may include persistent hemorrhage manifested as an expanding flank mass and shock. Renal angiography defines parenchymal injuries, traumatic arteriovenous fistulae, thrombosis or occlusion of the main renal artery or its branches, and discontinuity of the renal parenchyma with a major renal laceration. Angiography also identifies acute renal vein occlusion, an uncommon injury that may be recognized by an enlarged kidney.[2] Although the use of angiography for renal trauma has decreased, it does provide the opportunity for selective embolization of uncontrollable renal hemorrhage (see Figs. 7-3, 7-4, and 7-6).

Ultrasonography does not identify the extent of renal injury as well as the CT scan, but it does provide information about certain renal and perirenal abnormalities. Since the reliability curve is user-dependent, in the setting of acute trauma it is not recommended as a first-line examination.

Unstable patient. In the unstable trauma patient, plain radiographs of the chest and pelvis generally are also obtained because both provide significant information in the differential diagnosis of shock. In the presence of either gross hematuria or microhematuria and shock, evaluation of the kidneys should be performed but only after the patient is stabilized to a mean arterial blood pressure of at least 80 to 90 mm Hg. The likelihood of radiographic visualization of the kidneys will be increased if the patient's mean arterial blood pressure can be maintained at a level of 80 to 90 mm Hg or greater. Below that level glomerular filtration is significantly decreased and will preclude the excretion of contrast material in visible amounts.[2] The IVP may be modified to include a one-shot radiograph, in which a bolus of 150 ml of contrast material is administered after the plain radiograph is obtained. The rapid contrast excretion may provide limited information about the status of the kidneys. If an immediate laparotomy is indicated, IVP may also be obtained at surgery if an unexpected retroperitoneal or perirenal hematoma is encountered.[6] It is important to realize that the one-shot IVP has marked limitations. Such a study is useful only if it demonstrates two normal kidneys; if abnormal kidneys are present, it rarely provides sufficient information to suggest proper therapy.

Penetrating renal trauma

Penetrating trauma to the abdomen, flank, or back results in renal injury in 6% to 15% of patients. Flank and abdominal wounds account for the most serious renal injuries, with 8% of abdominal gunshot and 6% of abdominal stab wounds resulting in renal injury.[38] Lumbar wounds are less often associated with serious renal trauma.[38,39] Anatomically, flank wounds are located between the anterior and posterior axillary lines, extending from the sixth intercostal space (ICS) to the iliac crest,[40] and lumbar wounds are located behind the posterior axillary line from the seventh ICS or tip of the scapula to the iliac crest.

In contrast to blunt renal trauma, the majority of renal injuries caused by penetrating trauma are major, with severe injury to the parenchyma, collecting system, or vessels.[4,41] Although both gunshot and stab wounds cause major renal injury, gunshot wounds cause more renal injuries and are more often associated with serious abdominal injury (91%) than are stab wounds (53%).[5,38,41]

Most studies on penetrating renal trauma combine data from both stab and gunshot wounds. Carroll and McAninch[38] found that both contributed equally to major renal and pedicle injury but that gunshot wounds were twice as likely to cause serious abdominal injury (91% vs. 53%). Mee and McAninch[4] studied 91 stab wounds and 47 gunshot wounds.[4] Of the total number of patients with penetrating injuries (138), 42% had major renal lacerations and another 8% suffered renal vascular injury; however, there was no combination of parameters (including presenting signs and symptoms or associated injuries) that was predictive of injury. Other researchers have also found that clinical findings are inconsistent in predicting injury.[4,38,41,42]

Hematuria. The presence and degree of hematuria is not predictive of injury. A review of the literature reveals great variation in the degree of hematuria from significant renal injuries. Although there may be significant renal injuries with minimal or no hematuria, Carroll[38] found either microscopic or gross hematuria in 100% of patients with penetrating trauma of the kidney.

Indications and recommendations for imaging. Based on the high incidence of major renal injuries associated with penetrating trauma, full radiographic evaluation of patients with penetrating trauma to the flank, back, and abdomen is recommended.

Stable patient. In contrast to blunt renal trauma, the IVP is unreliable in the screening of significant renal injuries caused by penetrating trauma,[42] with a false-negative result rate of up to 30%. In the Federle et al. study series of stab wounds, the IVPs performed suggested renal injury, but many contained nonspecific abnormalities that did not correlate with the CT findings.[42] Carroll and McAninch[38] reported that 23% of patients with documented major renal injuries had normal IVPs. The only findings on the IVP predictive of major injury were nonfunction and extravasation.[38] Although conventional tomograms improve the diagnostic accuracy of the IVP, they are often unavailable. Despite clear evidence that the IVP does not adequately assess the presence and extent of renal injury, there is some reluctance in eliminating the IVP as the initial screening examination for penetrating trauma. However, in the stable patient, when technically possible, a double-contrast enhanced CT scan should be the primary imaging study for the evaluation of renal injury resulting from penetrating trauma to the abdomen, back, or flank.[42]

Integration of imaging into the total clinical evaluation is especially critical with penetrating trauma. Anterior abdominal stab wounds may injure intraperitoneal organs as well as the kidney. In the stable patient, evaluation of a stab wound to the anterior abdomen usually begins with local stab wound exploration. If fascial penetration has occurred or the exploration is indeterminate (the wound track cannot be identified), a DPL should be performed. If hematuria is present, a CT scan should be done to evaluate for possible renal injury. Stab wounds to the flank or back, on the other hand, injure intra-abdominal structures less often although flank stab wounds result in a higher incidence of injury than do wounds to the back.[38,39,43] In the presence of stab wounds to the flank or back with hematuria, a CT scan should be performed to evaluate for potential renal injury. A triple-contrast enhanced CT scan (oral, intravenous, and rectal) has been proposed to delineate all retroperitoneal structures (especially the retroperitoneal colon) and may be useful for evaluating penetrating injuries to the back and flank.[44] Although the management of gunshot wounds is undergoing modification—from the practice of mandatory laparotomy to a more selective approach—the standard of care remains mandatory laparotomy for most patients. In the unusual instance in which a stable patient does not undergo a laparotomy, a CT scan should be done to evaluate for renal injury from gunshot wounds to the abdomen, back, or flank.

Unstable patient. Complex radiographic evaluation in the unstable patient with penetrating trauma generally is deferred; occasionally it is performed in the operating room. The chest radiograph and plain abdominal radiographs are exceptions; these radiographs should be obtained with markers to identify the potential trajectory of a missile.

Technique for the intravenous pyelogram

In the emergency department, a quick and thorough protocol should be established for the emergency IVP. A plain radiograph of the abdomen (KUB), before contrast injection, must be obtained in all patients. Contrast material should be injected by rapid bolus technique in a dose of 1.5 to 2.0 ml/kg. Initially AP abdominal radiographs should be obtained at 1 minute, 5 minutes, and 10 minutes after injection of IV contrast material. In selected patients, oblique radiographs of the kidneys and 15-minute and 30-minute radiographs of the abdomen after IV contrast injection may be useful. Conventional tomography enhances the detection of parenchymal injuries and should be obtained if necessary.

Radiographic findings

Intravenous pyelogram. Abnormal IVP findings include the following: diminished nephrogram, delayed or absent filling of the calyces, and incomplete visualization of the renal outlines. These findings, however, are nonspecific and may be present in injuries ranging from renal contusion to parenchymal laceration. Because of the nonspecific nature of the urographic findings, suspected abnormalities are best evaluated with a subsequent CT scan.

Extravasation of contrast material. This finding indicates the presence of a laceration that has extended into the collecting system unless a pre-existing abnormality exists (i.e., ureteropelvic junction obstruction). In some cases the actual laceration may be visualized as a cleft in the renal parenchyma (Fig. 7-1).

Partial nephrogram. The presence of a partial nephrogram suggests either a segmental renal infarction or a laceration that has devitalized a portion of the kidney. An irregular nephrogram suggests perfusion defects from a segmental infarction or multiple parenchymal injuries.[2]

Diminished excretion. Diminished excretion is common and nonspecific because it may be seen in a variety of conditions (Fig. 7-2).[10]

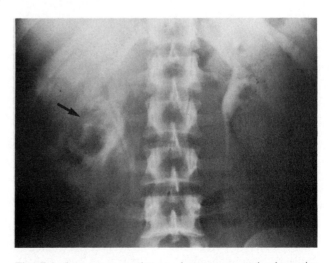

Fig. 7-1. Intravenous pyelogram demonstrates major laceration of the right kidney with contrast material extravasation *(arrow)* extending into the collecting system.

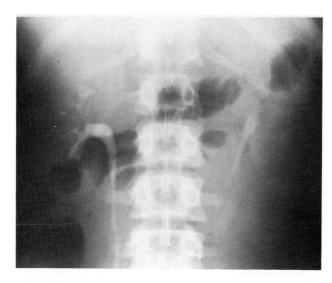

Fig. 7-2. Intravenous pyelogram demonstrates left renal contusion with diminished nephrogram and decreased calyceal filling of the left kidney.

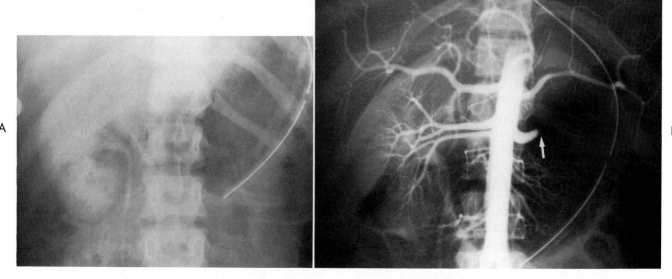

A

B

Fig. 7-3. Intravenous pyelogram and angiogram of traumatic renal artery occlusion. **A,** IVP shows no function of the left kidney. **B,** Angiogram shows thrombosis of the left renal artery *(arrow)*. Two right renal arteries are noted.

Unilateral nonvisualization. Unilateral absence of excretion is highly suggestive of either a renal pedicle injury or renal rupture. Unilateral nonvisualization may also be due to severe contusion, laceration, subcapsular hematoma, or pre-existing renal disease. The mechanism whereby a kidney with an intact renal artery fails to excrete contrast material is unclear.[2] Cass[9] studied unilateral nonvisualization and found that it was caused by a variety of renal injuries: contusion (15%), laceration (22%), renal rupture (22%) (see Fig. 7-6), and renal pedicle injury (40%) (Fig. 7-3). Regardless of the cause, the finding of unilateral nonvisualization on an IVP is an indication for further imaging studies to accurately define the extent of injury. Although renal rupture and renal pedicle injury are

well demonstrated on a CT scan, angiography may be required in patients with traumatic renal artery thrombosis if an attempt at renal revascularization is anticipated. In such a circumstance, the CT scan should be obtained only if it does not delay the angiographic procedure.

Computed tomography. The most common findings on the CT scan are perirenal hematomas (30%) (Fig. 7-4), intrarenal and subcapsular hematomas (25%) (Fig. 7-5), and parenchymal disruption (17%) (Fig. 7-6).[10] A CT scan is also useful in demonstrating traumatic renal infarction (Fig. 7-7).

Complications of contrast material administration. Major anaphylactic reactions have been reported with contrast material administration; therefore resuscitative equip-

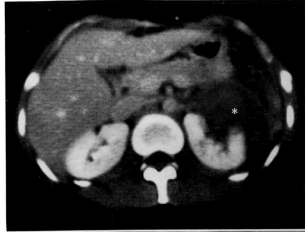

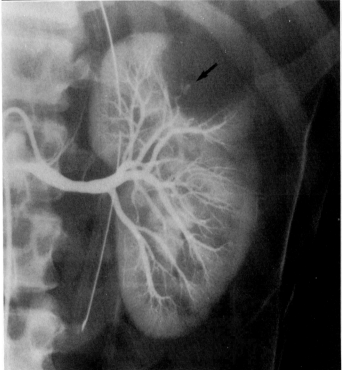

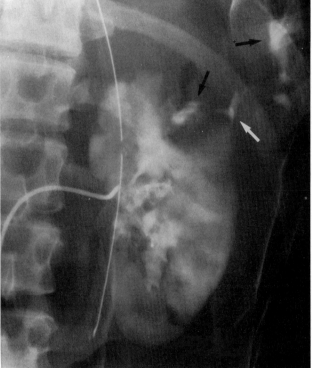

Fig. 7-4. A, CT scan of the left kidney demonstrating perirenal hematoma *(asterisk).* Arterial **(B)** and capillary **(C)** phase angiograms of left renal laceration with perirenal hematoma demonstrates contrast material extravasation *(arrows)* indicating active bleeding into the hematoma. Patient subsequently underwent embolization.

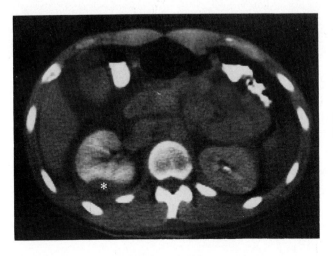

Fig. 7-5. CT scan of the right kidney demonstrates subcapsular hematoma *(asterisk).*

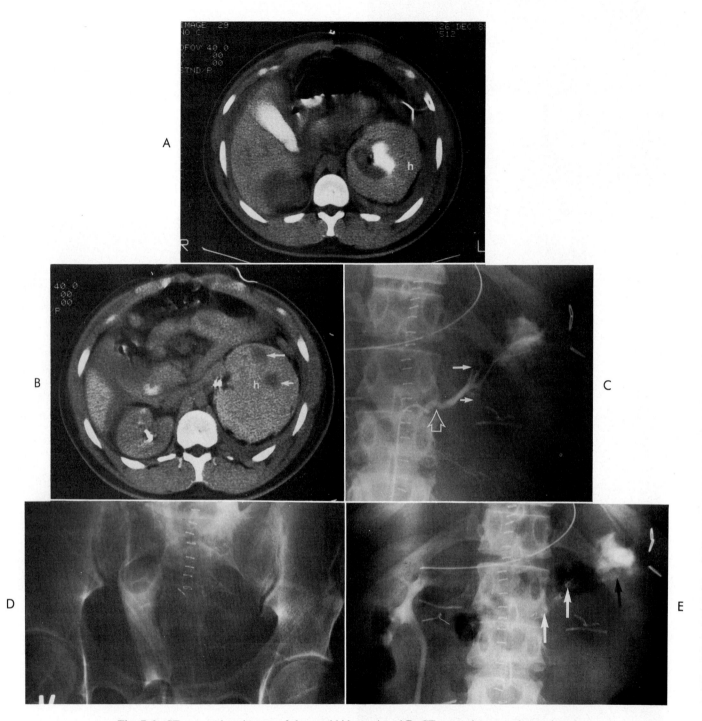

Fig. 7-6. CT scan and angiogram of shattered kidney. **A** and **B,** CT scans show massive perirenal hematoma *(h)* surrounding fragments of kidney *(white arrows)*. Extravasated contrast material from angiogram is seen in perinephric space. **C,** Angiogram demonstrates that only a small fraction of the kidney is perfused by the main renal artery. Multiple segmental thromboses, corresponding to multiple lacerations, are present *(arrows)*. Intimal flap in the renal artery is also seen *(open arrow)*. **D,** Plain radiograph of pelvis shows massive displacement of the bladder from left to right caused by large retroperitoneal hematoma. **E,** Following embolization with stainless steel coils *(white arrows)*, extravasation of contrast material in the renal parenchyma is still seen *(black arrow)*.

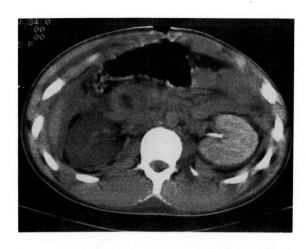

Fig. 7-7. CT scan of traumatic renal infarction demonstrates no contrast material enhancement of the right kidney.

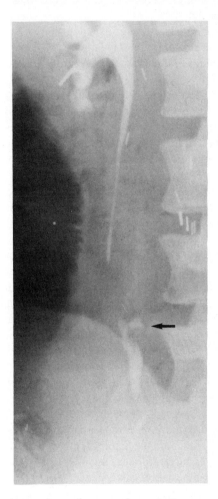

Fig. 7-8. Antegrade pyelogram of penetrating ureteral injury from a stab wound with contrast material extravasation from the right midureter *(arrow)*.

ment must be available.[29,45] Allergic or anaphylactoid reactions occur in about 2% of patients. Reported fatalities range from 1 in 14,000 to 1 in 117,000. Anaphylaxis is unpredictable, but the following represent reliable risk factors: patients who are younger in age (20 to 40) or who

have a history of allergy (seafood, shellfish, eggs, milk, or penicillin) or asthma. Prior anaphylactoid reactions are associated with a 30% risk of another similar reaction. Premedication with steroids and antihistamines appears to reduce the risk if these medications are begun 18 hours before the examination. Unfortunately, this is seldom practical in cases of acute trauma. The more expensive nonionic contrast materials should be considered for all patients at high risk for an anaphylactic reaction (see Chapter 25 and the Appendix for a further discussion).

URETERAL TRAUMA

Iatrogenic surgical trauma accounts for 95% of all ureteral injuries and usually occurs in association with gynecologic procedures, while penetrating trauma, primarily gunshot wounds, is the principal cause of the remaining 5%. Blunt trauma and stabbings rarely cause a ureteral injury.[47] Carlton[46] studied 1000 cases of stab wounds to the abdomen and found only two ureteral lacerations. Hematuria is usually present but may be absent in up to 36% of patients with ureteral injury.[31] The IVP findings are usually abnormal, generally revealing extravasation at the site of the injury while obstruction proximal to the injury is less often seen (Fig. 7-8). Carroll and McAninch[48] suggest that the IVP and initial urinalysis may not be reliable predictors of non-iatrogenic ureteral injury and suggest surgical exploration to confirm the diagnosis.[49] However, Pitts and Peterson[50] found that, although hematuria was present in only 77% of patients with documented ureteral injury, the IVP was diagnostic in 91%. There is significant morbidity—caused by urinary extravasation, hydronephrosis, and possible abscess formation—in cases in which the injury is missed, and surgical repair is mandatory.

BLADDER TRAUMA

Bladder trauma is most often associated with violent, blunt trauma (deceleration, auto-pedestrian and motor vehicle accidents, and falls) with only 15% of cases resulting from penetrating trauma. Of those bladder injuries caused by blunt trauma, two thirds are associated with a fractured

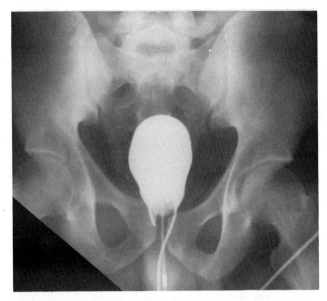

Fig. 7-9. Cystogram of perivesical hematoma compressing the bladder.

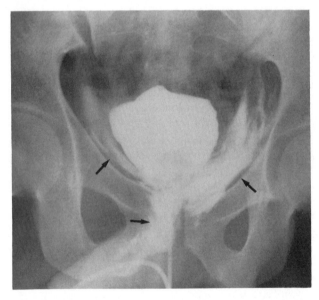

Fig. 7-10. Cystogram of extraperitoneal bladder rupture *(arrows).*

pelvis—most commonly fractures of the anterior arch, including pubic rami fractures and diastasis of the symphysis pubis.[48] Up to ten percent of patients with pelvic fractures have an associated bladder rupture.[51] Five to 10% of males with bladder injuries also have a posterior urethral tear. It must be emphasized that a pelvic fracture is associated with serious concomitant injuries and has a mortality rate of up to 25%.[48,51-55] There are sporadic reports of spontaneous rupture of the bladder in the pregnant patient who is near term. However, most "spontaneous" ruptures probably occur in patients whose mental status was altered so

that they do not recall the trauma or in patients with underlying pathologic conditions of the bladder.

Anatomy

The adult bladder is deep in the anterior pelvis, protected by the symphysis pubis and cushioned by perivesical fat, the colon, and muscles. The bladder is primarily an extraperitoneal organ, but the dome and upper posterior aspect are covered by the peritoneum.[56]

Signs and symptoms of bladder injury include difficulty voiding, gross hematuria, abdominal tenderness, and shock.[48,51]

Classification of bladder injuries

Bladder injuries may be classified as follows:
• Contusion
• Extraperitoneal rupture
• Intraperitoneal rupture
• Combined extraperitoneal and intraperitoneal rupture
Contusion of the bladder is the mildest and most common injury. The mechanism is usually that of blunt trauma to the lower abdomen. On cystogram, the perivesical spaces may fill with hematoma, causing extrinsic compression and deformity of the bladder outline, but there should be no extravasation of contrast material (Fig. 7-9).

Extraperitoneal rupture is the most common major injury to the bladder (70%) and nearly always occurs in association with a fractured pelvis. For many years it was thought that the tear was most often caused by direct penetration of the bladder by bone fragments. However, Carroll and McAninch[48] reported that the highest percentage of bladder lacerations were located in the bladder dome, and only 35% were noted to be in direct proximity to a pelvic fracture. Corriere and Sandler[57] confirmed these findings; in 65% of their patients, the laceration was not associated with the area of fracture. The most likely mechanism for extraperitoneal bladder rupture may be either a type of bursting injury or a shearing injury, resulting from the force of pelvic ring disruption.[57] Most often, urinary extravasation is limited to the perivesical space (Fig. 7-10). On occasion, a complex extraperitoneal rupture is seen in which the contrast material extends beyond the perivesical space into the scrotum, thigh, perineum, or penis.[58] This disruption of the fascial boundaries of the pelvis produces an extravasation pattern suggestive of an associated urethral tear. A urethral injury is commonly associated with a ruptured bladder and pelvic fracture. Controversy exists over the treatment of bladder injury based on recent reports of nonoperative management with catheter drainage and close clinical observation.[59] Corriere and Sandler[60] recently reported on a large series of patients with extraperitoneal bladder rupture who were managed with simple catheter drainage and close clinical observation.

Intraperitoneal rupture of the bladder accounts for

about 25% of major bladder injuries. It usually occurs after a blow to the lower abdomen in the presence of a distended bladder or after penetrating trauma to the lower abdomen. Rupture occurs at the dome, the weakest point of bladder, with urine and blood entering the peritoneal cavity. Initial extravasation of urine into the peritoneal cavity may cause little or no peritoneal irritation. Hematuria is a nearly universal finding, and the cystogram is diagnostic. Contrast material may be seen outlining the abdominal viscera, loops of bowel, or the paracolic gutters (Fig. 7-11). Standard treatment includes early surgical exploration, debridement, wound closure, and suprapubic catheter drainage.

Combined intraperitoneal-extraperitoneal bladder rupture occurs most often in the presence of a pelvic fracture and represents about 5% of major bladder injuries. Combined rupture may also be seen in penetrating trauma (Fig. 7-12). Both patterns of extravasation may be seen on cystograms. Gunshot wounds that result in bladder injury are often associated with concomitant vascular and bowel injuries, whereas stab wounds usually cause only bowel injuries.[61] Surgical intervention is dictated by the mechanism of injury and the patient's clinical status.

Indications for imaging

In patients with multisystem trauma, it is often impossible to clinically distinguish the source of hematuria. A urethrogram and cystogram should be obtained on any male who has sustained a pelvic fracture. A cystogram should also be done for patients with blunt or penetrating trauma to the lower abdomen associated with hematuria. If persistent hemorrhage is thought to be due to a pelvic fracture, angiographic examination should precede contrast material–enhanced studies of the lower tract.[54,62] Applying the guidelines discussed earlier for renal trauma, an IVP or a CT scan may be indicated to complete the evaluation.

Technique for cystography

Cystography is the only reliable method of identifying a bladder tear and has an accuracy rate approaching 100%.[58] However, false-negative cystographic findings can occur when an inadequate amount of contrast material is used or if the post-drainage radiograph is omitted (the post-drainage radiograph is the only view in which the diagnosis can be made in 10% of cases). Occasionally penetrating injury caused by small caliber (low-velocity) bullets or stab wounds may be missed on the initial cystogram.[56]

An initial plain radiograph of the abdomen should be obtained (KUB), and a Foley catheter should be inserted into the bladder. In males with a pelvic fracture, urethral injury should be excluded before insertion of the Foley catheter. The bladder should be filled by gravity infusion with 300 to 400 ml of 30% water-soluble contrast material. A 300-ml bottle of standard infusion contrast material (25% to 30%) and a similar amount of saline solution run

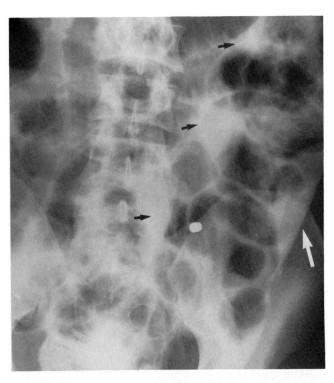

Fig. 7-11. Cystogram of intraperitoneal bladder rupture caused by gunshot wound. Contrast material is seen outlining bowel loops *(small arrows)* and in the left paracolic gutter *(large arrow)*. Bullet overlies the left iliac crest.

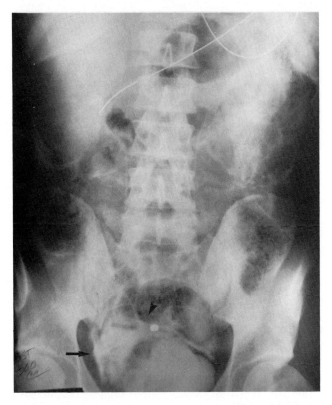

Fig. 7-12. Cystogram of extraperitoneal *(arrow)* and intraperitoneal *(arrowhead)* bladder rupture caused by a gunshot wound.

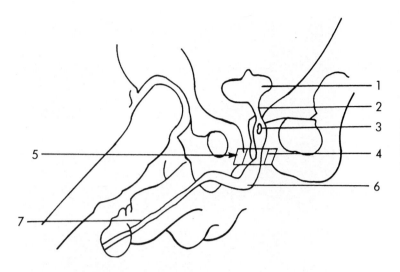

Fig. 7-13. Normal anatomy of the male urethra. *1*, bladder; *2*, prostatic urethra; *3*, verumontanum; *4*, membranous urethra; *5*, urogenital diaphragm; *6*, bulbous urethra; *7*, penile urethra.

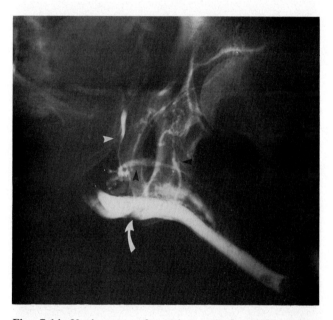

Fig. 7-14. Urethrogram of anterior urethral (straddle) injury demonstrating partial urethral disruption in the midbulbar urethra *(arrow)*. Extensive venous extravasation *(arrowheads)* is present.

through a Y connector should be infused simultaneously. After the first 100 ml of contrast material has been infused, a radiograph is obtained to assess for gross extravasation. If none is noted, the remainder of the contrast material is infused, and the catheter is clamped. Radiographs should be obtained in the AP, oblique (if the patient's condition permits), and lateral positions. The post-drainage radiograph should be taken after drainage of the contrast material from the bladder. The post-drainage radiograph permits visualization of small amounts of contrast extravasation that might be hidden by the distended, contrast–filled bladder. The amount of extravasation of contrast material does not necessarily correlate with the size of injury. Delayed or missed diagnoses may result in urinary ex-

travasation, peritonitis, sepsis, and death, although death is most often caused by associated injuries.

URETHRAL TRAUMA

Urethral trauma is a relatively uncommon injury associated with substantial morbidity. Any male with trauma to the perineum or pelvis should be suspected of having a urethral injury. The female urethra is short and rarely sustains significant trauma; therefore this topic is not addressed.

The anterior male urethra is comprised of the penile and bulbous urethra. The posterior urethra contains the membranous and prostatic urethra. The urogenital diaphragm is a 1.5-cm fascial layer between the ischial rami, traversed by the membranous urethra. It is clinically important because the urinary continence mechanism and autonomic nerve innervation responsible for erection are contained in the prostatic and membranous urethra. Because posterior urethral injuries usually involve the urogenital diaphragm, the potential exists for permanent loss of continence and sexual potency.

Anterior urethral injury

Blunt trauma to the anterior urethra is usually due to a straddle injury, sports injury, or sexual activity. Other causes include urethral instrumentation, indwelling catheters, and penetrating trauma (gunshot wounds). In most cases the bulbous urethra is compressed against the arch of the ischial rami. The injury may vary from a partial to a complete urethral tear. Signs and symptoms include blood at the urethral meatus, swelling, ecchymoses of the perineum, scrotum, or abdominal wall, and inability to void. If Buck's fascia is intact, extravasation of blood and urine are limited to the urethral epithelium. If Buck's fascia is torn, blood and urine pass into the penis, scrotum, and abdominal wall.[63] A retrograde urethrogram should be obtained if the diagnosis is suspected (Figs. 7-13 and 7-14).

Complete rupture of the anterior urethra is unusual, but,

if this is demonstrated on the urethrogram, urethral catheterization should not be attempted because catheterization may result in inoculation of the periurethral hematoma with bacteria.[64]

Treatment depends on the mechanism of injury, the extent of the injury, and local urologic treatment preferences. There are advocates of suprapubic catheterization with secondary repair and of immediate surgical repair.[64] Complications include chronic deep-bulbar urethral stricture and urinary tract infection.

Posterior urethral injury

Posterior urethral injury is seen in association with severe blunt trauma and is virtually always associated with a fractured pelvis.[65] Ten percent of individuals with a posterior urethral injury also have a concomitant ruptured bladder. Sandler and Phillips found that of males with pelvic fracture, up to 18% also had a posterior urethral injury. All had either fractures of the anterior arch, diastasis of the symphysis pubis, or a Malgaigne fracture (complex pelvic injury with separation or fracture of both the anterior and posterior pelvic arch).[66] Classically, the patient may complain of difficulty or inability to void. Examination may reveal gross hematuria or blood at the urethral meatus, an elevated or ill-defined prostate, and discoloration of the perineum or scrotum. However, none of these signs are diagnostic, and their absence does not preclude injury.

Posterior urethral injuries can be classified into three types[66]:

Type I: The prostatic urethra is stretched as the puboprostatic ligaments are ruptured, but the continuity of the urethra remains intact (Fig. 7-15).

Type II: The membranous urethra is ruptured above an intact urogenital diaphragm. On urethrographic examination, contrast material is extravasated into the pelvic extraperitoneal space. Type II was considered the "classic" urethral injury until recently (Fig. 7-16).

Type III: Now recognized as the most common pattern of injury; the membranous and proximal bulbous urethra are ruptured. The urogenital diaphragm is also disrupted, allowing for extravasation into the perineum (Figs. 7-17 and 7-18). Both types II and III urethral injuries may be partial or complete. With partial tears, some contrast material will be seen entering the bladder on urethrographic examination. With complete rupture, no contrast material will be demonstrated in the bladder.

Indications for imaging

In the presence of a pelvic fracture, a urethrogram must be obtained before attempts at catheterization. Any patient who complains of difficulty urinating after blunt trauma to the pelvis should also undergo urethrographic examina-

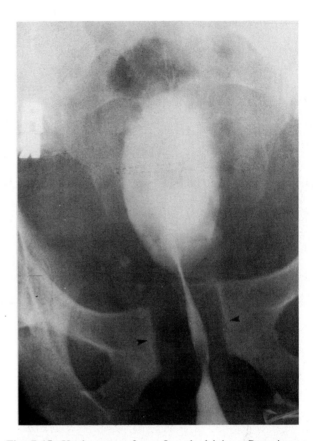

Fig. 7-15. Urethrogram of type I urethral injury. Posterior urethra is stretched and elongated, but no contrast material extravasation is present. There is diastasis of pubic symphysis *(arrowheads)*.

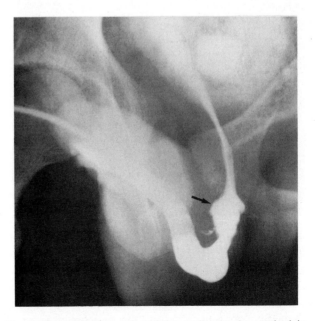

Fig. 7-16. Urethrogram of partial type II posterior urethral injury. Extravasation is present above the urogenital diaphragm, but continuity of the urethra *(arrow)* is maintained, indicating a partial injury.

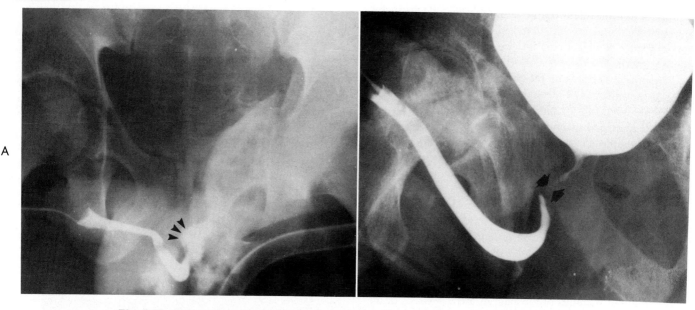

Fig. 7-17. Urethrogram of type III posterior urethral rupture. **A,** Urethrogram demonstrates type III extravasation *(arrowheads)*. **B,** Combined voiding cystourethrogram and retrograde urethrogram demonstrate complete 1-cm stricture *(arrows)* in posterior urethra after 6 months of suprapubic drainage.

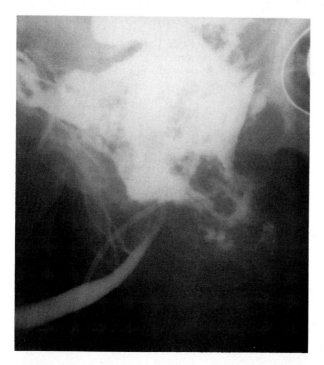

Fig. 7-18. Urethrogram of type III posterior urethral injury with massive contrast material extravasation.

tion. Because indications for a cystogram overlap with the indications for a urethrogram, the cystourethrogram is commonly performed. As mentioned earlier, in patients with multisystem trauma, either an IVP or a CT scan may also be indicated.

Hemodynamic instability is a frequent concern in the patient with multisystem blunt or penetrating trauma. In these patients special radiographic studies are usually contraindicated. However, instrumentation of the male urethra is a prerequisite to DPL. If the patient's condition permits a limited urethrographic examination, this may be performed before the insertion of a Foley catheter. If not, an open technique for DPL will be necessary.

Technique for the retrograde urethrogram

To obtain a retrograde urethrogram, it is necessary to insert, without lubricant, a no. 14 or no. 16 Foley catheter that is attached to an irrigating syringe. The syringe is filled with 30% contrast material. The catheter is inserted so that the balloon of the catheter is 2 to 3 cm proximal to the meatus. The balloon is then inflated with 1 to 2 ml of saline to "seat" it in the fossa navicularis of the penile urethra.[66] An oblique radiograph should then be obtained during the injection of 25 to 30 ml of contrast material. If the urethra is intact, the balloon should be deflated and the catheter advanced into the bladder for the cystographic examination. If the urethrogram shows extravasation, a suprapubic cystotomy may be done and a cystogram performed via this route. If angiography is planned, it should be performed before urethrography to avoid potential obscuring of angiographic details by the instilled contrast material.

The treatment of posterior urethral injuries is controversial. Treatment options include retention catheter realignment, primary reconstruction, or immediate suprapubic diversion with delayed repair.[63,67] Because this injury occurs most often in conjunction with significant pelvic trauma, the initial diagnosis and management may be of secondary concern in light of more life-threatening injuries. [65] Immediate suprapubic diversion with delayed repair (6 to 9 months after the injury) is the easiest initial method and yields the lowest morbidity.[63,67,68] The bladder may be inspected at the time of suprapubic tube placement, or a cystogram through the suprapubic tube may be obtained to rule out an associated bladder injury. A posterior urethral injury may result in serious, debilitating, lifelong complications, including severe strictures, sexual impotence, and urinary incontinence. These complications may occur as a result of the original injury or if the injury is complicated by initial mismanagement.[63,65,67] Repeated attempts at inserting rigid instruments into an injured urethra (e.g., catheters) may result in converting a partial tear into a complete tear, with subsequent increased morbidity.

SUMMARY

In summary, the essential aspects of genitourinary trauma, with a specific focus on radiographic evaluation, have been discussed. Pertinent anatomy, common injury patterns, classification of injury, and indications for imaging were integrated into the discussion of trauma management priorities. Our approach permits integration of the assessment of genitourinary system injuries into the general approach to management of trauma with special emphasis on rational application of the principles of radiographic imaging.

REFERENCES

1. Cass AS: Immediate radiologic and surgical management of renal injuries, *J Trauma* 22(5):361, 1982.
2. Pollack HM, Wein AJ: Imaging of renal trauma, *Radiology* 172:297, 1989.
3. Bretan PN, McAninch JW: Evaluation of renal trauma: indications for computed tomography and other diagnostic techniques. In *Advances in urology,* Chicago, 1988, Year Book Medical Publishers.
4. Mee SL, McAninch JW, Robinson AL et al: Radiographic assessment of renal trauma: a 10-year prospective study of patient selection, *J Urol* 141:1095, 1989.
5. Sagalowsky AI, McConnell JD, and Peters PC: Renal trauma requiring surgery: an analysis of 185 cases, *J Trauma* 23(2):128, 1983.
6. Cass AS, Bubrick M, Luxenberg BE et al: Renal trauma found during laparotomy for intra-abdominal injury, *J Trauma* 25(10):997, 1985.
7. Cox EF: Blunt abdominal trauma: a 5 year analysis of 870 patients requiring celiotomy, *Ann Surg* 199(4):467, 1984.
8. Sturm JT, Perry JF: Injuries associated with fractures of the transverse processes of the thoracic and lumbar vertebrae, *J Trauma* 24(7):597, 1984.
9. Cass AS, Luxenberg M: Unilateral nonvisualization on excretory urography after external trauma, *J Urol* 132:225, 1984.
10. Bretan PN, McAninch JW, Federle MP et al: Computerized tomographic staging of renal trauma: 85 consecutive cases, *J Urol* 136:561, 1986.
11. Federle MP, Kaiser JA, McAninch JW et al: The role of computed tomography in renal trauma, *Radiology* 141:455, 1981.
12. Lang EK, Sullivan J, and Frentz G: Renal trauma: radiological studies, *Radiology* 154:1, 1985.
13. Sclafani SJA, Becker JA: Radiologic diagnosis of renal trauma, *Urol Radiol* 7:192, 1985.
14. Sclafani SJA, Goldstein AS, Panetta T et al: CT diagnosis of renal pedicle injury, *Urol Radiol* 7:63, 1985.
15. Ertruk E, Sheinfeld J, DiMarco PL et al: Renal trauma: evaluation by computerized tomography, *J Urol* 133:946, 1985.
16. Sandler CM, Toombs BD: Computed tomographic evaluation of blunt renal injuries, *Radiology* 141:461, 1981.
17. Cass AS, Bubrick M, Luxenberg et al: Renal pedicle injury in patients with multiple injuries, *J Trauma* 25(9):892, 1985.
18. Turner WW, Snyder WH, and Fry WJ: Mortality and renal salvage after renovascular trauma, *Am J Surg* 146:848, 1983.
19. Brown MF, Graham JM, Mattox KL et al: Renovascular trauma, *Am J Surg* 140:802, 1980.
20. Lowe P, Hardy BR: Isolated bilateral blunt renal trauma with pelviureteric disruption, *Urology* 19:4:420, 1982.
21. Ryner P, Federle MP, and Jeffrey RB: CT of trauma to the abnormal kidney, *AJR* 142:747, 1984.
22. Bee DE, James GP, and Paul KL: Hemoglobinuria and hematuria: accuracy and precision of laboratory diagnosis, *Clin Chem* 25(10):1696, 1979.
23. Kennedy TJ, McDonnell JD, and Thal ER: Urine dipstick vs. microscopic urinalysis in the evaluation of abdominal trauma, *J Trauma* 28(5):1988.
24. Goldner AP, Mayron R, and Ruiz E: Are urine dipsticks reliable indicators of hematuria in blunt trauma patients? *Ann Emerg Med* 14(6):580, 1985.
25. Bright TC, White K, and Peters PC: Significance of hematuria after trauma, *J Urol* 120:455, 1978.
26. Guice K, Oldham K, Brock E et al: Hematuria after blunt trauma: when is pyelography useful? *J Trauma* 23(4):1983.
27. Griffen WO, Belin RP, Ernst CB et al: Intravenous pyelography in abdominal trauma, *J Trauma* 18(6):387, 1978.
28. Hardeman SW, Husmann DA, Chinn HKW et al: Blunt urinary tract trauma: identification of those who require radiologic diagnostic studies, *J Urol* 138:99 1987.
29. Nicolaisen GS, McAninch JW, Marshall GA et al: Renal trauma: re-evaluation of the indications for radiographic assessment, *J Urol* 133:183, 1985.
30. Stalker, HP, Kaufman RA: The significance of hematuria in children after blunt abdominal trauma, *AJR:* 569, 1990.
31. Halsell RD, Vines FS, Shatney CH et al: The reliability of excretory urography as a screening examination for blunt renal trauma, *Ann Emerg Med* 16(11):75, 1987.
32. Lang EK: Imaging examinations in the management of renal trauma, *Semin Ultrasound CT MR* 6(2):100, 1985.
33. McAninch JW, Federle MP: Evaluation of renal injuries with computerized tomography, *J Urol* 128:456, 1982.
34. Fabian TC, Mangiante EC, White TJ et al: A prospective study of 91 patients undergoing both computed tomography and peritoneal lavage following blunt abdominal trauma, *J Trauma* 26(7):602, 1986.
35. Peitzman AB, Makaroun MS, Slasky BS et al: Prospective study of computed tomography in initial management of blunt abdominal trauma, *J Trauma* 26(7):585, 1986.
36. Goldstein AS, Sclafani SJA, Kupferstein NH et al: The diagnostic superiority of computerized tomography, *J Trauma* 25(10):938, 1985.
37. Marx JA, Moore EE, Jorden RC et al: Limitations of computed tomography in the evaluation of acute abdominal trauma: a prospective comparison with diagnostic peritoneal lavage, *J Trauma* 25(10):933, 1985.
38. Carroll PR, McAninch JW: Operative indications in penetrating renal trauma. *J Trauma* 25(7):587, 1985.
39. Peck W: Posterior abdominal stab wounds, *J Trauma* 21:298, 1981.
40. Coppa, GF, Davalle M, Pachter HL, et al: Management of penetrating wounds of the back and flank, *Surg Gynecol Obstet* 159:514, 1984.
41. McAninch JW: *Urogenital trauma, Urol Clin North Am,* Philadelphia, 1989, WB Saunders.

42. Federle MP, Brown TR, and McAninch JW: Penetrating renal trauma: CT evaluation, *J Comput Assist Tomogr* 11(6):1026, 1987.

43. Bernath AS, Heinrich S, Fernandez RRD et al: Stab wounds of the kidney: conservative management in flank penetration, *J Urol* 129:468, 1982.

44. Hauser CJ et al: Triple contrast CT in the evaluation of penetrating posterior abdominal wounds, *Arch Surg* 122:1112, 1987.

45. Choyke PL, Meranze S, Pahira JJ et al: *Imaging of urinary tract disease: current approaches, Med Clin North Am,* Philadelphia, 1984, WB Saunders.

46. Carlton CE Jr.: *Injury to the ureter, Urol Clin North Am* Philadelphia, 1977, WB Saunders.

47. Boileau MA, Corriere JN, and Benson GS: Urologic trauma. In Wolfson A, Harwood-Nuss AL, eds: *Renal and urologic emergencies,* vol 8, New York, 1986, Churchill-Livingstone.

48. Carroll PR, McAninch JW: Major bladder trauma: mechanisms of injury and a unified method of diagnosis and repair, *J Urol* 132:254, 1984.

49. Presti, JC, Carroll, PR, and McAninch, JW: Ureteral and renal pelvic injury from external trauma, *J Trauma* 29(3):370, 1989.

50. Pitts JC, Peterson NE: Penetrating injuries of the ureter, *J Trauma* 21(11):978, 1981.

51. Palmer JK, Benson GS, and Corriere JN: Diagnosis and initial management of urological injuries associated with 200 consecutive pelvic fractures, *J Urol* 130:712, 1983.

52. Cass AS: The multiply injured patient with bladder trauma, *J Trauma* 24(8):731, 1984.

53. Grieco JG, Perry JF: Retroperitoneal hematoma following trauma: its clinical importance, *J Trauma* 20(9):733, 1980.

54. Mucha P, Farnell MB: Analysis of pelvic fracture management, *J Trauma* 24(5):379, 1984.

55. Murr PC, Moore EE, Lipscomb R et al: Abdominal trauma associated with pelvic fracture, *J Trauma* 20(1):919, 1980.

56. Guerriero WG: Bladder trauma. In *Urologic injuries,* Norwalk, CT, 1984, Appleton-Century-Crofts.

57. Corriere, JN, Sandler CM: Mechanism of injury, patterns of extravasation and management of extraperitoneal bladder rupture due to blunt trauma, *J Urol* 139:43, 1988.

58. Sandler CM, Hall JT, Rodriguez MD et al: Bladder injury in blunt pelvic trauma, *Radiology* 158:633, 1986.

59. Hayes EE, Sandler CM, Corriere JN: Management of the ruptured bladder secondary to blunt abdominal trauma, *J Urol* 129:946, 1983.

60. Corriere JN, Sandler CM: Management of ruptured bladder: seven year experience, *J Trauma* 26(9):830, 1986.

61. McConnell JD, Wilkerson MD, and Peters PC: *Rupture of the bladder, Urol Clin North Am,* Philadelphia, 1982, WB Saunders.

62. Gilliland MG, Ward RE, Flynn TC et al: Peritoneal lavage and angiography in the management of patients with pelvic fractures, *Am J Surg* 144:744, 1982.

63. Guerriero WG: Posterior urethral disruption. In *Urologic Injuries,* Norwalk, CT, 1984, Appleton-Century-Crofts.

64. Pontes JE, Pierce JM: Anterior urethral injuries: four years of experience at the Detroit general hospital, *J Urol* 120:563, 1978.

65. Cass AS: Urethral injury in multiply injured patients, *J Trauma* 24(10):901, 1984.

66. Sandler CM, Phillips JM: *Radiology of the bladder and urethra in blunt pelvic trauma, Radiol Clin North Am* Philadelphia, 1981, WB Saunders.

67. Morehouse DD, Mackinnon KJ: Management of prostatomembranous urethral disruption: 13 year experience, *J Urol* 123:173, 1980.

68. Weems WL: Management of genitourinary injuries in patients with pelvic fractures, *Ann Surg* 189(6):717, 1979.

Musculoskeletal Trauma

Kenneth C. Jackimczyk
Wolfgang Goy

Musculoskeletal injuries affect a significant portion of patients in the emergency department and primary care population. Commonly, the emergency physician must determine the need for diagnostic imaging, interpret the studies, provide the initial care, and determine those situations in which an orthopedic consultant is needed on an emergent basis. This chapter will attempt to summarize the diagnostic approach to patients with musculoskeletal trauma, the proper selection of diagnostic imaging studies, and the initial treatment and interpretation as well as follow-up of these problems. The musculoskeletal areas will be discussed separately in a cephalad to caudad anatomic order.

SHOULDER AND HUMERUS
Normal anatomy and radiographic views

A standard radiographic series of the shoulder in most hospitals consists of two views: an anteroposterior (AP) view and an AP in internal rotation (Figs. 8-1 and 8-2). The AP view allows for atraumatic positioning of the patient but does not give good visualization of nondisplaced acromioclavicular (AC) separations or posterior shoulder dislocations. The AP view in internal rotation (20-degree posterior oblique angle) can be obtained without causing the patient discomfort but gives little additional information about traumatic injuries. Either the lateral transthoracic or axillary view is a better second view for evaluation of traumatic injuries.

The lateral transthoracic view, or Y view (45-degree anterior oblique angle), is not painful for the patient but may be technically difficult to obtain since the shoulder must be accurately positioned to have the x-ray beam parallel to the scapula (Fig. 8-3). One may also have difficulty interpreting this view and visualizing fractures of the glenoid rim. The upper lines of the Y on the transthoracic view are formed by the acromion and coracoid process of the scapula while the body of the scapula forms the base. The glenoid fossa is at the junction of the Y.

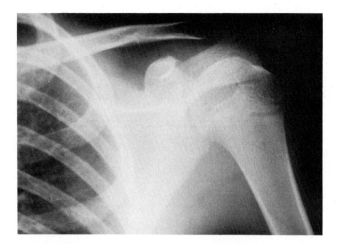

Fig. 8-1. Normal shoulder, anteroposterior (AP) view in external rotation, of a 14-year-old male showing normal epiphyses.

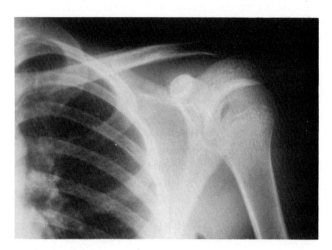

Fig. 8-2. Normal shoulder, AP view in internal rotation, of a 14-year-old male.

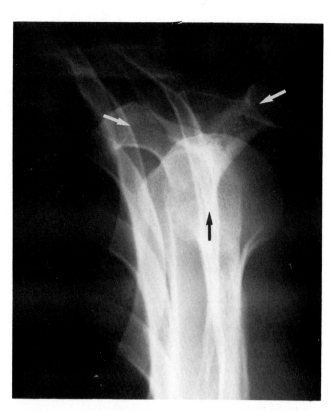

Fig. 8-3. Normal Y view of shoulder. The humeral head is shown in its normal position relative to the glenoid fossa, at the junction of the Y formed by the acromion *(arrow on right)*, coracoid process *(arrow on left)*, and the body of the scapula *(dark arrow)*.

The axillary view (Fig. 8-4) is an alternative to the lateral transthoracic view. This view may be more difficult to obtain because the patient's arm must be abducted approximately 45 degrees, which can be painful if not done slowly and carefully. Once the arm is abducted, the film is placed superior to the shoulder, and the x-ray beam is directed from the ipsilateral hip through the axilla. The axillary view is easy to interpret. Anterior and posterior dislocations are readily seen, and fractures not evident on frontal views may be demonstrated.

Acromioclavicular joint separation

The relationship between the acromion, coracoid process, and clavicle in the acromioclavicular joint (AC) is maintained by two sets of ligaments (Fig. 8-5) The coracoclavicular (CC) ligament is a strong, two-part ligament connecting the coracoid process of the scapula and the midportion of the clavicle. The acromioclavicular (AC)

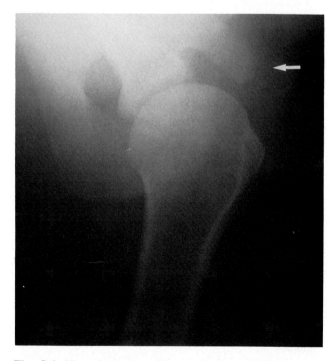

Fig. 8-4. Normal craniocaudal projection or axillary view of shoulder. This projection allows for easy visualization of anterior or posterior dislocations. The coracoid process of the scapula *(arrow)* identifies the anterior direction. The humeral head is seated normally in the glenoid fossa.

ligament is a weaker ligament that joins the acromion and the distal clavicle.

The AC joint is usually disrupted by either a direct blow to the shoulder while the arm is adducted or by a blow from above on the acromion. A fall that results in an indirect force across the AC joint can also rupture the ligaments. All patients with AC separation have point tenderness over the AC joint space.

A first-degree separation results in an incomplete tear of the ligaments. All radiographs, including stress films, are normal. Delayed radiographs, obtained several weeks after injury, may demonstrate periosteal reaction at the AC joint.

A second-degree separation (Fig. 8-6) involves complete disruption of the AC ligament, but the CC ligament remains intact. Radiographs show subluxation of the clavicle (less than 50% of its diameter), but the coracoid-to-clavicle (C-C) distance is maintained. Stress radiographs with weights may be used to demonstrate the subluxation; however, some authors question the efficacy of such stress radiographs in uncovering occult AC separations.[1]

A third-degree separation (Fig. 8-7) disrupts both the AC and CC ligaments. The C-C distance is increased on the injured side, and the distal clavicle is displaced superiorly (more than 50% of its diameter). On patient examination, obvious tenting of the skin is present over the distal clavicle.

Treatment for patients with AC joint separation injuries usually consists of immobilization in a sling, although surgical reconstruction may be performed for third-degree tears with a more cosmetic result. Most injuries heal without sequelae.

Shoulder dislocation

The glenohumeral joint is a ball-and-socket joint. The relatively large humeral head articulates with the relatively small and shallow glenoid fossa, allowing a wide range of motion but providing only limited stability. Approximately half of all dislocations occur at the shoulder.

More than 95% of shoulder dislocations are anterior, occurring during forced abduction and external rotation. Anterior dislocations are usually subcoracoid but may be subglenoid (inferior) or, rarely, subclavicular. Radiographic evaluation consists of an AP view (Fig. 8-8) and either a lateral transthoracic or axillary view (Fig. 8-9). Obtaining the axillary view is more difficult since the physician may need to abduct the arm slowly if motion is uncomfortable to the patient. However, the axillary view is easy to interpret and may reveal fractures of the coracoid process or glenoid rim.

A Hill-Sachs lesion is a hatchet-shaped impaction fracture of the posterolateral humeral head caused by the anterior rim of the glenoid during anterior shoulder dislocations. This fracture is most often seen with recurrent dislocations. Both the axillary and internal rotation views will usually reveal the defect.

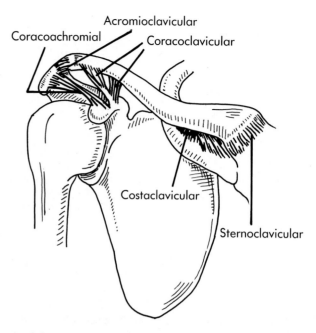

Fig. 8-5. Normal ligaments of the acromioclavicular (AC) joint.

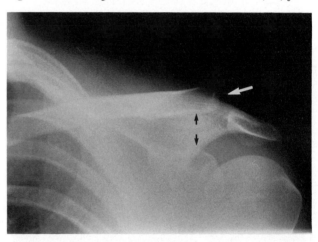

Fig. 8-6. Acromioclavicular joint, second-degree AC separation. Coracoclavicular (C-C) distance *(dark arrows)* is maintained while distal clavicle is subluxed less than 50% of its diameter *(arrow)*.

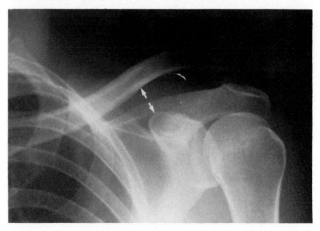

Fig. 8-7. Acromioclavicular joint, third-degree AC separation *(arrows)*. Coracoclavicular (C-C) distance is increased *(arrows)* while distal clavicle is subluxed more than 50% of its diameter.

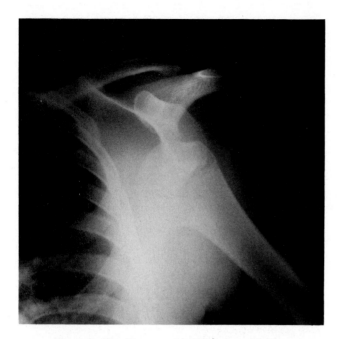

Fig. 8-8. Shoulder, anterior dislocation, AP view.

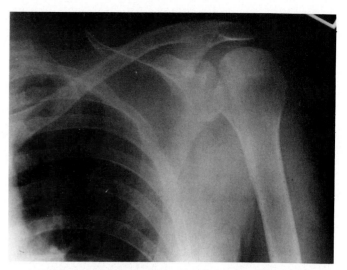

Fig. 8-10. Shoulder, posterior dislocation, AP view. No marked distortion of the joint is apparent. Note the humeral head defect. (From Crenshaw AH: *Campbell's operative orthopaedics,* ed 7, St Louis, 1987, CV Mosby.)

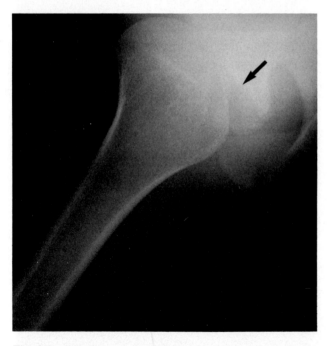

Fig. 8-9. Shoulder, anterior dislocation, axillary view. Note the humeral head is anterior to the anterior rim of the glenoid fossa *(arrow).*

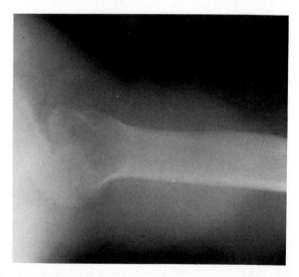

Fig. 8-11. Shoulder, posterior dislocation, axillary lateral view. There is posterior displacement of the humeral head and the posterior margin of the glenoid in the humeral head defect. (From Crenshaw AH: *Campbell's operative orthopaedics,* ed 7, St Louis, 1987, CV Mosby.)

Posterior glenohumeral dislocations account for less than 5% of shoulder dislocations but present a special problem because they may be easily missed. Posterior dislocations occur with a forced adduction, internal rotation, and flexion injury, such as occur with falls, electroconvulsive therapy, and seizures.[2] The patient with a posterior dislocation holds the arm internally rotated and abducted and vigorously resists external rotation and abduction. This makes obtaining an axillary view difficult. Interpretation of the AP view is difficult and on casual observation may be called normal. The following findings are useful in making the radiographic diagnosis of a posterior glenohumeral dislocation on the AP view[3] (Fig. 8-10):

- The distance between the articular surface of the humeral head and the anterior lip of the glenoid may be increased.
- The greater tuberosity is internally rotated.
- The humeral head does not fill the glenoid fossa.
- The humeral head is superimposed on the posterior glenoid rim.

If the AP view looks normal on initial inspection, it is essential to obtain a radiograph in a second projection. An axillary or lateral transthoracic view (Fig. 8-11) should be obtained if a posterior dislocation is suspected.

Luxatio erecta (Fig. 8-12), an inferior dislocation with the arm held in complete abduction above the head, occurs infrequently and does not present a diagnostic problem. This dislocation occurs with forceful hyperabduction during which the rotator cuff is disrupted as the shoulder dislocates.

All glenohumeral joint dislocations should be reduced in a timely manner. Radiographs should be obtained before and after reduction. The axillary nerve is the nerve most often involved in shoulder dislocation; its status and the neuromuscular function of the distal extremity should be assessed before and after reduction. Following reduction, the shoulder should be immobilized with a shoulder immobilizer or sling and swathe dressing. The patient should be given follow-up referral to an orthopedic surgeon or primary care physician.

Fractures

Fracture of the humeral shaft. Humeral shaft fractures (Figs. 8-13 and 8-14) usually are caused by a fall or a direct blow to the humerus. The radial nerve, which is in proximity to the humerus, may be injured; injury of this nerve results in a wrist-drop. Radial nerve injury is usually

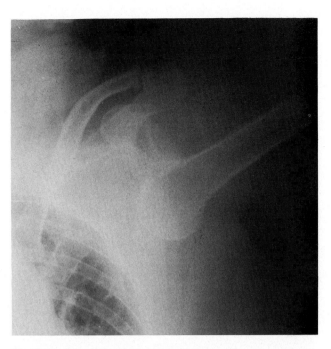

Fig. 8-12. Shoulder, luxatio erecta. Inferior dislocation with arm held above head in abduction.

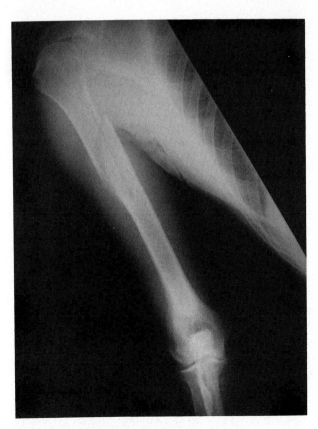

Fig. 8-13. Humerus, spiral fracture.

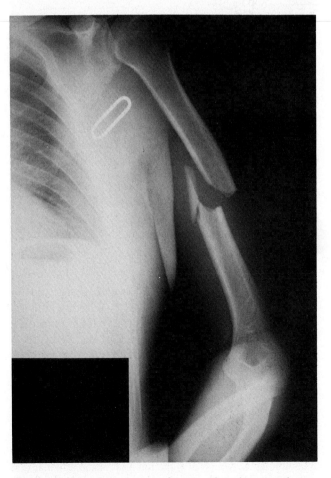

Fig. 8-14. Humerus, transverse fracture. Note that several comminuted fracture fragments are present.

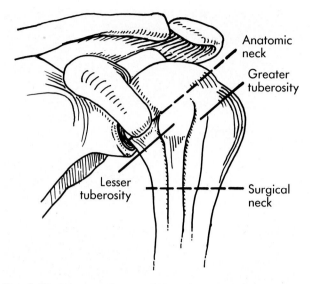

Fig. 8-15. Locations for fractures of the anatomic and surgical neck of the humerus.

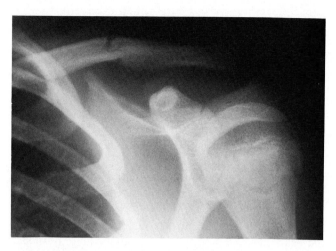

Fig. 8-17. Fracture through middle third of the clavicle.

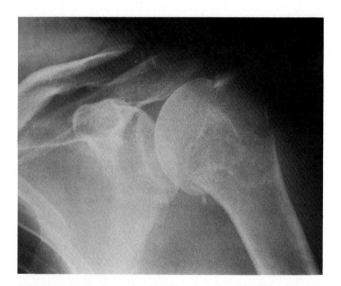

Fig. 8-16. Comminuted fracture of the surgical neck of the humerus.

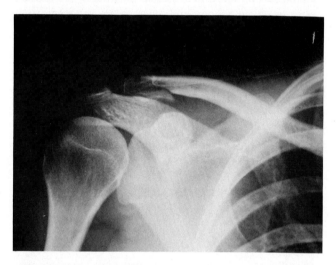

Fig. 8-18. Fracture through distal portion of clavicle. The fracture is nondisplaced and the ligaments remain intact.

only a contusion and should be observed over time for gradual resolution. Vascular injuries associated with humeral shaft fractures, on the other hand, require immediate surgical repair. Long-term complications such as stiffness and nonunion may also occur.

Treatment initially consists of immobilization in a sling and swathe. The patient should be told to obtain early orthopedic consultation since long-term treatment varies among orthopedic surgeons.

Fractures of the anatomic and surgical neck of the humerus. The neck of the humerus is divided into (1) the anatomic neck, which is at the junction of the articular and nonarticular surfaces of the humeral head, and (2) the sur-

gical neck, which is just distal to the greater and lesser tuberosities (Fig. 8-15).

Fractures of the humeral neck often occur in elderly patients who fall. Occasionally these fractures can result from a direct blow to the shoulder. Anatomic humeral neck fractures occur after a fall on the outstretched hand. Prepubescent children can sustain a proximal humeral epiphyseal injury, which is subject to avascular necrosis. Surgical humeral neck fractures are usually held in place by the supporting joint and muscle structures of the shoulder. One-segment fractures usually have minimal fragment displacement. Patients with fractures of multiple segments (Fig. 8-16) are more likely to have neurovascular injuries or delayed problems with mobility.

Treatment of these injuries consists of reduction, if displacement or angulation is present, and immobilization in a sling and swathe or hanging cast. Open reduction is

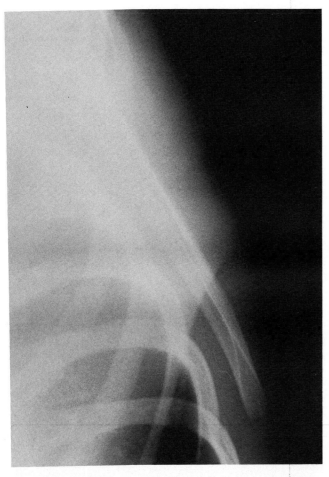

Fig. 8-19. Scapula, normal axial (tangential) view. The scapula is projected away from the chest wall.

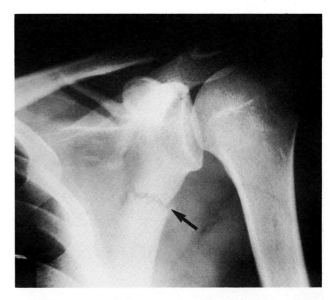

Fig. 8-20. Scapula, AP view of body fracture *(arrow).*

rarely indicated. Early range-of-motion exercises are employed, especially in elderly patients, so that shoulder stiffness does not occur.

Fracture of the clavicle. The clavicle is the bone most often fractured by children. Its superficial location and its position on the lever arm of the upper extremity make the clavicle especially vulnerable to injury.

Approximately 80% of clavicular fractures occur in the middle one third of the bone as the result of an indirectly transmitted force (Fig. 8-17). These fractures are easily seen on radiographs. Nondisplaced fractures usually heal without problems, but if significant displacement is present, care must be taken to evaluate the patient for subclavian vessel injury. Treatment with a sling or figure-of-8 bandage is usually adequate, but all displaced fractures should be followed by an orthopedic surgeon to ensure that adequate reduction is maintained.

Fractures of the medial one third of the clavicle occur only in about 5% of these patients and imply a significant direct blow to the clavicle. The force associated with a medial clavicular fracture may also cause damage to the subclavian vessels or chest structures, and this possibility must be considered when these fractures are seen. If a child is diagnosed as having a medial clavicular fracture, nonaccidental trauma (NAT) must also be considered. These fractures may be difficult to visualize because of overlying bony structures, and an apical lordotic view directed 45 degrees cephalad may be necessary. Treatment in a sling or figure-of-8 strap is usually adequate.

Distal fractures account for approximately 15% of clavicular fractures and are the result of direct trauma. They are graded as type I, II, or III based on the status of the AC and CC ligaments. Type I distal clavicular fractures (Fig. 8-18) have intact ligaments and are nondisplaced. Type II fractures have ruptured CC ligaments and clavicular displacement. Type III fractures involve the articular surface of the AC joint. Fractures that involve the articular surface of the AC joint are prone to arthritis. Generally, distal clavicular fractures can be treated with a sling, but displaced fractures may require open reduction and internal fixation.

Fracture of the scapula. The scapula is well protected by the muscles of the posterior shoulder girdle, and scapular fractures usually require a violent, direct blow. Since high-energy forces are necessary to produce a scapular fracture, the patient with a fracture must be carefully evaluated for other associated chest injuries, such as pneumothorax, vascular injuries, or brachial plexus damage.[4] Localized pain, tenderness, and crepitus are the usual clinical findings.

Standard scapular radiographs include an axial (tangential) view, which projects the scapula away from the chest wall and makes fractures more easily visible (Fig. 8-19)

The scapula may fracture through the body (Figs. 8-20 and 8-21), the coracoid process (Fig. 8-22), or the acro-

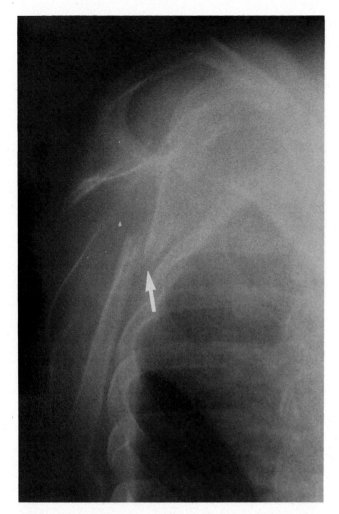

Fig. 8-21. Scapula, tangential view of body fracture *(arrow)*.

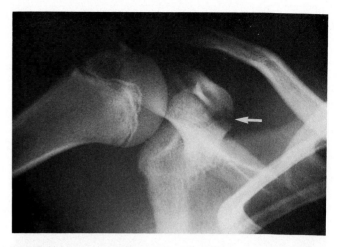

Fig. 8-22. Scapula, AP view showing fracture of coracoid process *(arrow)*.

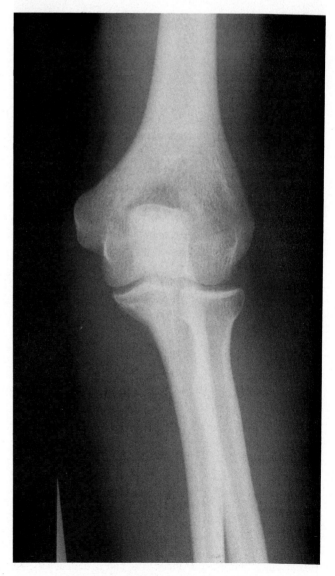

Fig. 8-23. Normal elbow, AP supination.

mion. Acromial fractures are often associated with AC joint and clavicular injuries and late development of bursitis.

Treatment of scapular fractures is sling and swathe immobilization maintained for 2 to 3 weeks for comfort once the possibility of associated chest injuries has been addressed. Acromial injuries are kept immobilized somewhat longer.

ELBOW AND FOREARM
Normal anatomy and radiographic views

The elbow is a complex joint. The humeroulnar joint is a hinge joint, and the radiohumeral joint is a pivot joint. Evaluation of suspected elbow fractures depends on obtaining well-positioned radiographs. The standard elbow series consists of an AP view with the elbow in a neutral position, AP view with elbow in supination (Fig. 8-23), and lateral view with elbow in 90% flexion (Fig. 8-24). Difficulty occurs when the patient is unable to extend or supinate the elbow because of pain or when the patient has difficulty fully flexing the elbow. Unless care

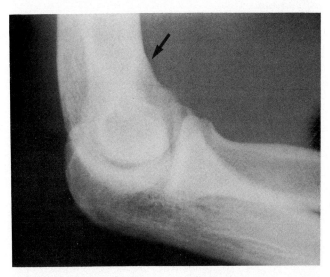

Fig. 8-24. Normal elbow, lateral view. A small anterior fat pad *(arrow)* may normally be present.

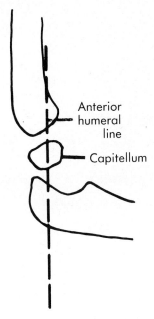

Anterior
humeral
line

Capitellum

Fig. 8-25. Anterior humeral line. This line, seen in the lateral view of the elbow, aids in diagnosis of displaced supracondylar fracture.

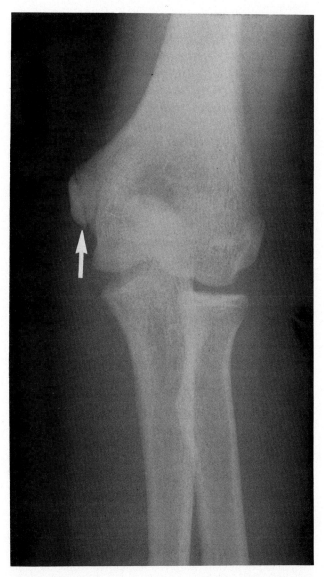

Fig. 8-26. Normal elbow of child, AP view in supination. The normal carrying angle between the humerus and ulna should be 5 to 25 degrees. Note the normal medial epicondylar epiphysis *(arrow)*.

is taken in positioning for the lateral view so that the two condyles are superimposed, subtle injuries may be missed. Once well-positioned radiographs have been obtained, they must be carefully scrutinized not only for fractures, but also for the presence of fat pads. In the lateral view a small anterior fat pad may be seen (Fig. 8-24) in the normal elbow, but a posterior fat pad should not be visualized, since it is hidden in the olecranon fossa.

Normal pediatric anatomy and radiographic views

Radiographs of a child's elbow may be difficult to interpret because of the numerous ossification centers about the elbow, and comparison views may be necessary. Determination of several normal alignments may be helpful in interpreting the radiographs. The anterior humeral line (Fig. 8-25) is seen on the lateral view; this line runs along the anterior surface of the humeral shaft and should pass through the middle third of the capitellum. Supracondylar fractures may displace the distal humerus by decreasing the normal anterior tilt in an extension injury or, less frequently, by increasing the normal anterior tilt in a flexion injury. The carrying angle is measured on the AP view of the elbow in supination (Fig. 8-26). The angle between a line drawn along the shaft of the humerus and a line drawn down the shaft of the ulna should measure 5 to 25 degrees.

Elbow dislocation

Dislocation at the elbow is a typical type of joint dislocation.[5] Usually the elbow dislocates posteriorly (Fig. 8-27). The injury results from a fall on the hand with the elbow extended or from a direct blow to the posterior humerus. Anterior elbow dislocations rarely occur; they result from a direct blow to the anterior humerus while the elbow is flexed.

Lateral radiographs readily demonstrate the dislocation. It is important to look for associated fractures about the elbow. Anterior dislocations may cause an avulsion fracture of the coronoid process of the olecranon. There may be associated injury to the ulnar or median nerve.

Reduction should be performed as soon as possible to minimize the development of vascular complications and edema. Once reduction has been accomplished, the elbow is splinted in flexion. Rarely, when closed reduction is unsuccessful, open reduction is required.

After successful reduction, hospital admission for observation and repeated evaluation of the patient's vascular status is required.[3]

Fractures

Fracture of the distal humerus. Distal humeral fractures are most often seen in children and usually result from a fall on the outstretched hand. The indirect force transmitted to the elbow results in posterior displacement of the distal humerus. A direct blow to the flexed elbow

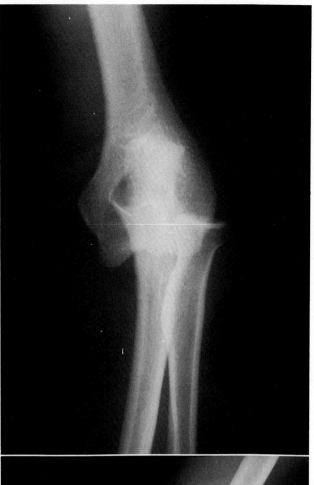

A

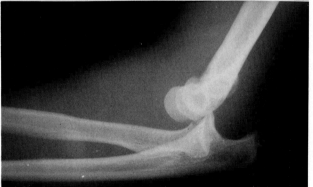

B

Fig. 8-27. Posterior dislocation of elbow. **A,** AP view. **B,** lateral view.

can also cause a fracture with anterior displacement of the distal fragment.

Examination of the anterior humeral line in these patients will demonstrate any posterior (Fig. 8-28) or anterior displacement. A fat pad sign should raise suspicion of a fracture even if the fracture is only minimally angulated. Bowman angle, which is between a line drawn across the condyles and a line drawn down the humeral shaft, should also be determined. This angle normally measures 70 to 90 degrees.

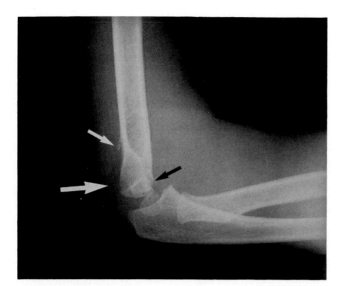

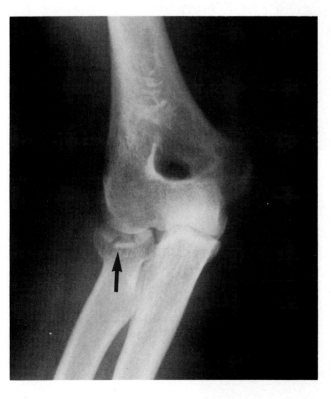

Fig. 8-28. Supracondylar fracture of humerus with posterior displacement *(small arrows)*, lateral view. Note the disruption of the anterior humeral line and the presence of a posterior fat pad *(large arrow)*.

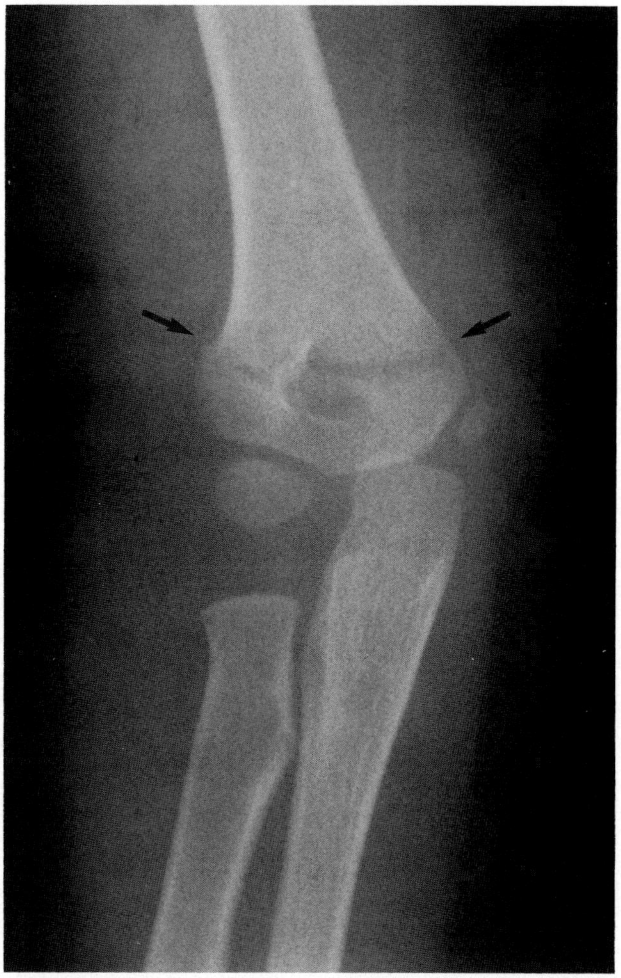

Fig. 8-29. Transcondylar fracture of humerus *(arrows)*, AP view.

Fig. 8-30. Comminuted radial head fracture *(arrow)*, oblique view.

Transcondylar fractures result from a direct blow to the elbow in flexion and are usually visualized on the AP view (Fig. 8-29).

Clinicians must be aware that distal humeral fractures may cause arterial compromise or compartment syndrome, resulting in ischemic contractures of the forearm. These fractures may also injure the median or ulnar nerve.

An orthopedic surgeon should be consulted immediately to reduce the fracture, and the patient should be admitted for observation.[6] The emergency physician should only reduce these fractures when displacement of the fracture is causing vascular compromise and immediate orthopedic consultation is unavailable.

Fracture of the radial head. Radial head fractures usually result from a fall onto the outstretched hand. The patient has tenderness over the radial head, pain with supination and pronation of the forearm, and possibly a palpable joint effusion. Radial head fractures may be nondisplaced, displaced, simple, or comminuted (Fig. 8-30).

Radial head fractures can be difficult to visualize on standard views, and oblique views may be necessary to demonstrate the fracture line. It is also helpful to scrutinize the lateral radiograph for the presence of a posterior fat pad (see Fig. 8-27). A joint effusion or hemarthrosis will displace the posterior fat pad, which is usually hidden in the olecranon fossae. As the posterior pad is pushed backward, it becomes visible on the lateral radiograph. The anterior fat pad, which may be visible on normal elbows, is also displaced anteriorly by joint effusion.

Radial head fractures usually do not result in long-term complications, but the patient must be carefully examined for associated forearm or wrist injuries.

Most patients with these fractures can be treated with a posterior splint or long arm cast for about 3 weeks. If the fracture is severely comminuted, or if chronic pain develops, the radial head may need to be exercised. All patients should have timely primary care or orthopedic follow-up.

Fracture of the olecranon. The olecranon articulates with the trochlea and may be injured by a direct or indirect force. If a patient falls on the forearm with the elbow in flexion, a nondisplaced fracture usually occurs (Fig. 8-31). A direct blow to the posterior elbow can cause a fracture fragment that may become displaced from the traction exerted by the triceps tendon. Posterior elbow dislocations

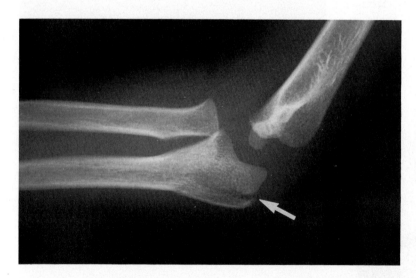

Fig. 8-31. Olecranon fracture, lateral view. This radiograph demonstrates an avulsion fracture of the olecranon process *(arrow)* with moderate dehiscence of the fracture fragment. It is not grossly displaced.

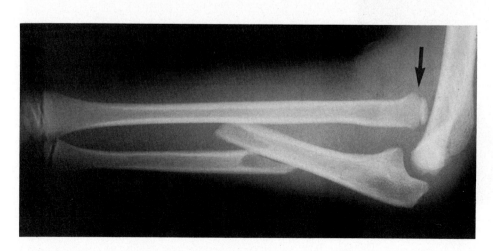

Fig. 8-32. Monteggia fracture, lateral view. A fracture of the proximal ulna is demonstrated along with anterior dislocation of the radial head *(arrow).*

may result in coronoid process fracture of the olecranon when the trochlea forcibly strikes the coronoid process.

Olecranon fractures are usually well visualized on standard radiographs and are best seen on the lateral view.

When an olecranon fracture is recognized, it is important to look for other fractures about the elbow. Ulnar nerve injury may also be associated with this fracture.

Nondisplaced fractures are immobilized in a long arm splint or cast. Displaced fractures require surgical fixation.

Monteggia fracture. The forearm should be thought of as a ringlike structure composed of the radius and ulna and joined by strong ligaments on each end. When a fracture occurs in a ring structure with displacement or change in length at the fracture site, a second break in the ring is likely. A Monteggia fracture involves the proximal third of the ulna associated with an anterior (80%) or posterior (20%) dislocation of the radial head (Fig. 8-32). Monteggia fractures result from a direct blow over the posterior ulna or from a fall onto the pronated forearm.

The key to radiographic diagnosis of a Monteggia fracture is to look for a dislocated radial head on all patients with a proximal ulnar fracture. Elbow radiographs must be obtained on any patient with a proximal ulnar fracture to determine if a dislocation of the radial head is present. The radiocapitellar line, a line passing through the center of the radial shaft and radial head, should pass through the capitellum in all standard elbow views. If the radiocapitellar alignment is lost, a radial head dislocation should be suspected.

Patients with Monteggia fractures typically have associated radial nerve palsy. Patients are usually admitted for closed reduction under anesthesia or for internal fixation of the ulnar fracture if reduction is not easily maintained.

Galeazzi fracture. A Galeazzi fracture involves the junction of the middle and distal third of the radius with subluxation or dislocation of the distal radioulnar joint (Fig. 8-33). This fracture results from a direct blow to the shaft of the radius or from a fall onto the hand. When a radius fracture is seen at the junction of the middle and distal third of the radius, a wrist radiograph must be obtained to check for a Galeazzi fracture.

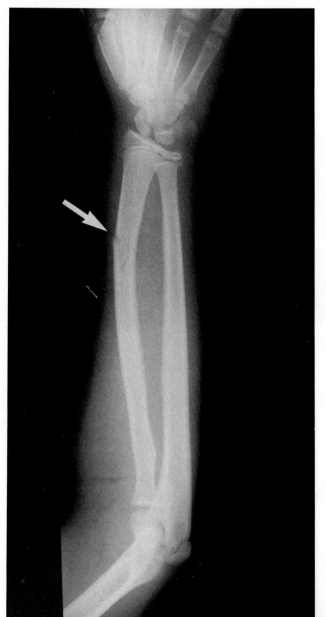

A

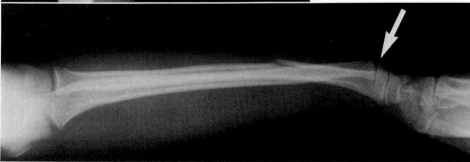

B

Fig. 8-33. Galeazzi fracture. **A,** AP view. This fracture involves a break at the junction of the middle and distal thirds of the radius *(arrow)* with disruption of the distal radioulnar ligaments. **B,** Lateral view. Note subluxation of distal radioulnar joint *(arrow)*.

Complications are rare with this fracture, and definitive treatment is surgical reduction with internal fixation.

Nightstick fracture of the distal ulna. A direct blow to the distal ulna may cause a nightstick fracture (Fig. 8-34). This fracture is so named because it may occur when the forearm is held up to protect the face from the blow of a club or stick. Complications rarely occur; however, care must be taken to differentiate this isolated fracture from fractures associated with ligamentous injury to the wrist or elbow. If displacement or shortening is seen on an isolated ulnar fracture, radiographs of the elbow and wrist should be obtained. The patient with a nightstick fracture is treated with immobilization in a long arm cast.

WRIST AND CARPAL BONES
Normal anatomy and radiographic views

The wrist joint consists of the distal radius and ulna, which are strongly bound together by ligaments, and the eight carpal bones, which are aligned in proximal and distal rows of four bones each (Figs. 8-35 and 8-36).

Several angles should be measured on the AP and lateral views of the wrist. The normal ulnar angulation of the distal radius is 15 to 30 degrees. This angle is measured between a line drawn across the distal ends of the radius and ulna and a line drawn across the tips of the radial and ulnar styloids. Loss of this angle from a fracture limits ulnar mobility. On the lateral view the palmar (volar) incli-

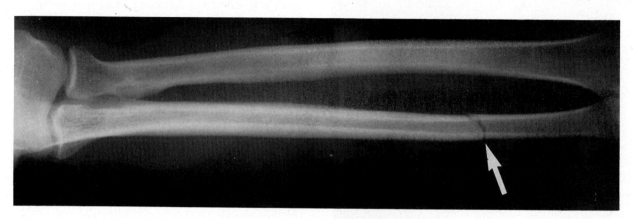

Fig. 8-34. AP view of forearm demonstrating nightstick fracture of distal ulna *(arrow)*.

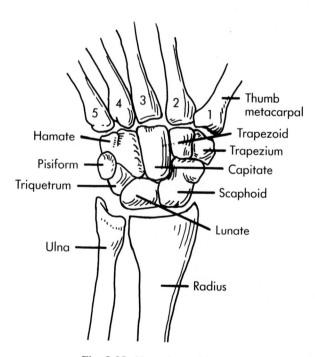

Fig. 8-35. Normal carpal bones.

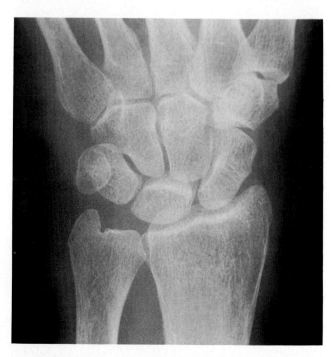

Fig. 8-36. Normal carpal bones, AP view.

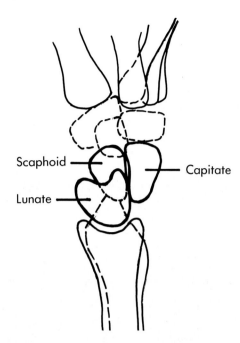

Fig. 8-37. Perilunate dislocation. Dislocation of the capitate with the lunate maintaining its normal alignment to the distal radius.

nation is described by the angle of a line drawn down the shaft of the radius and a line drawn across the articular end of the radius. This angle is normally 10 to 15 degrees.

The quadrate pronator shadow should also be examined on the lateral view. The quadrate pronator muscle stretches from the volar surface of the ulna to the radius. Hemorrhage caused by distal radius or ulnar fractures may displace the soft tissue volarly and provide a clue to an otherwise occult fracture.

Lunate and perilunate dislocations

Perilunate and lunate dislocations are subtle yet potentially debilitating hyperextension injuries of the wrist.

Perilunate dislocations occur more frequently and involve a dorsal dislocation of the capitate, with the lunate bone maintaining its normal alignment with the distal radius (Fig. 8-37). In the AP projection the carpal bones appear foreshortened, and the proximal capitate and distal lunate bones are superimposed (Fig. 8-38, *A*). The key view is the true lateral view, on which dorsal dislocation of the capitate can be seen (Fig. 8-38, *B*).

Lunate dislocations, which occur less often, are hyperextension injuries with the distal lunate bone rotating volarly. On the AP view the lunate has a triangular shape and overlaps the scaphoid bone. On the lateral view the C part of the lunate opens in a palmar direction (Fig. 8-39).

Both these injuries may be subtle and can be missed. The crucial element in making the diagnosis is to obtain a true lateral view and to check that the axis of the distal radius and the axis of the capitate pass through the center of

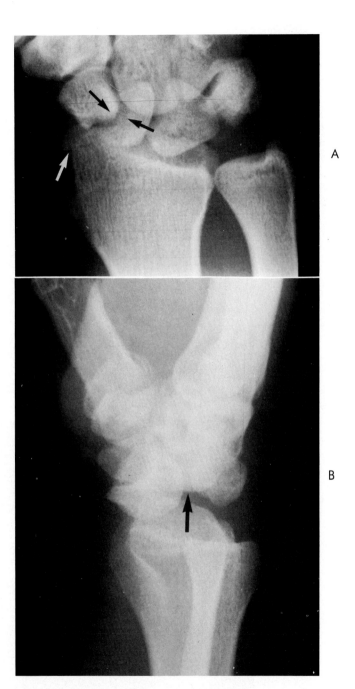

Fig. 8-38. Perilunate dislocation. **A,** AP view. The proximal carpal bones appear superimposed. Note the associated carpal scaphoid and radial styloid fractures *(arrows)*. **B,** Lateral view. The dorsal dislocation of the capitate is seen *(arrow)*. The lunate has begun to rotate volarly. Further volar rotation would transform it into a lunate dislocation.

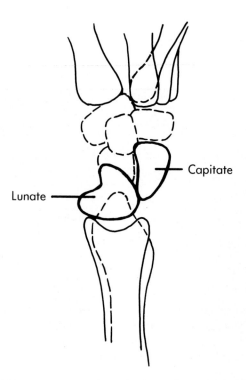

Fig. 8-39. Lunate dislocation. The lunate is rotated in a palmar direction and loses its normal alignment to the distal radius.

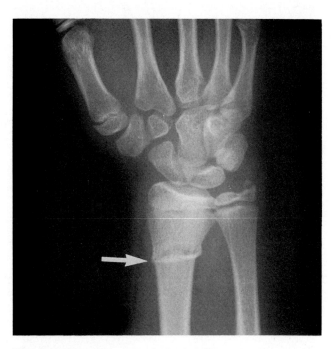

Fig. 8-40. Torus fracture of distal radius, AP view *(arrow)*. Buckling of the cortex of the distal radius is demonstrated in this radiograph.

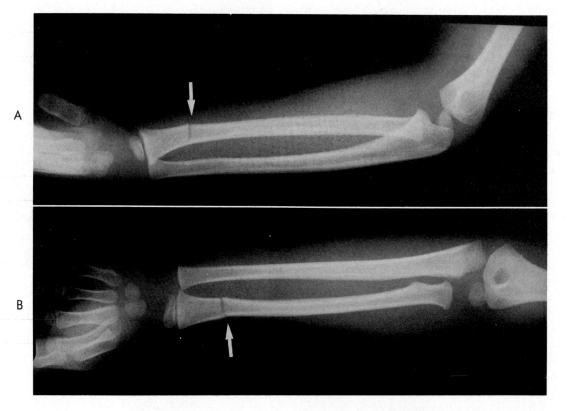

Fig. 8-41. Green-stick fracture of distal radius, AP view **(A)** and lateral view **(B).** There is incomplete cortical disruption of the distal radius *(arrows)*.

the lunate bone. The cup of the distal radius must fit into the lunate, and the cup of the lunate must fit into the capitate.

Treatment consists of initial closed reduction by an orthopedic surgeon, usually followed by open ligamentous repair. Wrist stiffness and arthritis may be seen as long-term complications.

Fractures

Torus and green-stick fractures. The developing bones of a child are more flexible than the mature bones of an adult, and traumatic injuries to the extremity in a child may cause an incomplete or partial fracture of the bony cortex.

A torus fracture is a wrinkling or buckling of the cortex without cortical disruption (Fig. 8-40). Torus fractures may be difficult to visualize unless the proper projection is obtained, and varying oblique views may be necessary to demonstrate a fracture. Complications are rare with a torus fracture, which is easily treated with plaster immobilization.

A green-stick fracture occurs when one cortex is broken and angulated but the opposite cortex remains intact (Fig. 8-41). These fractures usually result from a fall on the outstretched hand. The patient has localized tenderness, minimal swelling, and no deformity. It is called a green-stick fracture because the break is similar to the type seen if one

would bend and snap a growing twig. Green-stick fractures are treated by reduction and plaster immobilization. Complications rarely occur.

Colles' fracture. A Colles' fracture is a common injury sustained from a fall onto the extended wrist. This fracture usually occurs in adults over age 40 and is manifested by an obvious deformity with extreme swelling and tenderness (Fig. 8-42). The Colles' fracture accounts for about two thirds of distal radius fractures. In this fracture the distal radius is shortened and the articular surface of the radius is displaced or angled dorsally.

Complications often occur with Colles' fractures. Associated radiocarpal or radioulnar joint injuries sometimes are present, and ulnar styloid fractures occur in approximately 60% of these patients.[7] Median nerve compression leading to carpal tunnel syndrome often develops, and ulnar nerve injuries are also seen. The patient must be carefully followed once reduction has been accomplished, since gradual loss in range of motion may occur. Chronic stiffness at the wrist may ultimately develop.

Immediate orthopedic surgery referral and reduction and immobilization in a long arm cast should be accomplished as soon as possible for the patient with a Colles' fracture.

Smith fracture. A Smith (reverse Colles') fracture occurs as a result of a fall onto a flexed wrist or from a direct blow to a clenched and flexed fist. Volar displacement of the distal radius fragment occurs (Fig. 8-43). Smith fractures occur infrequently but are readily visualized on standard radiographs. The patient with this fracture is usually treated with closed reduction and immobilization in a long arm cast. Chronic stiffness may develop at the wrist.

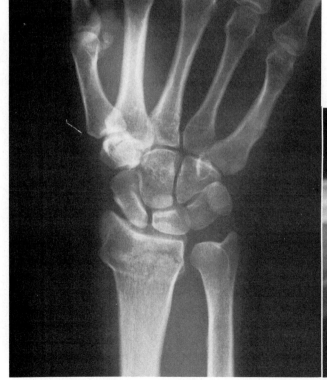

A

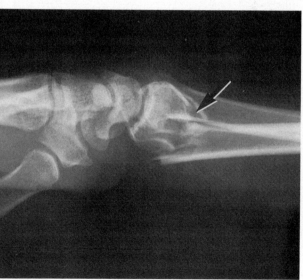

B

Fig. 8-42. Colles' fracture. **A,** AP view. **B,** Lateral view. The lateral view shows a fracture with comminuted fragments. The typical dorsal concave angulation is readily apparent *(arrow).*

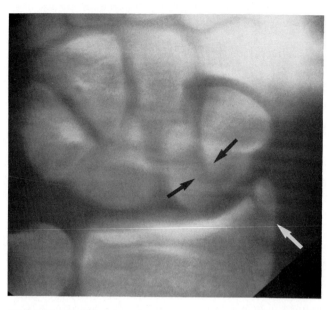

Fig. 8-44. Radial styloid fracture, conventional tomographic AP view. This radiograph shows the radial styloid fracture *(arrow)* with an associated carpal scaphoid fracture *(dark arrows)*.

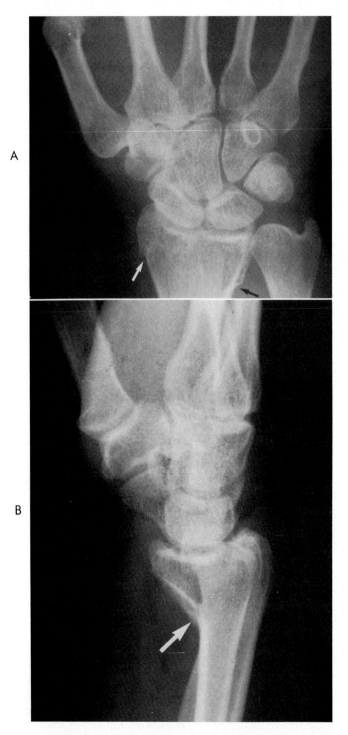

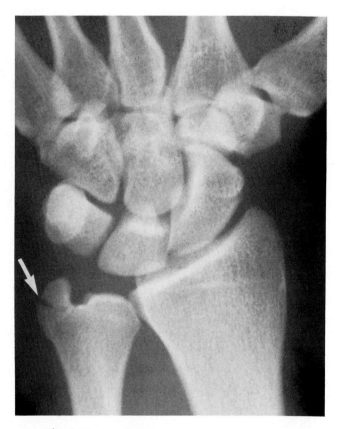

Fig. 8-43. Smith fracture. **A,** AP view *(arrows)*. **B,** Lateral view. Note the volar displacement of the distal radius fragment *(arrow)* giving the appearance of a reverse Colles' fracture.

Fig. 8-45. Ulnar styloid fracture *(arrow)*, AP view.

Fractures of the radial styloid and ulnar styloid processes. A radial styloid fracture occurs with forced hyperextension at the wrist (Fig. 8-44). This injury is easily seen on standard radiographs.

Ulnar styloid fractures usually occur in association with distal radius fractures (Fig. 8-45). An occult radius fracture should be sought when an isolated ulnar styloid fracture is seen.

Patients with both these fractures have localized tenderness with minimal swelling and no deformity. They are treated with cast immobilization. Complications rarely occur unless other injuries are present.

Fracture of the carpal scaphoid. The carpal scaphoid (navicular) is the most frequently injured carpal bone, accounting for about 60% of carpal fractures, but it remains a frequently misdiagnosed injury. Fractures usually occur from a fall onto the outstretched hand, resulting in pain in the wrist and anatomic snuffbox (the hollow on the radial aspect of wrist when thumb is fully extended). The diagnosis is made by a correlation of the clinical and radiographic findings. Even though the radiographs appear normal, if snuffbox tenderness is present, the presence of a scaphoid fracture must be assumed.[8]

Scaphoid fractures may be difficult to visualize, even with multiple views (Fig. 8-46). The fat stripe, which is normally present along the radial aspect of the scaphoid,

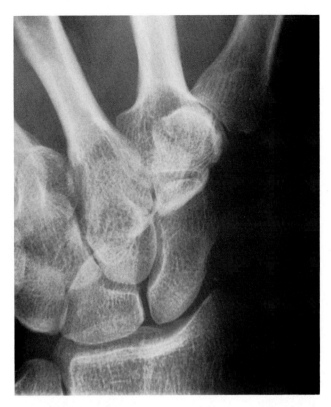

Fig. 8-46. Normal carpal scaphoid, navicular view.

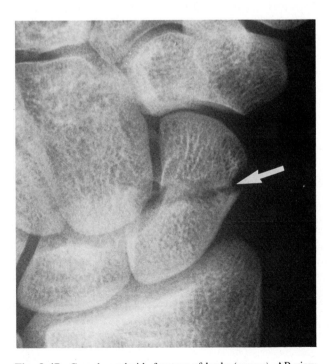

Fig. 8-47. Carpal scaphoid, fracture of body *(arrow)*, AP view.

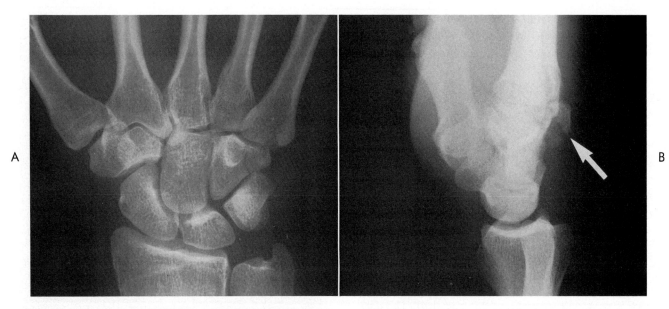

Fig. 8-48. Hamate fracture. Nondisplaced fracture of the medial aspect of the hamate bone is seen. **A,** Oblique view. **B,** Lateral view *(arrow)*.

should be examined. A scaphoid fracture may obliterate this fat stripe[9] (Fig. 8-47). If snuffbox tenderness is present and the radiographs are normal, the patient's wrist and thumb should be splinted for 10 to 14 days, at which time delayed radiographs are obtained. At 2 weeks a radiolucent fracture line with sclerotic margins may become more apparent.

Since the sole blood supply to the scaphoid bone enters distally, missed fractures, especially to the proximal portion, may result in nonunion. If the fracture is not immobilized, nonunion may become apparent several months after the injury. Nonunion is evidenced by cystic and degenerative changes at the fracture margins and as a persistent gap between the two fragments.

Initially, splinting may be done by the emergency physician, but, since complications can occur even with optimal treatment, close follow-up by an orthopedic surgeon is essential.

Fracture of the hamate. Fractures of the hamate bone occur infrequently and result from direct or indirect trauma (Fig. 8-48). Potential morbidity is secondary to the development of arthritis or ulnar nerve damage. Standard carpal views reveal most fractures, but a carpal tunnel view may be necessary to demonstrate fractures of the hamate hook. Patients with hamate fractures are managed by immobilization in a short arm cast for 4 to 6 weeks.

HAND
Normal anatomy and radiographic views

A high-quality hand radiograph is essential for the diagnosis of bony injuries. This radiograph should be ordered if the patient has localized tenderness and pain over the metacarpal bones or metacarpophalangeal joints. AP, lat-

eral, and oblique views usually are taken in a standard series (Figs. 8-49 to 8-51). Most injuries can be evaluated with a standard series of radiographs.

Fractures

Boxer fracture of the fifth metacarpal neck. The boxer fracture, or fracture of the neck of the fifth metacarpal bone, is the most common metacarpal fracture. It results from direct trauma to the metacarpal heads with the fist clenched, a mechanism seen when a punch is delivered to a hard object.

Standard radiographs reveal a fracture of the metacarpal head with volar angulation of the distal fragment (Fig. 8-52,*A*). Oblique views may be necessary to demonstrate the fracture if the other metacarpal heads are superimposed on the fracture site. A true lateral view allows the fracture angle to be measured (Fig. 8-52,*B*).

No significant complications usually occur from a closed boxer fracture. Open boxer fractures are associated with a high risk of infection. If the fracture is not properly aligned, rotation of the finger may occur with flexion, but the normal mobility of the metacarpal head will compensate for most of the deformity.

Treatment consists of closed reduction followed by immobilization in an ulnar gutter splint. Rarely, surgical reduction and internal fixation are necessary.

Fracture of the distal phalangeal tuft. Approximately half of hand fractures occur at the distal phalanx. Tuft fractures are the most common distal phalangeal fracture (Fig. 8-53) and result from direct trauma. The problem with this injury is usually not the fracture, which is easily treated, but the recognition and proper repair of the nailbed and soft tissue injury that may accompany the fracture.

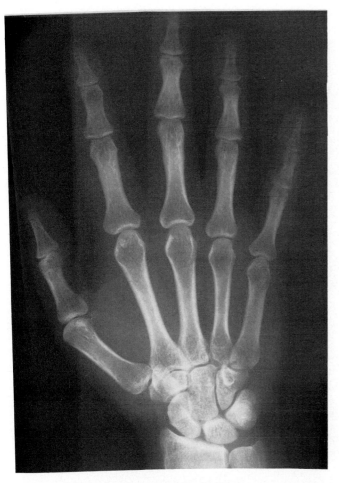

Fig. 8-49. Normal hand, AP view.

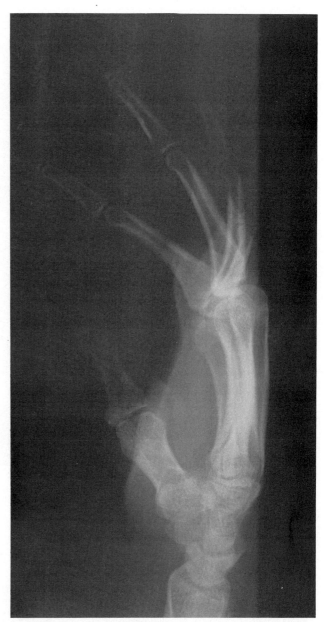

Fig. 8-50. Normal hand, lateral view.

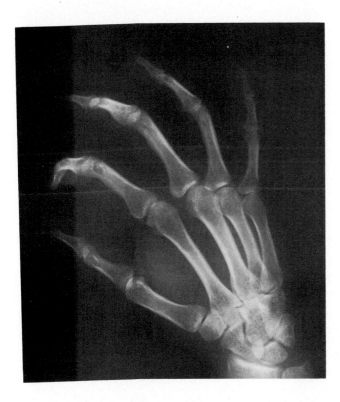

Fig. 8-51. Normal hand, oblique view. The hand is routinely examined in three different planes to identify fractures that cannot be identified in two views because of overlapping bony structures.

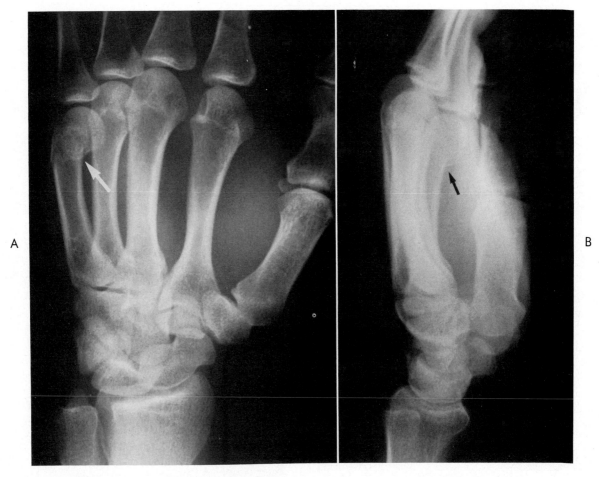

Fig. 8-52. Boxer fracture of fifth metacarpal. **A,** AP view *(arrow).* The distal fragment is angulated palmarly. **B,** Lateral view *(arrow).* The exact fracture angle can be measured in this projection.

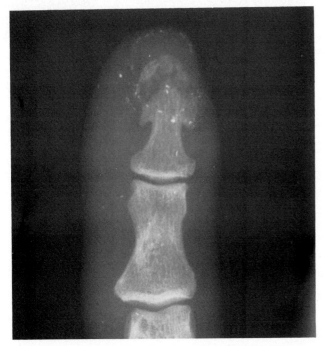

Fig. 8-53. Tuft fracture of distal phalanx, thumb, AP view. This radiograph reveals the comminuted displaced fracture fragments as well as some radio-opaque foreign material on the substance of the nail.

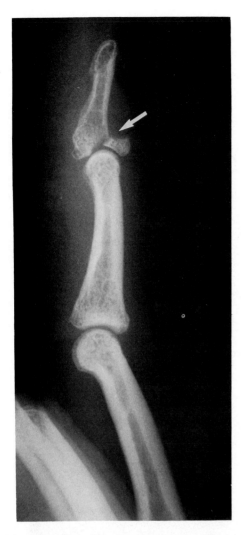

Fig. 8-54. Mallet finger fracture, lateral view. This is an intra-articular avulsion of the dorsal surface of the distal phalanx *(arrow)*.

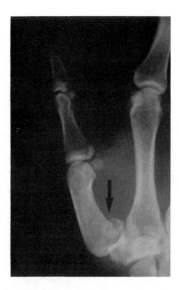

Fig. 8-55. Bennett fracture, AP view *(arrow)*. Avulsion fracture of the articular surface of the first metacarpal with subluxation at the carpometacarpal joint.

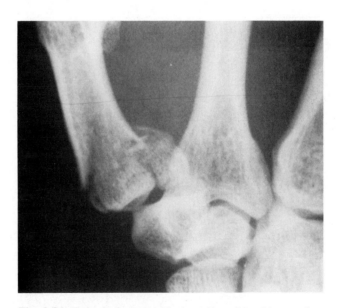

Fig. 8-56. Rolando fracture, AP view. Comminuted intra-articular fracture of the base of the first metacarpal.

Treatment consists of drainage of any subungual hematoma and meticulous repair of any significant nailbed injury. The finger is then splinted in anatomic position for 3 to 4 weeks. Stiffness of the joint and cosmetic deformity of the fingernail are long-term complications.

Mallet finger fracture (intra-articular avulsion fracture). The term *mallet finger fracture* has been given to intra-articular avulsion fractures of the dorsal surface of the distal phalanx, which cause loss of full extension at the distal interphalangeal (DIP) joint. The fracture results from a direct blow on the extended finger, which forcibly flexes the DIP joint and ruptures the attachment of the extensor tendon. Lateral radiographs of the finger easily demonstrate the avulsion fracture (Fig. 8-54).

Treatment of patients with mallet finger fracture consists of splinting the DIP joint in full extension for 6 to 8 weeks. Some orthopedic surgeons advocate internal fixation. Since joint stiffness and loss of full extension may occur, all patients should be referred to an orthopedic surgeon.

Bennett fracture. A Bennett fracture is an oblique avulsion fracture of the base of the articular surface of the first metacarpal bone, with radial subluxation or dislocation of the carpometacarpal joint (Fig. 8-55). The injury typically occurs from an axial force on the metacarpal of the partially flexed thumb.

Surgical reduction and internal fixation are required to repair this fracture. Arthritis at the base of the first metacarpal bone is a typical sequela.

Rolando fracture. A Rolando fracture is a comminuted intra-articular fracture of the base of the first metacarpal bone (Fig. 8-56). Rolando and Bennett fractures

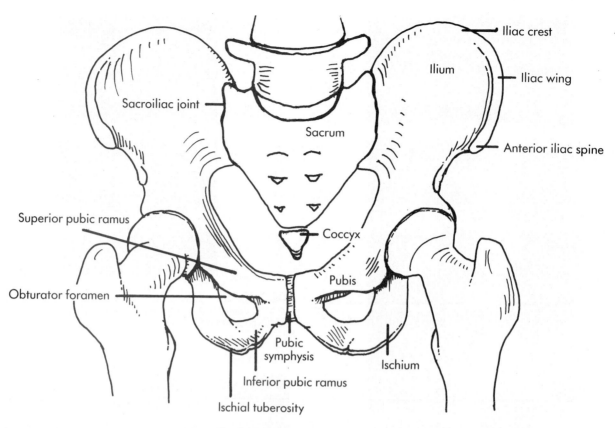

Fig. 8-57. Normal bones of the pelvis.

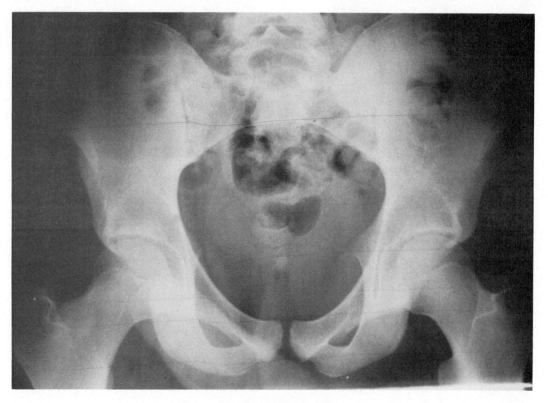

Fig. 8-58. Pelvis, normal AP view.

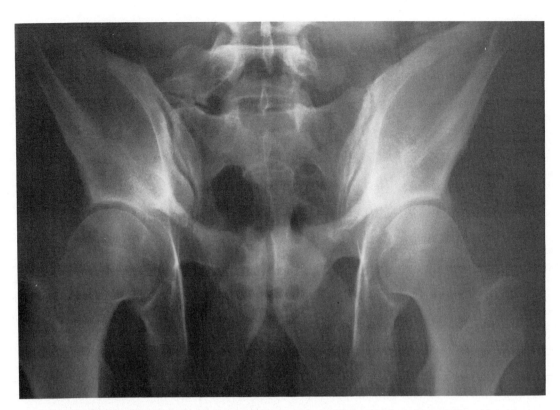

Fig. 8-59. Pelvis, inlet view. This caudad projection provides an en face view of the pubic and ischial bones and may be helpful when a standard AP view does not clearly delineate a fracture.

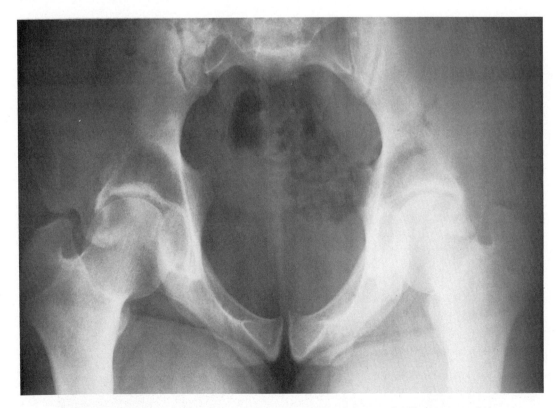

Fig. 8-60. Pelvis, outlet view. This cephalad projection demonstrates the iliac bones en face and the pubic bones in profile. Suspected fractures of the anterior pelvic rim and the integrity of the sacroiliac (SI) joints can be further elucidated with this view.

share the same mechanism of injury, but Rolando fractures occur less often. Surgical intervention is necessary for repair of this fracture. Arthritis and joint stiffness typically occur, even with optimal treatment.

PELVIS
Normal anatomy and radiographic views

The pelvis is a rigid bony structure that provides protection for the lower abdominal organs and serves as a support structure for ambulation. This ring structure is composed of the ilium, ischium, and pubis, held tightly together by three strong ligaments (Fig. 8-57). The two innominate bones are joined anteriorly at the pubic symphysis, and the sacrum is connected to the innominate bones at the sacroiliac (SI) joints. Each innominate bone is composed of an ilium, ischium, and pubis.

The standard AP radiograph of the pelvis is used for initial assessment of pelvic trauma and should be obtained for all patients with high-impact, blunt multiple trauma[10] (Fig. 8-58). This radiograph provides good visualization of most anterior structures and is usually adequate to detect most pelvic injuries. Posterior elements may be difficult to visualize on the AP view and may require special views. Inlet (25 degrees caudad) and outlet (35 degrees cephalad) views better demonstrate the SI joints and pelvic rim (Figs. 8-59 and 8-60). Judet (internal and external oblique) views should be obtained if a more detailed view of the acetabulum is needed to allow for better visualization of nondisplaced acetabular fractures (Fig. 8-61).

Fractures of the pelvis

Pelvic fractures can occur from a variety of mechanisms. Most (60%) are the result of high-impact forces sustained in motor vehicle accidents. Falls in the elderly (30%), crush injuries, and stress from overuse may also cause pelvic fractures. Mortality rates can be high in patients with such fractures because of associated injuries and blood loss.

Several classification systems have been devised to allow the clinician to categorize pelvic fractures. The following system, described by Rockwood and Green,[11] is widely used and is discussed here.

Type I pelvic fractures involve a single bone, and the continuity of the pelvic ring is maintained (Fig. 8-62). These fractures are subdivided into four categories. *Type IA* fractures are avulsion fractures secondary to vigorous muscle contraction that tend to occur in young athletic individuals. The avulsion may be from the anterosuperior iliac spine (contraction of the sartorius muscle), the ischial tuberosity (contraction of the hamstrings), or the anteroinferior iliac spine (contraction of the rectus femoris muscle). Type IA fractures are readily visualized on the standard AP view, but there may be some difficulty distinguishing avulsion fractures from the normal apophyses. Comparison with the opposite side is helpful. Type IA avulsion

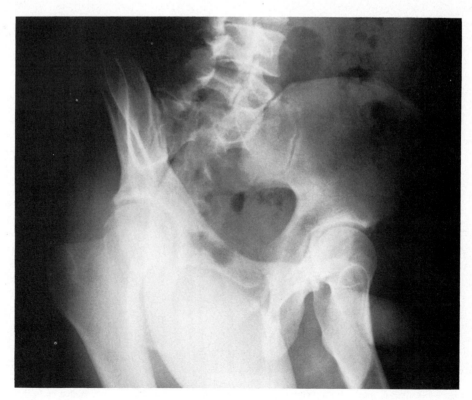

Fig. 8-61. Judet view. This view demonstrates both acetabula in different projections and is useful for evaluation of suspected acetabular fractures.

fractures usually heal without sequelae. All patients with type IA fractures are treated with analgesics, non-weight–bearing, and bed rest.

Type IB fractures result from falls or overuse stress and involve a single pubic ramus or the ischium. They are one of the most common types of pelvic fractures and usually heal without sequelae. *Type IC* fractures are iliac wing fractures that result from a direct blow to the side of the pelvis. Both type IB and IC fractures are easily seen on AP views. *Type ID* fractures are horizontal fractures of the sacrum or coccyx resulting from a direct blow. They should be distinguished from vertical fractures of the sacrum, which may disrupt the integrity of the pelvic ring. The standard AP view of the pelvis does not demonstrate type ID fractures well, and an outlet view of the pelvis or special sacral views may be necessary.

Type II pelvic fractures are stable breaks in the pelvic ring and account for approximately 20% of such fractures. No displacement of fracture fragments occurs. *Type IIA* fractures occur most often and involve both ipsilateral rami (Fig. 8-63). They result from direct trauma and are easily seen on the standard AP view of the pelvis. With these fractures one must clinically evaluate for ipsilateral SI joint involvement. If pain or tenderness at the SI joint is found, radiographic evaluation is necessary to rule out a more serious type III fracture. Treatment of patients with type IIA fractures consists of non-weight–bearing until pain resolves, then progressive ambulation.

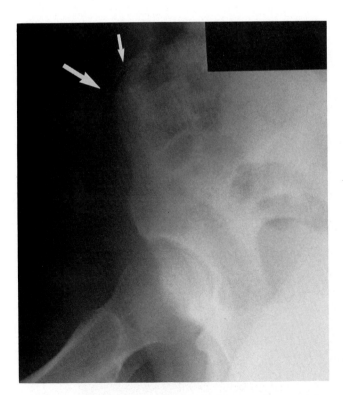

Fig. 8-62. Pelvis, type IA fracture. AP view reveals an avulsion fracture *(small arrow)* with lateral displacement *(large arrow)* of the nonfused iliac crest.

Type IIB fractures represent injuries near the pubic symphysis or disruption of the pubic symphysis. They are rare injuries and are often associated with trauma to the genitourinary system. Standard radiographs are usually adequate to make the diagnosis. Treatment consists of bed rest and analgesics. The urethra and bladder must be evaluated for injury with type IIB fracture (see Chapter 7). Patients with type IIB injuries should be hospitalized.

Type IIC fractures are rare injuries from a direct force that causes a fracture near the SI joint without displacement. The standard AP view of the pelvis may not demonstrate this fracture well, and outlet views may be necessary to better define it. It is important to look for a second disruption in the anterior section of the pelvic ring when a type IIC injury is suspected. Treatment consists of analgesics and bed rest.

Type III pelvic fractures are serious, unstable injuries and represent a double break in the pelvic ring. They account for approximately one third of pelvic fractures. *Type IIIA* fractures (butterfly fractures) are a double vertical break in the anterior portion of the pelvic ring (Fig. 8-64). They result from a straddle injury or a direct blow from the side and are associated with genitourinary damage in about one third of patients. Type IIIA fractures are easily demonstrated on the AP view. Type IIIA fractures require a diligent search for other injuries since associated abdominal and genitourinary injuries as well as other fractures are often seen in patients sustaining the force required to cause this degree of pelvic trauma. All these patients should be admitted for observation. Unstable fractures require fixation.

Type IIIB fractures, often referred to as *Malgaigne fractures,* are a double vertical fracture in the pelvic ring. One fracture is anterior and usually occurs at the pubic symphysis or through both ipsilateral pubic rami. The second fracture occurs at or near the ipsilateral SI joint and is unstable. If the segments of the pelvis are significantly displaced, the leg on the involved side may shorten. AP views reveal widening of the SI joint and displacement of the anteriorly disrupted segment. Patients with IIIB fractures should be admitted for observation and surgical fixation. Radiographic evaluation of the lower genitourinary system should be performed, and the patient should be examined for other fractures.

Type IIIC fractures are severe multiple fractures that occur from a crush injury (Fig. 8-65). The pelvic ring is very unstable, and the mortality rate is high in these patients. As with all type III injuries, the primary responsibility of the emergency physician is to ensure adequate volume resuscitation for patients and to search diligently for associated injuries. The patient should be admitted to the intensive care unit and observed closely for progressive retroperitoneal hemorrhage. Severe ongoing hemorrhage may necessitate selective pelvic embolization and external fixation. Surgical fixation is ultimately required.

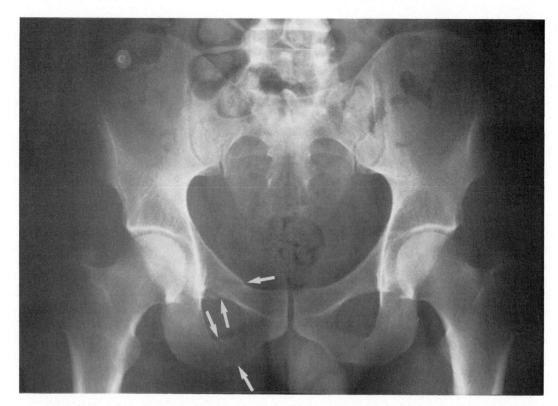

Fig. 8-63. Pelvis, type IIA fracture. There are nondisplaced fractures of both the superior and inferior pubic rami *(arrows)*.

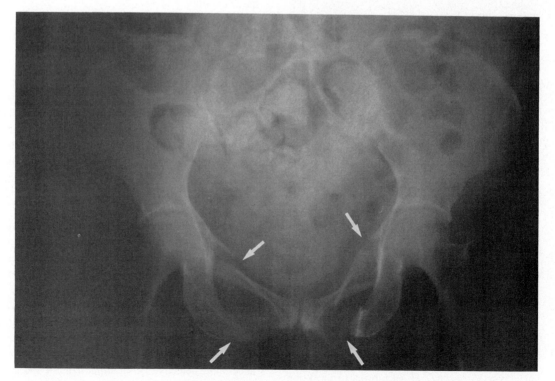

Fig. 8-64. Pelvis, type IIIA, butterfly fracture. This straddle injury fracture includes bilateral fractures of the superior and inferior pubic rami *(arrows)*. The fracture fragments are displaced.

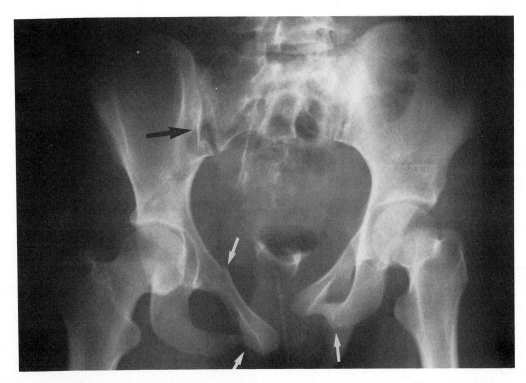

Fig. 8-65. Pelvis, type IIIC, crush injury. Fractures of both pubic rami *(small arrows)* and disruption of the ipsilateral SI joint *(large arrow)* are typical of a Malgaigne fracture. Additionally there is dehiscence of the pubic symphysis. A Foley catheter is present.

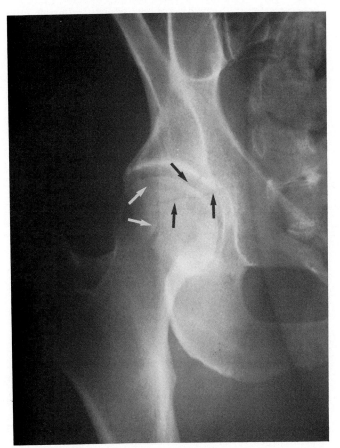

Fig. 8-66. Pelvis, type IV acetabular fracture. Multiple vertical and transverse nondisplaced fractures *(arrows)* of the posterior and superior acetabulum are demonstrated in this view.

Type IV pelvic fractures are injuries involving the acetabulum and account for approximately 15% of pelvic fractures (Fig. 8-66). They occur from an indirect blow to the greater trochanter or flexed knee and may be difficult to visualize on standard views. Therefore Judet views (Fig. 8-61) may be necessary to demonstrate the fracture. Acetabular fractures may be associated with damage to the ipsilateral hip, femur, and knee, as well as to the sciatic nerve; careful examination is necessary to rule out these injuries. Patients with type IV acetabular fractures are admitted to the hospital for immobilization. Surgical fixation may ultimately be required. Long-term development of avascular necrosis of the femoral head or arthritis may occur.

HIP AND FEMUR
Normal anatomy and radiographic views

The hip is a ball-and-socket joint designed for weight bearing and mobility (Fig. 8-67). A routine radiographic series of the hip consists of AP and lateral views (Figs. 8-68 and 8-69).

The normal angle between the axis of the shaft and neck of the femur is 120 to 130 degrees. A smooth curve should be described by the medial surface of the shaft and the inferior aspect of the neck of the femur. This curve continues uninterrupted along the inferior border of the superior pubic ramus. The trabecular meshwork of the femoral neck must also be closely inspected for any subtle disruption that might indicate a nondisplaced fracture.

The lateral radiograph is taken horizontally across the table with the patient supine. Although it is somewhat

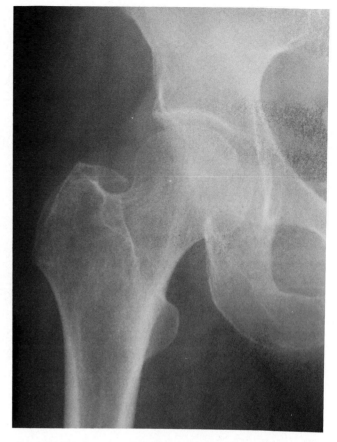

Fig. 8-68. Normal hip, AP view. The inferior border of the femoral neck forms a smooth curve with the inferior margin of the superior pubic ramus.

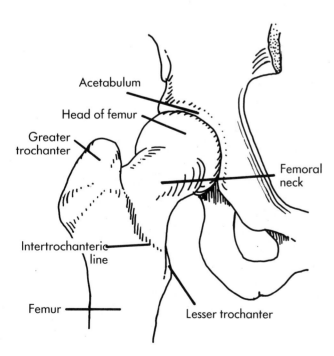

Fig. 8-67. Normal hip structures. Note that the angle between the shaft and neck of the femur is normally 120 to 130 degrees.

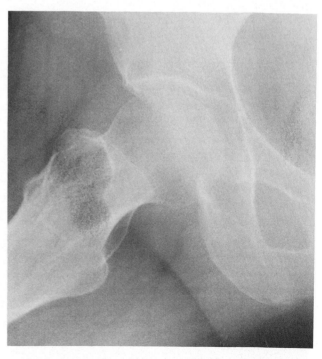

Fig. 8-69. Normal hip, lateral view. Note the continuity of the trabecular meshwork.

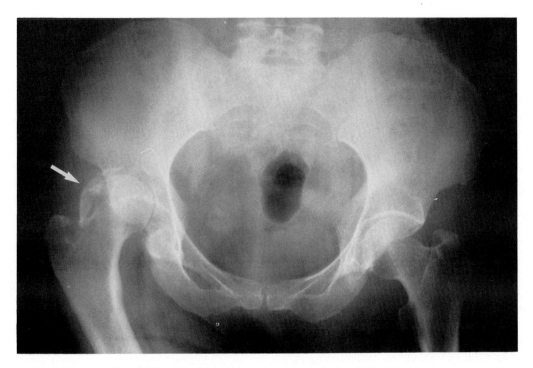

Fig. 8-70. Right hip, posteriorly and superiorly dislocated. An avulsion fracture of the posterior margin of the acetabulum is also present with gross displacement of the avulsed fracture fragment *(arrow)*.

more difficult to interpret, the lateral view may display displaced fractures or confirm disruption of the bony trabecular pattern.

Hip dislocation

The hip joint is relatively stable, and a large force must be applied for a dislocation to occur. This injury usually is caused by high-speed motor vehicle or auto-pedestrian accidents.

Posterior hip dislocations occur most often (85%) and result from a high-energy force impacting the flexed knee, a mechanism duplicated by the knee striking a dashboard. The patient has the hip flexed, adducted, and internally rotated.

Posterior dislocations are usually readily visualized on standard radiographs (Fig. 8-70), but it is also important to look for associated femoral neck or posterior acetabular lip fractures. Sometimes a patient with a posterior hip dislocation and femur shaft fracture is in traction, and the clues of abnormal leg posture are lost. In these patients the dislocation may only be discovered when a pelvic radiograph is obtained. All patients with femoral shaft fractures should have a pelvic radiograph done.

Complications of posterior hip dislocations include sciatic and peroneal nerve injury and late development of avascular necrosis of the femoral head or arthritis.[11]

Anterior hip dislocations occur much less often (15%) and result from either forced abduction or severe hyperextension with external rotation. The patient has the hip

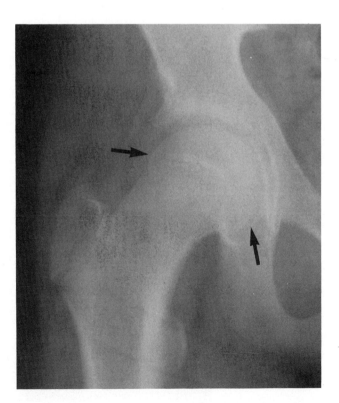

Fig. 8-71. Slipped capital femoral epiphysis, AP view. The femoral head has migrated in an inferior and posterior direction *(arrows)*.

flexed, abducted, and externally rotated. Nerve damage is much less frequent with anterior hip dislocations, but avascular necrosis may still occur.

Hip dislocations are an orthopedic emergency and must be rapidly reduced to minimize the risk of long-term complications, such as avascular necrosis. An orthopedic surgeon should be summoned immediately, and, if closed reduction cannot be easily performed, the patient should go to the operating room for reduction under general anesthesia.

Slipped capital femoral epiphysis

A slipped capital femoral epiphysis is the spontaneous movement of the growth plate of the femoral head in a posterior and downward direction (Fig. 8-71). It typically occurs in overweight males approaching adolescence. This slippage usually involves the gradual development of a deep aching pain in the hip, with subsequent development of a limp, but it occasionally occurs as an acute condition.[12]

Radiographic diagnosis may be difficult in the early stages of slipped capital femoral epiphysis, and "frog leg" views of the flexed abducted hips, as well as standard hip views, may be necessary. In early stages, radiographs may reveal a widened irregular epiphyseal plate. New periosteal bone may form later. As the slippage continues, the smooth line of the inferior aspect of the femur's head and neck is obscured, and the leg begins to rotate externally.

If the condition is not diagnosed early and referred to an orthopedic surgeon for treatment, permanent deformity and an abnormal gait may result.

Legg-Perthes disease

Legg-Perthes disease is an idiopathic, aseptic necrosis of the femoral head seen in childhood and most often occurring in preadolescent males. These children usually have a limp, hip pain, or knee pain.

The radiographic changes in Legg-Perthes disease parallel those seen with avascular necrosis of the femoral head (Fig. 8-72). Initially the radiographs appear normal, but as the process of revascularization occurs, the epiphysis becomes mottled. As reossification begins, gradual regeneration and sclerosis of the femoral head occurs, but with weight bearing the head flattens.

Legg-Perthes disease tends to be self-limited, but pain and deformity may persist. When the patient has pain, immobilization or traction may be helpful, but sometimes osteotomy is performed.

Fractures

Fracture of the femoral neck. Femoral neck fractures can present a difficult diagnostic problem because both the clinical presentation and the radiographic findings may be subtle. These fractures usually occur in elderly patients who fall and develop hip or groin pain, but sometimes the history of significant trauma may be lacking. The patient

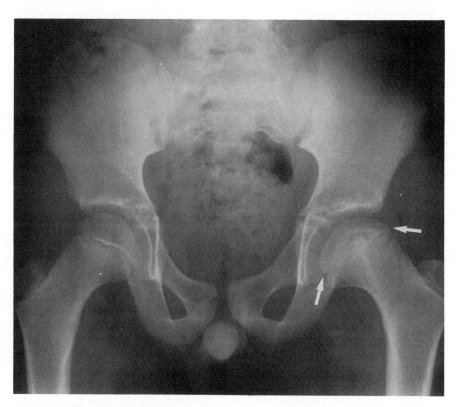

Fig. 8-72. Legg-Perthes disease, AP view. Involved femoral head is flattened and mottled *(arrows)*.

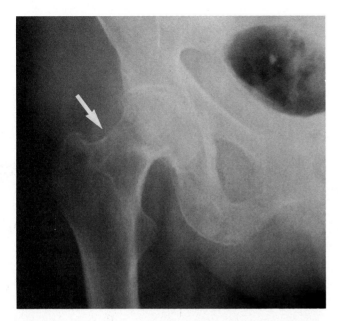

Fig. 8-73. Transcervical fracture of the femoral neck, AP view. The fracture line is not unequivocally demonstrated on this view although there is some suggestion of disruption of the cortex *(arrow).*

may be unable to ambulate or may have pain on ambulation. If the fracture is impacted or nondisplaced, no deformity occurs. Since the diagnosis may be easily missed, any elderly patient with hip pain after a fall or minor trauma should be suspected of having a femoral neck fracture, and hip radiographs should be obtained.

Interpretation of these radiographs may be difficult. Normally a subtle osteophytic lipping is seen at the femoral head and neck junction that is difficult to differentiate from a nondisplaced fracture, but on close examination some disruption of the trabecular latticework is usually apparent. If standard radiographs are inconclusive, additional views with the hip either slightly internally or externally rotated may demonstrate the trabecular disruption[6] (Fig. 8-73). If plain radiographs remain inconclusive, conventional tomograms may be necessary to differentiate the normal peripheral lip calcification from a fracture. Delayed radiographs taken 10 to 14 days after initial presentation usually show the sclerotic margins of a healing fracture, but the prolonged period of immobilization necessary for this method of diagnosis is neither practical nor desirable in the elderly patient.

When initial radiographs, including conventional tomograms, are inconclusive, a bone scan can be used to confirm the diagnosis of femoral neck fracture. At 72 hours after injury a bone scan demonstrates the fracture in approximately 95% of patients. A positive scan shows a band of increased uptake of radionuclide at the fracture site (Fig. 8-74). Long-term complications include avascular necrosis of the femoral head, nonunion, and arthritis.

Treatment of patients with femoral neck fracture con-

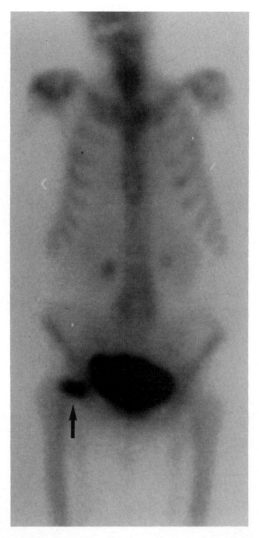

Fig. 8-74. Bone scan of patient in Fig. 8-73. The scan clearly shows a focus of increased activity in the region of the femoral neck *(arrow).*

sists of hospitalization and immobilization of the fracture site. Some orthopedic surgeons recommend bed rest with skin traction, but most recommend surgical fixation or a total hip replacement.

Extracapsular fractures. Extracapsular hip fractures occur often and are usually caused by falls in elderly patients or by high-speed motor vehicle accidents in younger patients. The patient has hip pain, and the leg is shortened and externally rotated.

Most extracapsular fractures are intertrochanteric but may be pertrochanteric or subtrochanteric. The fracture line extends between the greater and lesser trochanters (Fig. 8-75). Pertrochanteric fractures, the second most common type, are intertrochanteric fractures that extend into one or both trochanters (Fig. 8-76). Subtrochanteric fractures occur inferior to the greater and lesser trochanters.

Radiographic diagnosis is usually easily made with standard views of the hip.

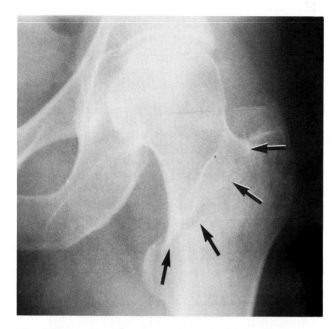

Fig. 8-75. Intertrochanteric fracture, AP view. Fracture line extends between the trochanters, disrupting the trabecular meshwork of the femoral head (arrows).

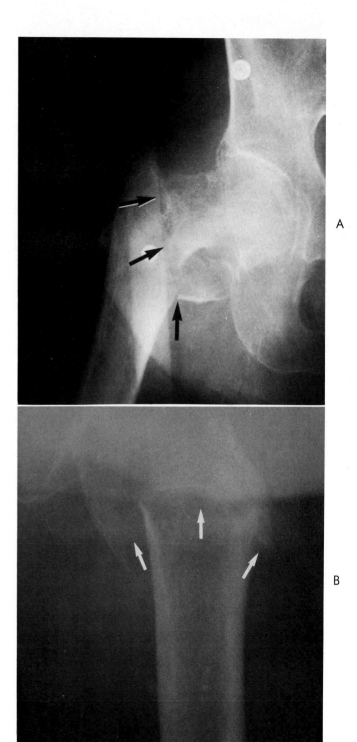

A

B

Fig. 8-76. Pertrochanteric fracture. **A,** AP view. Fracture line extends into both trochanters (arrows). **B,** Lateral view (arrows).

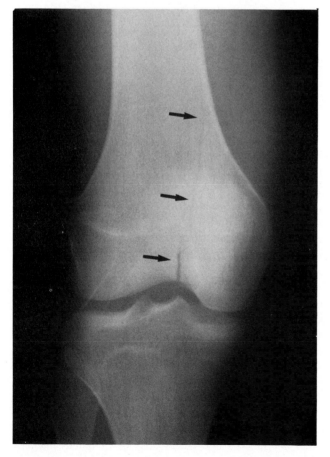

Fig. 8-77. Intra-articular fracture of the distal femur, AP view. Note that the fracture line extends superiorly into the supracondylar region (arrows).

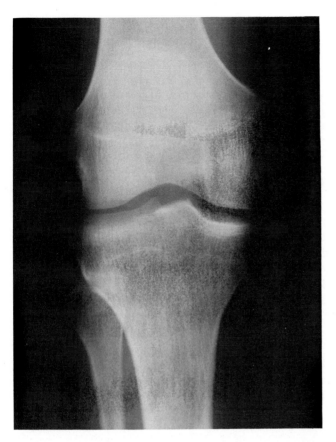

Fig. 8-78. Normal knee, AP view.

Young patients with isolated extracapsular fractures usually do well, in contrast to elderly patients, who are at high risk of developing deep venous thrombosis because of the long periods of immobilization often required to treat these fractures.

Most orthopedic surgeons recommend surgical repair of these fractures although some advocate bed rest if the fracture is stable.

Fracture of the distal femur. Supracondylar intra-articular fractures of the distal femur occur infrequently and result from a forceful direct blow (Fig. 8-77). Since a serious injury may be associated with significant damage to the popliteal artery or peroneal nerve, a careful neurovascular examination should be performed on all patients with a distal femur fracture. In addition, radiographs of the hip and entire femur should be obtained to rule out any related injury.

Patients with nondisplaced distal femur fractures are usually treated with plaster immobilization, whereas those with displaced fractures may require surgical fixation.

KNEE, TIBIA, AND FIBULA
Normal anatomy and radiographic views

The standard radiographic examination of the knee consists of AP and lateral views (Figs. 8-78 and 8-79). Two oblique views are sometimes included as part of a standard series. Special views, such as the axial view of the patella (Fig. 8-80) or tibial plateau views, may be added when specific injuries are suspected.

Although radiographs are essential in evaluation of knee trauma, most injuries are ligamentous and radiographic

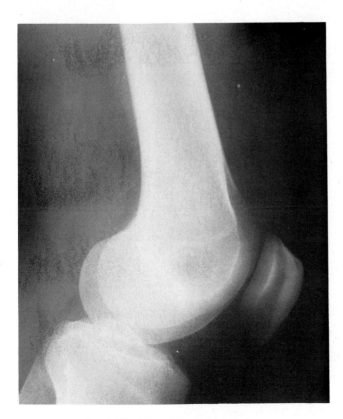

Fig. 8-79. Normal knee, lateral view.

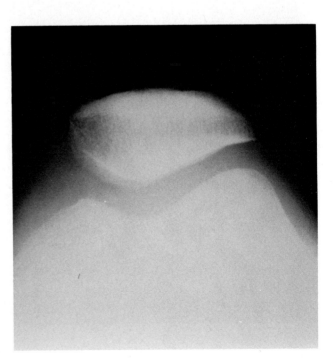

Fig. 8-80. Patella, sunrise (axial) view.

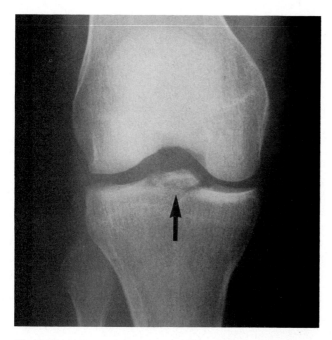

Fig. 8-81. Knee, AP view. Intercondylar spine fracture *(arrow)*. This fracture may be an indication of ligamentous damage to the knee.

findings may be subtle or absent, even when significant ligamentous damage is present.

Ligamentous injury may be suggested by several findings on plain radiographs. An anteriorly distended joint capsule, with displacement of the patella, may indicate hemarthrosis. Unilateral widening of a joint space may be seen as an indication of ligamentous instability. Avulsion fractures of the tibial spines or femoral condyles may provide an indication of a ligamentous injury (Fig. 8-81).

Knee dislocation

Knee dislocations occur infrequently. They result from a violent force and often have significant associated neurovascular and ligamentous injuries. Usually the tibia dislocates anteriorly (Fig. 8-82). Posterior, medial, lateral, and rotatory dislocations are extremely rare. Anterior dislocation results from a severe force in hyperextension that also ruptures the posterior capsule and cruciate ligaments.

Knee dislocation is usually obvious on clinical examination. Sometimes prehospital splinting and traction may spontaneously relocate the knee before the patient arives at the emergency department.

Anterior dislocation of the knee causes popliteal artery injury in approximately 40% of these patients. Therefore

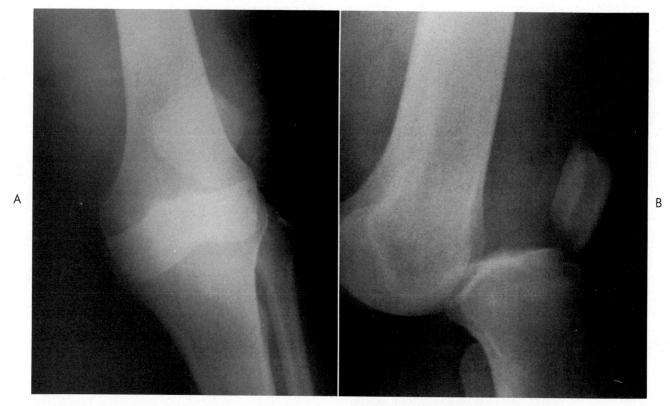

Fig. 8-82. Anterior dislocation of the knee. **A,** AP view. This view shows overlap of the femur and tibia, which is never seen under normal circumstances. The anteriorly dislocated tibia is magnified. **B,** Lateral view. Anterior dislocation of the tibia in relation to the femur is seen. The patella is also anteriorly dislocated.

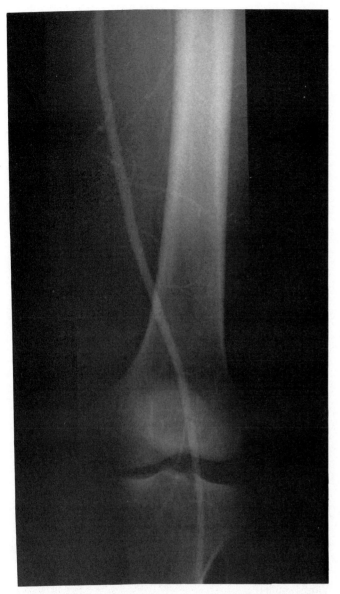

Fig. 8-83. Angiogram of popliteal artery. This angiogram (done on same patient as in Fig. 8-82, *B*) is normal. Popliteal artery injury results from a shearing force that results in occlusion of the vessel at or just distal to the joint line.

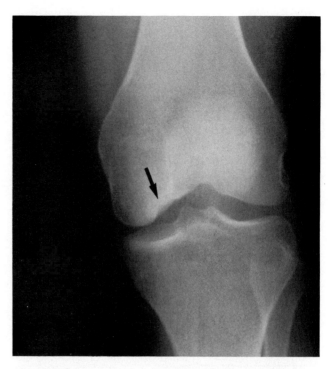

Fig. 8-84. Osteochondritis dissecans, AP view. A shallow concave defect is seen at the joint surface of the medial condyle of the distal femur *(arrow)*.

angiography of the popliteal vessels should be strongly considered as integral in the evaluation of these patients even if good pulses return immediately after reduction[13] (Fig. 8-83). Peroneal nerve injury is also seen in about one third of these patients and is usually manifested by foot-drop or weakness on dorsiflexion of the foot.

Knee dislocations are an orthopedic emergency. If vascular insufficiency is present, the emergency physician should immediately reduce the dislocation using longitudinal traction. If vascular compromise is not present, the orthopedic surgeon should be summoned immediately to reduce the dislocation. All patients should be admitted to the hospital after reduction has been accomplished.

Osteochondritis dissecans

Osteochondritis dissecans is a defect usually seen at the intercondylar aspect of the medial femoral condyle and is caused by a cartilaginous separation of the bone (Fig. 8-84). This defect is usually seen in older children or adolescents who have knee pain and tenderness, often without a history of previous trauma.[12] Once the cartilage separates, granulation tissue fills the defect, resulting in an irreuglar joint surface.

Radiographs reveal a shallow defect with irregular margins in the subchondral surface of the femur. Late in the disease a "joint mouse" or loose body may develop. Although the medial femoral condyle is classically involved, the lateral femoral condyle or patella may also be affected.

Treatment for patients with osteochondritis dissecans consists of immobilization and non-weight–bearing if the disorder is diagnosed in its early stages. If the diagnosis is delayed, surgical intervention may be required.

Fractures

Fracture of the patella. The patella may be fractured by either a direct blow or an indirect force transmitted via contraction of the quadriceps tendon. Fractures are usually transverse (Fig. 8-85) but may be comminuted (30%) or vertical (15%).

Standard AP and lateral views usually demonstrate the patellar fracture, but superimposed bony structures may obscure the fracture on the AP view. An axial (sunrise) view of

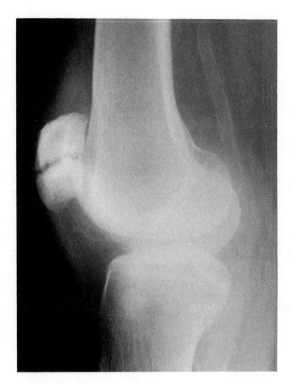

Fig. 8-85. Transverse fracture of patella, lateral view. The fracture margins are irregular with minimal distraction. Calcified popliteal vessels are also seen.

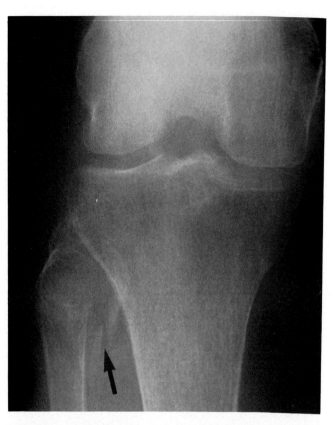

Fig. 8-87. Proximal fibular fracture *(arrow)*, AP view. This fracture in itself is not serious, but the ankle joint must be examined for injury when a proximal fibular fracture is discovered.

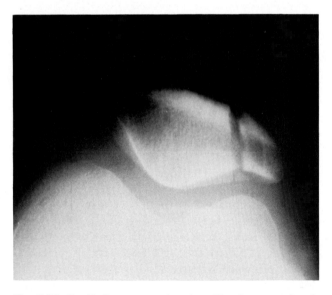

Fig. 8-86. Patella fracture, sunrise view. The sharp nonsclerotic margins identify this as an acute fracture and not a congenital finding.

the patella, obtained tangential to the patella with the knee in flexion, may aid in revealing these fractures (Fig. 8-86).

Complications are rare with patellar fractures unless there is associated quadriceps tendon injury. It is important to evaluate the pelvis, hip, and femur for injury when a patellar fracture is found. Traumatic chondromalacia may develop as a late complication.

Patients with nondisplaced patellar fractures can be treated by immobilization in a long leg cylindric cast and may be discharged. Patients with displaced, distracted, or badly comminuted patellar fractures are usually admitted for surgical reduction and internal fixation. Preservation of patellar fragments is desirable to minimize long-term knee joint pain and arthritis.

A bipartite patella results from nonunion of the two patellar ossification centers and can be confused with a fracture. The bipartite patella has smooth, sclerotic margins and is usually located in the superolateral portion of the patella.[14] If one is uncertain whether a patella is bipartite or fractured, comparison radiographs should be obtained since bipartite patella is usually a bilateral finding.

Fractures of the proximal fibula and the Maisonneuve fracture. An isolated proximal fibular fracture is not in itself a serious injury since the fibula is not a weight-bearing bone. When a proximal fibular fracture is detected, however, there must be a careful evaluation for associated injuries (Fig. 8-87).

A Maisonneuve fracture is a fracture of the proximal one third of the fibula associated with a rupture of the anteroinferior tibiofibular ligament (Fig. 8-88). This fracture results from forced external rotation and abduction of the foot or from a direct blow and may be associated with peroneal nerve injury.

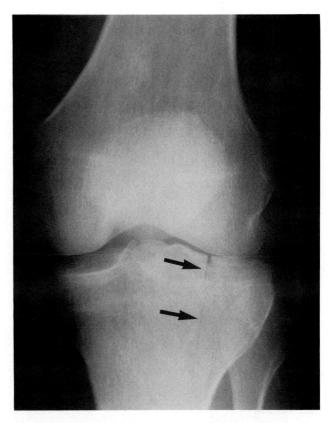

Fig. 8-89. Lateral tibial plateau fracture, AP view. The fracture *(arrows)* is demonstrated well in this projection even though minimal displacement has occurred.

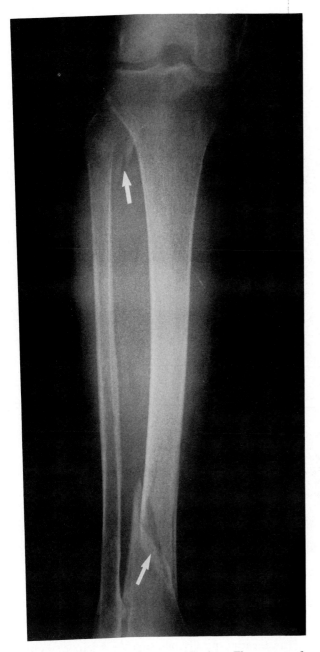

Fig. 8-88. Maisonneuve fracture, AP view. The rotatory force involved in this injury has caused fractures of the distal tibia as well as the proximal fibula *(arrows)*.

When a proximal fibular fracture is visualized on radiographs, it is essential to check for injury to the ankle ligaments.[15] Conversely, when ankle radiographs demonstrate an abnormal widening between the fibula and tibia, knee radiographs should also be obtained.

If the fibular fracture is initially missed, the patient is likely to develop arthritis at the ankle. Patients with a Maisonneuve fracture should be admitted to the hospital for surgical fixation.

Fracture of the tibial plateau. Tibial plateau fractures occur when a compressive force is transmitted from one of the condyles of the femur onto the medial or lateral tibial plateau. This may occur with a fall from a height or a direct blow to the side of the knee.

Tibial plateau fractures may be difficult to visualize on standard views if there is not significant displacement or depression (Fig. 8-89). Clues to the diagnosis on the lateral view include presence of a fat-blood interface anterior to the joint, indicating an intra-articular fracture or anterior displacement of the soft tissue line between the femur and quadriceps tendon. If standard views do not demonstrate the fracture, a tibial plateau view, obtained perpendicular to the angle of the plateau in a 14-degree caudad direction, may reveal the fracture. In some instances only conventional tomograms or a CT scan will demonstrate the fracture.

Ligamentous and peroneal nerve injury is often associated with tibial plateau fractures.

Patients with minimally displaced fractures may be treated by plaster immobilization. However, if they have significant pain or swelling, they should be admitted to the hospital and observed for the development of a compartment syndrome. Displaced fractures may require surgical fixation.

Fracture of the tibia and fibula. The tibia and fibula are often fractured together either by direct trauma, such as that occurring in auto-pedestrian accidents, or by indi-

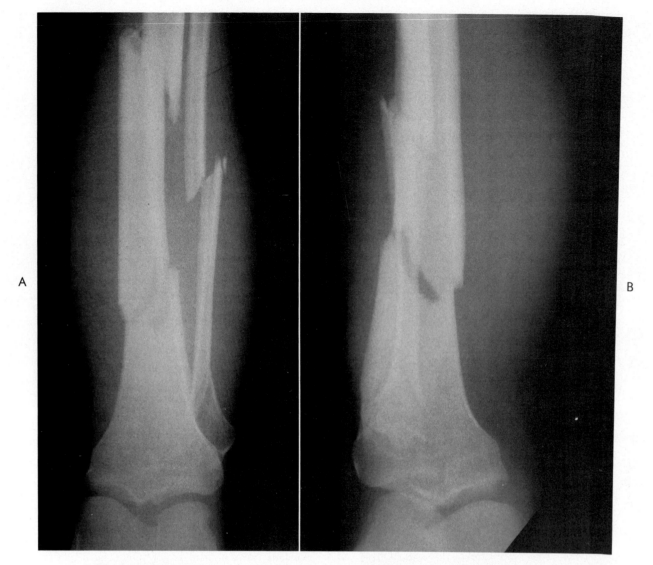

Fig. 8-90. Tibiofibular fracture. **A,** AP view. Comminuted fractures of the tibial and fibular shafts are present. Note the obliteration of the normal soft tissue planes due to edema or hemorrhage. **B,** Lateral view.

rect forces, such as those occurring in falls. Since the two bones are strongly connected by ligaments, a break with displacement or change in length requires careful evaluation of both the knee and the ankle.

Standard radiographs readily demonstrate tibiofibular fractures (Fig. 8-90). Radiographs of the knee and ankle should also be obtained to rule out associated injuries.

Tibiofibular fractures occur in a region with several muscular compartments, and patients with closed fractures should initially be admitted to the hospital and observed for development of a compartment syndrome. Since the tibia has very little protective covering anteriorly, open fractures often occur and should be surgically debrided. Treatment in the emergency department consists of protec-

tive splinting unless gross deformity occurs with vascular compromise. If vascular compromise is present, the fracture should be reduced anatomically until pulses return and then splinted. Maintenance of immobilization is important so that closed fractures are not converted into an open injury.

ANKLE
Normal anatomy and radiographic views

The standard radiographic series of the ankle consists of radiographs in three projections: AP, lateral, and mortise views (Figs. 8-91 to 8-93). The mortise view is taken obliquely (15 degrees of internal rotation) to rotate the lateral malleolus from a position superimposed on the talus.

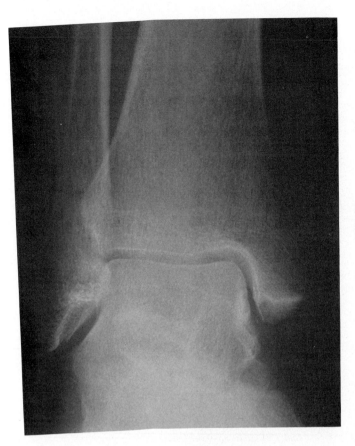

Fig. 8-91. Normal ankle, AP view. Note that there is overlapping of the distal tibia and fibula and a constant smooth joint margin.

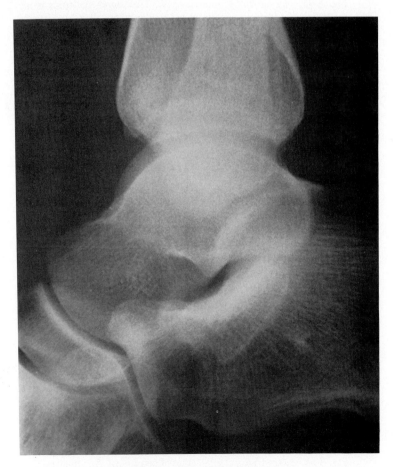

Fig. 8-92. Normal ankle, lateral view.

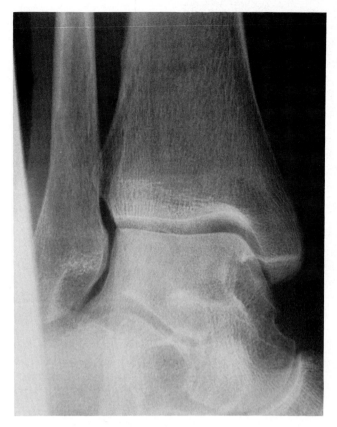

Fig. 8-93. Normal ankle, mortise view. The lateral malleolus is rotated so that it is not superimposed on the talus.

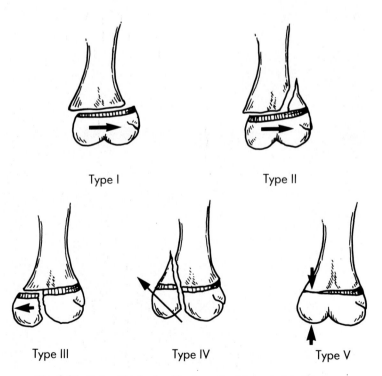

Type I   Type II

Type III   Type IV   Type V

Fig. 8-94. Salter-Harris classification of epiphyseal plate injuries.

Fractures generally are readily visualized, but patients may have significant ligamentous injury with normal ankle radiographs. The mortise view should be carefully examined for abnormal separation of the distal tibia and fibula and preservation of a constant joint space superior to the talus.

Salter-Harris fractures

The Salter-Harris classification of fractures is applied to injuries to or across the epiphyseal plate in children[16] (Fig. 8-94). The epiphyseal plate is the weakest and most vascular portion of the growing bone, and injuries may result in growth disturbances caused by vascular injury.

The Salter-Harris categories may be summarized as follows:

Type I: Injury to the epiphyseal plate. Radiographs may show soft tissue injury with swelling or widening of the epiphyseal space but are often normal. Diagnosis is often made on the basis of a normal radiograph and local tenderness over an epiphysis. Complications rarely occur.

Type II: Injury of the plate associated with a metaphyseal fracture. Complications rarely occur (Fig. 8-95).

Type III: Plate injury with an epiphyseal fracture extending into the articular surface. Epiphyseal growth disturbances may occur (Fig. 8-96).

Type IV: A fracture extending from the epiphysis through and including the metaphysis. Growth disturbances often occur.

Type V: A crush injury to the growth plate. The epiphyseal space may be widened, and growth disturbances usually occur.

Patients with Salter-Harris type I fractures require a clinical diagnosis and proper splinting or casting for immobilization. Patients with type II and III fractures are usually treated by casting with plaster immobilization. Type IV fractures may require surgical fixation. Patients with type V injuries have a poor prognosis and frequent loss of normal epiphyseal growth, regardless of the treatment. All patients should have timely orthopedic follow-up because of the potential morbidity associated with damage to the epiphysis.

FOOT
Normal anatomy and radiographic views

The foot consists of the tarsal bones, metatarsal bones, and phalanges. It can be divided into the hindfoot (talus and calcaneus), midfoot (navicular, cuboid, and cuneiform bones) and forefoot (metatarsals and phalanges). Trauma can result from direct or indirect forces or from overuse. Foot fractures account for about 10% of all fractures.

Standard radiographs consist of AP, lateral, and oblique views (Figs. 8-97 to 8-99). The AP view superimposes the

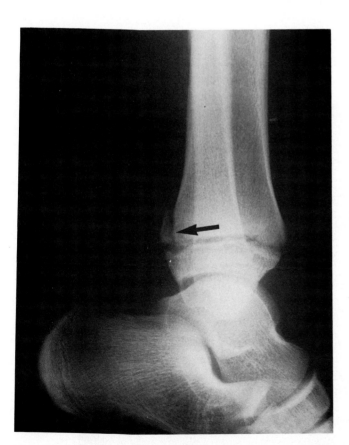

Fig. 8-95. Salter II fracture of distal tibia, lateral view. Fracture line extends into the metaphysis and is posteriorly displaced *(arrow)*.

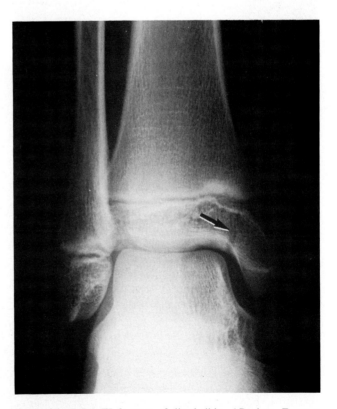

Fig. 8-96. Salter III fracture of distal tibia, AP view. Fracture line extends into the articular surface of the tibia *(arrow)*.

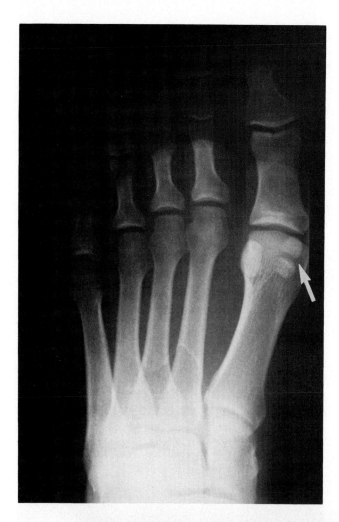

Fig. 8-97. Normal foot, AP view. Note that the second through fifth metatarsals are superimposed. Note incidental presence of bipartite sesamoid of great toe *(arrow).*

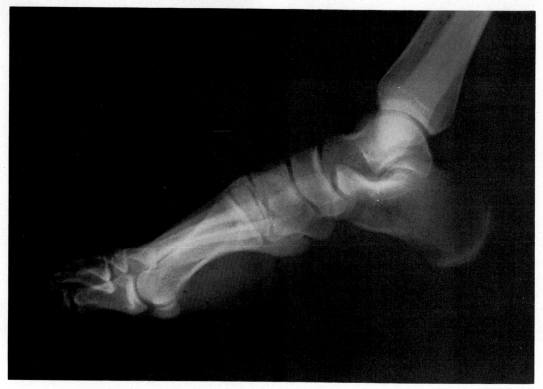

Fig. 8-98. Normal foot, lateral view.

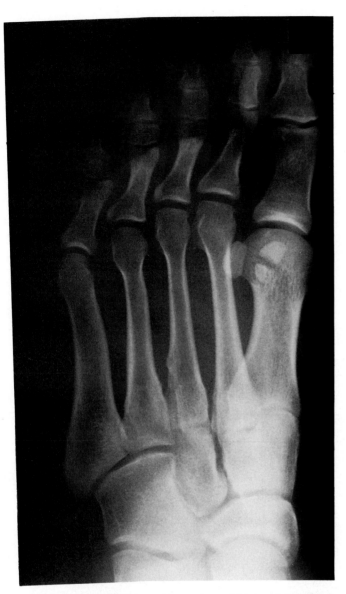

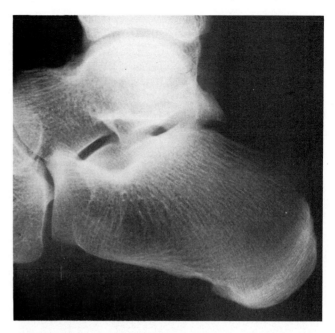

Fig. 8-100. Normal calcaneus, lateral view. Integrity of the trabecular structure should be closely examined in this view.

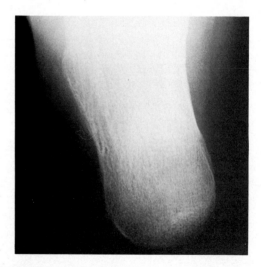

Fig. 8-101. Normal calcaneus, axial view. Medial and lateral walls of the calcaneus are well visualized on this view.

Fig. 8-99. Normal foot, oblique view. Metatarsal heads are more clearly seen in this projection.

second through fifth metatarsals and makes visualization of the third cuneiform and cuboid bones difficult. The oblique view provides a clearer picture of these areas.

Calcaneal views and Boehler angle

The standard calcaneal series consists of three views: AP, lateral, and axial (Figs. 8-100 and 8-101). The lateral view should be carefully examined for fracture lines and measurement of the Boehler angle, which is determined by lines drawn across the tuber line and the joint line of the calcaneus (Fig. 8-102). This angle normally measures 20 to 40 degrees, but disruption of the subtalar joint by a compressive force transmitted from the talus may result in a decreased angle. The axial view demonstrates the medial and lateral surfaces of the calcaneus as well as the sustentaculum tali.

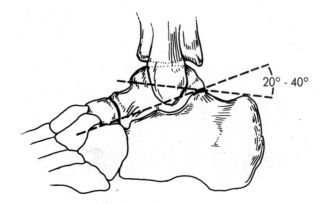

Fig. 8-102. Boehler angle. Disruption of the subtalar joint can decrease this angle.

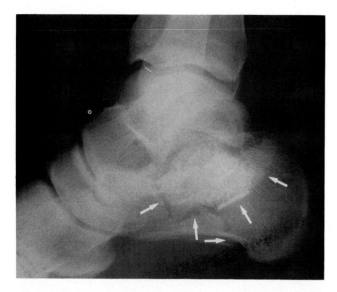

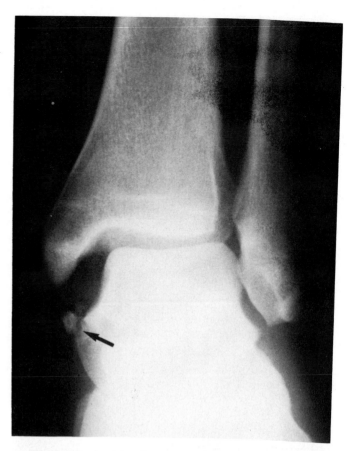

Fig. 8-103. Comminuted body fracture of calcaneus with subtalar involvement. Note the decrease in Boehler angle.

Fig. 8-105. Avulsion fracture of talus *(arrow)*, AP view.

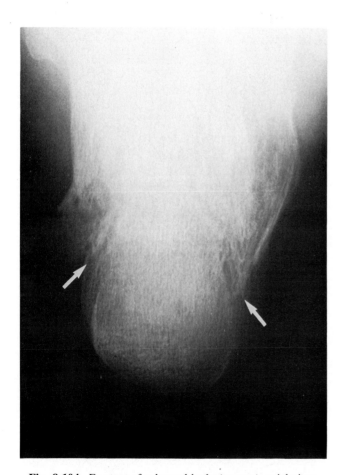

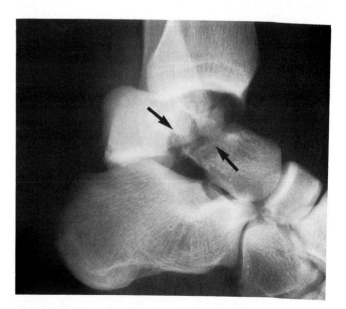

Fig. 8-104. Fracture of calcaneal body *(arrows)*, axial view.

Fig. 8-106. Comminuted fracture of body of the talus *(arrows)*, lateral view.

Fractures

Fracture of the calcaneus. The calcaneus is the largest and most frequently fractured tarsal bone. Injury usually occurs after a fall from a height. Misdiagnosis sometimes occurs when patients with this mechanism of injury are evaluated for ankle pain, and normal ankle views are obtained. Patients who fall from a height should be examined for heel tenderness by lateral and plantar compression; if tenderness is present, calcaneal views should be obtained. In addition, any patient found to have a calcaneal fracture must be closely examined for vertebral compression fractures and long bone fractures of the lower extremities, both of which are associated with calcaneal injuries.[17]

Most fractures involve the body of the calcaneus and are visualized with standard views (Figs. 8-103 and 8-104). This is a debilitating injury because subtalar joint involvement often results in chronic pain and arthritis. Avulsion fractures and fractures of the tuberosity or sustentaculum tali are less serious than calcaneal body fractures and usually heal without sequelae.

Treatment of patients with calcaneal fractures initially consists of elevation, ice packs, and immobilization in a bulky dressing. Some controversy exists regarding the optimal treatment of these patients. Most surgeons advocate a prolonged period of non-weight–bearing in a cast, whereas some recommend surgical fixation.

Fracture of the talus. The talus is the second most frequently fractured tarsal bone. These fractures may be difficult to visualize, and if a fracture is suspected on a standard foot or ankle series, additional views may be required.

The talus is most often fractured when forced dorsiflexion occurs at the ankle, resulting in an anterior avulsion fracture (Fig. 8-105). Posterior avulsion fractures occur with forced plantar flexion. Fractures of the body, neck, and head of the talus usually occur from axial compression secondary to a fall from a height (Figs. 8-106 and 8-107).

Patients with talus fractures are prone to long-term complications of arthritis and avascular necrosis. These patients are usually treated by reduction and immobilization. Surgical fixation may be necessary if closed reduction cannot be maintained.

Fractures of the cuneiform and cuboid. Cuboid and cuneiform fractures are secondary to direct crush injuries. Cuboid fractures are often associated with calcaneal fractures, whereas cuneiform fractures may be seen in association with metatarsal fractures (Fig. 8-108). If a cuboid fracture is demonstrated, the Lisfranc (tarsometatarsal)

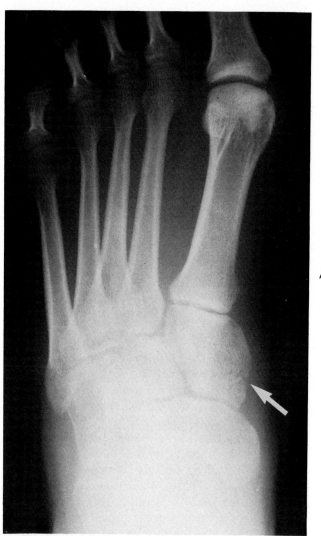

A

Fig. 8-108. Cuneiform fracture. **A,** AP view. The first cuneiform fracture can be easily seen *(arrow)*, but the metatarsal bases are overlapped in this view.   *Continued.*

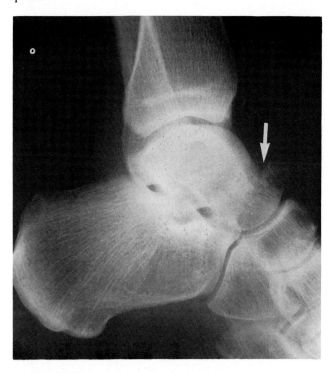

Fig. 8-107. Fracture, neck of talus *(arrow)*, lateral view.

B

Fig. 8-108, cont'd. **B,** Oblique view. This view not only reveals the cuneiform fracture *(arrow)* but demonstrates the normal position of the metatarsal bases and the integrity of the Lisfranc joint.

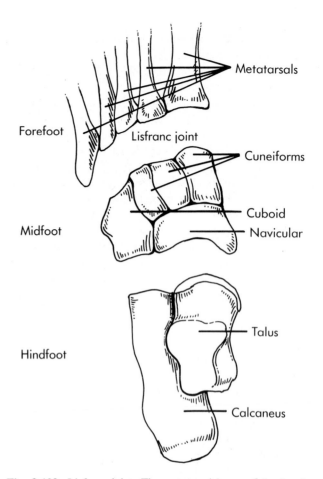

Fig. 8-109. Lisfranc joint. The metatarsal bases of the forefoot and distal margins of the bones of the midfoot mark the borders of the Lisfranc joint.

joint should be closely examined for fractures or dislocation.

Since superimposition of the midfoot bones is present, oblique views or comparison radiographs may be necessary to demonstrate cuboid or cuneiform fractures.

Patients with these fractures are treated by a short leg cast and usually heal without sequelae.

Lisfranc fracture (tarsometatarsal dislocation). The Lisfranc joint is located between the distal margins of the bones of the midfoot and the metatarsal bases (Fig. 8-109). This joint is normally maintained by strong ligamentous connections. The second through fifth metatarsal bases are tightly bound together by the transverse ligament. Ligaments also attach the second metatarsal base to the first and third cuneiform bones (Fig. 8-110).

A Lisfranc fracture or tarsometatarsal dislocation usually occurs when a violent, direct force is transmitted

along the metatarsals while the foot is in plantar flexion. This can occur during an auto accident as the foot strikes the brake pedal or with a fall from a height on the flexed foot.

Standard radiographs usually demonstrate the injury (Fig. 8-111). Patients with a Lisfranc fracture should be carefully examined for long bone and hip injuries on the same side. Arthritis and chronic foot pain are long-term complications.

Lisfranc fractures demand immediate orthopedic referral. These patients usually can be treated with closed reduction under general anesthesia, but surgical fixation may be required.

Fracture of the proximal fifth metatarsal. Radiographs of the proximal fifth metatarsal bone may present some difficulty to the inexperienced observer since the normal apophysis of the fifth metatarsal can simulate a fracture. However, the apophysis is longitudinally oriented rather than transversely, normally fuses at 16 years of age, and is present on comparison views of the opposite foot (Fig. 8-112). Two sesamoid bones may be confused with a

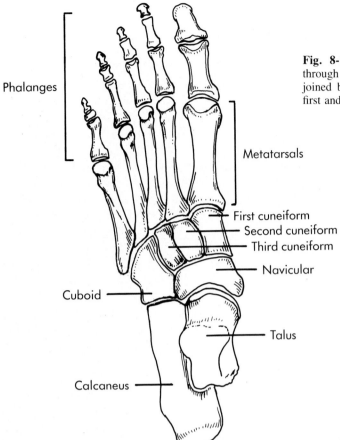

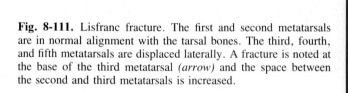

Fig. 8-110. Strong ligamentous connections hold the second through fifth metatarsals together. The forefoot and midfoot are joined by ligaments connecting the second metatarsal with the first and third cuneiforms.

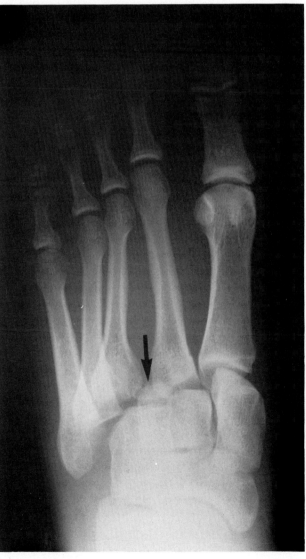

Fig. 8-111. Lisfranc fracture. The first and second metatarsals are in normal alignment with the tarsal bones. The third, fourth, and fifth metatarsals are displaced laterally. A fracture is noted at the base of the third metatarsal *(arrow)* and the space between the second and third metatarsals is increased.

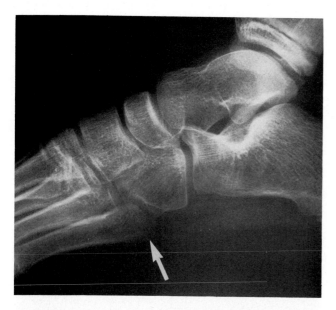

Fig. 8-112. Normal foot, lateral view. This radiograph of a 14-year-old male demonstrates the normal apophysis *(arrow)* of the fifth metatarsal.

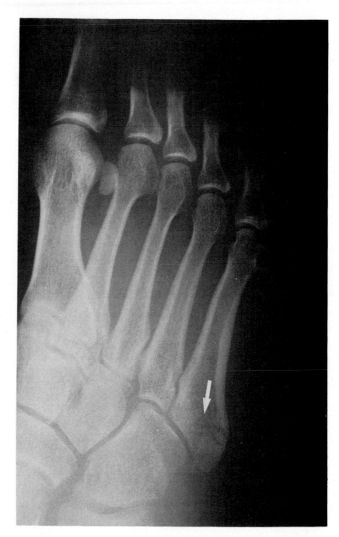

Fig. 8-113. Jones fracture (avulsion fracture of the fifth metatarsal base), AP view. Note the transverse fracture line *(arrow)*.

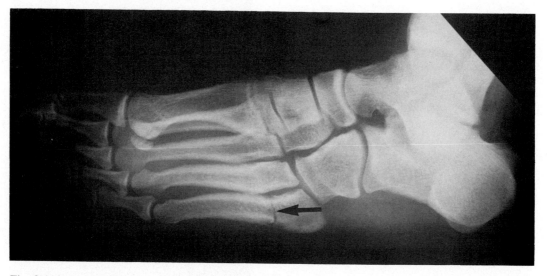

Fig. 8-114. Fracture of proximal shaft of the fifth metatarsal *(arrow)*. This diaphyseal injury must be differentiated from a Jones fracture.

fracture. The fibular and Vesalius accessory bone are located at the base of the fifth metatarsal but can be differentiated from a fracture by their smooth sclerotic margins. Comparison radiographs of the opposite extremity demonstrate bilateral accessory ossicles.

Jones fracture is an avulsion fracture of the base of the fifth metatarsal caused by the pull of the peroneus brevis tendon when the foot is forcibly inverted (Fig. 8-113). The fracture line is oriented transversely and has irregular margins. This allows differentiation of a fracture from an apophysis or accessory ossicle.

A *transverse fracture* of the proximal shaft of the fifth metatarsal may be the result of direct or indirect trauma or may be caused by recurrent stress (Fig. 8-114). This injury, which is a diaphyseal fracture, must be differentiated from the Jones fracture, which has a better prognosis.

Patients with a Jones fracture are treated by wearing a hard shoe or a walking cast and heal without complications. Proximal fifth metatarsal diaphyseal fractures are more problematic, since they have a high incidence of nonunion. These patients are treated with either a short leg cast or surgical fixation.

SUMMARY

In summary, orthopedic injuries are frequently encountered in the emergency department. Orthopedic consultation should be obtained immediately for those patients who have neurovascular compromise and for those who will have increased morbidity with a delay in treatment. Telephone consultation should be obtained whenever doubt exists concerning proper treatment or when several treatment options exist. Follow-up radiographs and a repeat neurovascular examination should be obtained for all patients who undergo reductions of dislocations or fractures. All patients must be referred for follow-up in a timely fashion.

ACKNOWLEDGMENTS

Special thanks to David Reedy, M.D., and Thomas Erickson, M.D., for assistance in obtaining radiographs and Kay Weitz for assistance in preparing the manuscript.

REFERENCES

1. Bossart PJ, Joyce SM, Manaster BJ et al: Lack of efficacy of weighted radiographs in diagnosing acute acromioclavicular separation, *Ann Emerg Med* 17(1):20, 1988.
2. Roberts JR, Hedges JR, eds: *Clinical procedures in emergency medicine,* Philadelphia, 1985, WB Saunders.
3. Harris JH, Harris WH, eds: *The radiology of emergency medicine,* Baltimore, 1975, Williams & Wilkins.
4. Thompson DA, Flynn TC, Miller PW et al: The significance of scapular fractures, *J Trauma* 25(10):974, 1985.
5. Simon RR, Koenigsknecht SJ, eds: *Emergency orthopedics: the extremities,* Norwalk, Conn, 1987, Appleton and Lange.
6. Neviaser RJ, Eisenfeld LS, Wiesel SW et al, eds: *Emergency orthopedic radiology,* New York, 1985, Churchill-Livingstone.
7. Prop DA, Chin H: Forearm and wrist radiology, Part I, *J Emerg Med* 7:393, 1989.
8. Waeckerle JF: A prospective study identifying the sensitivity of radiographic findings and the efficacy of clinical findings in carpal navicular fractures, *Ann Emerg Med* 16(7):733, 1987.
9. Terry DW, Ramin JE: The navicular fat stripe: a useful roentgen feature for evaluating wrist trauma, *AJR* 124(1):25, 1975.
10. Gillott A, Rhodes M, and Lucke J: Utility of routine pelvic x-ray during blunt trauma resuscitation, *J Trauma* 28(11):1570, 1988.
11. Rockwood CA, Green DP, eds: *Fractures in adults,* Philadelphia, 1984, JB Lippincott.
12. Swischuk LE, ed: *Emergency radiology of the acutely injured child,* Baltimore, 1986, Williams & Wilkins.
13. Walls RM, Rosen P: Traumatic dislocations of the knee, *J Emerg Med* 1:527, 1984.
14. Keats TE, ed: *Emergency radiology,* Chicago, 1984, Year Book Medical publishers.
15. Del Castillo J, Geiderman JM: The Frenchman's fibular fracture (Maisonneuve fracture), *JACEP* 8:404, 1979.
16. Salter RB, Harris WR: Injuries involving the epiphyseal plate, *J Bone Joint Surg* 45A(3):587, 1963.
17. Reynolds BM, Balsano NA, and Reynolds FX: Falls from heights: a surgical experience of 200 consecutive cases, *Ann Surg* 174(2):304, 1971.

Spinal Trauma

John G. Keene
Richard H. Daffner

Trauma involving the spine is seen commonly in every emergency department. The proper management and diagnosis of such trauma is crucial to the patient's well-being. Radiographic evaluation is frequently the key diagnostic step and often determines the therapeutic approach. A very careful and deliberate evaluation of the entire spinal column is necessary to prevent further injury to the spine-injured patient.

This chapter presents a thorough, systematic approach to dealing with spinal trauma, including sections on management of the spine-injured patient, indications for spinal radiography, the appearance of normal radiographic anatomy, and recognition of spinal injury patterns. Understanding the use of various diagnostic modalities in spinal trauma will assist the physician in optimizing emergency department evaluation and care of the trauma victim.

GENERAL APPROACH

The most critical step in handling the spinal trauma victim is for all members of the emergency health care team to assume that the patient has a life- or limb-threatening injury. It is incumbent on the emergency health care team to take the appropriate steps to protect the trauma patient. Initial steps include immobilizing the spine and following the ABCs of trauma care. All health care personnel must understand proper immobilization and transportation techniques to prevent unnecessary injury to the patient.

At whatever point a trauma victim enters the health care system, whether in the pre-hospital setting or the emergency department, as a patient the victim must be assessed and protected from the complications of spinal injury. All too often because a patient is walking at the scene or comes to the emergency department several days after an accident, neck or back pain is minimized and essential precautions are not taken. Also when concerns about the stability and integrity of a patient's spine are not properly communicated to all of the personnel handling the patient, errors omitting proper spinal protection can jeopardize the patient's well-being.

"Clearing the spine"—that is, determining that an unstable spinal injury is not present in a patient—is one of the most critical decisions in evaluating the trauma victim. Because the stakes are high and the patient may be at risk for quadriplegia or paraplegia, it is best to err on the side of being overprotective. This will help avoid inadvertent and unnecessary complications.

In general, if a patient exhibits neurologic deficits, complains of neck or back pain, or has a clinical presentation that suggests potential spinal injury, there are four basic steps that must be followed. The first step is to properly immobilize the patient to protect the spine from movement across unstable segments. The second step is to stabilize the patient in terms of other trauma that may compromise the patient hemodynamically. These first two steps should occur simultaneously following the ABCs of trauma care. The third step is to properly evaluate the pa-

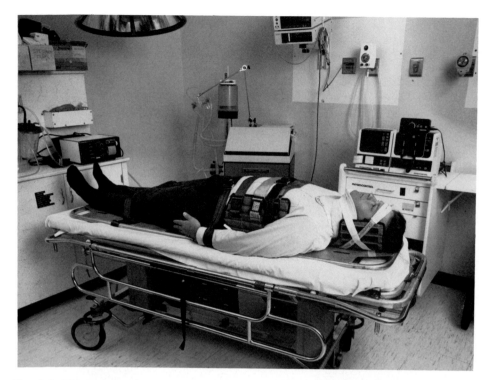

Fig. 9-1. This patient is fully immobilized on a long spine board. The vest-like extraction device provides some immobilization during extraction from a vehicle. The rigid cervical collar enhances the protection, and the straps prevent the patient from moving. Protected in this manner, the spine-injured patient can be safely transported.

tient's spine radiographically, and the fourth is to involve the proper specialists to provide definitive care for the injuries that are found.

TRANSPORTATION OF THE SPINE-INJURED PATIENT

Transporting the patient with a spinal injury or one who has the possibility of a spinal injury is potentially dangerous to the patient and must be approached with utmost caution. If a patient has an unstable spinal fracture or ligamentous tear, movement of the bony segments may result in permanent neurologic damage, particularly in the unconcious patient. Interdepartmental policies and procedures coordinating the efforts of the emergency department and the radiology department are necessary to ensure the proper handling of such patients. It is extremely important that all involved personnel understand both the risks and proper techniques for transporting a spine-injured patient.

The patient who is presumed to have a spinal injury based on the mechanism of injury or a complaint of neck or back pain should be handled with the same precautions as a patient with neurologic damage until the spine can be thoroughly evaluated radiographically. The process of ruling out vertebral injury involves both clinical assessment and radiographic examination. Only after thorough evaluation of all parameters can the patient be transported without fear of disabling injury. Until that point, the patient must be presumed to have an unstable injury that could result in paralysis.

The potentially spine-injured patient should be transported only after proper immobilization with straps on a long spine board (Fig. 9-1). To prevent motion of the cervical spine, the patient should have a rigid cervical collar in place with padding on either side to hold the head stationary, with tape or straps securing the head to the spine board. Soft cervical collars provide only minimal protection for the cervical spine and should not be used for stabilization.[1] After being immobilized on a spine board, the patient can be safely moved by lifting the board or by transporting the patient on a stretcher. When it is necessary to take radiographs, the straps and pads can be removed to clear the radiographic field; however, the patient must be able to lie perfectly still or personnel must be present to hold the patient still and protect the spine.

The patient should be maintained in spinal immobilization at all times, except when specific procedures are being performed, in order to prevent sudden unexpected movements that could cause neurologic compromise. In addition, spinal protection should firmly attach the patient to the board so that, should the patient become nauseated and vomit, the board can be tipped to prevent aspiration. This can be a problem with very large patients as even very secure strapping may not prevent motion of the spine. In these instances, someone should be standing by with suction available to clear the patient's airway.

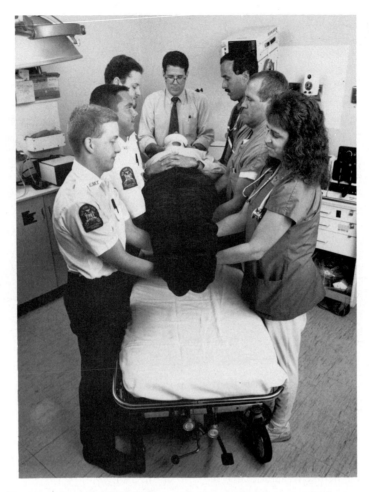

Fig. 9-2. The seven-person lift is ideal for transferring a patient from one device to another, such as from a spine board to a radiographic table. The lift provides sufficient manpower to ensure the patient's safety. Care must be exercised to coordinate all movements.

Should it be necessary to move the patient on or off a spine board for radiographic procedures or further treatment, the "seven-person lift" should be used. In this lift (Fig. 9-2), three staff members are placed on either side of the patient for lifting and the seventh member of the team is responsible for the patient's head. The person at the patient's head should be in charge of the lift to ensure that everyone is well positioned before any movement is begun. Movement should be kept to a minimum and all action should be taken in unison in order not to put stress across an unstable portion of the spine.

An alternate lift for lightweight patients, urgent situations, or when adequate personnel are not available and movement is essential for the patient's well-being is the "four-person lift" (Fig. 9-3). This lift is similar to the "seven-person lift" except that there are only three staff members lifting from a single side with the fourth member of the team at the patient's head. In either of these lifting techniques, additional help may be necessary to remove the stretcher, clothing, and other items that may impede easy movement.

In young children, the growth of the head outpaces the rest of the body. Because of this, placing a child on a flat spine board will cause some flexion of the head and neck. To prevent this, it has been suggested that pediatric spine boards be modified with a cutout to recess the occiput or that a mattress or pad be used to raise the trunk and maintain normal cervical spine alignment.[2]

The key points to remember when transferring or transporting a patient with known or potential spinal trauma are:

- Assume that all documented or potential spinal injuries are unstable until proved otherwise.
- Remember the spinal canal is only 2 cm wide on average, and motion of an unstable segment can result in spinal cord damage.

INDICATIONS FOR RADIOGRAPHY

Considerable controversy exists over when radiography is indicated to exclude vertebral injury after trauma. Because of the devastating effects of spinal cord injury, some authors advocate cervical spine radiography in all high-risk cases.[3-5] Neifeld et al.[6], however, in a prospective study of over 800 patients with blunt head trauma demonstrated that patients without pain or tenderness in the neck—who were alert, not under the influence of alcohol or drugs, and

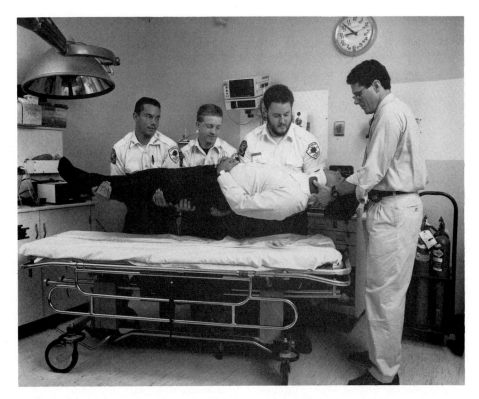

Fig. 9-3. The four-person lift is an alternative for small patients and in emergencies where fewer staff members are available. Caution must be observed because decreased lifting capacity may inadvertently jeopardize the patient.

who had no distracting injuries—did not have cervical spine injuries and could be spared cervical spine radiography. A number of authors support this conclusion.[7-14]

In general there is a consensus that spinal radiography should be performed only in trauma victims with a mechanism of injury that could cause spinal trauma, such as a motor vehicle accident or a fall, and in whom evaluation is complicated by unconsciousness, altered mental status, or major distracting injuries. Altered mental status can result from drug or alcohol intoxication, shock, or head injury. Severely painful injuries, such as a femur or pelvic fracture, may distract a patient, and a potentially grave spinal injury may go unnoticed or ignored.

The occurrence of painless cervical spine fractures has been suggested.[15-18] This, however, has been questioned, and reports of painless spinal injuries probably result from inebriation or poor documentation.[9,19] Therefore, because the risks to the patient are extremely serious, one should always act to protect the patient. Radiographs should be taken whenever there is any suspicion that the patient may have a spinal injury. The specific recommendations for obtaining spinal radiographs are summarized in the box opposite. These indications should be applied to the entire vertebral column.

RADIOGRAPHIC APPROACH

Historically, the cross-table or horizontal beam lateral cervical radiograph has been used to exclude spinal injury in head and neck trauma. This assumes that (1) the cervi-

---

Indications for radiography in spinal trauma

1. Acute neurologic deficit.
2. Altered mental status secondary to head injury or shock.
3. Intoxication from alcohol or other drugs.
4. Head or back pain.
5. Neck or back tenderness.
6. Unconsciousness.
7. High-risk mechanism of injury
   a. High-speed motor vehicle accident
   b. Fall from >10 feet
   c. Drowning
8. Severe associated injuries
   a. Head or face
   b. Multiple skeletal
9. Competitive pain from a nonspinal injury.

---

cal spine is the only area of concern, (2) the cross-table lateral view will reveal all of the serious injuries, and (3) plain radiographs will be sufficient to protect the patient.

A thorough examination of the entire vertebral column is necessary to evaluate the trauma victim. Because of the mobility of the cervical spine and the weight of the head that area is most vulnerable. However, depending on how the force vectors impinge on the spine and are dissipated, areas other than the cervical spine may be injured. When a trauma victim arrives in the emergency department, the entire spine must be considered when providing immobilization and ordering radiographs to evaluate for spinal injury.

Trauma radiographs for the thoracic and lumbar portions of the spine may need evaluation before the patient can be safely removed from immobilization devices. This is particularly true for a patient who is not fully alert or who is unconscious. It has been strongly recommended that the entire vertebral column be surveyed in the multiple trauma victim.[20] A victim of a motor vehicle accident, especially a motorcycle accident, fall, or diving incident, is particularly vulnerable to devastating spinal injuries, particularly multiple injuries. In the cervical area, multiple injuries occur 15% to 25% of the time, and, if cervical injuries are combined with thoracolumbar fractures, such injuries occur 5% to 17% of the time.[21-24]

Studies have shown that only 77% to 85% of cervical spine injuries can be detected using the cross-table lateral radiograph.[25-27] Bachulis et al.[10] found a 26% false negative rate in their review of lateral cervical radiographs in patients ultimately diagnosed with spinal injuries.[9] To "clear the spine," more views are necessary. Shaffer and Doris[25] suggest the use of three views—the lateral view, anteroposterior view, and modified odontoid view. In a subsequent study, these authors suggest the use of five views—the lateral view, anteroposterior view, odontoid view, and supine oblique views.[28] Addition of oblique views, conventional tomography, or computed tomography (CT scan) may also be necessary.[28,29]

The radiographic evaluation of the cervical spine should begin with a three-view trauma series that includes the cross-table lateral view, the anteroposterior view, and the modified odontoid view. In the thoracic region, the cross-table lateral and anteroposterior views will need to be supplemented by a modified swimmer's view. In the lumbar region, virtually all acute injuries are visible on the lateral and anteroposterior views.[20] If there are any questionable findings, oblique views or CT scans should be added.[28]

Plain radiographs may sometimes appear normal, failing to reveal serious spinal injuries.[30] Several authors have demonstrated significant numbers of spinal injury cases not detected by normal trauma series that later required conventional tomography or CT scans to detect the fractures.[26,31-33]

Adequate cross-table lateral views may be difficult to obtain. In a very large individual, if portable equipment is used, the cross-table lateral view of the thoracic and lumbar areas may be suboptimal. The CT scan may be useful for such cases, particularly when sagittal reformatting is performed. However, the plane of the CT scan will not demonstrate injuries to C7. In the cervical region, in a patient with a short, stocky neck, muscular shoulders, or shoulder injuries, it may also be difficult to demonstrate C7.

The preferred technique for moving the shoulders away from the lower cervical spine is gentle axial traction on the upper extremities. If this is unsuccessful, a modified swimmer's view, performed without moving the patient's spine, can reveal C7 and the upper thoracic vertebrae, which are typically not visualized on a lateral thoracic radiograph.

RADIOGRAPHIC ANATOMY

The key to interpreting spinal radiographs is to have a clear understanding of the anatomy involved. It is frequently helpful to have an anatomy atlas available for reference. Also, when examining spinal radiographs, it is important to use a systematic approach to evaluate all structures and signs on every radiograph. Missing a spinal injury can be devastating to the patient, so it is necessary that the clinician make a thorough and disciplined evaluation in every case.

The spine is a semiflexible column that provides structural support and mobility for the trunk. The spine can be functionally divided into anterior and posterior elements. The anterior elements consist of cylindric vertebral bodies with interposed cartilaginous disks that are held together by a variety of ligaments. These anterior elements provide the main structural support for the trunk. In addition to these anterior elements, the posterior elements consist of arch-like rings with protruding processes. The bony arches serve to protect the spinal cord, while the processes provide anchor points for the various muscles that move the vertebral column as well as act as articular surfaces that facilitate movement between each of the vertebrae.

The vertebrae of the spinal column can be separated into five groups, each with characteristics in common (Fig. 9-4). The seven cervical vertebrae provide structural support and mobility for the neck. The twelve thoracic vertebrae provide the same functions for the chest, but, in addition, provide posterior points of attachment for the rib cage. The five lumbar vertebrae are much larger because of the greater weight that they must bear. The sacral and coccygeal vertebrae are fused and form the posterior portion of the pelvic girdle.

Cervical spine

Seven vertebrae form the cervical spine. The first cervical vertebra, or atlas, is a circular structure that supports the skull. The second cervical vertebra, or axis, begins to take on more of the shape of the classic vertebra with a cylindric body; however, it has a vertical process—the odontoid process or dens—that forms a joint with the atlas. The remaining five vertebrae are similar in configuration with slightly increasing size caudally.

Fig. 9-5, A, illustrates an axial view of an isolated atlas. This photograph clearly depicts the ring structure with its large lateral masses and articular condyles that form joints with the occipital bone. The lateral masses are connected by an arch of bone anteriorly and posteriorly. Small transverse processes extend laterally. They are each perforated by a passage, the foramen transversarium, that con-

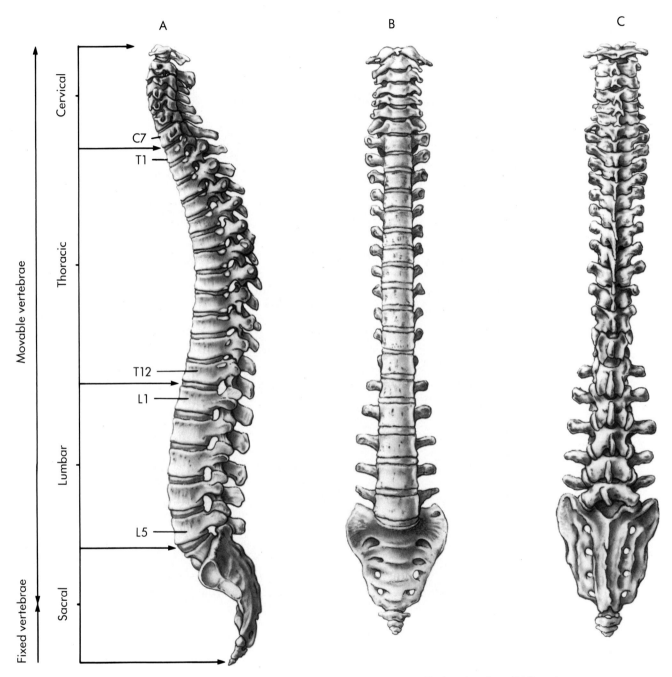

Fig. 9-4. Segmentation of the vertebral column. **A,** Lateral view. **B,** Anterior view. **C,** Posterior view. (From Daffner RH: *Imaging of vertebral trauma*, Rockville, Md, 1988, Aspen Publishers. Reproduced with permission.)

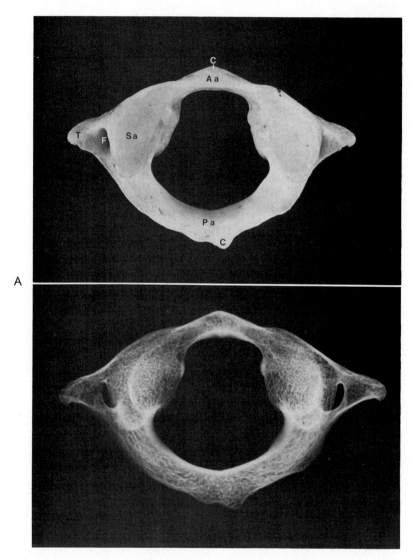

Fig. 9-5. A, Atlas vertebra (C1) from above. *T,* transverse process; *F,* foramen transversarium; *Sa,* superior articular facet; *C,* central tubercle of atlas; *Aa,* anterior arch of atlas; *Pa,* posterior arch of atlas.

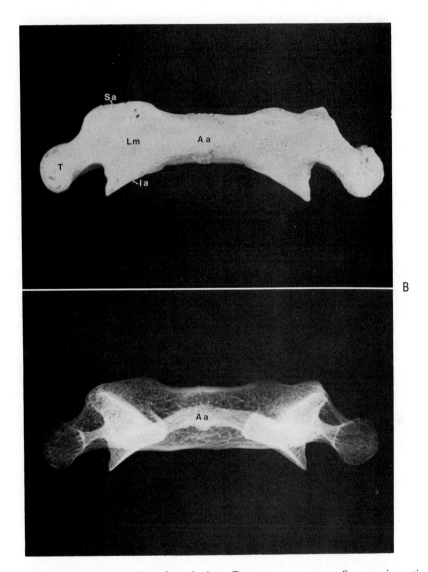

Fig. 9-5, cont'd. B, Atlas vertebra, frontal view. *T,* transverse process; *Sa,* superior articular facet; *Lm,* lateral mass; *Ia,* inferior articular facet; *Aa,* anterior arch of atlas.   *Continued.*

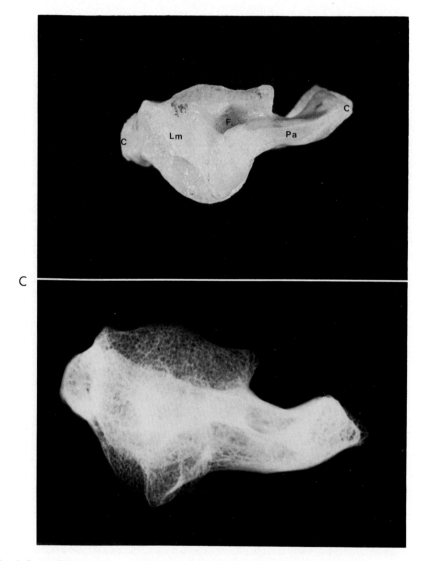

Fig. 9-5, cont'd. C, Atlas vertebra, lateral view. *C,* central tubercle of atlas; *Lm,* lateral mass; *F,* foramen transversarium; *Pa,* posterior arch of atlas. (From Daffner RH: *Imaging of vertebral trauma,* Rockville, Md, 1988, Aspen Publishers. Reproduced with permission.)

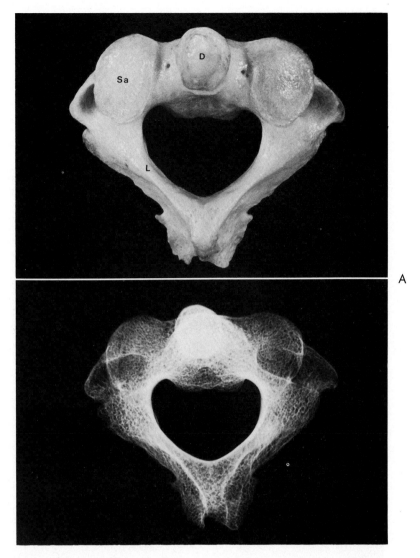

Fig. 9-6. A, Axis vertebra (C2) from above. *Sa,* superior articular facet; *L,* lamina; *D,* dens.

Continued.

tains the respective vertebral artery. There is a small tubercle located posteriorly instead of a spinous process. On the inner aspect of the anterior arch, the small depression for the joint with the odontoid process can be seen.

Viewed from the anteroposterior aspect, the atlas takes on the appearance of a bow tie. This can be seen in Fig. 9-5, *B,* and should be compared to the "open-mouth view" (see Fig. 9-36) used to visualize the odontoid process. The transverse processes protruding laterally from each of the lateral masses serve as "handlebars" on which the cervical muscles can attach and turn the atlas.

The lateral aspect of the atlas seen in Fig. 9-5, *C,* displays the superimposed lateral masses and transverse processes with the anterior and posterior arches curving away from them. The ease with which this ring of bone can be broken—for example, from axial loading as a result of a diving injury forcing the skull between the lateral masses—can be appreciated on this view, which shows how thin the bone is that makes up the posterior arch.

With its cylindric body and odontoid process (Fig. 9-6), the axis completes the transition from the skull to the vertebral column. The articular facets on its superior aspect are similar to the condyles on the atlas and skull; however, inferiorly, the articulation has developed into an articular pillar with an obliquely positioned facet. The bony arch protecting the spinal cord consists of the pedicles, articular pillars, laminae, and the spinous process.

The spinous processes of the cervical vertebrae are bifid and begin with the short spinous process of the axis. These protrusions provide additional points of attachment for the posterior cervical muscles, allowing for greater control of motion of the head and neck.

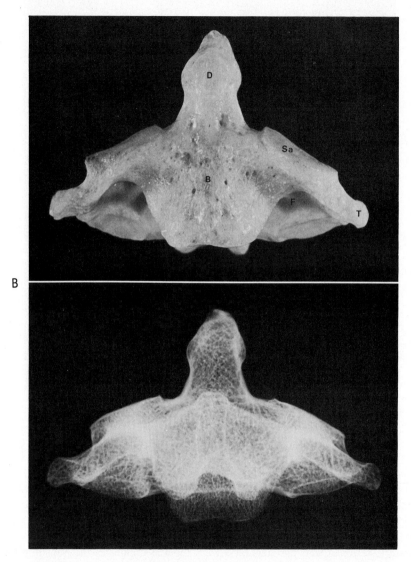

Fig. 9-6, cont'd. B, Axis vertebra, frontal view. *D,* dens; *B,* body; *Sa,* superior articular facet; *F,* foramen transversarium; *T,* transverse process.

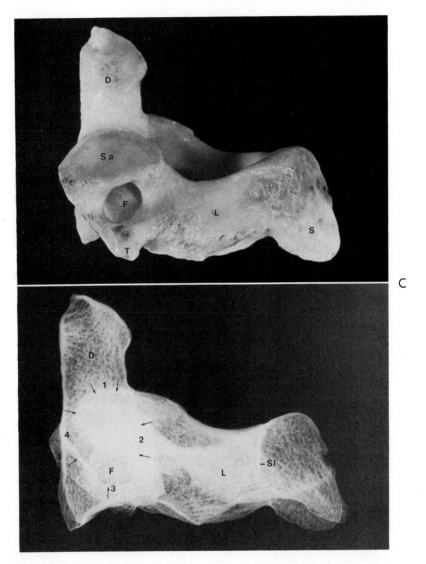

Fig. 9-6, cont'd. C, Axis vertebra, lateral view. *D,* dens; *Sa,* superior articular facet; *F,* foramen transversarium; *T,* transverse process; *L,* lamina; *S,* spinous process. "Harris's ring" is outlined by arrows on the radiograph. This is a composite of radiographic images composed of the following structures: *(1)* upper arc is the superior articular facet, *(2)* posterior arc is the posterior aspect of the body of C2, *(3)* inferior arc is the inferior border of the foramen transversarium, *(4)* anterior arc is formed by the anterior portion of the body of C2. (From Daffner RH: *Imaging of vertebral trauma,* Rockville, Md, 1988, Aspen Publishers. Reproduced with permission.)

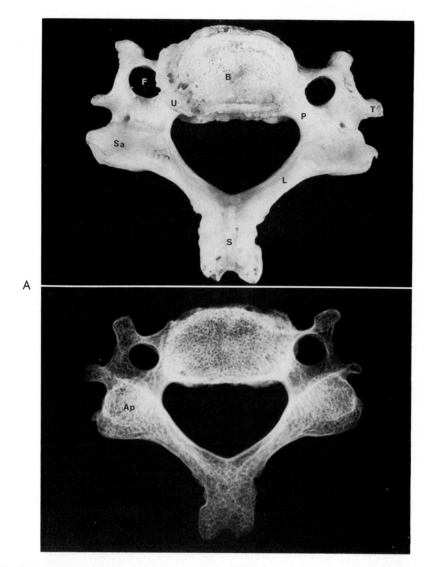

Fig. 9-7. A, Typical cervical vertebra (C5) from above. *Sa,* superior articular facet; *F,* foramen transversarium; *U,* uncinate process; *B,* body; *S,* spinous process; *L,* lamina; *P,* pedicle; *T,* transverse process; *Ap,* articular pillar.

The third to seventh cervical vertebrae are similar in configuration, varying only slightly in size. Their characteristics are detailed in Fig. 9-7.

Thoracic spine

The thoracic portion of the vertebral column consists of twelve similar vertebrae that increase slightly in size caudally. They possess all of the features of typical vertebrae as illustrated in Fig. 9-8.

The thoracic vertebrae are similar to the cervical vertebrae except the spinous processes are longer, there are no transverse foramina, and articular facets exist for the attachment of the ribs. The first, eleventh, and twelfth thoracic vertebrae have complete circular facets on the sides to accommodate the heads of their corresponding ribs. The other thoracic vertebrae have only demi-facets to articulate

the heads of their ribs. These semi-circular facets are located on the upper and lower margins of the vertebral bodies. In addition, the ten upper thoracic vertebrae have articular facets on the transverse processes that also connect with tubercles on the ribs.

Lumbar spine

The lumbar portion of the vertebral column consists of five large, rugged vertebrae. Occasionally, there can be a sixth lumbar vertebra (which is, in fact, "lumberization" of S1) as a normal variant. In addition, there may be "sacralization" or fusion of the fifth lumbar vertebra with the sacrum.

These variant findings occur in approximately 3.2% of patients in a normal series of 500 patients but in 16.4% of patients undergoing laminectomy for herniated

Text continued on p. 228.

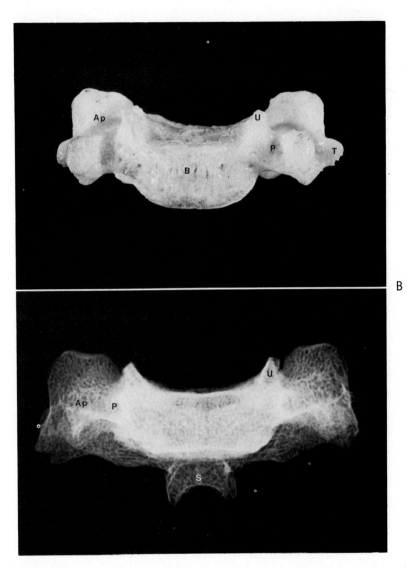

Fig. 9-7, cont'd. B, C5 vertebra, frontal view. *Ap,* articular pillar; *B,* body; *U,* uncinate process; *P,* pedicle; *T,* transverse process; *S,* spinous process. *Continued.*

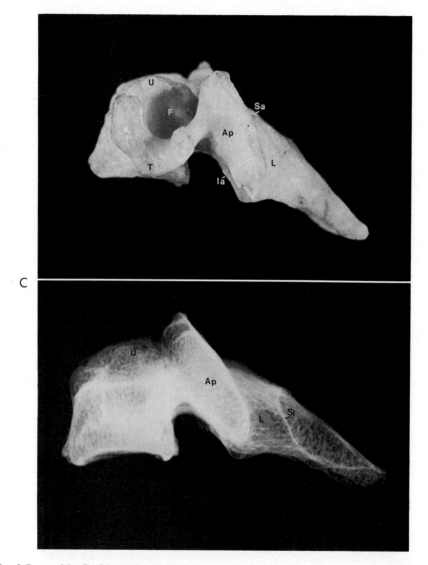

Fig. 9-7, cont'd. C, C5 vertebra, lateral view. *U,* uncinate process; *F,* foramen transversarium; *T,* transverse process; *Ap,* articular pillar; *Ia,* inferior articular facet; *Sa,* superior articular facet; *L,* lamina; *Sl,* spinolaminal line. (From Daffner RH: *Imaging of vertebral trauma,* Rockville, Md, 1988, Aspen Publishers. Reproduced with permission.)

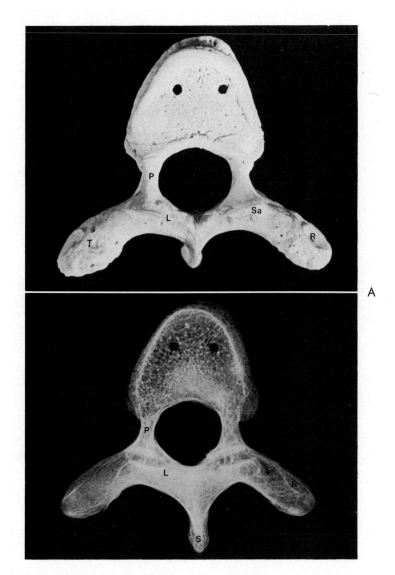

Fig. 9-8. A, Typical thoracic vertebra (T7) from above. *T*, transverse process; *P*, pedicle; *L*, lamina; *Sa*, superior articular facet; *R*, rib facet; *S*, spinous process.   *Continued.*

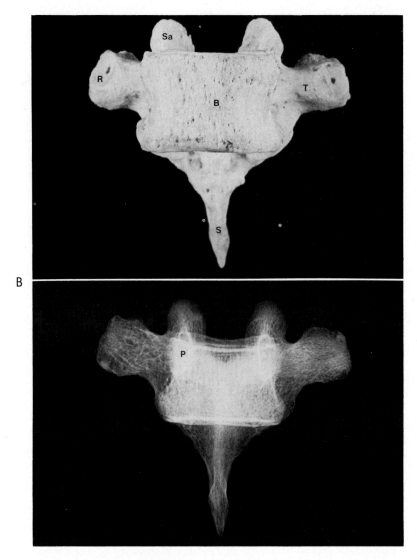

Fig. 9-8, cont'd. B, T7 vertebra, frontal view. *R,* rib facet; *Sa,* superior articular facet; *B,* body; *S,* spinous process; *T,* transverse process; *P,* pedicle.   *Continued.*

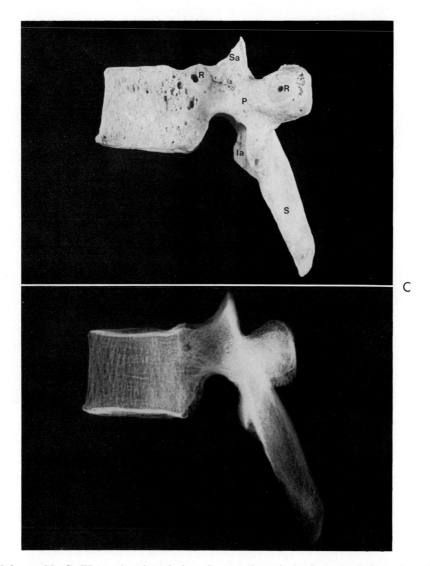

Fig. 9-8, cont'd. C, T7 vertebra, lateral view. *Sa,* superior articular facet; *R,* rib facet; *P,* pedicle; *Ia,* inferior articular facet; *S,* spinous process. (From Daffner RH: *Imaging of vertebral trauma,* Rockville, Md, 1988, Aspen Publishers. Reproduced with permission.)

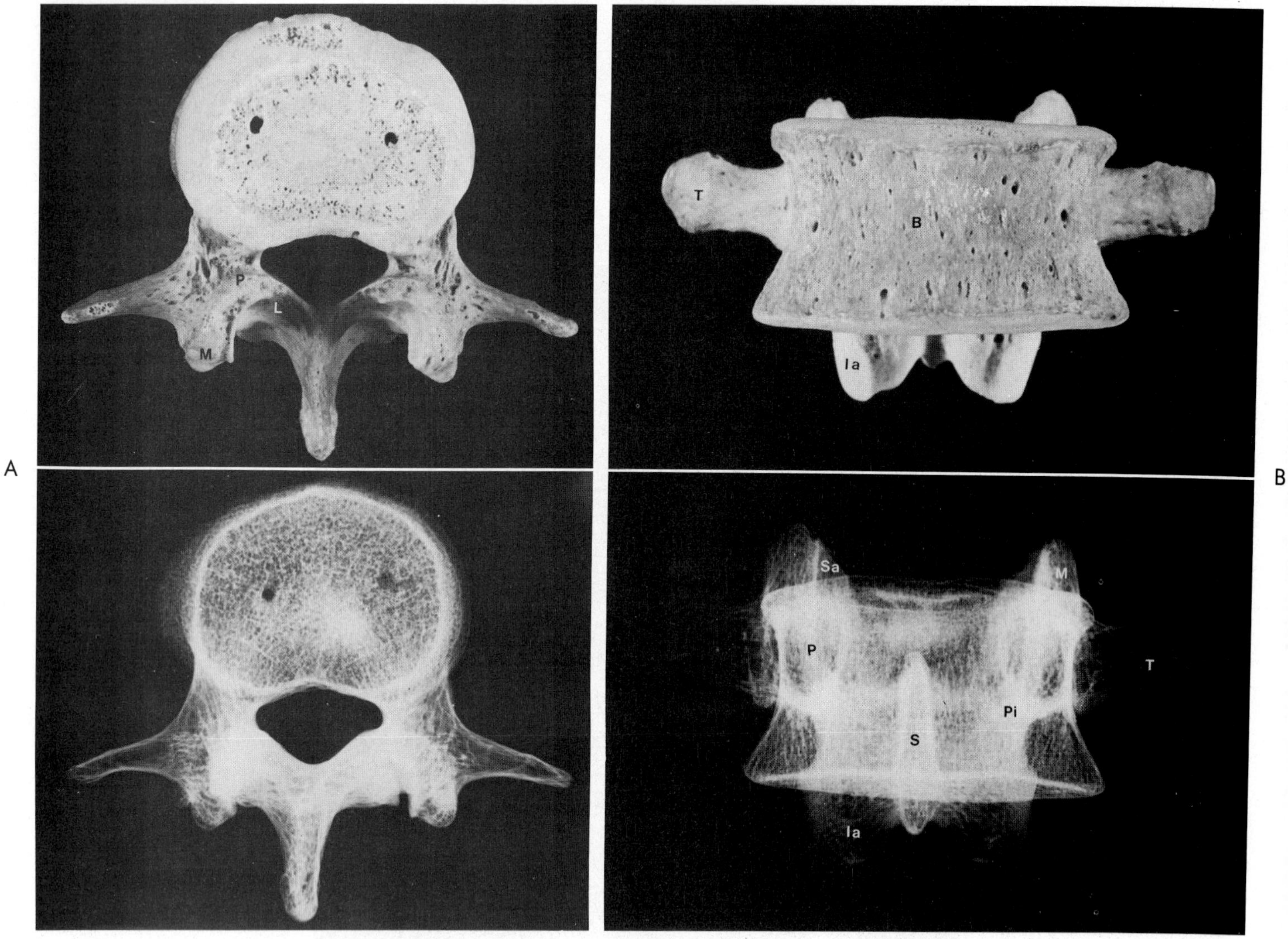

Fig. 9-9. A, Typical lumbar vertebra (L3) from above. *P,* pedicle; *L,* lamina; *M,* mammillary process. **B,** L3 vertebra, frontal view. *T,* transverse process; *B,* body; *Ia,* inferior articular facet; *Sa,* superior articular facet; *P,* pedicle; *S,* spinous process; *Pi,* pars interarticularis.   *Continued.*

disks.[34] The spinous process and transverse processes of the lumbar vertebrae are broad and thick. They provide attachments for the large segments of the erector spinae muscle. These large bones and muscles carry the weight of and support the entire trunk. Because of their size and construction, significant force is necessary to damage this portion of the spine. Fig. 9-9 illustrates their structure.

The superior and inferior articular facets are much larger than they are in other regions. They are located on large articular processes that are slightly curved and that interlock.

EVALUATION OF RADIOGRAPHS

A systematic approach should be used in evaluating the spine. Emphasis should be on (1) thoroughness of interpre-

tation, (2) recognition of normal structures, and (3) understanding examples of traumatic abnormalities. The importance of developing a systematic approach cannot be overemphasized.

Just as there are ABCs of trauma management that systematize and prioritize the care of multiple trauma victims, ABCs of assessment of vertebral trauma have been developed.[35] These ABCs provide the clinician with a logical system for reviewing the plain film radiographs that are a critical part of the diagnostic armamentarium in the emergency department setting.

The ABCs of radiographic assessment of vertebral trauma are listed in the box on p. 231. This system should be applied to all regions of the spine. Thorough evaluation of each of these categories should help the emergency physician avoid missed or delayed diagnoses.

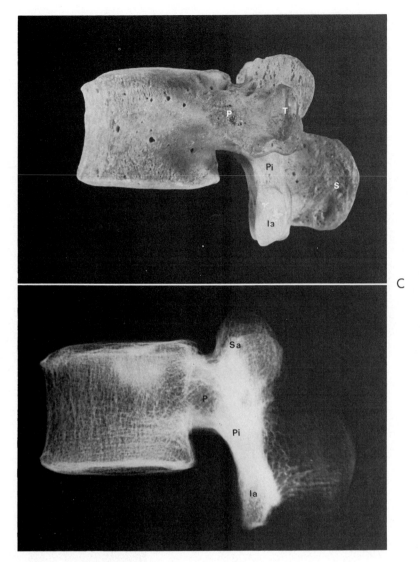

C

Fig. 9-9, cont'd. C, L3 vertebra, lateral view. *P,* pedicle; *T,* transverse process; *Pi,* pars interarticularis; *Ia,* inferior articular facet; *S,* spinous process; *Sa,* superior articular facet.   (From Daffner RH: *Imaging of vertebral trauma,* Rockville, Md, 1988, Aspen Publishers. Reproduced with permission.)

ALIGNMENT AND ANATOMY ABNORMALITIES

A number of important points should be noted in assessing for abnormalities of alignment and anatomy. Disruptions of the anterior or posterior vertebral body lines may indicate instability with subluxation (Fig. 9-10) or encroachment on the spinal cord (Fig. 9-11). Malalignment of the spinolaminal line indicates displacement. This may occur as the result of degenerative disease as well as trauma. In a patient with this latter condition, active flexion and extension views are needed for further evaluation. Widening of the interpediculate distance is an important hallmark of fracture (Fig. 9-12) as seen on the AP view.

Other alignment abnormalities in this category include rotation of the spinous process, jumped or locked facets, and unusual curvature or angulation of the spine. Abrupt

widening of the laminar space has been described as a sign of unilateral facet dislocation.[36]

Bony integrity abnormalities. Problems of bony integrity can be readily identified. Interruption of the cortex and abnormal trabecular patterns are generally clear indications of a fracture. In the thoracic and lumbar areas, however, fractures may be difficult to discern. Two signs must be scrupulously sought—widening of the interpediculate distance[20] (Fig. 9-12) and disruption of the posterior vertebral body line.[37]

Cartilage and joint space abnormalities. Abnormalities of cartilage and joint spaces can be deceiving. Narrowing of intervertebral disk spaces from degenerative arthritis is an extremely common finding. Traumatic narrowing may result from flexion injuries. Widening of the inter-

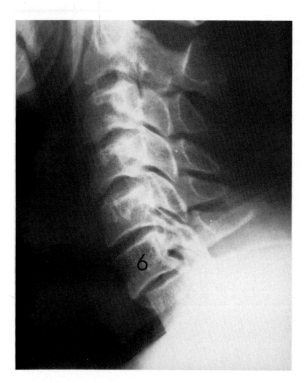

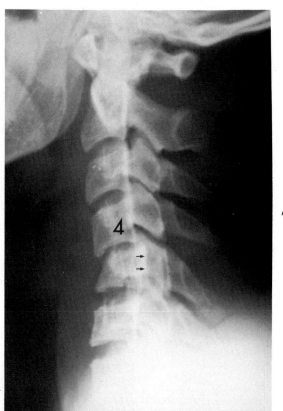

A

Fig. 9-10. Anterior subluxation of C6 on C7 in a patient with previous flexion sprain.

Fig. 9-11. Burst fracture of C5. **A,** Lateral radiograph shows anterolisthesis of C4 on C5. There is encroachment of the vertebral canal from a fragment of bone from the posterior vertebral body line of C5 *(arrows).* **B,** CT scan shows the retropulsed fragment on the left narrowing the vertebral canal. **C,** MRI scan at gradient echo parameters shows the encroachment of the spinal cord *(arrows).*

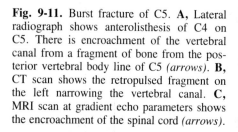

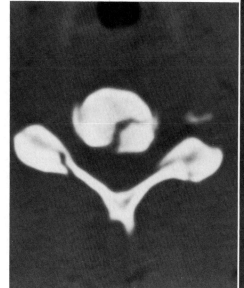

B

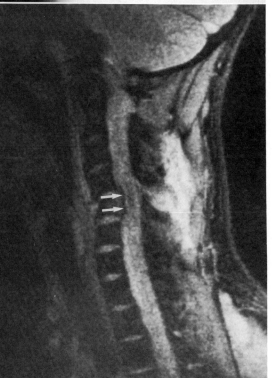

C

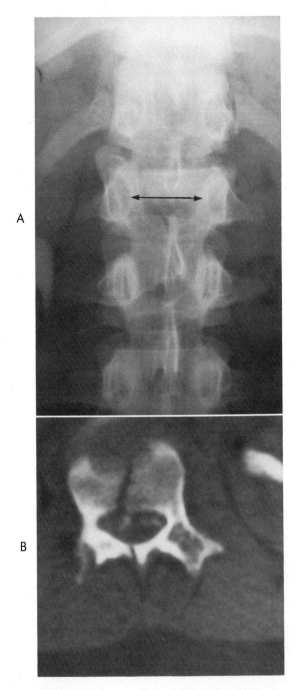

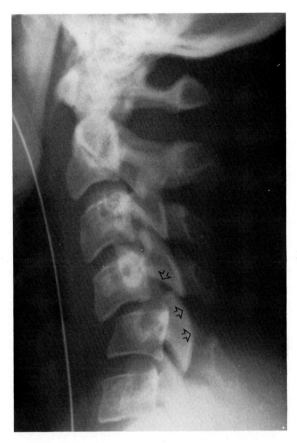

Fig. 9-13. Abnormal facet joints in a patient with unilateral locked facets at C4/C5. There is anterolisthesis of C4 on C5. Note the abnormal facet joint at C4/C5 *(arrows)*. The facet of C5 is almost "naked."

ABCs of radiographic assessment of vertebral trauma

Look for abnormalities of:
A = Alignment and anatomy
B = Bony integrity
C = Cartilage or joint space
S = Soft tissues

From Daffner RH: *Imaging of vertebral trauma*, Rockville, Md, 1988, Aspen Publishers.

Fig. 9-12. Burst fracture of L1. **A,** AP radiograph shows widening of the interpediculate distance of L1 *(double arrow).* There is loss of height of the body of L1. **B,** CT scan shows the fractures in the axial plane through the body and lamina of L1. There are retropulsed bone fragments within the vertebral canal.

vertebral disk space occurs when there is significant disruption of the intervertebral attachments and suggests an unstable injury.

In the thoracic and lumbar regions the facets can be easily seen on the AP radiograph. When there is a fracture of the articular pillar or facet, the facet joint may appear widened (Fig. 9-13). If the facet from the lower vertebrae is displaced, "naked facet"[20,35] is produced (Fig. 9-14).

Soft tissue abnormalities. Soft tissue signs have long been appreciated for their diagnostic value, especially in the cervical area. Widening of soft tissue shadows is the result of hemorrhage or hematoma. In the thoracic area, this may appear as widening of the mediastinum or as a paraspinal mass (Fig. 9-15). Loss of the psoas line may be the result of bleeding from a fracture in the lumbar area (Fig. 9-16).

By developing a disciplined approach to examining the plain film radiographs of the spine in the trauma patient and following the ABCs of radiographic assessment of vertebral trauma, the clinician can do much to avoid

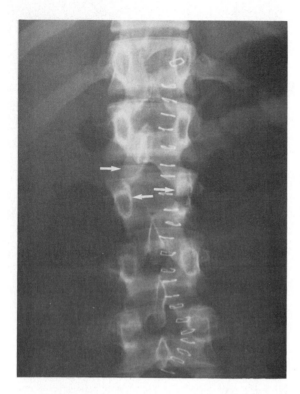

Fig. 9-14. "Naked" facets at L1/L2 in a patient with a distraction injury. There is widening of the interspinous space between L1 and L2. In addition, there is loss of continuity of the facet joints, which produces "naked" facets *(arrows)*.

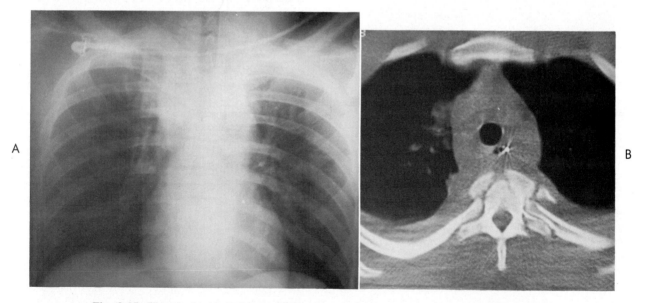

A   B

Fig. 9-15. Paraspinal widening in a patient with a T4 fracture/dislocation. **A,** AP chest radiograph shows widening of the mediastinum. **B,** CT scan through the area shows multiple bone fragments and bilateral pleural effusions. Note the widening of the paraspinal soft tissues although the aortic contour is normal.

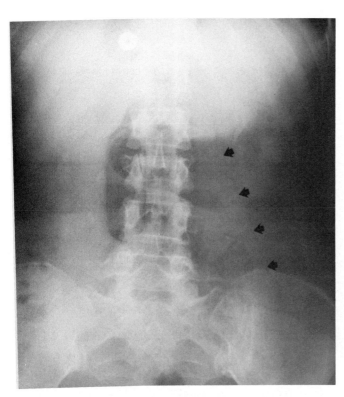

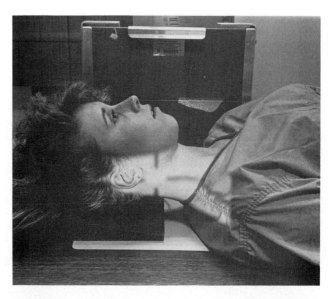

Fig. 9-17. Radiographic positioning for horizontal beam lateral radiograph of the upper cervical region. (From Daffner RH: *Imaging of vertebral trauma,* Rockville, Md, 1988, Aspen Publishers. Reproduced with permission.)

Fig. 9-16. There is loss of the psoas stripe on the right in a patient with a compression fracture of L3. Note the normal psoas stripe on the left *(arrows).*

missed and delayed diagnoses. It is also important to remember that there is a high incidence of multiple vertebral fractures in spinal trauma.[22] An undetected second or third fracture may contribute significantly to patient morbidity.

Cervical spine

Lateral view. Fig. 9-17 illustrates the technique for obtaining a horizontal beam lateral radiograph of the cervical spine. The normal lateral view of the cervical spine in Fig. 9-18 identifies important anatomic structures. Photographs of the different views of the individual vertebrae should be examined in order to develop a clear mental picture of the three-dimensional structures being viewed on the two-dimensional radiograph.

To analyze the technical adequacy of a lateral radiograph, the number of vertebrae should be counted. Fig. 9-19 illustrates a lateral view of the cervical spine that, on first glance, might appear adequate. However, the repeat view in Fig. 9-19 underscores the importance of visualizing all seven cervical vertebrae. Not doing this is a common error that may lead to significant patient morbidity. Also, the radiograph must be adequately exposed in order to visualize the trabecular pattern of the bones and to demonstrate the soft tissue markings. An underpenetrated film may obscure a fracture line while an overpenetrated film may obscure abnormal soft tissue findings.

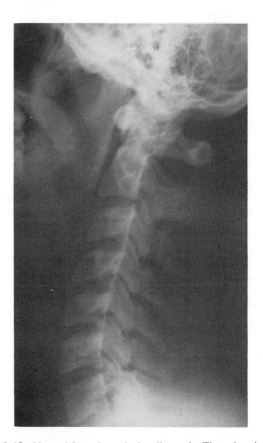

Fig. 9-18. Normal lateral cervical radiograph. There is minimal reversal of lordosis at C2/C3 and anterior and posterior vertebral body lines are intact. Note the alignment of the spinolaminal line. The facet joints are uniform and the predental space is normal.

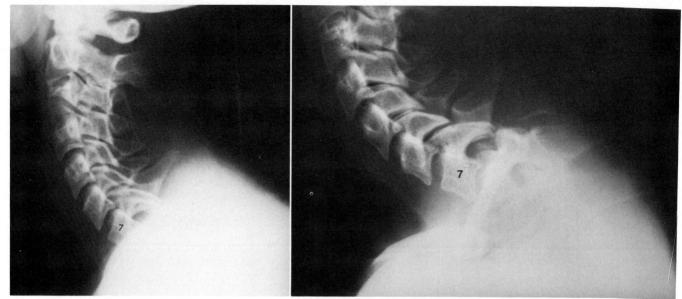

Fig. 9-19. Hazards of inadequate cervical radiography. **A,** Lateral radiograph fails to demonstrate the inferior portion of C7. **B,** Follow-up radiograph shows complete dislocation of C7 on T1. There is a fracture of the spinous process of C7. The importance of obtaining complete studies of the cervical vertebrae cannot be overemphasized.

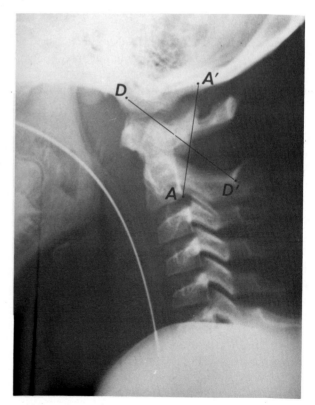

Fig. 9-20. Relationships of occiput to atlas and axis using Lee lines in a lateral radiograph of a child with an atlanto-occipital dislocation. A line is drawn from the basion to the midpoint of the spinolaminal line of C2 *(D-D', the descending limb)*. A second line is drawn from the opisthion to the posteroinferior corner of the body of C2 *(A-A', the ascending limb)*. Under normal circumstances, the descending limb should touch the dens or be within 5 mm of it as is the case in this radiograph. The ascending limb should pass through the spinolaminal line of C1, which, in this case, does not occur. This indicates that the head is dislocated anteriorly on C1.

In order to protect the spinal cord, a lateral radiograph should be analyzed to determine the integrity of the spinal column and, in particular, the spinal canal. This canal should be considered to be a tube beginning at the foramen magnum and lying protected within the bony arch of the cervical, thoracic, and lumbar vertebrae. The foramen magnum can be located by identifying its anterior and posterior margins. The posterior margin can be found by following the inner and outer tables of the occipital bone forward to a point where they come together, giving the appearance of a small beak (opisthion).

The anterior aspect can be located by finding the sella turcica. The clivus should be followed inferiorly and posteriorly from the sella turcica to a point forming a beak similar to the posterior margin of the foramen magnum (basion). To determine if the occiput and the atlas are in proper alignment, a line should be drawn from the basion to the midpoint of the spinolaminal line of C2 (descending limb). A second line (ascending limb) should be drawn from the opisthion to the posteroinferior corner of the body of C2. Under normal circumstances, the descending line should touch the dens or be within 5 mm of it whereas the ascending limb should pass through the spinolaminal line of C1 (Fig. 9-20).

Harris[51] has recently made an observation on normal occipito-atlanto-axial relationships. Under normal circumstances, a line drawn along the posterior margin of the dens and extended cephalad should be within 6 mm of the basion. Any deviation from this distance should be considered evidence of occipito-atlantal subluxation.

After the base of the skull has been evaluated, the atlas should be examined for injury. The lateral masses are difficult to see as there are many overlapping bones; however, they usually can be identified as hazy trapezoidal shadows. It is important to note whether they are malpositioned. The anterior arch can be seen as a bony D-shaped structure positioned anterior to the odontoid process.

The odontoid process is held in place against the anterior arch of the atlas by the transverse ligament of the atlas. The joint between these bones is seen radiographically as the "predental space." This space is normally no greater than 3 mm in the adult. Four mm is considered equivocal, and 5 mm or larger is pathognomonic for a rupture of the transverse ligament of the atlas (Fig. 9-21). In children, because of the elasticity of this ligament, 5 mm is considered normal; anything greater is considered pathologic. With rupture of the transverse ligament of the atlas, the atlas can sublux anteriorly. This can result in significant and potentially fatal damage to the spinal cord.

The posterior elements of the atlas should be assessed for signs of trauma. Disruption of the bony framework of the atlas can be seen as a disruption of the margins of the

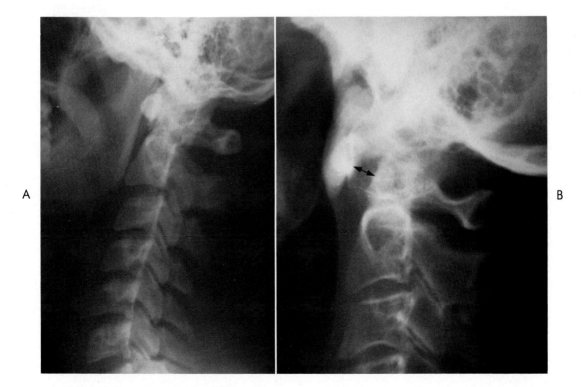

Fig. 9-21. Atlanto-axial relationships. **A,** Normal lateral radiograph with a normal predental space. This should measure no more than 3 mm in an adult or 5 mm in a child. **B,** Radiograph widened predental space *(arrows)* in a patient with rheumatoid arthritis. Note the disruption of the spinolaminal line as well.

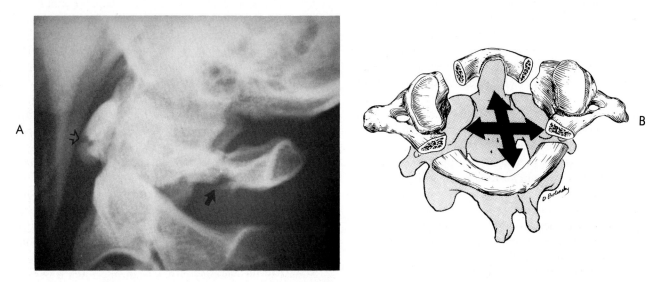

Fig. 9-22. Jefferson fracture. **A,** Lateral radiograph shows fractures of the anterior arch *(open arrow)* as well as the posterior arch *(solid arrow).* **B,** Schematic drawing of Jefferson fracture.

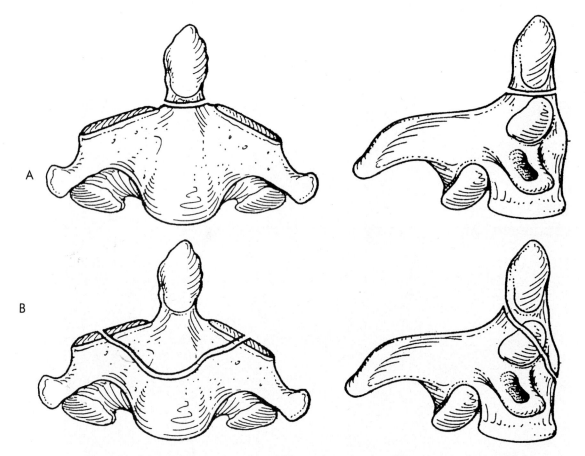

Fig. 9-23. AP and lateral schematics of C2 vertebra, showing different sites of odontoid fractures. **A,** Fracture at junction of odontoid process and body of C2 cervical vertebra. **B,** Fracture through upper body of vertebra. (Redrawn from Anderson LD, D'Alonzo RT: *J Bone Joint Surg* 56(A):1663, 1974.)

Chapter 9 Spinal trauma 237

bone, particularly in the posterior arch. In addition, there may be a displacement of the spinolaminal line of the atlas.

A Jefferson fracture is the classic fracture of the atlas. It results from axial loading, such as occurs when a diver strikes the head on the bottom of a pool or a hidden rock. Downward forces push the occipital condyles into the lateral masses of the atlas, disrupting it at two or more points (Fig. 9-22).

With the evaluation of the atlas completed, the odontoid process should be examined closely for fracture lines. These fractures occur at one of two levels: (1) transversely at the base or (2) obliquely through the body, avulsing a portion of C2, giving the appearance of "a tooth with a root" (Fig. 9-23). On the lateral view, these can occasionally be identified as small offsets in the anterior margin of the odontoid, as seen in Fig. 9-24. There is frequently a small depression in the anterior surface of the axis where the odontoid attaches to the body. This should not be confused with a fracture (Fig. 9-25).

Hyperextension can result in a fracture of the axis through both of the pedicles. This can be seen on a lateral radiograph either as an oblique fracture line running across the pedicles superimposed on the body or as a subluxation

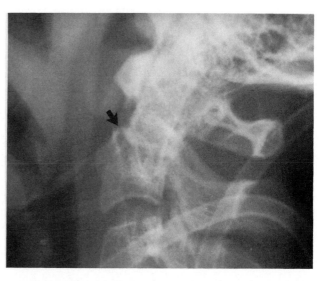

Fig. 9-24. Fracture at the base of dens. Lateral radiograph shows a disruption of the anterior margin of C2 at the base of the dens *(arrow)*.

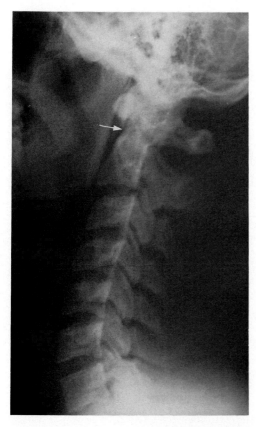

Fig. 9-25. Normal lateral radiograph of the cervical spine. Note the normal anterior depression at the point of fusion of the dens with the body *(arrow)*.

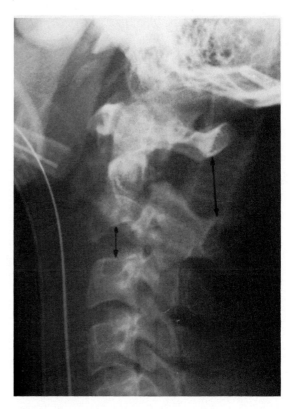

Fig. 9-26. Hangman-type fracture. Lateral radiograph shows disruption of the posterior arch of C2 extending into the body. There is widening of the disk space *(short double arrow)* and also widening of the interspinous space between the posterior arch of C1 and the spinous process of C2 *(long double arrow)*.

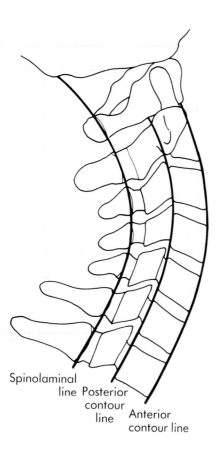

Fig. 9-27. Normal structural relationships of the lateral cervical spine. This lateral schematic illustrates the anterior longitudinal (contour) line, posterior longitudinal (contour) line, and the spinolaminal line. (From Rosen P, Baker FJ II, Barkin R et al, eds: *Emergency medicine: concepts and clinical practice,* ed 2, St Louis, 1988, CV Mosby.)

Fig. 9-28. Unilateral locked facet at C5/C6. Lateral radiograph shows slight anterolisthesis of C5 on C6. There is widening of the interspinous space between C5 and C6. Note the point of locking of the facets *(arrow).*

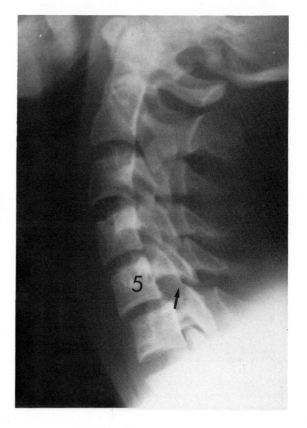

anteriorly of C2 on C3. This has been dubbed the "hang-man fracture" because it is the mechanism of injury that occurs with hanging. Fig. 9-26 illustrates the typical findings of this fracture. Just as with the atlas, displacement of the spinolaminal line of the axis from a line drawn between the spinolaminal lines of the first three cervical vertebrae indicates an unstable disruption in the bony arch.

After the first two cervical vertebrae have been closely inspected, the overall integrity of the bony column should be evaluated by looking for disruptions of the ligamentous connections. Fig. 9-27 is a schematic drawing depicting these ligaments.

The anterior longitudinal ligament is a tough fibrous band that holds the vertebral bodies together anteriorly. While examining a lateral radiograph, one should be able to draw a line along the anterior surfaces of the vertebral bodies without any steps or indentations. The anterior margins of the bodies should match within 1 mm. An exception to the strict alignment of these margins of the vertebral bodies is the pseudosubluxation seen in children. Pseudosubluxation is most common and most prominent (up to 3 mm) with overriding of C2 on C3.[38] It can be seen to a lesser degree at C3/C4 and C4/C5. Because of the flexibility of the ligaments, there can also be overriding of the atlas on the odontoid.[38] These findings are common below the age of 8, but pseudosubluxation has been seen in older children and teens. The key to proper diagnosis is normal alignment of the spinolaminal line.

Likewise, the posterior longitudinal ligament runs as a thick strap along the posterior aspects of the vertebral bodies. One should be able to draw a similar imaginary line as was done in evaluating the anterior longitudinal ligament. If there are any steps or mismatches of the vertebral mar-

gins, a ligamentous or bony disruption is indicated (Fig. 9-28). If there is a question of instability because of a minor discrepancy, flexion and extension views should be obtained to determine if an instability actually exists. This should be done only in a patient who is neurologically intact and who can actively flex and extend the neck. Under no circumstances should the patient's neck be passively moved.

A third line should be drawn joining the spinolaminal lines as seen in Fig. 9-27. This should be a gently curving arc. A fourth arcing line can be drawn joining the tips of the spinous processes. Irregularities in either of these latter two lines may indicate a bony disruption in the posterior elements and occasionally an isolated injury, such as a fractured spinous processes or a "clay shoveler" fracture. This fracture is illustrated in Fig. 9-29 and results from either a direct blow, an extraordinarily strong muscular contraction that rips the spinous process from its attachment, an avulsion fracture associated with another fracture dislocation, or a whiplash injury with hyperflexion-hyperextension.[39] Isolated spinous process fractures have been sustained in football accidents.[40]

The vertebral bodies of the third through seventh cervical vertebrae are similar in contour, with slightly increasing size caudally. The shapes, cortical margins, and trabecular patterns should be examined closely for fracture lines. Small compression fractures can result from hyperflexion injuries. They are seen as flattening of either the anterosuperior margin or anteroinferior margin of a vertebral body (Fig. 9-30).

Occasionally a wedge of bone, usually from the anteroinferior margin, can be fractured by the compressive forces of a hyperflexion injury[41] or pulled free as the bone

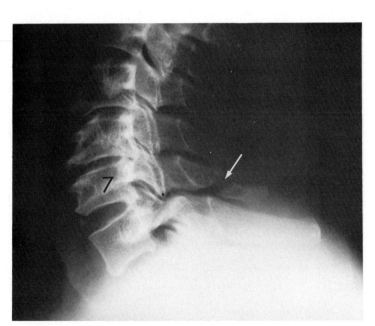

Fig. 9-29. "Clay shoveler" fracture of the spinous process of C7 *(arrow).*

fragment is torn in a hyperextension injury (Fig. 9-31). This is known as a "tear-drop" fracture because of the appearance of the fragment of bone. Other triangular fractures can occur at all four corners of the vertebral body and are frequently associated with damage to the posterior elements.[42] Because the amount of force required to create a tear-drop fracture is substantial, there is usually significant ligament damage, resulting in instability (Fig. 9-32).

The posterior elements should be examined closely for

evidence of disruption or displacement. The articular facets and their supporting pillars can be seen as a series of nearly quadrilateral structures immediately posterior to the vertebral bodies. These will appear as a "row of shingles" with even spacing and a slight overlap. In a true lateral view the pillars on opposite sides of a vertebra will be superimposed and appear as a single structure. If there is a slight rotation they will be offset with both pillars visible as if one were "seeing double" (Fig. 9-33).

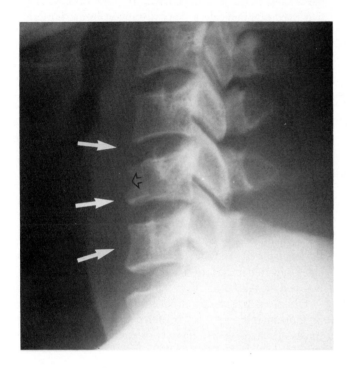

Fig. 9-30. Compression fracture of C5. Lateral radiograph shows buckling of the anterior cortex of C5 *(open arrow)*. Note the displacement of the prevertebral fat stripe *(solid arrows)*.

Fig. 9-31. "Tear-drop" fracture of the anteroinferior margin of C2.

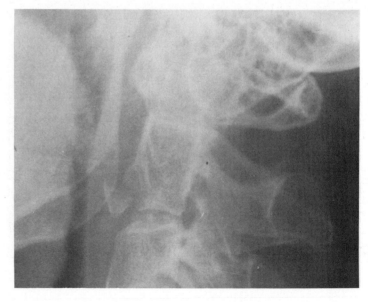

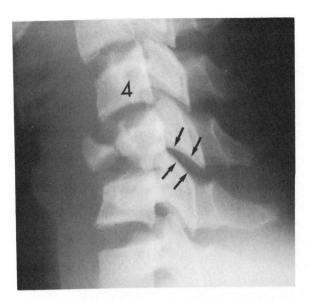

Fig. 9-32. Fracture of C5 in a diving accident. Lateral radiograph shows a large anterior "tear-drop" fragment. There is buckling of the posterior vertebral body line and retropulsion into the vertebral canal. Note the widening of the facet joints *(arrows)*.

When there is ligamentous disruption with instability, there may be a dislocation of the facet joints with one or both of the inferior facets of a more cephalad vertebra sliding forward and off the face of the superior facet of a vertebra below. Because there is a notch just anterior to the face of the joint, the edge of the facet will drop into the notch and become "locked." This can occur unilaterally (Fig. 9-34, *A*) or bilaterally (Fig. 9-34, *B*).

When examining a lateral radiograph for a facet dislocation, the alignment of the vertebral bodies as well as articular pillars will be a clue. In a unilateral facet dislocation, there will be a slight rotation and anterolisthesis of the vertebra above the disruption with respect to the vertebra below. This will cause the articular pillars above and below the dislocation to have different degrees of overlap[43] (Fig. 9-34, *A*). In both facet dislocations, an interruption of the overlap or "row of shingles" appearance of the facets can be seen.

The *s* or soft tissue in the ABCs of radiographic assessment of vertebral trauma plays an important role in the initial radiographic survey of the trauma victim. The widening of the retropharyngeal soft tissues is a valuable indica-

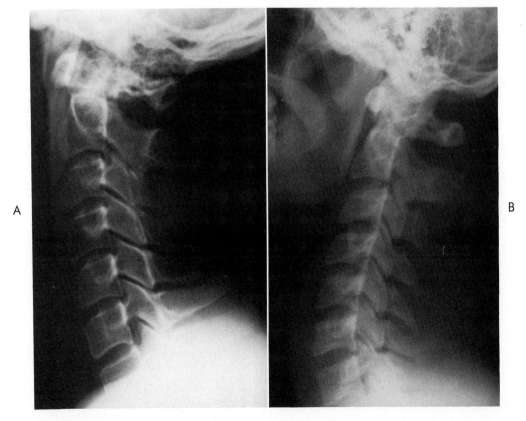

Fig. 9-33. Normal lateral radiographs of the cervical spine. **A,** Lateral radiograph shows perfect overlap of the articular pillars and facet joints. **B,** When slightly rotated, there is an offset of articular pillar images and facet joints. This radiograph is acceptable as long as the observer notes that the patient is slightly rotated.

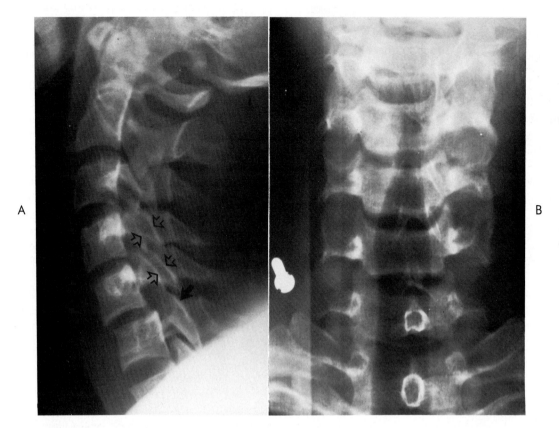

Fig. 9-34. A, Unilateral jumped and locked facet at C5/6. Left lateral view demonstrates overlapping pillar shadows at C6 and below *(solid arrow)*. There is duplication of pillar shadows from C5 upward *(open arrows)*. **B,** Right AP view shows spinous processes from C5 and above rotated toward the left, indicating the lock is on that side.

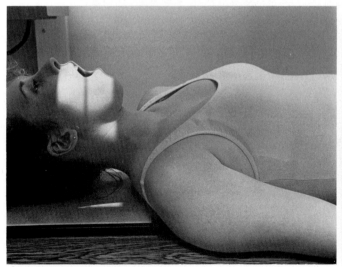

Fig. 9-35. Radiograph positioning for occipito-atlanto-axial ("odontoid") view. (From Daffner RH: *Imaging of vertebral trauma*, Rockville, Md, 1988, Aspen Publishers. Reproduced with permission.)

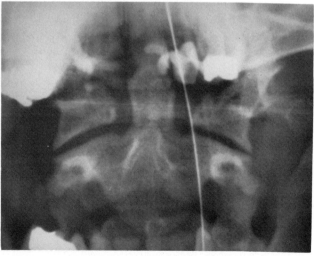

Fig. 9-36. Normal atlanto-axial view. The dens is perfectly centered between the lateral masses of C1. There is no overlap of the lateral masses of C1 on the lateral portions of C2.

tor of injury.[44-47] These tissues are tightly applied to the vertebral column and are usually less than 10 mm wide to the level of C4. At this point, the esophagus is interposed increasing the width of the soft tissues to 20 mm.[42] There is, however, considerable variation in the retropharyngeal soft tissues with the tissues appearing of normal width in approximately 70% of fractures.[47]

Odontoid view. The odontoid or "open-mouth" view is an AP radiograph of the first and second cervical vertebrae. It is named for the odontoid process, which is in the center of the radiograph, and for the position the patient must assume in order that the structure can be visualized (Fig. 9-35).

Fig. 9-36 is an example of an odontoid view. This radiograph affords an excellent view of the structures of C1, including the lateral masses, the transverse processes, and the two arches. C2 is also well visualized, displaying the body, superior articular facets, and the spinous process.

Following the ABCs of radiographic assessment of vertebral trauma, alignment and anatomy should be analyzed first. The space between the lateral masses and the odontoid process may not be equal depending on the rotation of the head and neck. In order to assess the alignment of C1 and C2, the margins of the articular facets should be examined. They should match within 1 mm.

The inferior edge of the occipital bone should be identified in order to avoid confusion with the arches or a fracture line. Also, the interface between the central incisors and air may mimic a fracture or obscure the details of the odontoid process.

Bony abnormalities can be identified, including subtle fracture lines through the lateral masses of C1 and in the

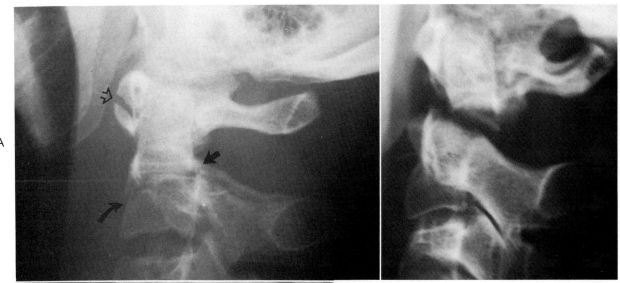

Fig. 9-37. A, Fracture of the base of the dens and body of C2 *(curved arrow)*. There is also a fracture of the anterior arch of the atlas *(open arrow)*. Note the disruption of the posterior vertebral body line at the base of the dens *(straight arrow)*. **B,** Fracture at the base of the dens with retrolisthesis of the proximal fragments. **C,** Subtle fracture of the base of the dens and the body of C2. Several abnormalities are present including widening of the transverse diameter of C2 *(small straight arrows)*—the so-called fat "C2" sign or disruption of Harris's ring inferiorly *(squiggly arrow)*. There is also duplication of the posterior vertebral body line *(arrowheads)* and disruption of the spinolaminal line with anterolisthesis of C1 on C2 *(open arrows)*.

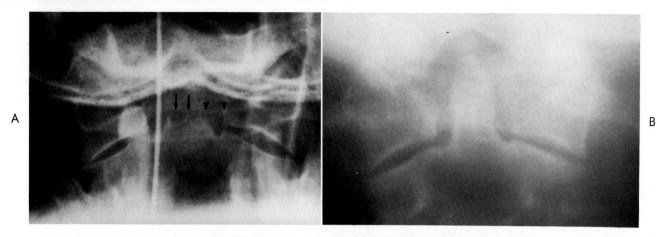

Fig. 9-38. Pseudofracture (Mach band phenomenon) of the dens. **A,** AP atlanto-axial radiograph shows a lucency across the dens *(arrows)*. This is due to the overlap of the image of the posterior arch of C1 on the dens. Note the continuity of the image of the arch *(arrowheads)* with the lucency. **B,** AP conventional tomogram shows no evidence of fracture.

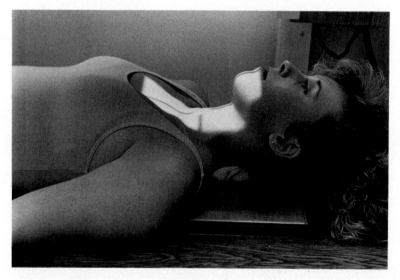

Fig. 9-39. Radiographic positioning for AP view of the cervical spine. (From Daffner RH: *Imaging of vertebral trauma*, Rockville, Md, 1988, Aspen Publishers. Reproduced with permission.)

body of C2. Odontoid process fractures typically appear at these locations (see Fig. 9-23). Examples of these fractures can be seen in Fig. 9-37. The posterior arch of the atlas or the edge of the occipital bone overlying the dens can mimic an odontoid fracture (Fig. 9-38). This pseudofracture is due to the Mach band phenomenon, which results when superimposed bony edges are radiographed.

Anteroposterior view. Positioning for an AP radiograph of the cervical spine can be seen in Fig. 9-39. Though difficult to interpret because of the many overlapping structures, the AP radiograph can provide valuable data. On this radiograph the vertebral bodies, spinous pro-

cesses, and the articular pillars can be evaluated. The vertebral bodies and vertebral spaces can readily be identified. The normal AP radiograph (Fig. 9-40) demonstrates the configuration of the vertebral bodies with their concave superior surface and convex inferior surface. The margins, trabecular pattern, and shape of the vertebral bodies should be evaluated for disruptions and asymmetries.

The spinous processes can be seen lining up vertically in the center of the AP view. When a single spinous process is out of alignment with the other spinous processes, there may be a fracture of that spinous process with displacement. The typical appearance of a unilateral facet dis-

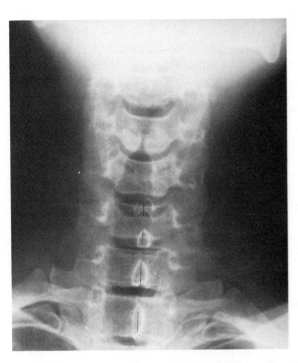

Fig. 9-40. Normal AP radiograph of the cervical spine. Note the alignment of the spinous processes, uncinate processes, and lateral margins of the vertebrae.

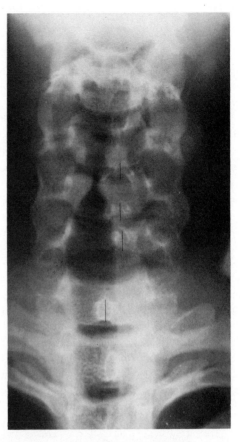

Fig. 9-41. Unilateral facet lock of C6/C7 (same patient as Fig. 9-34, *B*). There is widening of the interspinous space between C6 and C7 *(straight lines)*. Furthermore, the spinous processes do not align.

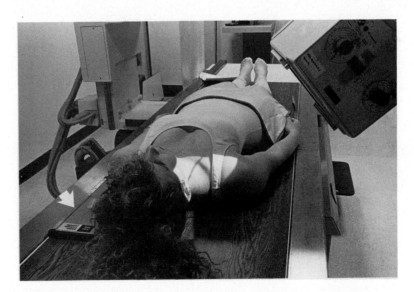

Fig. 9-42. Radiographic positioning for "trauma oblique" views of the cervical spine. The patient is supine. The film is placed adjacent to the patient's head and neck *(arrow)* and the x-ray tube is angled 35° to 40° off the horizontal with a 15° cephalad tilt. (From Daffner RH: *Imaging of vertebral trauma*, Rockville, Md, 1988, Aspen Publishers. Reproduced with permission.)

location shows the spinous processes from the dislocation and above lined up and the spinous processes below lined up, but these two rows do not intersect because of the rotation caused by the facet dislocation[43] (Fig. 9-41).

The pedicles and articular pillars protrude laterally from the vertebral bodies. Because of the many overlapping structures in this area, the vertebral body is seen as a bony density with a gently undulating margin. This portion of the radiograph should be analyzed for disruptions of the margin and appearance of fracture lines. The cartilage and joints, soft tissues, mandible, and first rib should also be carefully examined.

Oblique views. Oblique views of the cervical spine display the bony arch of the posterior vertebral elements. In the traumatized patient who is immobilized, an oblique view can be obtained in the modified fashion shown in Fig. 9-42. Because of the distance of the film from the bony structures, there is some magnification and distortion. Fig. 9-43, A, which is a standard oblique view, should be compared to Fig. 9-43, B, which was obtained using the modified technique depicted in Fig. 9-42.

With oblique views the laminae and articular pillars are clearly demonstrated and should be evaluated for fractures and dislocations. Just as on the lateral view, the articular facets should overlap as a row of shingles. Both oblique views should be obtained in order to evaluate for unilateral injury.

Thoracic spine

Lateral view. Just as with the cervical spine, it is important to visualize *all* of the thoracic vertebrae. Because of the density of structures in the region of the shoulders, the upper thoracic vertebrae are frequently difficult to visualize unless specialized views are taken. The normal positioning for the swimmer's view rotates the shoulders so that they do not overlie the vertebrae (Fig. 9-44). This view reveals the upper thoracic vertebrae as seen in Fig. 9-45, A. In the traumatized patient, this rotation of the shoulders may not be advisable and a modified swimmer's view should be used. In this case, the x-ray tube is angled rather than the patient's arms being rotated (Fig. 9-45, B). The swimmer's view, in combination with cross-table lateral and anteroposterior radiographs, demonstrates the thoracic vertebrae, allowing the clinician to employ the ABCs of radiographic assessment of vertebral trauma.

The shape and appearance of the vertebral bodies should be assessed for alignment and fractures. When a patient falls on the upper back and shoulders, the normal curvature of the thoracic spine tends to concentrate the forces in the areas of T5 and T6. Compression and tear-

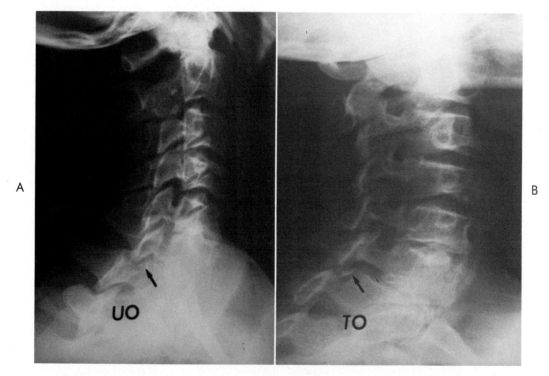

Fig. 9-43. Comparison of standard and "trauma oblique" radiographs in a patient with unilateral facet lock of C6 on C7. **A,** Standard oblique radiograph shows the abnormality *(arrow).* **B,** "Trauma oblique" radiograph obtained without moving the patient. There is improved demonstration of the vertebral foramina. There is also elongation of the vertebral bodies. In this instance, the point of locking *(arrow)* is equally well demonstrated. However, there is a small fragment of a facet located near the end of the arrow. This is not visible on the standard radiograph.

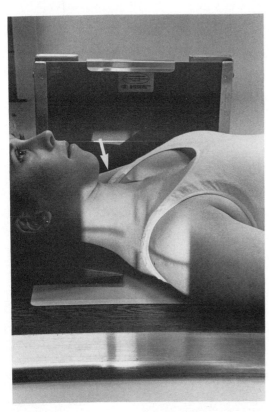

Fig. 9-44. Radiographic positioning for swimmer's view of the cervicothoracic region. The patient is supine with the arm closest the film *(arrow)* elevated. (From Daffner RH: *Imaging of vertebral trauma,* Rockville, Md, 1988, Aspen Publishers. Reproduced with permission.)

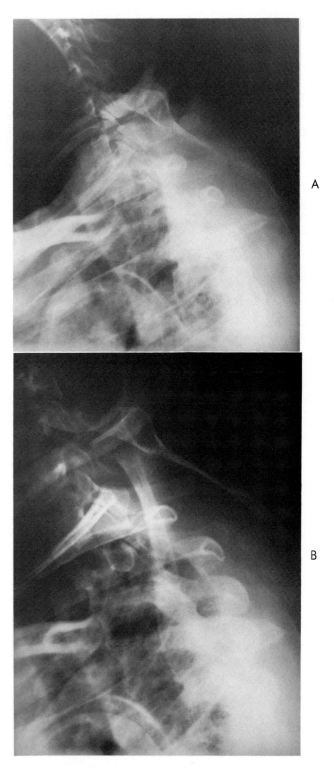

Fig. 9-45. A, Standard swimmer's view of the cervicothoracic junction. This view is sometimes useful for showing this region although a CT scan is preferable. **B,** Modified swimmer's view. The increased angulation projects the shoulder girdle higher on the radiograph. Compare with **A.**

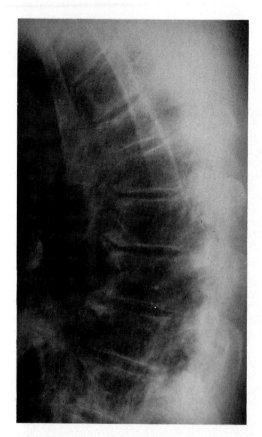

Fig. 9-46. Compression fractures at T4/T6. There is degenerative change in the spine as well.

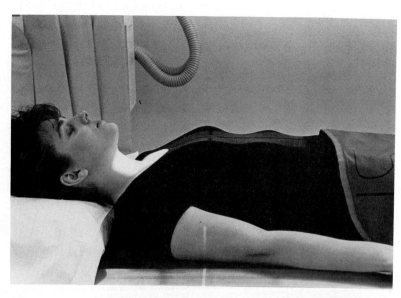

Fig. 9-47. Radiographic positioning for an AP view of the thoracic spine. (From Daffner RH: *Imaging of vertebral trauma*, Rockville, Md, 1988, Aspen Publishers. Reproduced with permission.)

Fig. 9-48. Normal AP radiograph of the thoracic spine. The pedicles, spinous processes, and lateral margins of the vertebrae align. There is no widening of the interpediculate distance.

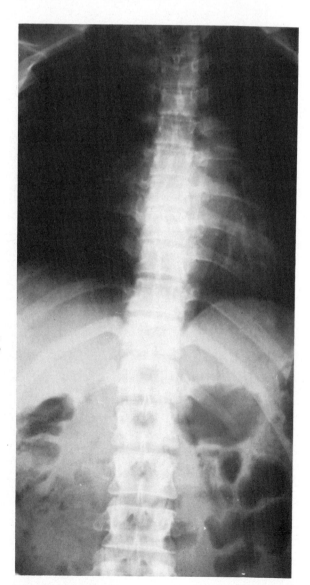

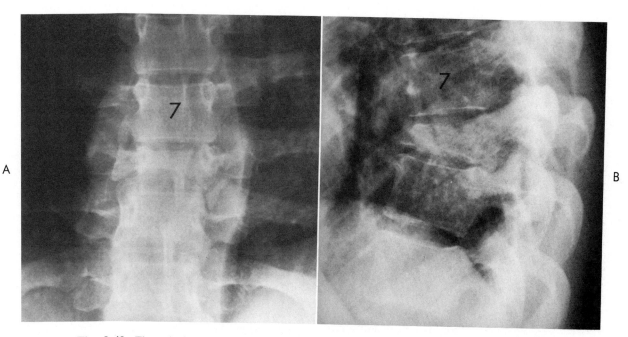

Fig. 9-49. Thoracic fracture subluxation of T8. **A,** AP radiograph shows compression of T8 and left laterolisthesis of T8 on T9. Note the paraspinal tissue widening. **B,** Lateral radiograph shows the compression of T8.

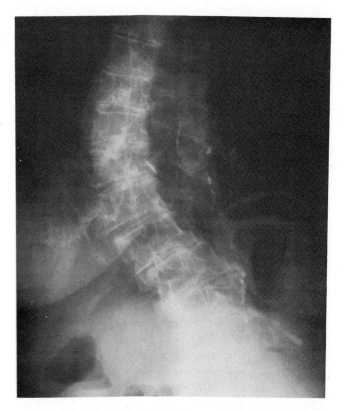

Fig. 9-50. Classic dextroscoliosis.

drop fractures can result from this type of injury (Fig. 9-46).

Anteroposterior view. In the AP view of the thoracic spine, all of the thoracic vertebral bodies should be visualized. Positioning for this radiograph is seen in Fig. 9-47. Fig. 9-48 illustrates a normal AP radiograph of the thoracic spine. The vertebrae should be inspected for symmetry, comparing each vertebra to the adjacent one above and below. The vertebral height, contour, cortices, and trabecular pattern should be evaluated. Particular attention to angulations in the spinal column is important as this malalignment may be evidence of a compression fracture. In Fig. 9-49, the abrupt angulation that occurs marks a compression fracture. It should not, however, be confused with scoliosis as seen in Fig. 9-50.

The spinous processes can be seen overlying the vertebral bodies and should form a straight row. The thoracic vertebrae do not have bifid spinous processes. Because of the large masses of the erector spinae muscles in the thoracic vertebrae, the spinous processes are well protected. However, they can be fractured by a direct powerful blow, sheared during hyperflexion in the high-speed deceleration of a motor vehicle accident in which only a lapbelt is worn, or avulsed in a rotational injury such as a fall. The posterior portions of the ribs, the transverse processes, and the costovertebral junctions should also be inspected. The ribs can help stabilize a thoracic spine fracture; however, the same precautions should be observed when dealing with thoracic injuries as with cervical spine injuries. Even the logroll transport can shift an unstable segment causing

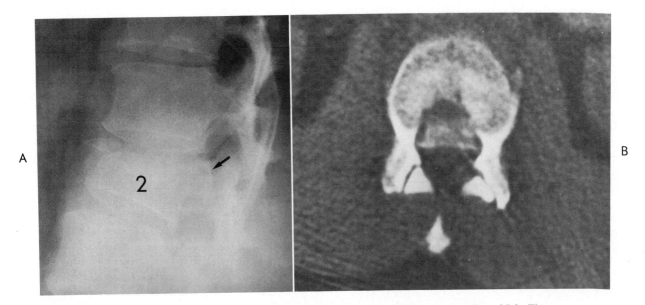

Fig. 9-51. Burst fracture of L2. **A,** Lateral radiograph shows anterior compression of L2. There is retropulsion of a bone fragment into the vertebral canal *(arrow).* **B,** CT scan shows the retropulsed fragment narrowing the vertebral canal by 50%.

potential neurologic damage. It should be used with utmost caution.

It is important to note that when there is axial loading from a fall or other trauma, the forces are dissipated along the vertebral column and will be concentrated where there is a change in the curvature of the spine. This is particularly true in the midthoracic region if the patient falls on the head or shoulders, or, at the thoracolumbar junction, if the patient undergoes a folding of the trunk or other scissor-like action on the spine. In a patient who falls or jumps from a height and lands on the feet or buttocks, the force of the impact is transmitted up to the spine and frequently results in a fracture. Particular attention should be paid to these areas with such mechanisms of injury.

When evaluating the AP view of the thoracic spine, information about the ribs, lungs, mediastinum, and the heart should also be noted. Apical capping, subtle pneumothoraces, and fractures may be visualized.

Oblique views. Oblique views of the thoracic spine are not performed since they are rarely useful. If additional information is needed, a CT scan of the thoracic spine should be done (Fig. 9-51).

Lumbar spine

Lateral view. It is extremely important when the patient complains of low back pain in a trauma center to perform a horizontal beam lateral radiograph as one of the early diagnostic steps. The patient should remain immobilized with the spine protected during this procedure. Fig. 9-52 demonstrates proper positioning. Fig. 9-53 is a typi-

cal horizontal beam lateral radiograph of the lumbar spine. Just as in the cervical spine, this view can provide valuable information in early assessment of the trauma victim. However, the lateral radiograph alone is insufficient because of the limitations of the technique. In a patient where there is a strong clinical suggestion of a fracture additional views or a CT scan will be necessary.

All five lumbar vertebrae must be visualized. There can occasionally be a sixth lumbar vertebra or sacralization of the fifth lumbar vertebra as normal variations. Because of the high incidence of fractures in the thoracolumbar area, it is essential to include the lower thoracic vertebrae in the horizontal beam lateral radiograph or to obtain a lateral thoracic radiograph as well. The same guidelines and thoroughness in evaluating this portion of the spine should be used as those applied in the cervical and thoracic regions.

The lateral lumbar radiograph in Fig. 9-53 illustrates normal radiographic anatomy. When viewing such a radiograph, the ABCs of vertebral trauma should be assessed. The anterior and posterior margins of the vertebral bodies should be aligned within 1 mm. Wider discrepancies may signal subluxation and disruption of the anterior and posterior longitudinal ligaments. In some patients arthritic changes may make this evaluation more difficult.

To complicate matters, 5% of patients have spondylolisthesis secondary to chronic occult stress fractures and, even more rarely, due to a congenital anomaly.[48] This usually occurs at the L5/S1 junction. There can be marked subluxation without neurologic compromise. One must distinguish these conditions from a traumatic change by historic and clinical parameters.

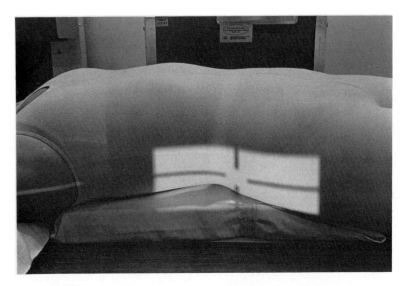

Fig. 9-52. Radiographic positioning for a cross-table lateral view of the lumbar spine. (From Daffner RH: *Imaging of vertebral trauma,* Rockville, Md, 1988, Aspen Publishers. Reproduced with permission.)

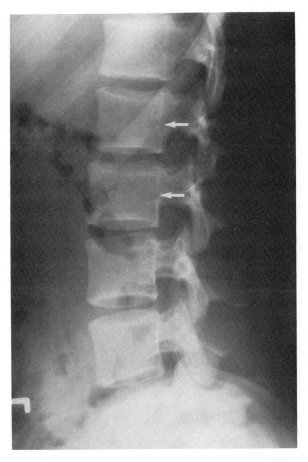

Fig. 9-53. Normal lateral radiograph of the lumbar spine. There is normal alignment anteriorly and posteriorly. The posterior vertebral body lines are either solid or interrupted centrally by a nutrient canal *(arrows).*

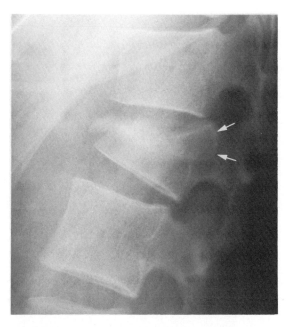

Fig. 9-54. Burst fracture of L2. Lateral radiograph shows the marked compression of the body of L2 and bowing of the posterior vertebral body line of L2 *(arrows).*

Particular attention should be paid to the integrity of the posterior vertebral body line.[37] Disruption of this line as shown in Fig. 9-54 demonstrates encroachment of bony fragments on the spinal canal.

The posterior elements should be viewed with the same scrutiny. Smith[49] and Chance[50] fractures are variations of a flexion fracture in which the vertebra is literally torn apart by forces of distraction (Fig. 9-55).

The burst fracture is the most common vertebral injury, comprising 36% of thoracic and lumbar injuries.[20] In this injury the intensity of flexion forces shatters the vertebral body (Fig. 9-56).

A simple compression fracture of a lumbar vertebra (Fig. 9-57) also results from a flexion mechanism. It occurs in 25% of cases.[20]

Anteroposterior view. The anteroposterior view provides a wealth of information about the lumbar spine, including the vertebral bodies, articular facets, articular pillars, and spinous processes. In addition, this view is easily performed without jeopardizing the patient's spinal cord by movement or removal of immobilizing devices. Fig. 9-58 illustrates the proper positioning for this radiograph. The AP radiograph in Fig. 9-59 clearly displays the normal anatomy of this region. When analyzing these radiographs, particular attention should be paid to rotation of the spinous process, widening of the interpediculate distances, alignment of the bodies, facet appearance, joint spaces, and the transverse processes.

COMPUTED TOMOGRAPHY AND MAGNETIC RESONANCE IMAGING

Advances in computed tomography (CT scan) and magnetic resonance imaging (MRI) have added significantly to

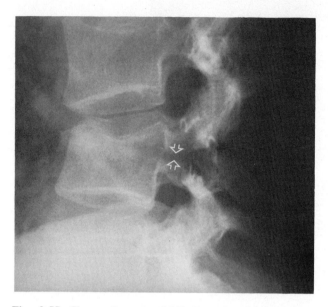

Fig. 9-55. Chance fracture of L2. Lateral radiograph shows compression of the anterior portion of the body of L2. Fracture lines are seen extending through the pedicles *(arrows)*.

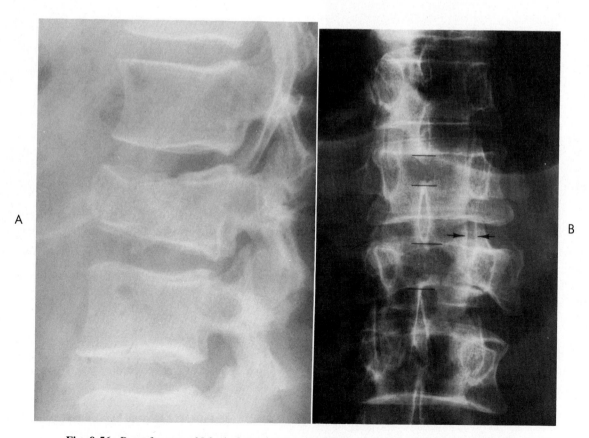

Fig. 9-56. Burst fracture of L2. **A,** Lateral radiograph shows compression of the body of L2 and disruption of the posterior vertebral body line. **B,** AP radiograph shows widening of the facet joints at L1/L2 *(arrows)*. Note the widening of the interspinous space between L1 and L2 compared with that of T12 and L1 *(lines)*.

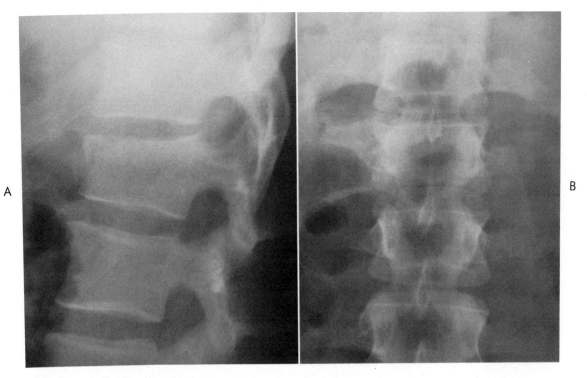

Fig. 9-57. Simple compression fracture of L1. **A,** Lateral radiograph shows buckling of the anterior cortex of L1 and narrowing of the T12 disk space. The posterior vertebral body line is intact. **B,** AP radiograph shows buckling of the body of L1 superiorly on the right side. The interspinous space and interpediculate distances are normal.

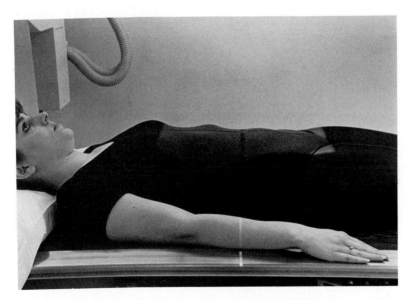

Fig. 9-58. Radiographic positioning for an AP view of the lumbar spine. (From Daffner RH: *Imaging of vertebral trauma,* Rockville, Md, 1988, Aspen Publishers. Reproduced with permission.)

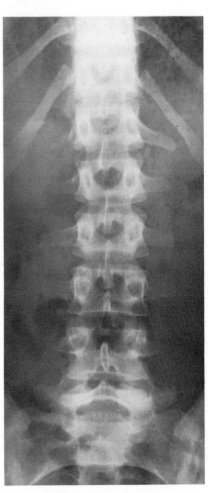

Fig. 9-59. AP radiograph of the lumbar spine. Note the uniformity of the interpediculate distances and interspinous spaces.

the evaluation of the spine-injured patient. Conventional tomography has been a useful adjunct.[51] However, the newer technologies provide far superior images and are not limited in their orientation.

Computed tomography

The CT scan has gained wide acceptance in the evaluation of trauma because it provides excellent visualization of the complex structures of the spine. This is particularly useful in evaluating the posterior elements comprising the bony canal. The newer generation of CT scanners have reduced the imaging time, making the CT scan a primary tool for use in the emergency setting.

Currently, a plain film radiographic survey is used to guide the clinician in selecting focused areas for CT scan evaluation. There have been recommendations for universal applications of this technology in the assessment of spinal trauma.[52] However, it is felt that evaluation of the spine in the trauma victim should begin with plain film radiography.[20,35,53] One study added cervical spine CT scans to

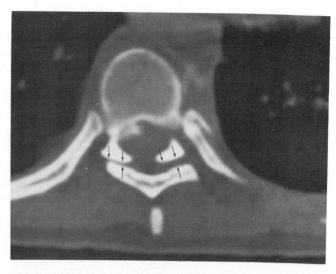

Fig. 9-60. CT scan showing paraspinal hematoma and disruption of facet joints *(arrows)* in a patient with T8/T9 fracture dislocation (same patient as Fig. 9-49).

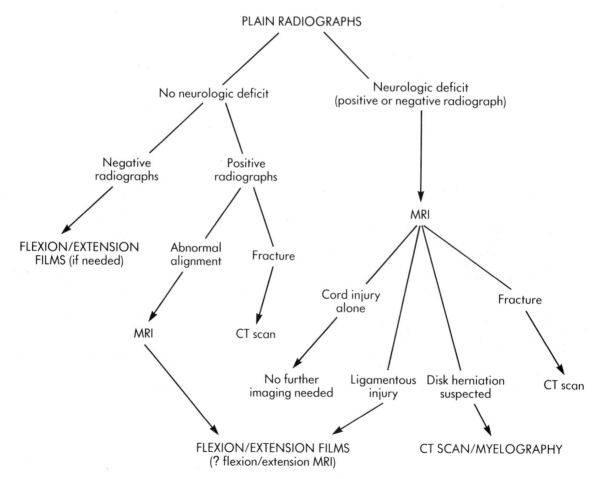

Fig. 9-61. Algorithm for the radiographic evaluation of acute vertebral injury. (From Goldberg AL et al: *Skel Radiol* 17:89, 1988.)

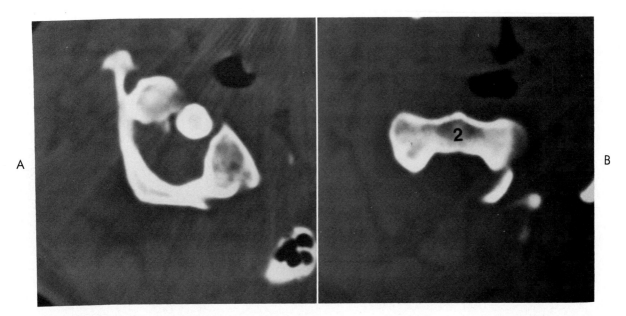

Fig. 9-62. Rotary fixation of C1 on C2. **A,** CT scan through the atlas shows it to be rotated to the left. **B,** CT scan through the axis shows it to be in a normal position.

head CT scans in cases of severe head injury and in 50 cases found four upper cervical fractures not demonstrated on the plain radiographs.[54] A CT scan also provides the distinct benefit of simultaneous imaging of the chest and abdomen when the thoracic and lumbar areas are scanned.

In a patient with a strong clinical presentation of a spinal fracture involving the thoracic or lumbar regions or when there are neurologic deficits and the patient is at significant risk from movement, cross-table lateral views are frequently limited in quality. A CT scan is invaluable in that it provides clear images of these sections of the spine as well as visualization of paravertebral hematomas and important details of thoracic and abdominal cavities (Fig. 9-60).

The limitations of the CT scan in the emergency setting are primarily technical. The CT scanner is frequently at some distance from the emergency department. Transportation of the patient to the radiology suite may be difficult and time-consuming, especially if the patient is intubated and requires significant resuscitation. Management during the CT scan may be difficult if the trauma team is remote from the patient because of radiation hazard. Time may become a factor in the unstable patient. An uncooperative patient, whether from alcohol, shock, or head trauma, is difficult to manage for plain radiographs and CT scans. Depending on the clinical setting, such a patient may require sedation, constant reassurance, or restraint. There is also the technical limitation that the typical CT table can only support 300 to 350 pounds when extended into the CT scan gantry.[20]

The CT scan is indicated to evaluate the patient with equivocal radiographs, to further define known fractures, to complete an inadequate plain film radiographic survey, and as an additional step in evaluating the patient with normal radiographs but in whom the clinical picture suggests a fracture. Fig. 9-61 provides an algorithm for the integration of plain radiographs, CT scans, and MRI in the evaluation of spinal trauma patients.

Rotatory subluxation (Fig. 9-62), facet fractures (Fig. 9-63), malalignment (Fig. 9-64) and narrowing of the spinal canal (Fig. 9-65), and encroachment of the lateral recess or neural foramen (Fig. 9-66) are all effectively displayed by CT scans.[35,55] Jefferson fractures of C1 with multiple fragments and distortion are also well defined (Fig. 9-67).

Epidural hematoma can be visualized with a CT scan but is better delineated by MRI. Unfortunately, most institutions are not set up to perform an MRI on an unstable trauma patient, and the clinician will be forced to rely on neurologic observation and repeat CT scans since progression of an epidural hematoma can result in further neurologic deficit. Frequent neurologic assessment and repeat CT scans are invaluable.

Nondisplaced fractures may not be visualized on plain radiographs. Fig. 9-68 is an illustration of a hangman fracture that was not seen on the initial plain radiograph yet was demonstrated on a CT scan.

Horizontal fractures that do not lie in the plane of the CT scan may not be visualized. An example would be an odontoid fracture. Also some compression fractures may be missed by a CT scan.

Soft tissue injuries such as disk herniation may be visualized by CT scans (Fig. 9-69). Damage to the cord and nerve roots can also be demonstrated using CT scans but are usually better visualized with MRI. Intrathecal contrast material enhances CT scan imaging, but this may be impractical in the emergency setting.

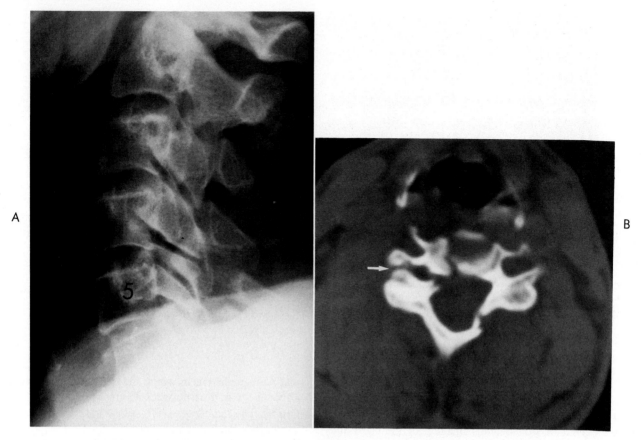

Fig. 9-63. Anterolisthesis of C5 on C6 with facet fracture. **A,** Lateral radiograph shows anterolisthesis of C5 on C6. **B,** CT scan at the level of the C5 disk space shows a fracture through the body of C6 on the right, fractures through the pedicle at C6 on the right, and through the lamina on the left. There is also a fracture through the facet *(arrow)*.

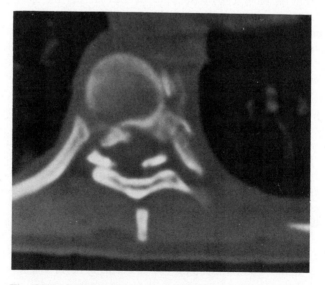

Fig. 9-64. CT scan demonstrates malalignment (same patient as in Figs. 9-49 and 9-60).

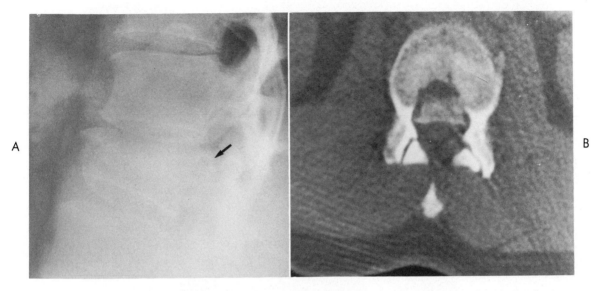

Fig. 9-65. Burst fracture of L2. **A,** Lateral radiograph shows anterior compression of the body of L2. There is retropulsion of a bone fragment into the vertebral canal *(arrow).* **B,** CT scan shows the retropulsed bone fragment within the vertebral canal.

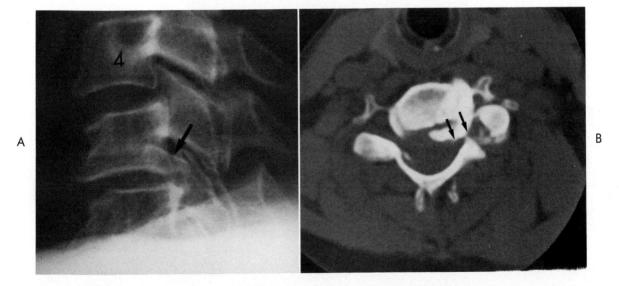

Fig. 9-66. Encroachment of the neural canal by a bone fragment. **A,** Lateral radiograph shows a bone fragment from the superior articular facet of C6 *(arrow).* The fragment overlies the area forming the neural foramen. **B,** CT scan shows fragmentation of the superior articular facet of C6. A large bone fragment from that facet narrows the neural canal *(arrows).*

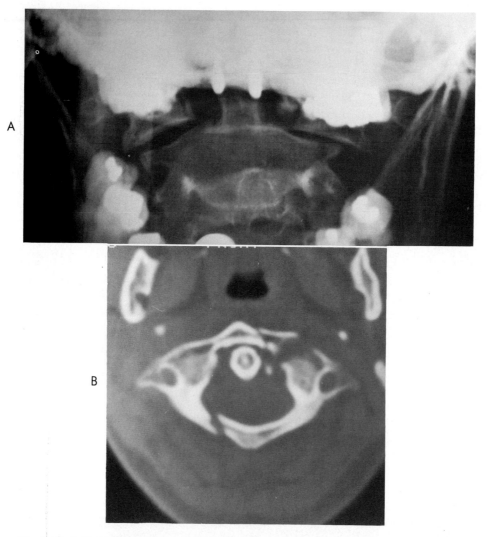

Fig. 9-67. Jefferson fracture of C1. **A,** AP radiograph shows bilateral lateral atlanto-axial offset. Note widening of the space between the dens and the lateral masses of C1. **B,** CT scan shows fractures through the anterior and posterior aspects of C1.

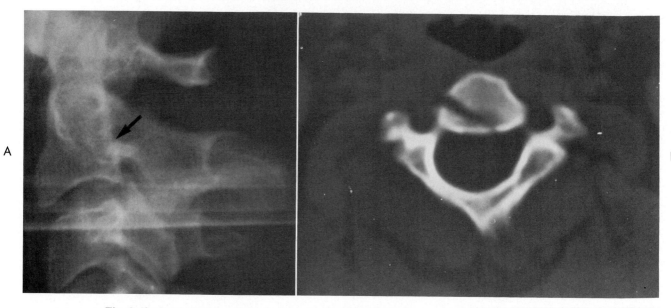

Fig. 9-68. Subtle fracture of C2. **A,** Lateral radiograph shows disruption of the posterior vertebral body line of C2 *(arrow)*. **B,** CT scan shows the fracture through the lower aspect of the body of C2. In this instance, the CT scan demonstrates the fracture more clearly than the plain radiograph.

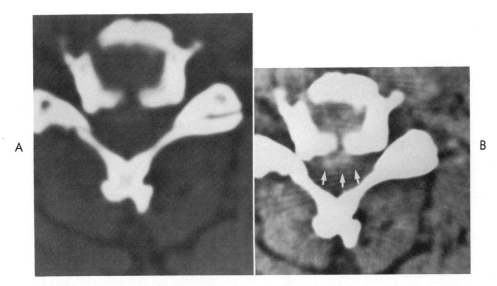

Fig. 9-69. Herniated intervertebral disk associated with a vertebral fracture. **A,** CT scan at bone window shows fractures of vertebral body anteriorly on the right and posteriorly centrally. **B,** CT scan at soft tissue windows shows herniated disk material *(arrows)* encroaching on the vertebral canal.

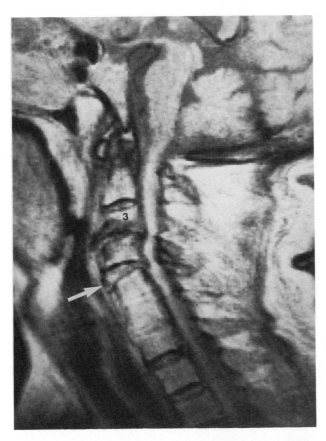

Fig. 9-70. Extension injury at C4/C5 in a patient with diffuse idiopathic skeletal hyperostosis (DISH). T_1-weighted MRI scan shows rupture of the anterior longitudinal ligament *(arrow)*. Note the marked narrowing of the vertebral canal at the C3 and C4 disk levels. There is herniated disk material at each of these levels. The patient was quadriplegic.

Magnetic resonance imaging

Magnetic resonance imaging (MRI) has become one of the key modalities in evaluating spinal trauma because of its unique ability to provide clear pictures of the spinal cord and soft tissues as well as its advantage of multiplanar imaging.[20,56-58] Demonstration of ligamentous injury (Fig. 9-70), disk herniation (Fig. 9-71), epidural hematoma[59,60] (Fig. 9-72), bony compression (Fig. 9-73), and vertebral artery occlusion may significantly impact treatment.[60-63]

The delineation of spinal cord injury patterns by MRI provides significant diagnostic and prognostic capabilities not previously available. Three patterns of cord injury have been defined: hemorrhage into the substance of the spinal cord (Fig. 9-74), edema or contusion of the spinal cord (Fig. 9-75), and mixed injuries[64,65] (Fig. 9-76). Spinal cord edema tends to resolve with neurologic improvement while hemorrhage into the spinal cord is a grave prognostic sign.

Post-traumatic MRI evaluation may be helpful in managing patients, particularly if there is new or progressive neurologic impairment. Spinal cord cysts and syringomyelia (Fig. 9-77) may be revealed.[20,66,67]

The disadvantages of MRI include standard contraindications, such as metallic aneurysm clips, metallic prostheses, pacemakers, and metallic foreign bodies. In addition, unstable patients or patients requiring intensive, hands-on care cannot be left alone in the MRI scanner. Life-support equipment, cardiac monitors, and cervical traction devices also interfere with MRI scanning. MRI-compatible respirators have been developed but technical problems still exist.

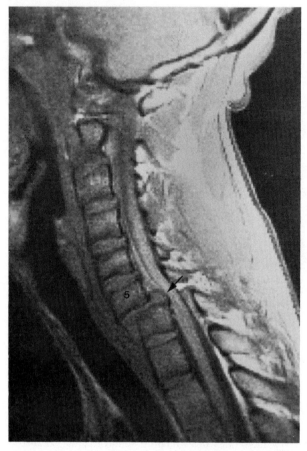

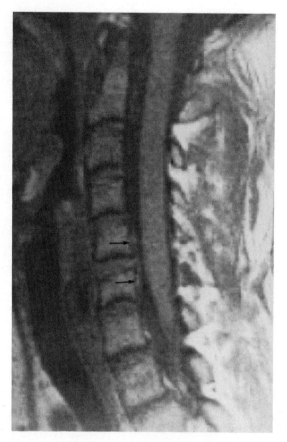

Fig. 9-71. T_2-weighted image of herniated intervertebral disk at C5/C6 *(arrow)*.

Fig. 9-72. Epidural hematoma in a patient with an extension injury at C5/C6. This T_2-weighted image shows bright area of hemorrhage in the epidural space posterior to C5 and C6 *(arrows)*.

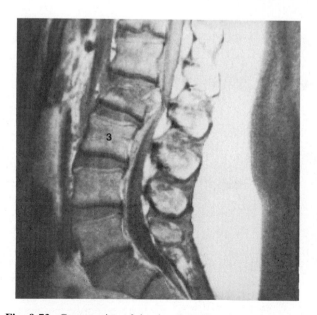

Fig. 9-73. Compression of the thecal sac by a bone fragment in a patient with a burst injury of L2. Note the bowing of the thecal sac at L2 by the large bone fragment within the vertebral canal on this T_1-weighted image.

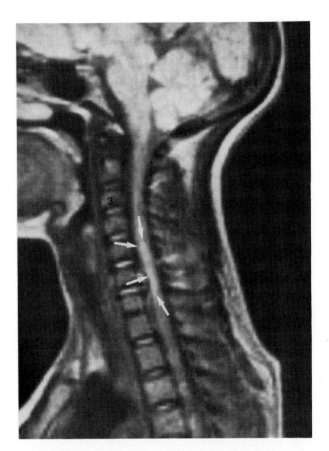

Fig. 9-74. Hemorrhage in the spinal cord at C5 and C6 secondary to a burst fracture of C5. This sagittal T_2-weighted image shows an area of increased signal *(brightness)* extending from C5 down to C7 *(arrows)*. The patient was quadriplegic.

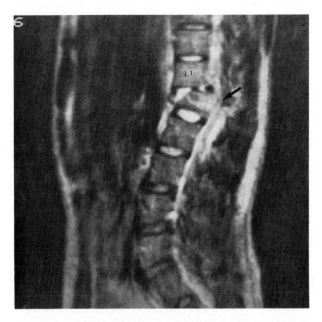

Fig. 9-76. Fracture dislocation at T11/T12. This sagittal T_1-weighted scan shows anterior dislocation of T11 on T12. There is complete transection of the thecal sac *(arrow)*. The bright area behind T12 and L1 represents hemorrhage. This image demonstrates multiple abnormalities present.

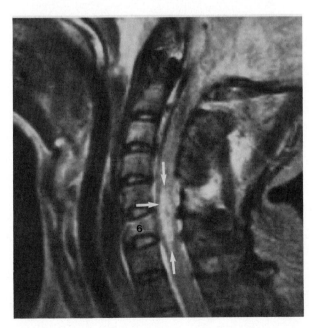

Fig. 9-75. Myelomalacia secondary to cord contusion at C5/C6 in a patient with burst fracture of C6. There is a central area of increased signal *(brightness) (arrows)* in the C5/C6 region on this T_2-weighted image. The patient was quadriplegic.

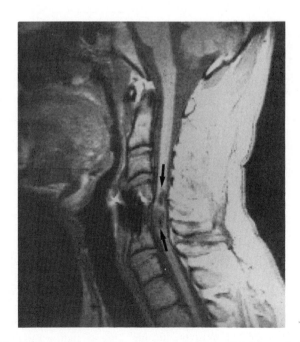

Fig. 9-77. Post-traumatic cord cyst (syringomyelia) in a patient with a healed fracture dislocation at C4/C6. Note the cystic areas of low signal within the substance of the spinal cord *(arrows)*.

Table 9-1. "Fingerprints" of the different mechanisms of vertebral trauma

Mechanism	"Fingerprints"
Flexion	Compression, fragmentation, burst vertebral bodies
	"Tear-drop" fragments
	Wide interspinous space
	Anterolisthesis
	Disrupted posterior vertebral body line
	Locked facets
	Narrow disk space
	Abrupt angulation of vertebral column
Extension	Wide disk space
	Triangular avulsion fracture
	Retrolisthesis
	Neural arch fracture
	Anterolisthesis with normal interspinous space and spinolaminal line
Shearing	Lateral distraction
	Lateral dislocation
	Transverse process fractures
	"Windswept appearance"
	Linear array of fragments
Rotation	Rotation
	Dislocation
	Facet and pillar fractures
	Transverse process fractures
	"Grinding of vertebrae"
	Circular array of fragments

From Daffner RH et al: *Skel Radiology,* 15:518, 1986.

Table 9-2. Mechanism and location of vertebral injuries in 1000 cases

| Level | Mechanism | | | | |
	Flexion	Extension	Shear	Rotation	Total
Cervical	511	124	0	11	646
Upper thoracic	87	0	0	0	87
Lower thoracic	25	0	0	0	25
Thoracolumbar	216	2	12	2	232
Lower lumbar	10	0	0	0	10
Total	849	126	12	13	1000

From Daffner RH: *Imaging of vertebral trauma,* Rockville MD, 1988, Aspen Publishers.

MECHANISMS OF INJURY

There are four basic mechanisms of injury to the spinal column: flexion, extension, rotation, and shearing.[35] These can occur in isolation or in combination. The exact nature of an injury depends on the architecture of the spine and the way in which the forces are applied. The injuries produced have very predictable patterns radiographically (Table 9-1).

The results of a study of 1000 vertebral injuries[35] are summarized in Table 9-2. The vast majority are flexion in-

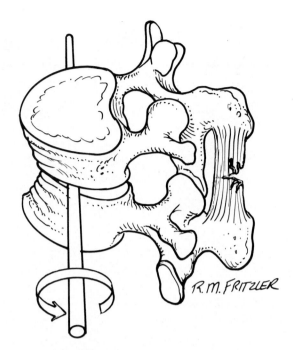

Fig. 9-78. Mechanism of flexion injury.

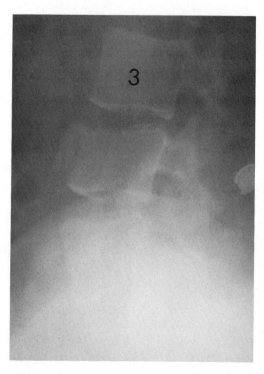

Fig. 9-79. Simple flexion injury of L4. There is fragmentation anteriorly. The posterior vertebral body line is intact.

juries, but, because of its mobility, the cervical spine is also exposed to extension injuries.

Flexion injuries

Flexion injuries, regardless of their location, all occur as a forward rotation of one vertebra on another (Fig.

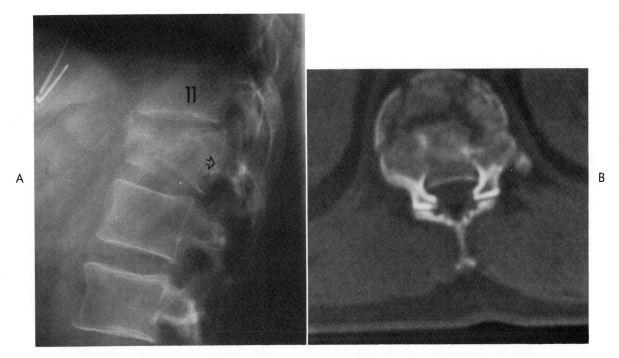

Fig. 9-80. Burst fracture of T12. **A,** Lateral radiograph shows anterior compression of T12, fragmentation of the vertebral body, and posterior bowing of the posterior vertebral body line *(arrow).* **B,** CT scan shows the comminution of the body and retropulsion of the bone fragment so it encroaches on the vertebral canal.

9-78). Flexion injuries can be divided into four groups. Simple flexion injuries result in compression of the bone of the vertebral body below the point of injury (Fig. 9-79). This can occur with or without narrowing of the disk space above. The ligaments and posterior arch remain intact.

Burst injuries are a progression of the simple flexion injury to the point where there are forces sufficient to shatter the vertebral body. There may be retropulsion of a fracture fragment into the spinal canal. This can be observed on a lateral radiograph as a disruption of the posterior vertebral body line[37] (Fig. 9-80). In this mechanism of injury, the anterior effect is compression and the posterior effect is distraction. The latter results in tearing of the interspinous ligaments and may include the ligamentum flavum and the posterior longitudinal ligament. Burst injuries almost always involve the ligaments and bony damage to the posterior elements.

Distraction injuries appear as separation of the spinous processes, widening of facets, and occasionally tearing of the bone (Fig. 9-81). There is no dislocation, but frequently there is neurologic damage.[20]

The last group of flexion injuries are dislocations. Ligamentous and bony attachments are completely disrupted, and the spine is mobile at this level. This results in a subluxation or facet dislocation (Fig. 9-82).

Extension injuries

Extension injuries can occur with falls, such as when a driver strikes the chin on a steering wheel, with the hyper-

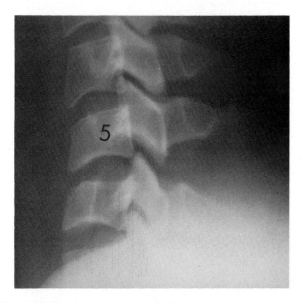

Fig. 9-81. Distraction injury at C5/C6. There is kyphotic angulation at C5/C6, widening of the facet joints, and widening of the interspinous space.

extension whiplash in a rearend collision, and with other similar mechanisms. These injuries are chiefly cervical injuries but can occur elsewhere in the spine.

Extension injuries can also be grouped. Simple extension injuries involve an avulsion fracture from the antero-

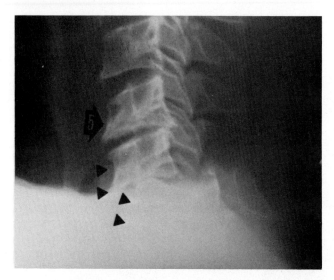

Fig. 9-82. Cervical dislocation of C6 on C7 with fractures through the posterior elements of C6 and the anterior subluxation of C6 on C7. Anterior margins of C6 and C7 are noted *(arrowheads)*.

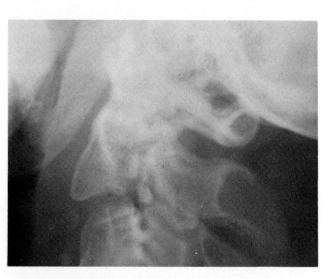

Fig. 9-84. Hangman fracture of C2. A lateral radiograph shows disruption of the posterior aspect of the body of C2. There is slight anterolisthesis of the body of C2 on C3.

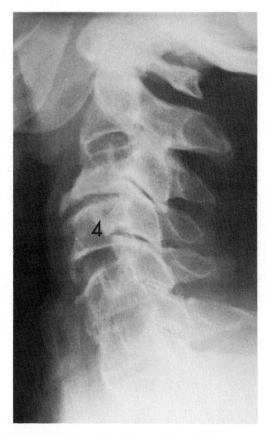

Fig. 9-83. Extension injury C4/C5 (same patient as Fig. 9-70). Note the widening of the C4 disk space. There is slight retrolisthesis of C4 on C5. There are severe degenerative changes present as well as changes of DISH.

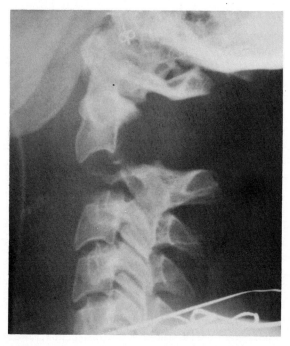

Fig. 9-85. Extension dislocation. Lateral radiograph shows a cervical hangman fracture of C2. There is gross distraction of C2 cephalad. This patient was ejected from a motorcycle and literally hung himself on power lines. This is the typical radiographic appearance that would be encountered in a patient following a judicial hanging.

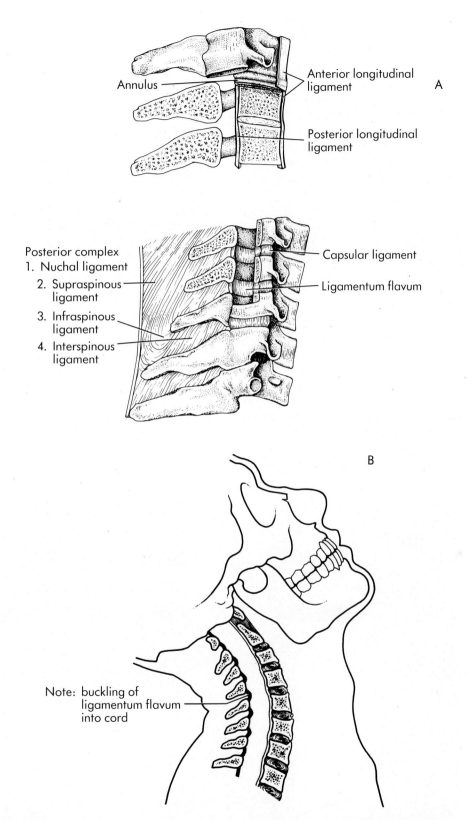

Fig. 9-86. A, Ligaments of the anterior column. **B,** Ligaments of the posterior column. (From Rosen P, Baker FJ II, Barkin R et al, eds: *Emergency Medicine: concepts and clinical practice,* ed 2, St Louis, 1988, CV Mosby.)

superior surface of the vertebral body or widening of the intervertebral disk space (Fig. 9-83). In distraction-type extension injuries there is loss of integrity between vertebral bodies and a widening of the disk space. The hangman fracture (Fig. 9-84) is typical of this category. Dislocations, as the name implies, result in severe neurologic damage because of the complete loss of attachment that results in movement of the spinal segments (Fig. 9-85). In elderly patients who suffer extension injuries, the spinal cord is damaged by impingement from osteophytes and thickening of the ligamentum flavum (Fig. 9-86). There may be no abnormalities demonstrated on plain radiographs in these cases.

Rotational injuries

Rotational injuries involve a severe blow or fall that twists the upper body while the lower body is fixed. There is usually a flexion component in most cases of these injuries (Fig. 9-87). The radiograph will show significant crushing or grinding of the vertebrae as well as the transverse processes or rib fractures (Fig. 9-88). A typical concentric pattern of bony fragments can be seen on the CT scan.

Shearing injuries

A mechanism involving shearing can be seen in Fig. 9-89. This causes a radiographic finding that has been dubbed "windswept appearance."[20,35] Fig. 9-90 demonstrates the fragmentation that follows the force vector in a shearing injury. These uncommon injuries are usually the result of a severe horizontal blow with lateral flexion.

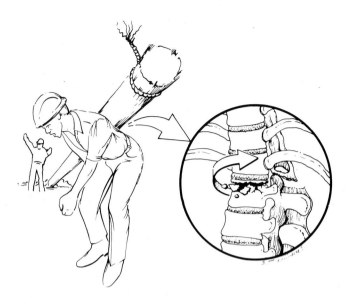

Fig. 9-87. Mechanism of rotary injuries with flexion. (From Daffner RH: *Imaging of vertebral trauma*, Rockville Md, 1988, Aspen Publishers. Reproduced with permission.)

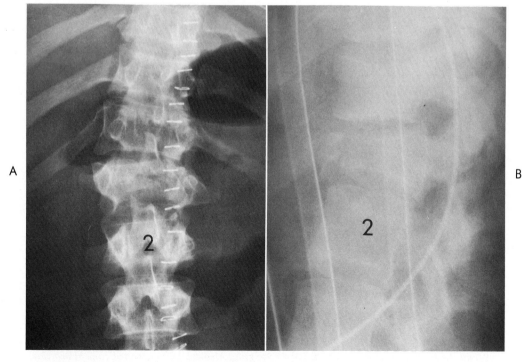

Fig. 9-88. Rotary injury of L1. **A,** AP radiograph shows distortion of the anatomy of L1 by fragmentation and compression. **B,** Lateral radiograph is deceptive because of its similarity to a burst fracture.

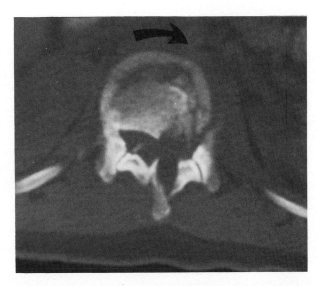

Fig. 9-88, cont'd. C, CT scan shows the rotary arrangement of bone fragments *(arrow).* Compare these findings to those demonstrated in Fig. 9-80, *B*.

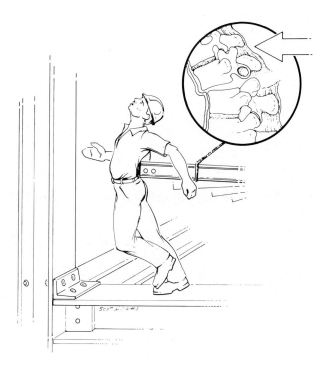

Fig. 9-89. Mechanism of shearing injury. (From Daffner RH: *Imaging of vertebral trauma,* Rockville, Md, 1988, Aspen Publishers. Reproduced with permission.)

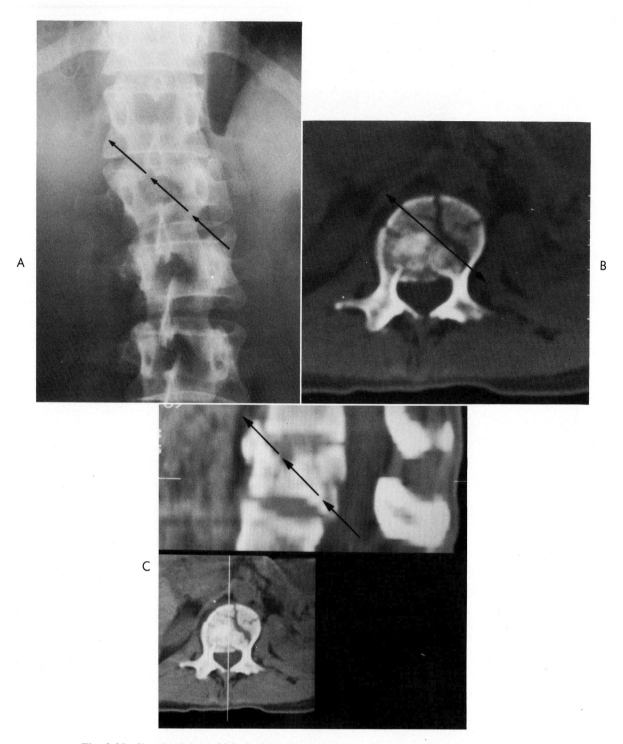

Fig. 9-90. Shearing injury of L2. **A,** AP radiograph shows a "windswept appearance" to L2. The vector of injury is demonstrated *(arrows)*. **B,** CT scan shows the same appearance of the bone fragments of L2 *(double arrow)*. **C,** Sagittal reconstruction of the CT scan also shows the typical "windswept appearance" *(arrows)*.

SUMMARY

A thorough evaluation of the entire vertebral column of the trauma victim is necessary to prevent overlooking a severe injury. Proper immobilization, transfer, and following the ABCs of radiographic assessment of vertebral trauma can assist the clinician in this process. A thorough understanding of the anatomy and mechanisms of injury will alert the trauma team to potential problems.

REFERENCES

1. Chilton J, Dagi TF: Acute cervical spinal cord injury, *Am J Emerg Med* 3(4):340, 1985.
2. Herzenberg JE, Hensinger RN, Dedrick DK et al: Emergency transport and positioning of young children who have an injury of the cervical spine, *J Bone Joint Surg* 71A(1):15, 1989.
3. Williams CF, Bernstein TW, and Jelenko C: Essentiality of the lateral cervical spine radiograph, *Ann Emerg Med* 10(4):198, 1981.
4. Mahoney BD, Ruiz E: Acute resuscitation of the patient with head and spinal cord injuries, *Emerg Med Clin North Am* 1:583, 1983.
5. Reid DC, Henderson R, Saboe L et al: Etiology and clinical course of missed spine fractures, *J Trauma* 27(9):980, 1987.
6. Neifeld GL, Keene JG, Henesy G et al: Cervical injury in head trauma, *J Emerg Med* 6(3):203, 1988.
7. Fischer RP: Cervical radiographic evaluation of alert patients following blunt trauma, *Ann Emerg Med* 13(10):905, 1984.
8. Wales LR, Knopp RK, and Morishima MS: Recommendations for evaluation of the acutely injured cervical spine: a clinical radiologic algorithym, *Ann Emerg Med* 9(8):422, 1980.
9. Gattrell CB: Asymptomatic cervical injuries: a myth? *Am J Emerg Med* 3(3):263, 1985.
10. Bachulis BL, Long WB, Hynes GD et al: Clinical indications for cervical spine radiographs in the traumatized patient, *Am J Surg* 153(5):473, 1987.
11. Bayless P, Ray VG: Incidence of cervical spine injuries in association with blunt head trauma, *Am J Emerg Med* 7(2):139, 1989.
12. McNamara RM, Heine E, and Esposito B: Cervical spine injury and radiography in alert, high risk patients, *J Emerg Med* 8(2):177, 1990.
13. Rigenberg BJ, Fisheer AK, Urdaneta LF et al: Rational ordering of cervical spine radiographs following trauma, *Ann Emerg Med* 17(8):792, 1988.
14. Roberge RJ, Wears RC, Kelly M et al: Selective application of cervical spine radiography in alert victims of blunt trauma: a prospective study, *J Trauma* 28:784, 1988.
15. Maull KI, Sachetello CR: Avoiding a pitfall in resuscitation: the painless cervical fracture, *South Med J* 70(4):477, 1977.
16. Bohlman HH: Acute fractures and dislocations of the cervical spine, *J Bone Joint Surg* 61A(8):1119, 1979.
17. Bresler MJ, Rich GH: Occult cervical spine fracture in an ambulatory patient, *Ann Emerg Med* 11(8):440, 1982.
18. Walter J, Doris PE, and Shaffer MA: Clinical presentation of patients with acute cervical spine injury, *Ann Emerg Med* 13(7):512, 1984.
19. Morales JE: Analysis of cervical spine injury, *Ann Emerg Med* 15(10):1247, 1986.
20. Daffner, RH: Thoracic and lumbar vertebral trauma, *Orthop Clin North Am* 21(3):463, 1990.
21. Berquist TH: *Imaging of orthopedic trauma and surgery*, Philadelphia, 1986, WB Saunders.
22. Calenoff L, Chessare JW, Rogers LF et al: Multiple level spinal injuries: importance of early recognition, *AJR* 130:665, 1978.
23. Gehweiler JA, Osborn RL, and Becker FG: *The radiology of vertebral trauma*, Philadelphia, 1980, WB Saunders.
24. Berquist TH: Imaging of adult cervical spine trauma, *Radiographics* 8(4):667, 1988.
25. Shaffer MA, Doris PE: Limitation of the cross table lateral view in detecting cervical spine injuries: a retrospective analysis, *Ann Emerg Med* 10(10):508, 1981.
26. Streitweiser DR, Knopp R, Wales LR et al: Accuracy of standard radiographic views in detecting cervical spine fracture, *Ann Emerg Med* 12(9):538, 1983.
27. Ross SE, Schwab CW, Eriberto TD et al: Clearing the cervical spine: initial radiologic evaluation, *J Trauma* 27(9):1055, 1987.
28. Doris PE, Wilson RA: The next logical step in the emergency radiographic evaluation of cervical spine trauma: the five view trauma series, *J Emerg Med* 3(5):371, 1985.
29. Karbi OA, Caspari DA, and Tator CH: Extrication, immobilization and radiologic investigation of patients with cervical spine injuries, *CMAJ* 139(10):617, 1988.
30. Djang WT: Radiology of acute spinal trauma, *Crit Care Clin* 3(2):495, 1987.
31. Maravilla KR, Cooper PR, and Sklar FH: The influence of thin section tomography on the treatment of cervical spine injuries, *Radiology* 127:131, 1978.
32. Binet EF, Moro JJ, Marangola JP et al: Cervical spine tomography in trauma, *Spine* 2:163, 1977.
33. Acheson MB, Livingston RR, Richardson ML et al: High-resolution CT scanning in the evaluation of cervical spine fractures: comparison with plain film examinations, *AJR* 148:1179, 1987.
34. Zimmer EA: *Borderlands of the normal and early pathologic in skeletal roentgenology*, New York, 1968, Grune & Stratton.
35. Daffner RH: *Imaging of vertebral trauma*, Rockville, Md, 1988, Aspen Publishers.
36. Young JWR, Resnik CS, DeCandido P et al: The laminar space in the diagnosis of rotational flexion injuries of the cervical spine, *AJR* 152:103, 1989.
37. Daffner RH, Deeb ZL, and Rothfus WE: The posterior vertebral body line: importance in the detection of burst fractures, *AJR* 148:93, 1987.
38. Cattell HS, Filtzer DL: Pseudosubluxation and other normal variations in the cervical spine in children, *J Bone Joint Surg* 17A(7):1295, 1965.
39. Meyer, PG, Hartman JT, and Leo JS: Sentinal spinous process fractures, *Surg Neurol* 18:174, 1982.
40. Nuber GW, Schafer MF: Clay shovelers' injuries: a report of two injuries sustained from football, *Am J Sports Med* 15(2):182, 1987.
41. Kim KS, Chen HH, Russell EJ et al: Flexion teardrop fractures of the cervical spine: radiographic characteristics, *AJR* 152:319, 1989.
42. Lee C, Kim KS, and Rogers LF: Triangular cervical body fractures: diagnostic significance, *AJR* 136:1123, 1982.
43. Scher AT: Unilateral locked facet in cervical spine injuries, *Am J Roentgenol* 129:45, 1977.
44. Shmueli G, Herold ZH: Prevertebral shadow in cervical trauma, *Israel J Med Sci* 16(9-10):698, 1980.
45. Penning L: Prevertebral hematoma in cervical spine injury: incidence and etiologic significance, *AJR* 136:553, 1981.
46. Gopalakrishnan KC, El Masri W: Prevertebral soft tissue shadow widening: an important sign of cervical spine injury, *Injury* 17:125, 1986.
47. Templeton PA, Young JWR, Mirvis Se et al: The value of retropharyngeal soft tissue measurements in trauma of the adult cervical spine, *Skeletal Radiol* 16:98, 1987.
48. Resnick D: *Bone and joint imaging*, Philadelphia, 1989, WB Saunders.
49. Smith WS, Kaufer H: Patterns and mechanisms of lumbar injuries associated with lap seatbelts, *J Bone Joint Surg,* 51A:239, 1969.
50. Chance GQ: Note on a type of flexion fracture of the spine, *Br J Radiol* 21:452, 1948.
51. Harris JH, Edeiken-Monroe B: *The radiology of acute cervical spine trauma*, Baltimore, 1987, Williams & Wilkins.
52. Mace SE: Emergency evaluation of cervical spine injuries: CT versus plain radiographs, *Ann Emerg Med* 14(10):973, 1975.

53. Kaye JJ, Nance EP: Cervical spine trauma, *Orthop Clin North Am* 21(3):449, 1990.

54. Kirshenbaum KJ, Nadimpalli SR, Fantus R et al: Unsuspected upper cervical spine fractures associated with significant head trauma: role of CT, *J Emerg Med* 8(2):183, 1990.

55. Mark LP, Haughton VM: CT Scanning of the spine. In Haaga JR, Alfidi RJ, eds: *Computed tomography of the whole body,* St Louis, 1988, CV Mosby.

56. Haughton VM: MR imaging of the spine, *Radiology* 166:297, 1988.

57. Miller GM, Forbes GS, and Onofrio BM: Magnetic resonance imaging of the spine, *Mayo Clin Proc* 64:986, 1989.

58. Murphey MD, Batnitzky S, and Bramble JM: Diagnostic imaging of spinal trauma, *Radiol Clin North Am* 27(5):855, 1989.

59. Pan G, Kulkarni M, MacDougall DJ et al: Traumatic epidural hematoma of the cervical spine: diagnosis with magnetic resonance imaging, *J Neurosurg* 68:798, 1988.

60. Garza-Mercado R: Traumatic extradural hematoma of the cervical spine, *Neurosurgery* 24(3):410, 1989.

61. Goldberg AL, Rothfus WE, Deeb ZL et al: The impact of magnetic resonance on the diagnostic evaluation of acute cervicothoracic spinal trauma, *Skeletal Radiol* 17:89, 1988.

62. Beers GJ, Raque GH, Wagner GG et al: MR imaging in acute cervical spine trauma, *J Comput Assist Tomogr* 12(5):755, 1988.

63. Quencer RM: The injured spinal cord: evaluation with magnetic resonance imaging and intraoperative sonography, *Radiol Clin North Am* 26(5):1025, 1988.

64. Kulkaeni MV, McArdle CB, Kopanicky D et al: Acute spinal cord injury: MR imaging at 1.5T, *Radiology* 164:837, 1987.

65. Kulkarni MV, Bondurant FJ, Rose SL et al: 1.5 Tesla magnetic resonance imaging of acute spine trauma, *Radiographics* 8(6):1059, 1988.

66. Goldberg AL, Deeb ZL, Rothfus WE et al: Magnetic resonance imaging in evaluation of acute spine trauma, *Spine: State Art Rev* 3(2):339, 1989.

67. Quencer RM, Sheldon JJ, Post MJ et al: Magnetic resonance imaging of the chronically injured cervical spinal cord, *AJNR* 7:457, 1986.

68. Daffner RH, Deeb ZL, and Rothfus WE: "Fingerprints" of vertebral trauma: a unifying concept based on mechanisms, *Skeletal Radiol* 15:518, 1986.

PART THREE

Presenting Complaints

C H A P T E R *10*

Shortness of Breath

Steven M. Barrett
Thomas H. Johnson

Patients presenting in the emergency department with acute dyspnea and shortness of breath or with an acute exacerbation of chronic stable dypsnea generally require radiographic examination. The radiographic findings are occasionally diagnostic, but more often they are suggestive of differential diagnostic considerations. Patients presenting with dyspnea of unknown cause minimally require a chest radiograph; those with stridor, dysphagia, or throat or neck pain may only require a soft tissue cervical radiograph.

CHEST RADIOGRAPHY

The chest radiograph serves as the primary imaging modality in evaluating patients with shortness of breath. A systematic approach to evaluating the study must incorporate specific aspects of anatomy and technical considerations.

Anatomy

Interpretation of radiographs must incorporate a thorough knowledge of pulmonary structures. Normally, the right lung is slightly larger than the left and is divided into three lobes and ten segments. The left lung has two lobes and eight segments (Fig. 10-1). Certain lung disorders, such as pneumonia, atelectasis, and pulmonary embolism, may follow a segmental distribution. Lobes and segments are surrounded by connective tissue sacs that form fissures. The minor or horizontal fissure separates the right upper lobe from the right middle lobe and can frequently be visualized on the posteroanterior (PA) and lateral chest radiographs. The major or oblique fissures travel diagonally in both lungs and are best seen on lateral radiographs. Fissures, blood vessels, and the cross-sectional walls of occasional bronchi are the only radiographically identifiable structures within the normal lung.

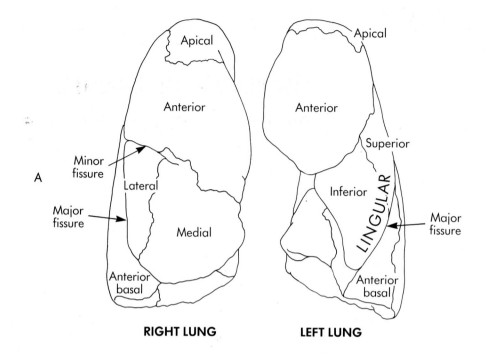

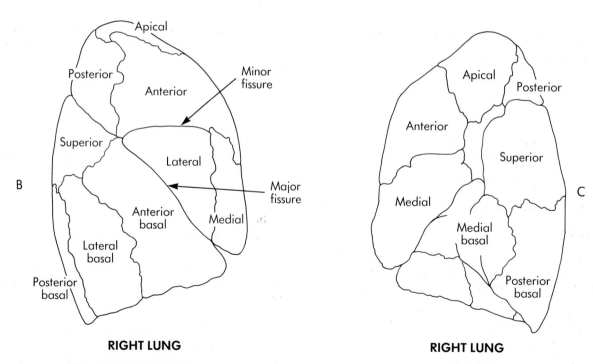

Fig. 10-1. Bronchopulmonary segments. **A,** Anterior view, both lungs. **B,** Lateral view, right lung. **C,** Medial view, right lung.   *Continued.*

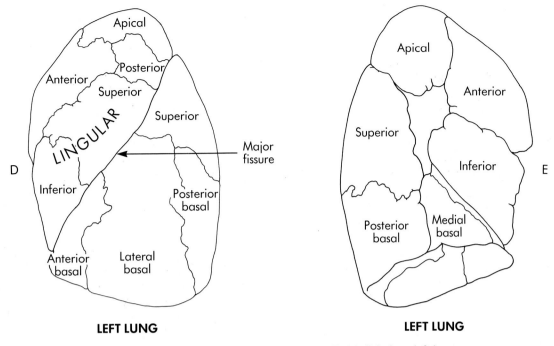

Fig. 10-1, cont'd. D, Lateral view, left lung. **E,** Medial view, left lung.

The "azygous lobe fissure" is a finding that results from incomplete migration of the azygous vein from the chest wall to its usual position within the mediastinum at the right tracheobronchial angle. The invaginated visceral and parietal pleura persist and form the fissure, which contains the azygous vein at its inferior end. However, the normal segmental anatomy of the lung is not changed in patients with an azygous lobe fissure; therefore the term *lobe* is a misnomer.

The mediastinum contains the trachea, esophagus, aorta, central pulmonary arteries and veins, hilar lymph nodes, and the heart. Pleural reflections form the lateral borders of the mediastinum. From birth to 2 years of age, the thymus gland can be visualized on the chest radiograph. It is generally located in the anterior mediastinum and may simulate a pathologically widened or enlarged mediastinum. The normal thymus often has a prominent lobe, frequently on the right side, which appears larger than the contralateral lobe and may resemble a sail (the characteristic "sail shape"). The normal thymus may also simulate cardiomegaly but has characteristic wavy or scalloped borders that represent contour effects caused by the internal portion of the anterior chest wall.[1]

Systematic approach to interpretation

In evaluating the chest radiograph, it is essential to develop a very distinct systematic routine to ensure that all components of the pulmonary, cardiac, soft tissue, and chest wall anatomy are examined.[2] The following components should be assessed:

- Film quality and radiographic technique.

- Neck (for soft tissue asymmetry or swelling, calcifications, and airway abnormalities).
- Trachea and bronchi.
- Shoulders, humeri, clavicles, scapulae, sternum, spine, and ribs (for symmetry, deformities, fractures, dislocations, and lytic or blastic lesions).
- Soft tissues, including breasts (for symmetry, calcifications, masses, and irregularities).
- Subphrenic areas (for free or loculated air, calcifications, and soft tissue or hollow organ abnormalities).
- Diaphragm (for position, contour, and calcifications).
- Pleural surface (for free or loculated effusion, adhesions, calcifications, and pneumothorax).
- Mediastinum and hilar areas (for contour, position, density, and free air).
- Major, minor, or accessory fissures (for position and appearance).
- Lung fields, including apices and regions around the hila and superior mediastinum (for consolidation, interstitial changes, hyperlucency, atelectasis, infiltrates, cavities, nodules, masses, calcifications, and vascular markings).

Technical considerations

The interpretation of the chest radiograph requires some awareness of the technical aspects of imaging.

The upright, standing patient faces the film cassette during the posteroanterior (PA) radiograph exposure of the chest. The x-rays travel through the patient in the posterior-to-anterior direction. If the PA examination is taken with a tube-film distance of greater than or equal to 6 feet, distortion caused by the magnification of structures is reduced.

Anterior structures are positioned farther from the film cassette and therefore may be magnified with the anteroposterior (AP) projection in comparison to the PA chest radiograph. For example, there is an apparent increase in cardiac size on the portable AP chest radiograph of the upright sitting patient.

On the AP radiograph of the supine patient, the mediastinum widens and the transverse diameter of the cardiac shadow increases. Filling and dilatation of upper lobe pulmonary vessels, which are recognized on the upright chest radiograph of the patient with congestive heart failure, can occur in the normal supine patient because gravitational effects on blood flow are applied more evenly. A pleural effusion or hemothorax may be layered posteriorly and be indiscernible or appear as a diffuse unilateral haziness on the supine or semiupright portable AP radiograph. Likewise, a pneumothorax may rise anteriorly and be undetectable.

For interpretability, the PA chest radiograph of the upright, standing patient is preferable over the AP radiograph of the upright, sitting patient, which in turn is preferable over the AP radiograph of the supine patient. However, the patient's condition may preclude optional positioning for the study.

The lateral chest radiograph allows for confirmation of the presence and location of pulmonary and pleural abnormalities and mediastinal masses, provides the best view of the posterior lung bases and retrosternal area, and allows for further evaluation of cardiac size and configuration.

In infants and children, oblique radiographic projections of the chest can aid in the detection of lower lobe densities that otherwise may be obscured by the cardiac shadow on the PA radiograph and by the thoracic spine and ribs on the lateral view.

A PA chest radiograph taken during forced expiration may aid in the detection of a small pneumothorax, but the lung markings and cardiac silhouette will be distorted.

A lateral decubitus chest radiograph is taken with the patient in the side-lying position. This view is useful for evaluation in the dependent side of free pleural fluid (see Fig. 10-51) and air trapping and for pneumothorax, air-fluid levels, and basilar infiltrates hidden behind the diaphragm in the nondependent side. Furthermore, if a pleural effusion obscures the lung, a lateral decubitus view with the abnormal side up permits detection of an otherwise hidden pulmonary infiltrate. The bedfast patient should be positioned on a spine board for these views.

The apical lordotic PA chest radiograph projects the clavicles and anterior first ribs above the lung fields to allow for visualization of subtle apical lesions obscured on the PA view.

If the abdomen of a pregnant patient is well shielded during chest or neck radiography, little or no radiation should reach the fetus. Nevertheless, all radiographs ordered for a pregnant patient should be medically indicated and justifiable, and appropriate shielding must be used.

Technical difficulties

Difficulties in imaging techniques may affect the ability of the radiologist to intepret the radiograph.

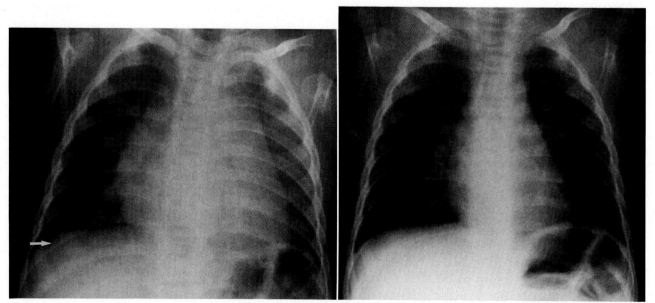

Fig. 10-2. Respiratory changes on chest radiographs. **A,** Expiratory chest radiograph of 11-month-old child appears to show congestive heart failure changes. Ninth rib is indicated *(arrow)*. **B,** Inspiratory chest radiograph taken a few minutes later is within normal limits.

A properly penetrated PA chest radiograph shows a clearly visible trachea, thoracic spine margins visible through the cardiac shadow, and thoracic spinal disk spaces barely visible through the cardiac shadow.[2] An underpenetrated chest radiograph may show undue prominence of vascular and parenchymal markings, which may suggest pulmonary interstitial disease. Abnormalities may be obscured by bone or mediastinal shadows on an underpenetrated view.

Overpenetration, patient motion, or poor patient-film contact may obscure small or poorly defined pulmonary or cardiovascular abnormalities.

On a frontal (PA or AP) chest radiograph with the patient in rotation, lesions may be hidden from view, a normally positioned trachea may appear deviated, and a normal mediastinal contour may be misjudged to be abnormal or widened. On a correctly centered PA or AP radiograph, the medial clavicular surfaces are both approximately the same distance from the midline spinous process.

Maximum patient inspiration during radiographic exposure allows for optimal evaluation of the lung fields, hilar and vascular shadows, mediastinal contour, and heart size. A poor inspiratory effort may cause radiographic misinterpretations (such as cardiomegaly) and basilar parenchymal densities, suggesting atelectasis or pneumonia (Fig. 10-2). The degree of inspiratory effort is deemed adequate if most of the posterior portion of the right ninth rib is visible above the diaphragmatic surface.[3]

On the frontal (PA or AP) chest radiograph, the shadow of a well-developed pectoral muscle mass may produce a hazy density that resembles an infiltrate. Likewise, the breast shadow may cause an ill-defined haziness at either base that suggests an infiltrate. A pneumothorax may be simulated by a skinfold or by the medial scapular border superimposed on the peripheral third of the hemithorax.

Male or female nipple shadows on the PA radiograph may be misinterpreted as metastatic nodules. To confirm that the density is caused by a nipple shadow, the PA radiograph can be repeated after application of a barium marker to the nipple. Healing and healed rib fractures can be mistaken for pulmonary nodules. Costochondral junctions and calcifications may resemble lung densities. The first costochondral junction can be hyperplastic, irregular, and asymmetric, thus simulating pulmonary abnormalities such as carcinoma and tuberculosis.

LOWER AIRWAY AND OTHER THORACIC ABNORMALITIES

A variety of conditions produce dyspnea, either from lower airway or upper airway pathologic conditions (see box at right).

Consolidation

The term *infiltrate* is used by some authorities to indicate any abnormal lung density or shadow and by others as a synonym for consolidation. A consolidation is a localized process that is due to the accumulation of abnormal material within alveolar (air) or interstitial (connective tissue) spaces. The term *consolidation* is preferable to *alveolar* because severe, diffuse interstitial disease can mimic the radiographic findings of alveolar filling and appear as consolidation. This effect is possible because confluent thickening of the interstitium can force air out of intervening alveoli. Consolidation may also result from mixed alveolar filling and interstitial disease. In fact, alveolar filling or collapse can mask interstitial disease.[2] The categorization of diffuse shadowing into alveolar or interstitial compartments is often difficult, and many disorders affect both compartments.

Characteristics of consolidation, which is due primarily to alveolar or air-space filling, include the following:[2]
- Confluence within areas of involvement.
- Indistinct margins, unless the density abuts a peripheral pleural surface or fissure.
- Dense and homogeneous or patchy and nonhomogeneous areas.
- Frequent air bronchograms.

Common causes of shortness of breath (dyspnea)

Lower airway and other thoracic causes

Consolidation
Pneumonia
Congestive heart failure
    Intravascular congestion
    Interstitial edema
    Alveolar pulmonary edema
Noncardiogenic pulmonary edema and adult respiratory distress syndrome
Aspiration
Pulmonary embolism
Fat embolism
Amniotic fluid embolism
Interstitial lung disease
Sarcoidosis
Collagen vascular disease
Hyperlucency and air trapping
Asthma
Chronic obstructive pulmonary disease
Atelectasis
Air-containing sacs and cavities
Nodules and masses
Neoplasms
Pediatric entities
    Bronchiolitis
    Cystic fibrosis

Upper airway causes

Croup
Epiglottitis
Retropharyngeal abscesses
Bacterial tracheitis
Foreign body

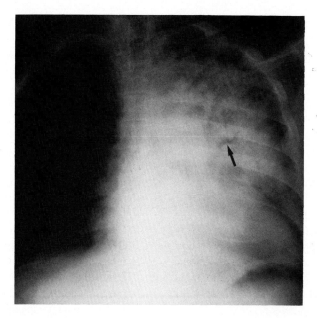

Fig. 10-3. Mixed flora pneumonia (monilia and *Streptococcus pneumoniae*). There are nodular and confluent air-space consolidations throughout the left lung. Air bronchogram is present *(arrow)*.

- Obliteration of "vascular" shadows.
- Presence of the "silhouette sign."

Normal intrapulmonary airways are invisible unless they are positioned end on with respect to the x-ray beam. However, if the airways pass through a zone of increased radio-opacity caused by reduction or replacement of surrounding alveolar air, they become visible as linear, branching radiolucencies. This abnormal visualization of lower airways is called an *air bronchogram* and is a reliable indicator of intrapulmonary pathologic conditions (Fig. 10-3). Consolidation is by far the most common cause of an air bronchogram.[4]

The pattern of consolidation is most often caused by exudate, edema, or hemorrhage and occasionally results from neoplasm or other disorders. A useful mnemonic list of causes of consolidation is "blood, pus, water, protein, or cells".[2] Causes of localized consolidation include the following:[11]

- *Lobar or segmental:* pneumonia and infarction.
- *Patchy:* infection, aspiration, edema, neoplasm, allergic reaction, radiation damage, contusion, vasculitis, and collagen vascular disease.
- *Mass-like:* infection, infarction, neoplasm, hematoma, and radiation damage.
- *Diffuse:* edema, infection, aspiration, hemorrhage, respiratory distress syndrome, neoplasm, allergic reaction, and alveolar proteinosis.

An algorithm is presented to suggest the differential diagnosis of consolidation that appears to be primarily alveolar in nature (Fig. 10-4).

As the weight of the lung/unit volume (density) approaches that of soft tissue, the normally visualized line of demarcation between the heart or diaphragm and the contiguous lung becomes obscured, thus creating the "silhouette sign."[5] A corollary of the "silhouette sign" is a consolidation that lies posterior to the heart if it is superimposed on but does not obscure the heart border.[6] Some examples of the clinical usefulness of the "silhouette sign" and its corollary are discussed in the following paragraphs.

A consolidation in the medial segment of the right middle lobe obliterates the right heart border (Fig. 10-5). Lung tissue in the right costophrenic angle on the PA chest radiograph represents the lateral basilar segment of the lower lobe, which is not involved with a right middle lobe consolidation. On the lateral radiograph, a right middle lobe density appears between the minor and major fissures and is superimposed on the cardiac shadow.

Consolidation of the lateral segment of the right middle lobe silhouettes neither the right heart border nor the right hemidiaphragm.

Consolidation of the lingula of the left upper lobe is characterized by visual loss of the left heart left margin.

A right lower lobe consolidation results in a "silhouette sign" at the right hemidiaphragm but preservation of the right heart border (Fig. 10-6). Right lower lobe consolidation may have a contour that simulates the normal appearance of the diaphragmatic surface on the PA radiograph. The lateral radiograph often demonstrates a well-demarcated major fissure anterosuperior to the lower lobe infiltrate.

Obliteration of the left hemidiaphragm with preservation of the left heart left border indicates a left lower lobe consolidation. Furthermore, the posterior basilar segment of the left lower lobe is involved if the density is superim-

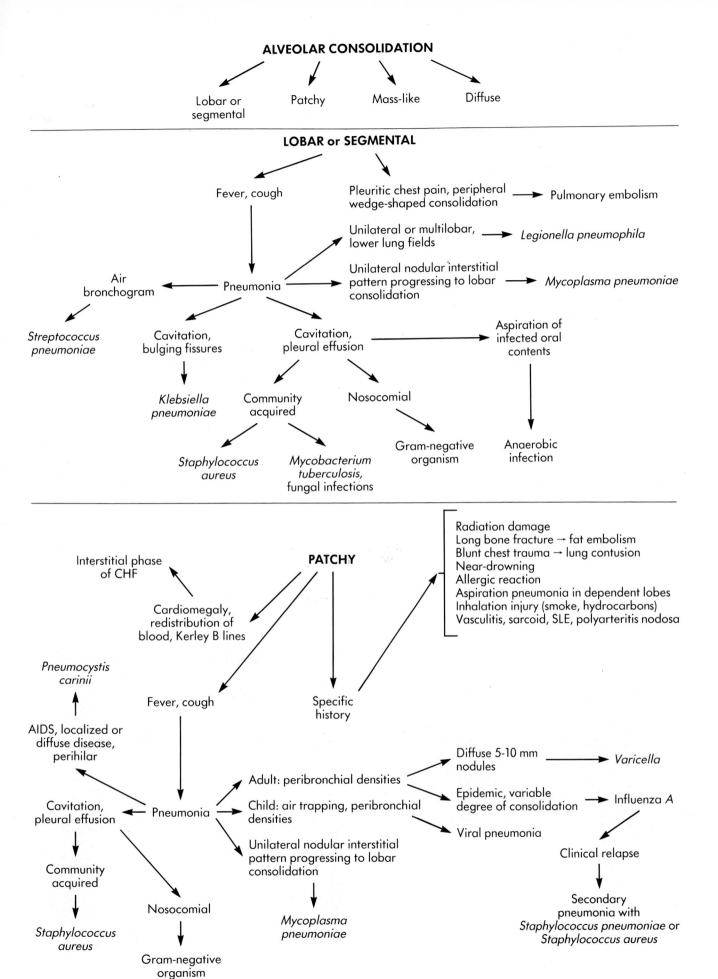

Fig. 10-4. Algorithmic approach to the cause of alveolar consolidation.

Continued.

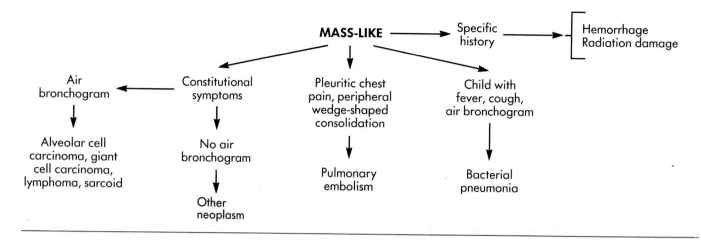

MASS-LIKE → Specific history → [Hemorrhage
Radiation damage]

Air bronchogram ← Constitutional symptoms

Air bronchogram ↓ Alveolar cell carcinoma, giant cell carcinoma, lymphoma, sarcoid

Constitutional symptoms ↓ No air bronchogram ↓ Other neoplasm

Pleuritic chest pain, peripheral wedge-shaped consolidation ↓ Pulmonary embolism

Child with fever, cough, air bronchogram ↓ Bacterial pneumonia

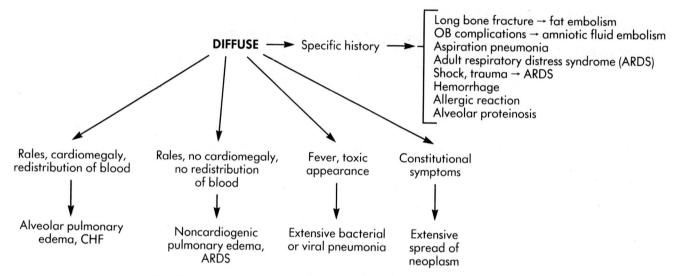

DIFFUSE → Specific history → [Long bone fracture → fat embolism
OB complications → amniotic fluid embolism
Aspiration pneumonia
Adult respiratory distress syndrome (ARDS)
Shock, trauma → ARDS
Hemorrhage
Allergic reaction
Alveolar proteinosis]

Rales, cardiomegaly, redistribution of blood ↓ Alveolar pulmonary edema, CHF

Rales, no cardiomegaly, no redistribution of blood ↓ Noncardiogenic pulmonary edema, ARDS

Fever, toxic appearance ↓ Extensive bacterial or viral pneumonia

Constitutional symptoms ↓ Extensive spread of neoplasm

Fig. 10-4, cont'd. Algorithmic approach to the cause of alveolar consolidation.

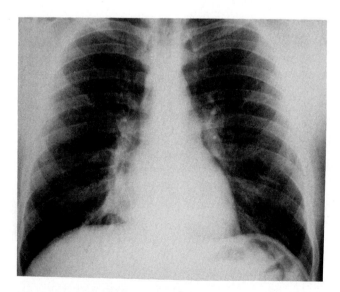

Fig. 10-5. Right middle lobe consolidation. This pneumonia has silhouetted much of the right heart border.

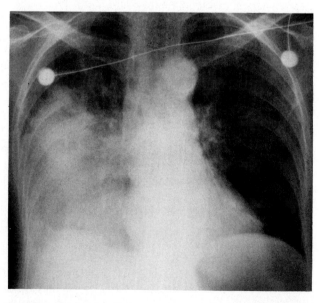

Fig. 10-6. Right lower lobe consolidation. The right heart border is visually preserved, but the lateral margin of the right hemidiaphragm cannot be discerned.

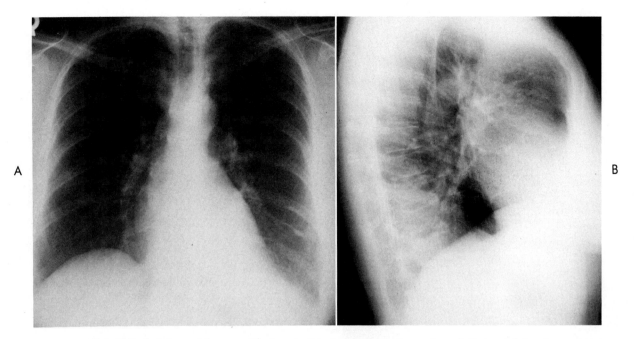

Fig. 10-7. Left lower lobe consolidation. **A,** PA chest radiograph reveals an indistinct left hemi-diaphragm. **B,** On lateral projection, pneumonia is evident posteriorly as a density over the lower thoracic vertebral bodies.

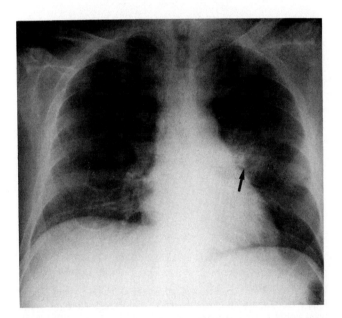

Fig. 10-8. Left lower lobe superior segment consolidation. This density *(arrow)* does not obliterate the left heart border and therefore is located in the lower lobe. (Corollary to the "silhouette sign").

posed on the lower thoracic vertebral bodies on the lateral radiograph (Fig. 10-7).

A left midlung consolidation with preservation of the left heart margin suggests involvement of the superior segment of the lower lobe (Fig. 10-8), which is visualized in a posterior location on the lateral radiograph.

On the lateral radiograph, lower thoracic vertebral bod-

ies should normally have less overlying tissue density and therefore should be darker than the upper thoracic vertebrae. A white density over these lower vertebrae is caused by a consolidation or other abnormality in a lower lobe. This finding is often useful, along with the "silhouette sign" and its corollary, for the localization of consolidation (Fig. 10-7).

On the PA radiograph, the juxtacardiac portion of the right lower lung (right cardiophrenic angle) contains overlapping vessels of the anteriorly placed middle lobe and the posteriorly placed lower lobe. This superimposition of vascular structures may simulate an infiltrate. Furthermore, a pericardial fat pad often occupies the right cardiophrenic angle. However, despite the presence of either of the above causes of increased density, the right cardiac and diaphragmatic margins usually remain visible. A large, sharply defined density in this area may represent a pericardial cyst.

Pneumonia

Lobar pneumonia appears as a homogeneous consolidation, whereas bronchopneumonia is characterized by nonhomogeneous, patchy consolidation (Fig. 10-9). In infants and children, lobar or segmental consolidation and atelectasis are characteristic of bacterial infections. However, bacterial pneumonia occasionally appears spheric in children and may resemble a hilar, pulmonary, or mediastinal mass.[1]

Streptococcus pneumoniae pneumonia (pneumococcal pneumonia) occurs at any age and is the most common community-acquired bacterial pneumonia in young adults

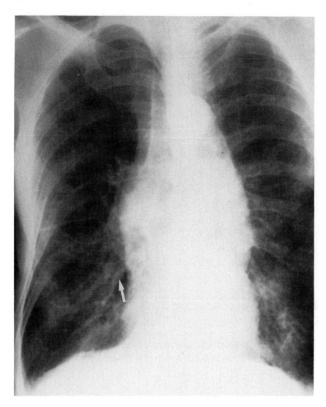

Fig. 10-9. Bronchopneumonia. There are ill-defined, small alveolar consolidations in the mid and lower lungs. Peribronchial thickening is seen in right infrahilar area *(arrow)*. Emphysematous changes are also present.

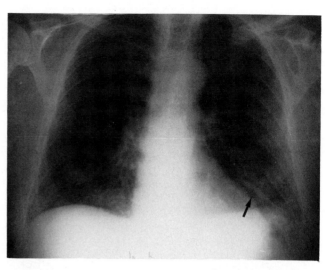

Fig. 10-10. Staphylococcal bronchopneumonia. There are ill-defined areas of alveolar consolidation with round lucencies that may represent pneumatoceles *(arrow)* in the left lower lung. Staphylococcal bronchopneumonia may follow influenza.

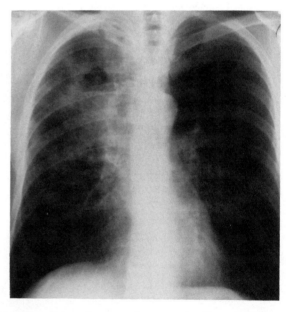

Fig. 10-11. Lung abscess and pneumonia. There is right upper lobe pneumonia with cavitation and a fluid level. Culture results were positive for anaerobes.

It typically presents as a sublobar or lobar consolidation containing an air bronchogram (see Fig. 10-3). On occasion, the density is spheric. Cavitation, effusion, and empyema are unusual, but bulging of fissures may be noted.

Staphylococcus aureus pneumonia occurs in pediatric, geriatric, and debilitated patients and presents initially as a bronchopneumonia that can be bilateral (Fig. 10-10). Air bronchograms are unusual, but volume loss, cavitation, effusion, empyema, and pneumatoceles (especially in children) are common findings. A cavity or pneumatocele may rupture into the pleural space and produce a pneumothorax. Hematogenous dissemination of *S. aureus,* such as in drug addicts, can cause multifocal, nodular, and sometimes cavitary consolidations.[7] A pleural effusion with pneumonia in children who are less than 1 year of age usually indicates *S. aureus* infection. Furthermore, the presence of an abscess within a consolidation, along with a pleural effusion or pneumothorax, is highly suggestive of staphylococcal pneumonia in children.[3]

Gram-negative pneumonias are the most common nosocomial pneumonias. The radiographic patterns can be similar to those caused by *S. aureus* infections in adults. Several gram-negative organisms can induce pneumonias with distinctive characteristics. *Klebsiella pneumoniae* pneumonia can be acquired outside the hospital by middle-aged or elderly men with alcoholism or chronic illness. Radiographically, it can resemble a *Streptococcus pneumoniae* pneumonia and has a predilection for the upper lobes and the right lung. Characteristic features include bulging of fissures, followed by rapid cavitation. *Legionella pneumophila* is a gram-negative organism that can cause a pneumonia typified by a unilateral, peripheral (and occasionally spheric) consolidation of the lower lungs. The infection commonly spreads to other lobes and both lungs and may

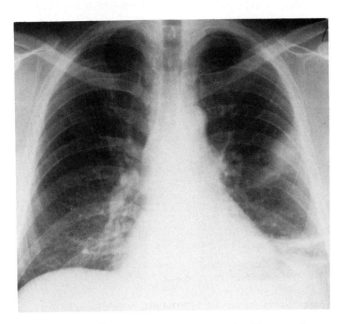

Fig. 10-12. Viral or mycoplasmal pneumonia. Changes of consolidation are present in left midlung, and platelike atelectasis is evident at the left costophrenic angle.

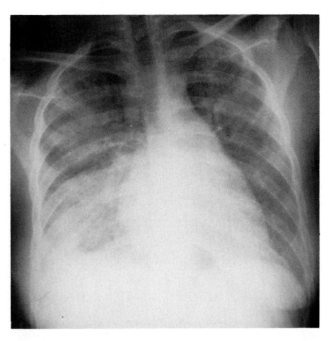

Fig. 10-13. Viral pneumonia. There is extensive homogeneous consolidation throughout the lungs. Patient presented with fever, chills, pleuritic pain, and sputum production.

present as multiple spheric consolidations.[8] In children, whooping cough caused by *Bordetella pertussis* may cause radiographic findings that simulate viral pneumonia patterns.

Anaerobic pneumonias usually result from aspiration of infected oral contents. Consolidation is often cavitary but may be homogeneous. An empyema is a frequent finding, lung abscess can occur, and both may be detected with or without radiographic evidence of an associated pneumonia (Fig. 10-11). Hilar adenopathy often develops if lung abscess is present.[8]

Mycoplasma pneumoniae is the major nonbacterial cause of community-acquired pneumonia in the 20- to 40-year-old age group and is a frequent cause of pneumonia in children over 5 years of age. Radiographic findings are variable, but the most common pattern is a unilateral, patchy, nodular, peribronchial infiltrate in a lower lobe that progresses to a homogeneous sublobar or lobar consolidation (Fig. 10-12). Occasionally, the initial pattern is an interstitial process with linear shadows and small, irregularly shaped, rounded nodules. Progression of this interstitial pattern to a consolidation is very suggestive of a *M. pneumoniae* infection. Pleural effusions may form. Development and resolution tend to occur more slowly than with bacterial pneumonias, and striking radiographic findings may be present, along with relatively minor clinical signs and symptoms.[7]

Viral pneumonia is common in infants and children. Hyperinflation caused by air trapping, bilateral, patchy or streaky infiltrates, and peribronchial thickening typify viral

disease in children. For example, diffusely scattered, streaky densities representing atelectasis may appear, interspersed with focal areas of obstructive hyperinflation. Another common pattern is represented by peribronchial infiltrates, which extend from the hila and are often prominent as a result of lymphadenopathy. However, on occasion, the only radiographic abnormalities in viral pneumonia may be a small pleural effusion and Kerley B lines.[3]

Influenza A is the most common cause of viral pneumonia in adults. Consolidation ranges from minor and evanescent to extensive (Fig. 10-13). In the latter case a significant mortality risk exists, especially in debilitated or pregnant patients. Clinical relapse, occurring about 1 to 2 weeks after the onset of the influenza illness, suggests a secondary bacterial pneumonia, often caused by *Streptococcus pneumoniae* or *Staphylococcus aureus*.

Varicella causes pneumonia more frequently in adults than in children. This illness can be serious, with a significant mortality risk, particularly during pregnancy. Radiographically, 5- to 10-mm nodules occur diffusely and may regress or become confluent. These nodules usually resolve within a week but can persist for months and may calcify.[7] Severe pneumonia in children, especially those caused by viruses such as varicella or influenza in the immunosuppressed patient, may progress to a diffuse pulmonary opacification that is indistinguishable from pulmonary edema.

A *Pneumocystis carinii* infection in the patient with acquired immunodeficiency syndrome can cause localized

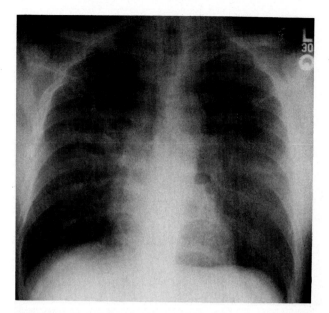

Fig. 10-14. *Pneumocystis carinii* pneumonia in an immunosuppressed 37-year-old patient with AIDS. There is a characteristic perihilar reticular and granular pattern early in the process, which may progress to extensive consolidation.

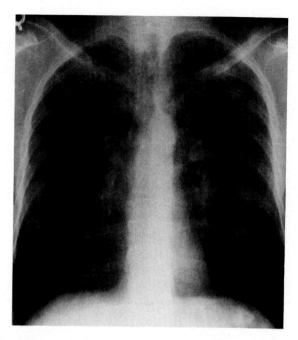

Fig. 10-15. Tuberculosis. Upper lung and apical fibronodular consolidation is typical of tuberculosis. Other granulomatous diseases, such as fungal infection, can also develop this appearance.

disease, but more commonly the infection spreads to a bilateral, ill-defined, mixed alveolar and interstitial perihilar infiltration pattern (Fig. 10-14). The radiographic appearance may simulate pulmonary edema; both lungs may become involved, with some sparing of the periphery, and pneumothorax can develop.[9] Infection with *Mycobacterium tuberculosis* classically causes apical lung densities (Fig. 10-15) with cavity formation, but it may assume any appearance.

Incomplete resolution of a pneumonia with appropriate therapy should suggest a co-existing problem (e.g., bronchial obstruction from neoplasm or a foreign body) or an alternative diagnosis (e.g., alveolar cell carcinoma). Some pneumonias disappear gradually; however, if a pneumonia has not resolved on radiographic examination within 6 weeks, evaluation for a concomitant disorder is indicated. Recurrent pneumonia may indicate underlying disorders such as altered immunity, cystic fibrosis in children, or an anatomic abnormality such as bronchiectasis.

Radiation therapy for chest malignancy can induce an acute pneumonitis with dry cough and dyspnea, which develops soon or up to 6 or more months after treatment. Radiographically, a patchy or homogeneous density appears, which may have linear borders that match the radiation ports or, in some cases, may extend beyond the area of radiation. Radiographic changes may be apparent before symptoms begin. The lung injury may resolve or progress to diffuse interstitial fibrosis.[10]

Congestive heart failure

A frequently used method to determine heart size is to compare the maximum cardiac diameter to the thoracic diameter (C:T ratio). The largest transverse diameter of the

heart is measured horizontally from the apex to the right heart border. The widest thoracic diameter is measured horizontally from the inner rib margins. A C:T ratio of greater than 0.5 (50%) supports the diagnosis of cardiomegaly. However, the body habitus and degree of inspiration by the patient may distort the baseline measurements. Furthermore, serial C:T ratios over time are valid as comparisons only if the inspiratory volume of the chest radiographs is consistent. Values between 0.45 and 0.55 and small changes in the ratio are not diagnostic. For example, small differences in the C:T ratio are often caused by exposure of comparison radiographs during different times of the cardiac cycle. In fact, the cardiac diameter may change 2 cm between systole and diastole. The diagnosis of cardiomegaly therefore should be confirmed with other evidence, such as the cardiac contour on the chest radiograph and findings from physical examination, electrocardiogram, or ultrasonography.[2]

In left ventricular enlargement, the apex of the heart is pointed downward to the left and the ascending aorta may appear enlarged on the frontal (PA or AP) radiograph. Furthermore, the left heart border frequently extends posteroinferiorly on the lateral radiograph. In right ventricular enlargement, rounding and elevation of the apex of the heart and enlargement of the pulmonary arteries on the frontal (PA or AP) radiograph are suggestive findings. Furthermore, the right heart border extends anterosuperiorly (retrosternally) into the lower half of the anterior clear space on the lateral radiograph.

Left atrial enlargement often causes a double-density

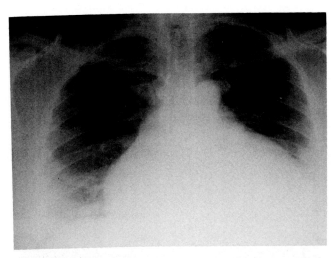

Fig. 10-16. Pericardial effusion. There is enlargement of the cardiopericardial silhouette. The shape is equal bilaterally and resembles a "water bottle." Hila are partially submerged. Occasionally, cardiomyopathy can give a similar appearance, except that the hila remain visible.

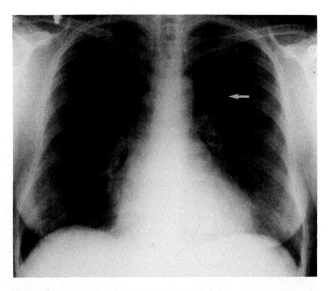

Fig. 10-17. "Cephalization" or redistribution of blood flow to the upper lungs. There is an increase in the caliber of the upper lung-zone vessels *(arrow)* as a first sign of congestive heart failure. This represents early pulmonary venous hypertension and stage I left ventricular failure.

Stages of left ventricular failure

Stage I: Intravascular congestion
Stage II: Interstitial edema
Stage III: Alveolar pulmonary edema

---

visible through the right side of the heart and may eventually displace the left main bronchus superiorly on the frontal (PA or AP) radiograph.

Impingement of the barium-filled esophagus by the atrium on lateral and oblique radiographs provides evidence of left atrial enlargement. A convexity at the junction of the middle and upper thirds of the left heart border on a frontal (PA or AP) radiograph often indicates an enlarged left atrial appendage, which is a characteristic finding in rheumatic heart disease. Right atrial enlargement is difficult to differentiate from right ventricular enlargement, although prominence of the superior right heart border may be present on the frontal (PA or AP) radiograph with right atrial enlargement. An enlarged cardiac shadow can also represent chronic pericardial effusion (Fig. 10-16).

Enlargement (greater than 10 mm in diameter) or increasing size of the azygous vein on serial frontal (PA or AP) radiographs may be caused by congestive heart failure (CHF) (especially right heart failure), cardiac tamponade, constrictive pericarditis, portal hypertension, or obstruction of the great veins with increased collateral blood flow through the azygous system.[2] The azygous vein travels cephalad, adjacent to the esophagus, and then arches anteriorly to join the superior vena cava. The anterior portion of this arch is often visualized to the right of the trachea just superior to the origin of the right main bronchus.

Radiographic evidence of CHF may precede clinical symptoms, especially in inactive individuals. Findings in the early stages of CHF may be difficult to interpret because changes in the pulmonary vasculature and interstitial markings may be influenced by radiographic techniques and patient-induced factors, such as inadequate inspiratory effort, obesity, and chronic obstructive pulmonary disease.

Right heart failure and cor pulmonale may cause pleural effusions and enlargement of the azygous vein and supe-

rior vena cava. Corroborative evidence includes enlargement of the right ventricle and pulmonary arteries; in addition, the patient often has a diffuse lung condition, such as chronic obstructive pulmonary disease.

Most episodes of CHF are left ventricular or biventricular in origin. At least three stages of left ventricular failure (LVF) exist (see box above). Progression through the first two stages to pulmonary edema may be rapid.

Stage I: intravascular congestion. In the normal, upright individual, most of the blood flow through the pulmonary arteries and veins is to the lower lung fields because of gravity. In early left ventricular failure, pulmonary venous pressure increases and upper lobe vessels become dilated on the upright chest radiograph. In addition, more of these cephalad vessels fill because of an increase in blood flow to the upper regions. Basal pulmonary emboli and basal emphysema also can cause redistribution of blood flow to the upper zones.[8] Cephalad blood flow redistribution occurs in the normal supine patient because the gravitational forces are applied more evenly throughout the posterior lung fields. Therefore it is important to compare radiographs of the same technique (i.e., supine or upright) over time if changes are to be reliably interpreted. Finally, fluid will leak into the lung interstitium centrally around the hilar structures during stage I. Therefore radiographic findings in stage I LVF (Fig. 10-17) include dilatation of

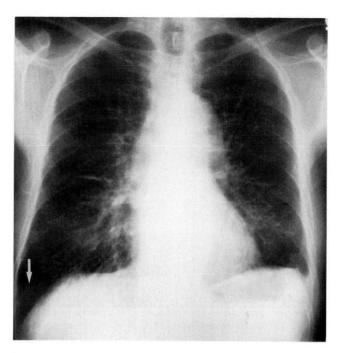

Fig. 10-18. Kerley B lines as a sign of stage II left ventricular failure. Short horizontal lines in the lower lung zones in the region of the costophrenic angles *(arrow)* are a common sign of interstitial edema and can also be due to conditions other than left ventricular failure, such as viral pneumonia or mitral valve disease.

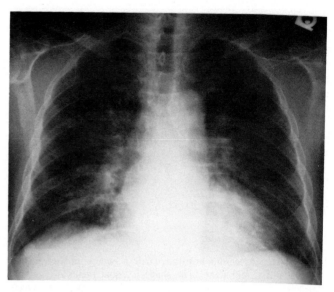

Fig. 10-19. Interstitial pulmonary edema. There is an increase in pulmonary vascularity with indistinct edges of the vessels and of the perihilar regions. This represents stage II left ventricular failure (compare with Figs. 10-17 and 10-18). Mild cardiomegaly is present.

upper lobe vessels to a size equal to or greater than the diameter of lower lobe vessels (compared vessels should be equidistant from the hilum), a hazy loss of definition of hilar and perihilar structures, and some loss of definition of lower lung-field vessels (especially behind the heart) caused by perivascular edema. The patient is often minimally symptomatic at this stage (e.g., easy fatigability) and physical examination of the chest generally reveals no signs of CHF.

Stage II: interstitial edema. In this stage, the intravascular hydrostatic pressure exceeds the ability of the vessels to retain the increased fluid load, so fluid leaks into the pulmonary interstitium. Interstitial edema causes thickening of interstitial tissue and is manifested radiographically by a reticular pattern and septal (Kerley) lines.

A reticular pattern is defined as fine, branching lines that follow many directions, including directions not possible for normal bronchi and vessels. Kerley B lines are dilated interlobular septa. In CHF, these septa are made visible by the exudation of fluid from the interlobular septal lymphatic channels into the perilymphatic spaces. Kerley B lines abut the pleura and extend medially into the lung for several millimeters. They are characteristically visible as horizontal, parallel, short (less than 2 cm), thin lines in the costophrenic angles (Fig. 10-18).

Kerley A lines also represent dilated interlobular septa (from distended or infiltrated lymphatic channels), but they

extend from the periphery to the hilum. Kerley A lines are difficult to differentiate from vessels and are never present without Kerley B lines or reticulations (also called Kerley C lines).[2]

The radiographic findings in stage II LVF include Kerley B lines (often with Kerley A lines), loss of definition of lower lung-field vessels and perihilar structures (Fig. 10-19), peribronchial cuffing that represents accumulation of interstitial fluid in the areas adjacent to the bronchi, irregular reticulations (Kerley C lines), small indistinct nodules that represent patchy areas of alveolar edema (especially in the lower lung fields), and, often, manifestations of right heart failure such as pleural effusions, fluid in the fissures, an enlarged and dilated azygous vein, and widening of the upper mediastinum caused by venous distention.

Stage III: alveolar pulmonary edema. In this most severe phase of left ventricular failure, the intravascular and interstitial fluid pressures exceed the intra-alveolar air pressure, and fluid flows into the alveoli. The radiographic findings in stage III LVF include consolidation (alveolar infiltrate in the perihilar regions ["butterfly" or "batwing" pattern]) or in the bibasilar areas or a diffuse distribution in severe cases (Fig. 10-20) with air bronchograms, loss of definition of vessels in all lung fields, septal lines and reticulations in those areas not involved with the consolidation (Fig. 10-21), thickened fissures, and unilateral or bilateral pleural effusions.[2] The consolidation pattern is not necessarily symmetric between lungs.

The "butterfly" or "batwing" pattern of alveolar pulmonary edema (Fig. 10-22) in the central perihilar regions also occurs in patients in renal failure who are overhy-

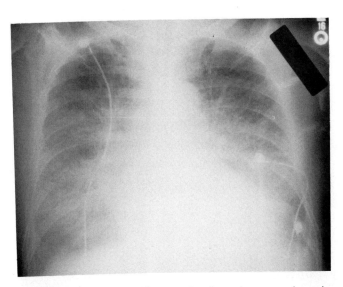

Fig. 10-20. Air-space filling or alveolar pulmonary edema in stage III left ventricular failure. There is total "white out" of structures, with indistinct outlines of all pulmonary vasculature. Moderate cardiomegaly is present.

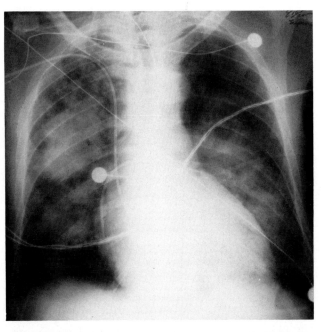

Fig. 10-22. "Butterfly" or "batwing" pulmonary edema. This is a specific manifestation of pulmonary edema, affecting the central but sparing the peripheral lung.

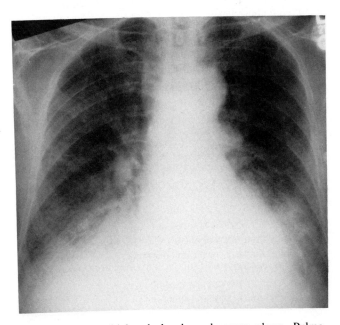

Fig. 10-21. Interstitial and alveolar pulmonary edema. Pulmonary vessels are indistinct, and reticulations are present as result of interstitial edema. There is a consolidation of alveolar pulmonary edema in the lower lung zones. These findings represent stages II and III left ventricular failure.

drated. Central perihilar pulmonary edema may be difficult to detect by physical examination. Pulmonary edema may also present with an unusual appearance (atypical pulmonary edema) because of structural defects in the lungs. For example, radiographic findings of CHF in a patient with emphysema may be most recognizable in the lung areas with the least amount of emphysematous damage. For this reason, pulmonary edema in a patient with emphy-

sema can assume a patchy distribution that simulates pneumonia.[11]

When an isolated pleural effusion develops in a patient with CHF, it is usually right-sided. When pleural effusions are bilateral, the larger effusion is also often on the right side. LVF may infrequently produce pleural effusions in the absence of radiographic findings of alveolar pulmonary edema.[3] Cardiomegaly may not be present in patients with acute LVF (e.g., following myocardial infarction or a ruptured papillary muscle). If a patient with pulmonary edema lies on one side for prolonged periods, the dependent side will accumulate more edema than the nondependent side.

Noncardiogenic pulmonary edema and adult respiratory distress syndrome

Many disparate noxious conditions and insults can damage the alveolar epithelium, the capillary walls, or both, causing increased permeability of the alveolar-capillary membrane and noncardiogenic pulmonary edema (NCPE) (see box on p. 288). The pulmonary parenchymal changes are similar to those in CHF, except that cephalad redistribution of blood flow in the upright patient, cardiomegaly, and pleural effusions do not develop. Narcotic drugs can cause NCPE after intravenous or oral use. Radiographic evidence of pulmonary edema appears several hours after drug administration (Fig. 10-23).

Inhalation of irritant gases and fumes (e.g., sulfur dioxide, ammonia, chlorine) may directly injure bronchial mucosa and alveoli, and NCPE typically appears within 4 to 24 hours after exposure. The risk of NCPE seems highest after inhalation of less soluble gases (e.g., nitrogen oxide,

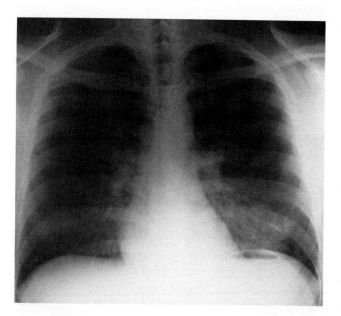

Fig. 10-23. Noncardiogenic pulmonary edema. There are indistinct pulmonary vessels with interstitial and early alveolar pulmonary edema. The heart is not enlarged. This case was due to drug overdose.

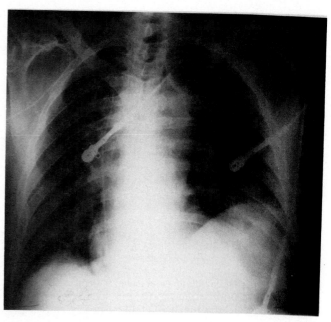

Fig. 10-24. Smoke inhalation pulmonary edema. Patient had second- and third-degree skin burns as well as smoke inhalation. Pulmonary interstitial edema and indistinct vascular changes did not develop immediately.

Major causes of noncardiogenic pulmonary edema

Narcotics use and overdose
Salicylate intoxication
Smoke inhalation
Toxic gas inhalation
Aspiration of noxious substances
Near-drowning
High-altitude pulmonary edema
Neurogenic pulmonary edema
Rapid lung re-expansion
Drug reactions
Poisonous snakebite
Diffuse bacterial or viral pneumonia
Transfusion reactions
Disseminated intravascular coagulation
Radiation pneumonitis
Severe hypoalbuminemia
Uremia
Shock lung
Cardiopulmonary bypass (pump lung)

Major causes of adult respiratory distress syndrome

Shock
Blunt trauma
Major burns
Sepsis
Severe bacterial or viral pneumonia
Fluid overload
Smoke inhalation
Near-drowning
Aspiration of noxious substances
Pulmonary thromboembolism
Fat, amniotic fluid, or air embolism
Acute pancreatitis
Disseminated intravascular coagulation
Cardiopulmonary bypass (pump lung)

---

phosgene) and metal fumes. Smoke inhalation may induce focal atelectasis, consolidation, or irregular patchy infiltrates 24 to 36 hours after injury. Furthermore, NCPE can develop soon after severe exposure or up to 96 hours after smoke inhalation (Fig. 10-24). However, in patients with inhalation injury, significant hypoxemia and carboxyhemoglobinemia can be present, despite an innocuous-appearing radiograph.[8] Rapid re-expansion of a collapsed lung after drainage of a large pleural effusion or pneumothorax may cause a unilateral NCPE. Both increased capillary permeability and a rapid rise in negative intrapleural pressure may be responsible for this form of NCPE.[12] It is most likely to occur if the lung has been collapsed for a number of days.

Adult respiratory distress syndrome (ARDS) is a severe form of NCPE that results from diffuse alveolar injury caused by a wide variety of insults (see box above). Certain types of lung injury characteristically progress from NCPE to ARDS. Damage to the alveolar epithelium, capillaries, or both causes a capillary leak, which, along with

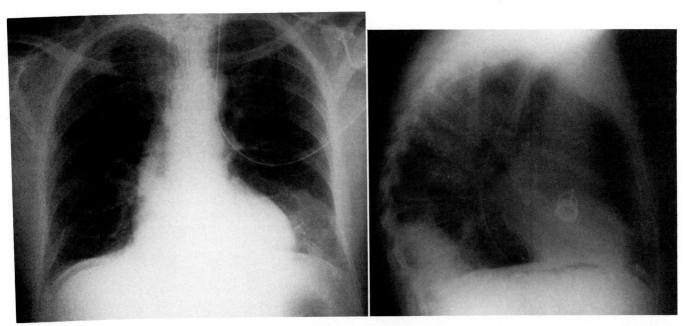

A   B

Fig. 10-25. "Hampton hump" pulmonary infarction. PA **(A)** and lateral **(B)** chest radiographs reveal a well-circumscribed consolidation in the left lower lobe. On lateral projection, the consolidation appears to be a truncated cone, projecting towards the hilum ("Hampton hump"). Free intraperitoneal air is also visible under both hemidiaphragms.

impairment of surfactant activity, leads to edema, atelectasis, an inflammatory reaction, and hyaline membrane formation (from denatured plasma proteins). Radiographically, an interstitial edema pattern is followed by a patchy, then confluent, alveolar edema with diffuse volume loss that occurs hours to days after the insult. A ground-glass pattern with homogeneous, smooth opacities and scattered lucencies often appears and is more distinctive than nonspecific consolidation. Clinical correlation and measurement of pulmonary capillary wedge pressure may help distinguish pulmonary edema caused by CHF from that caused by ARDS because the radiographic appearance of the two disorders can be similar.[2] Clinical symptoms and hypoxemia occasionally may be present before radiographic abnormalities are identified.

Aspiration

For a discussion of the lung response to aspiration, see Chapter 11.

Pulmonary embolism

The most common symptoms of pulmonary embolism (PE) are dyspnea, chest pain (usually pleuritic), apprehension, and cough. A concurrent or previous condition that predisposes the patient to PE or deep venous thrombosis may exist. These conditions include estrogen use, heart disease, cancer, obesity, previous PE or deep venous thrombosis, trauma, pelvic and lower extremity fractures, immobilization, pregnancy, hereditary clotting disorders, and the patient's post-operative status.

Fewer than 40% of patients with angiographically documented acute PE have a normal chest radiograph. Many of the remaining patients have one or more nonspecific findings, including patchy consolidations, pleural effusion, elevation of a hemidiaphragm, linear atelectasis, or signs of pulmonary artery hypertension or even cor pulmonale. Signs of lung-volume loss (such as hemidiaphragm elevation and linear atelectasis) may be related to pleural pain and resulting hypoventilation or to the effects of ischemia such as bronchoconstriction or surfactant loss. Nevertheless, the patient with a PE can have a completely normal chest radiograph. However, PE is strongly suggested by certain specific findings:

- A dense, peripheral wedge-shaped consolidation, especially if it is based on a pleural surface. These densities represent pulmonary infarctions or areas of focal hemorrhage. If the medial surface is convex to the heart, the finding is referred to as a "Hampton hump" (Fig. 10-25).
- An enlarged, amputated, or "pruned" major hilar pulmonary artery: this vessel appears to end abruptly and to have no branches continuing beyond it.[13]
- One or more segmental or regional areas of decreased vascularity not due to bullae, emphysema, or pulmonary hypertension; this finding of pulmonary oligemia is called "Westermark sign" and is often difficult to visualize.

If PE is suspected, a technetium 99m–labelled macroaggregated albumin or albumin microsphere perfusion (Q) scan should be performed (Fig. 10-26). A low probability

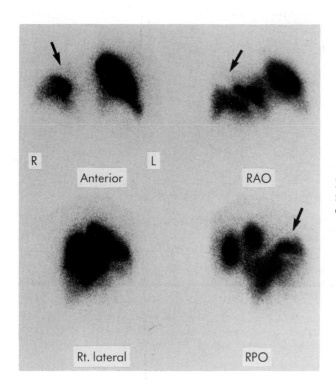

Fig. 10-26. Pulmonary embolism on perfusion (Q) scan. Radionuclide scan demonstrates decreased uptake *(arrows)*, indicating diminished blood flow to the right upper lobe caused by embolus.

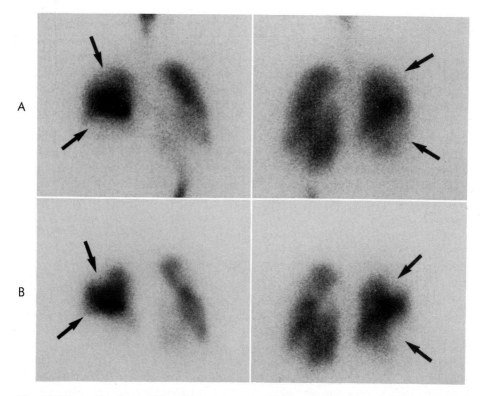

Fig. 10-27. A, Ventilation (V) scan, anterior and posterior views shows normal areas *(arrows)* that correspond with defects in the right lung on the perfusion (Q) scan. **B,** Perfusion (Q) scan, anterior and posterior views shows perfusion defects *(arrows)* in the right lung. Findings of such mismatched V/Q defects indicate a high probability of pulmonary embolism.

perfusion (Q) scan usually indicates that the patient does not have a clinically significant PE, and the workup for PE can be terminated. Perfusion defects can occur with disorders other than PE, such as acute or chronic obstructive pulmonary disease, pneumonia, atelectasis, pulmonary edema, and vasculitis. In fact, vasculitis can be associated with an abnormal Q scan and a normal chest radiograph. Therefore a Q scan that is abnormal only in areas of co-existing chest radiographic abnormalities is a nondiagnostic result that will not be resolved by a ventilation (V) scan (technetium 99m aerosol or xenon-133 gas). However, a Q scan that is abnormal in areas that are normal on the chest radiograph should be followed by a V scan.

When technetium and xenon are present within the lungs, radioactivity from both substances can be detected by the gamma camera. Therefore the most technically sound V scans are obtained either before the Q scan or several hours after the Q scan to allow for radioactive decay of the technetium. However, a normal Q scan obviates the need for a V scan; thus routine initial performance of a V scan results in a number of unnecessary ventilation studies. Furthermore, the Q scan results can determine the optimal projection for the xenon-133 ventilation study. Thus in some centers the V scan is performed immediately after the Q scan with the understanding that interpretation accuracy may be compromised to some extent. Other institutions prefer that the V scan be done initially and be followed immediately by a Q scan.

If the findings from the V scan are abnormal (revealing areas of inflow obstruction or air trapping) in areas corresponding to the Q-scan abnormalities (matched V/Q defects), then PE is unlikely. However, if the V scan is normal in areas that are abnormal on the Q scan (mismatched V/Q defects) (Fig. 10-27), the presence of a PE should be suspected. Although very small mismatched areas are non-specific, the presence of two or more segmental or larger mismatched defects indicates a high probability that PE has occurred (particularly when the chest radiograph is normal). The clinical likelihood of PE should be considered along with the V/Q scan results to estimate the clinical probability (low, intermediate, or high) that the diagnosis of PE is correct. A low probability V/Q scan is associated with a 10% to 15% incidence of PE. However, if PE is clinically likely, significant risk factors are present, and the scan is interpreted as "high probability," then the likelihood of PE exceeds 90%. The results of the chest radiograph and V/Q scan may be nondiagnostic (i.e., of a low or intermediate probability), especially in patients with CHF or chronic obstructive pulmonary disease. The decision to begin anticoagulant or more aggressive thrombolytic therapy must then be based on clinical criteria, noninvasive vascular studies of the lower extremities, or pulmonary angiography. If performed correctly, pulmonary angiography is a highly sensitive and specific test for PE (Fig. 10-28). Disadvantages of the procedure include expense, patient discomfort, and potential morbidity and

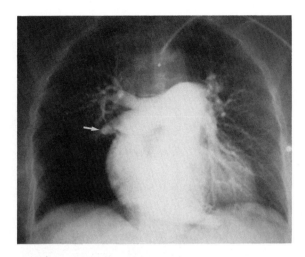

Fig. 10-28. Pulmonary angiogram revealing no contrast material circulating into the right lower lobe, confirming a right lower lobe embolus *(arrow)*.

mortality as a result of the required pulmonary artery catheterization.[2] Other potentially useful diagnostic tests, such as a contrast-enhanced CT scan of the thorax, magnetic resonance imaging, and digital subtraction angiography, have not been clinically validated at this time for general use in the diagnosis of PE.

Fat embolism

The syndrome of fat embolism appears 12 to 48 hours after a long bone fracture, especially fracture of the femur or tibia, and is almost invariably associated with respiratory distress. Widespread embolic fat droplets from bone marrow enter the venous circulation and ultimately lodge or deposit in the pulmonary parenchyma. Central nervous system dysfunction is present, and petechiae (especially over the anterior neck, shoulders, and chest) occur in at least half of the patients who have clinically evident disease. The radiographic findings of fat embolism are generally delayed until 24 to 48 hours after the trauma.[14] Patchy densities or the more diffuse alveolar edema (Fig. 10-29) of adult respiratory distress syndrome may appear.[6]

Amniotic fluid embolism

Amniotic fluid embolism (AFE) is an uncommon but potentially fatal obstetric emergency. The patient presents with respiratory distress followed by cyanosis, seizures, and cardiovascular collapse. AFE should be considered in a patient with the preceding symptoms who has experienced a difficult or prolonged labor, intrauterine fetal death, or operative delivery. In 50% of patients who survive the initial cardiovascular crisis, a life-threatening coagulopathy will develop. Pulmonary vascular obstruction from particulate matter in the amniotic fluid and possibly from fibrin formed intravascularly may lead to acute cor pulmonale.[15] Should the patient survive the acute episode with aggres-

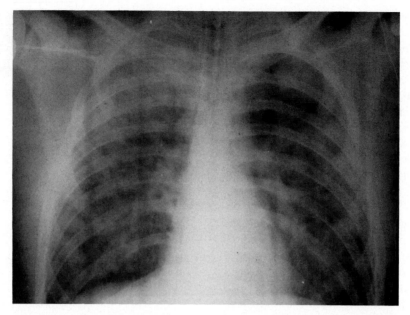

Fig. 10-29. Traumatic fat emboli. This patient sustained a fractured femur in a motor vehicle accident. Three days later, a chest radiograph demonstrated extensive irregular, ill-defined, nodular alveolar consolidations.

sive pulmonary and cardiovascular support, a diffuse pattern of patchy consolidation will often be evident on chest radiography. If aspiration of gastric contents has not occurred in these patients, the chest radiographic findings are most likely due to amniotic fluid embolism.[16,17]

Interstitial lung disease

The most typical radiographic signs of interstitial lung disease (abnormal thickening of pulmonary interstitium) are the reticular pattern (fine lines overlapping to form a meshwork pattern) and septal Kerley lines. Kerley B lines are sometimes the only sign of mild, diffuse interstitial thickening. Radiographic patterns of interstitial disease without reticulations or septal lines include amorphous scattered densities, small irregular shadows, small round nodules, vascular attenuation, and ground-glass shadowing. The term *ground-glass appearance* describes a generalized haziness of the lungs, as if a light veil had been drawn across the radiograph. Reticulations can co-exist with nodules to form a reticulonodular pattern. Mild interstitial thickening may be difficult to diagnose because normal blood vessels can be mistaken for a nodular or reticular pattern of disease. Severe interstitial thickening may cause the collapse of intervening air spaces, resulting in large, poorly marginated densities with air bronchograms; this presentation simulates alveolar consolidation.[2]

The most common cause of acute interstitial thickening is edema, especially CHF (see Figs. 10-18 and 10-19). Other causes of acute interstitial disease include infections (usually viral, mycoplasmal, or fungal) and drug or allergic reactions. Lymphangitic spread of carcinoma is an im-

portant cause of interstitial disease and may resemble edema. Interstitial disease is typically diffuse but may be asymmetric or localized. Chronic basilar disease is often caused by asbestosis, scleroderma, or rheumatoid disease. Plaquelike calcifications of both hemidiaphragms are pathognomonic for asbestosis. Upper lobe reticulonodular patterns are frequently caused by pneumoconiosis or eosinophilic granuloma. Interstitial diseases almost never have a distribution in specific bronchopulmonary segments, which, instead, is characteristic of atelectasis and consolidative diseases such as pneumonia.[2]

The most common cause of a chronic interstitial pattern is pulmonary fibrosis, which is idiopathic or can be induced by any disease that diffusely damages the lung. Other causes of a chronic interstitial pattern include residual changes of sarcoidosis, neoplasm, eosinophilic granuloma, pneumoconiosis, collagen vascular disease (especially rheumatoid disease and diffuse scleroderma), hemosiderosis, bronchiectasis, and bronchiolitis obliterans. The term *honeycomb lung* should be reserved to describe an end-stage scarring process and can be recognized by irregular interstitial thickening and cystic spaces that extend far into the lung periphery. If a typical reticular or honeycomb pattern is not in evidence, then the pattern should be termed *indeterminate* so that diffuse alveolar processes are not excluded.

A significant abnormality of the pulmonary interstitium may be present without radiographic findings. Evaluation of arterial blood gases sometimes allows for the detection of a diffusion abnormality caused by interstitial disease before radiographic signs appear.[2]

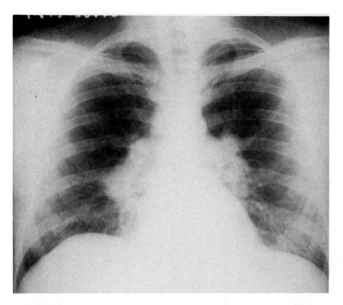

Fig. 10-30. Sarcoidosis. There is lobulated hilar lymph node enlargement. Patient is usually asymptomatic at this stage.

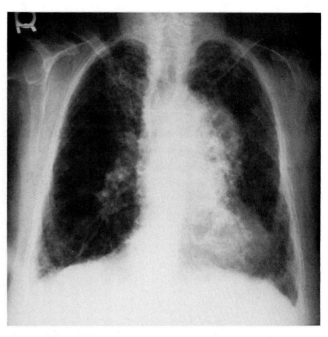

Fig. 10-31. Disseminated sarcoidosis. Sarcoid may progress to end-stage fibrosis in the lungs, with or without adenopathy. This radiograph demonstrates a reticular pattern of fibrosis and mediastinal adenopathy.

Sarcoidosis

Sarcoidosis is a multisystem granulomatous disorder that may represent a nonspecific, immunologically determined host response to one or more inhaled agents. Young adults, especially black women, are common victims. The lung interstitium and mediastinal nodes are the most commonly affected areas of the body. A characteristic radiographic finding is bilaterally symmetric, lobulated hilar enlargement caused by lymphadenopathy (Fig. 10-30). This pattern commonly presents without parenchymal lung disease. The enlarged hila "stick out" from the mediastinum and often have well-defined inferomedial borders. Another finding is small, diffuse, bilaterally symmetric parenchymal nodularity. Occasionally homogeneous cloudy opacities with ill-defined edges resembling consolidations are present. The chest radiograph often appears to display a far worse disease state than the patient's symptoms indicate; this incongruity represents a clue to the diagnosis. Severe involvement may produce consolidation with fluffy densities and air bronchograms. Pleural effusions and nodal compression of surrounding structures are uncommon.[18] The parenchymal abnormalities may progress to pulmonary fibrosis (Fig. 10-31).

Collagen vascular disease

The collagen vascular diseases have an autoimmune basis and present with major pulmonary involvement.

Systemic lupus erythematosus (SLE) is characterized by inflammatory changes in connective tissue, vessels, and serosal surfaces. The lungs and pleura are involved more often in SLE than in any other collagen vascular disease. The most common radiographic abnormality in SLE is pleural effusion, which is frequently bilateral, small in volume, and often associated with pleuritic chest pain. Pulmonary consolidation may result from secondary infection, pulmonary edema (caused by cardiac failure or renal disease), or lupus pneumonitis (caused by an acute vasculitis, hemorrhage, and a mononuclear infiltrate). Lung cavitation, pericardial effusion, diaphragmatic dysfunction, and diffuse interstitial fibrosis are other complications of SLE.

On chest radiographs, a frequent manifestation of rheumatoid arthritis is pleural effusion, which is often associated with subcutaneous nodules. Rheumatoid lung disease can also present with pulmonary nodules, which may cavitate and accompany pulmonary fibrosis and pleural changes. Diffuse interstitial disease can occur and may progress to pulmonary fibrosis.[9]

Progressive systemic sclerosis (diffuse scleroderma) can be associated with diffuse interstitial disease and pulmonary fibrosis. An extraskeletal manifestation of ankylosing spondylitis is upper lobe fibrosis with upward retraction of the hila and often with bullous or cavity formation and apical pleural thickening. Common radiographic manifestations of Sjögren syndrome are pleural effusions and diffuse bilateral reticulonodular shadowing. Furthermore, inspissated secretions in Sjögren syndrome can lead to secondary pneumonias or areas of segmental atelectasis. In patients with polymyositis or progressive systemic sclerosis, aspiration pneumonitis can occur because of dysfunction of pharyngeal or esophageal muscles.

Asthma is the most common presenting pulmonary

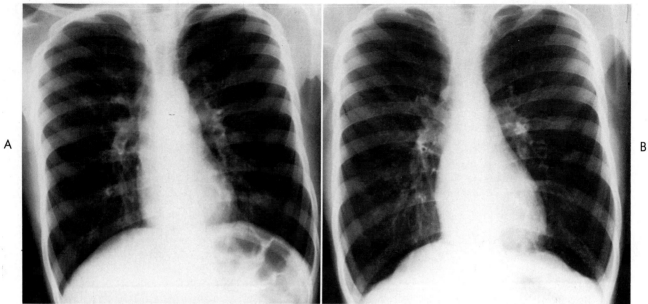

Fig. 10-32. Asthma. **A,** Chest radiograph of an 11-year-old child during a "normal" period. **B,** Chest radiograph during an asthma attack in the same patient. There is generalized hyperlucency caused by air trapping and hyperinflation. Diaphragms are depressed. Thickened bronchial walls are seen in the right lower lung and are usually a sign of repeated bouts of infection.

symptom in patients with allergic granulomatosis, a disorder closely related to polyarteritis nodosa. Furthermore, pulmonary consolidations (some caused by hemorrhage) may occur, and pulmonary edema can develop as a result of cardiac or renal failure. Finally, allergic granulomatosis may be associated with pulmonary nodules, which may cavitate. Wegener granulomatosis almost always involves the lung, with typical nodular granulomas that may cavitate. Furthermore, pleural effusions and alveolar densities representing pulmonary hemorrhage may develop in these patients.[9]

Hyperlucency and air trapping

Air trapping is one of the causes of lung hyperlucency (see box at right) and indicates an obstructive cause of hyperinflation. Air trapping can be detected by assessment of mediastinal and diaphragmatic movement on an inspiratory and expiratory pair of PA chest radiographs. On the expiratory radiographs, the mediastinum and diaphragm move away from the affected lung because the normal lung expels a greater amount of air during expiration.

Relative to the size of the trachea and bronchi, the peripheral airways are narrower in children who are under 5 years of age. Thus inflammatory edema, mucus, and debris may have significant obstructive effects on the airways. In addition, collateral air pathways are not as well developed in children. For these reasons, radiographic evidence of air trapping and atelectasis frequently accompanies pulmonary infections in children. In fact, opacities in children who have had few respiratory infections are more likely to represent atelectasis than consolidation.[1]

Causes of hyperlucency in the lungs[11]

Air trapping
    Ball-valve mechanism in a major bronchus
        Foreign body
        Intrinsic or extrinsic neoplasm
        Enlarged lymph nodes
        Broncholith
        Mucosal thickening (granulomatous disease, amyloid)
    Asthma
    Bronchitis
    Cystic fibrosis
    Emphysema
    Small airway inflammatory disease (bronchiolitis obliterans)
    Congenital lobar emphysema
Decreased vascularity
    Parenchymal or airway disease (emphysema)
    Pulmonary embolism
    Pulmonary arterial hypertension
    Neoplasm (primary or metastatic) involving pulmonary arteries
    Congenital cardiovascular or bronchial anomalies
Bullae, blebs, and pneumatoceles
Pneumothorax
Compensatory emphysema caused by volume loss in adjacent areas
Soft tissue asymmetry
    Mastectomy
    Poland syndrome (unilateral congenital absence of pectoral muscles)

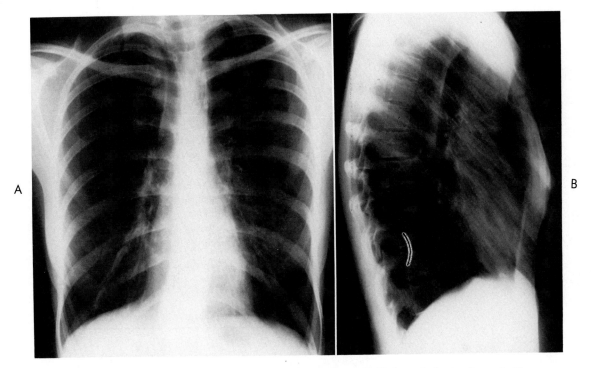

Fig. 10-33. Chronic recurrent asthma. **A,** PA chest radiograph. **B,** Lateral chest radiograph. Patient was not having an acute attack at the time the radiographs were taken; however, there was wheezing on auscultation. Radiographs reveal hyperinflation. There is fibrosis (centrally) in the lower lungs.

Asthma

In patients with asthma, a chest radiograph is ordered when clinically indicated to detect complications associated with the disorder and to recognize other causes of wheezing. A chest radiograph should not be obtained routinely, but it is useful in an acute asthma attack accompanied by fever, when a patient fails to respond to therapy in a quiet chest, or with findings of a pneumothorax or pneumomediastinum (i.e., unilateral decreased breath sounds or subcutaneous emphysema). The radiographic abnormality in acute asthma is diffuse bilateral pulmonary hyperlucency caused by air trapping. Spasm of the alveolar ducts and small bronchioles acts as a ball-valve obstruction to the effluence of air during expiration and thus leads to air trapping. The lungs become diffusely distended, the intercostal spaces may bulge, the diaphragms are depressed (Fig. 10-32), and the ribs may appear more horizontal (especially in infants). Diaphragmatic depression, a reliable indicator of hyperinflation, is often best appreciated on the lateral radiographic view.

Lobar or sublobar atelectasis caused by mucous plugs or pneumonia may also be present in acute asthma. Finally, asthma attacks can also precipitate pneumomediastinum or pneumothorax. In an acute asthma episode, pneumomediastinum is usually of no particular clinical significance.

When the acute episode has subsided, evidence of air trapping is no longer identifiable on the chest radiograph.

If bronchiolar spasm persists or is recurrent, muscular hypertrophy develops in the bronchial walls, which leads to continual air trapping, disruption of alveoli, and radiographic evidence of chronic obstructive pulmonary disease (Fig. 10-33).[3]

Chronic obstructive pulmonary disease

The radiographic diagnosis of chronic obstructive pulmonary disease (COPD; chronic bronchitis, emphysema, and asthma) is possible in only one half of the patients who have significant disease. Chronic bronchitis and emphysema are often present concurrently, although each can occur independently. Chronic bronchitis is diagnosed in patients who have coughed up sputum on most days for periods of at least 3 months during the last two consecutive years in the absence of other possible causes, such as tuberculosis or bronchiectasis. Uncomplicated chronic bronchitis without emphysema produces no specific abnormalities on plain chest radiographs.

Emphysema is defined as an abnormal increase in the size of air spaces distal to the terminal bronchioles that is caused by dilatation or destruction of air-space walls. The classic radiographic manifestations of advanced emphysema are diffuse air trapping and lung hyperinflation, decreased pulmonary vascularity, and bullae (Fig. 10-34). An increase in total lung volume is associated with a low, flat configuration of the hemidiaphragms, vertical elongation of the cardiac silhouette, an increased anteroposterior

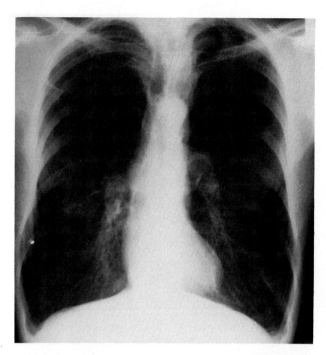

Fig. 10-34. Emphysema. There is upper lung hyperlucency (with compression of the more normal lung) and vascularity downward.

Causes of atelectasis

Total lung, lobar, or segmental

  Foreign body
  Neoplasm
  Mucous plugs
  Secretions
  Misplaced endotracheal tube
  Enlarged lymph nodes
  Endobronchial blood clots
  Broncholith
  Parenchymal scarring
  Pneumothorax
  Pleural effusion
  Bronchiectasis

Subsegmental (discoid, platelike)

  Pulmonary embolism
  Secretions
  Splinting during respirations (chest or abdominal pain)

---

diameter of the chest, and increased depth of the retrosternal and retrocardiac spaces. Portions of the lungs may herniate behind and in front of the heart (Fig. 10-35). On the lateral radiograph, the retrosternal space is measured from the back of the sternum to the anterior aspect of the proximal ascending aorta and normally is less than 4 cm.[19]

Bullae and areas of decreased vascularity (especially in the peripheral lung fields) are reliable indicators of severe parenchymal destruction caused by emphysema. Bullae and blebs have sharp, thin, often lobulated margins and are hyperlucent because parenchymal and vascular markings are absent within the air-filled sacs (Fig. 10-36). Although bullae and blebs may be present in patients who do not have generalized obstructive lung disease, multiple bullae are usually associated with advanced emphysema.[2] On the expiratory chest radiograph, the area with blebs remains hyperlucent relative to the rest of the lung because the diseased lung portion that contains blebs cannot expel the air within its walls. Large bullae can cause respiratory compromise.

In advanced emphysema, peripheral pulmonary vessels are attenuated in size and number. Furthermore, emphysematous bullae cause an abnormal spreading and a distorted, irregular pattern of the lung vasculature. The hilar vessels are larger than normal and taper abruptly because the normal smooth gradation in vessel size from the central hilum to the periphery is lost.[19] Widespread vascular damage in COPD can lead to pulmonary hypertension. In contrast to emphysema, pulmonary vascularity is not significantly decreased radiographically in chronic bronchitis.

When emphysematous changes predominate radio-

graphically in the lower lung fields, especially in a young person, α-1-antitrypsin deficiency disease should be considered in the differential diagnosis (Fig. 10-37). Congenital lobar emphysema can present as a life-threatening problem during the first year of life. It is more common in males than in females and usually involves the right upper lobe or right lower lobe. Air retention occurs following expirations as a result of the inability of the involved lobe to deflate. Symptoms include cough, tachypnea, respiratory distress, and cyanosis. Radiographic signs include marked hyperinflation of the abnormal lobe, compression of the adjacent lobes, depression of the ipsilateral hemidiaphragm, displacement of the mediastinum to the side opposite the involved lobe, and (on the lateral radiograph) herniation of the hyperinflated lobe into the retrosternal space. Definitive therapy is surgical resection of the abnormal lobe.[3]

Atelectasis

Atelectasis is the collapse or volume loss of an entire lung, lobe, segment, or subsegment (see box above). When an entire lung is collapsed, the diaphragm and mediastinum are displaced towards the involved lung unless either or both of these structures is fixed in position. A mediastinal shift is recognized by a change in the position of the tracheal air column, the aortic arch, the right heart border, and a nasogastric tube on the frontal (PA or AP) radiograph (Fig. 10-38).

With lobar atelectasis, the shift of the mediastinum and diaphragm is less marked than with collapse of the entire lung. However, characteristic displacement of fissures, hilar vessels, and persistent lung markers (such as granulomas or scars) occurs. For example, atelectasis of the left upper lobe or the right middle lobe causes anterosuperior displacement of the respective major fissure noted on the

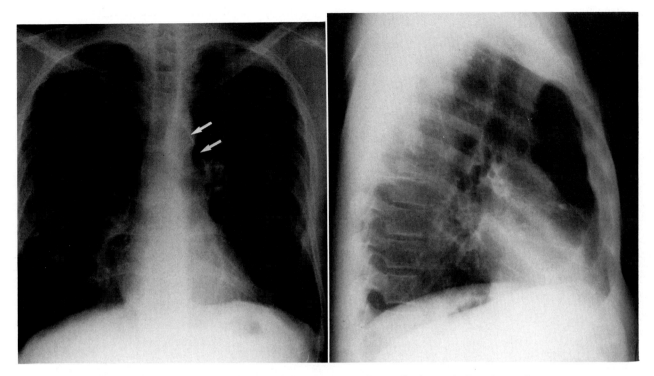

Fig. 10-35. Emphysema with lobe bulging across anterior mediastinum. **A,** PA chest radiograph shows emphysematous hyperlucency in the upper lungs. Anterior mediastinal line bulges to the left *(arrows)* because of lateral herniation of lung tissue. **B,** Lateral radiograph reveals an increased AP diameter; the anterior clear space is enlarged and hyperlucent.

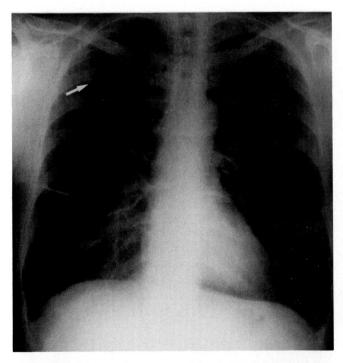

Fig. 10-36. Bullous emphysema. Radiograph demonstrates numerous curved lines in the parenchyma *(arrow)*, representing compressed tissue outlining air-filled spaces that do not participate in respiration.

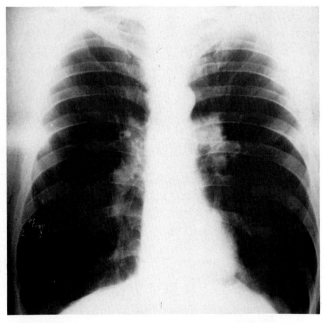

Fig. 10-37. α-1-antitrypsin deficiency emphysema. Disease occurs in younger individuals in their thirties and forties. Radiograph demonstrates hyperinflation in the lower lungs.

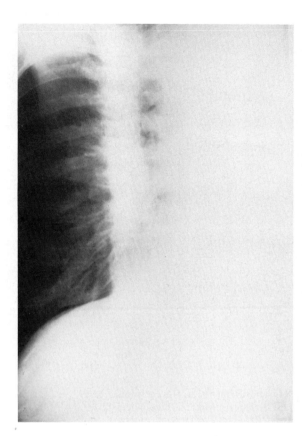

Fig. 10-38. Left lung atelectasis. Radiograph demonstrates complete opacification and collapse of the left lung with mediastinal shift to the left. This represents left main bronchus obstruction if left pneumonectomy has been excluded by history.

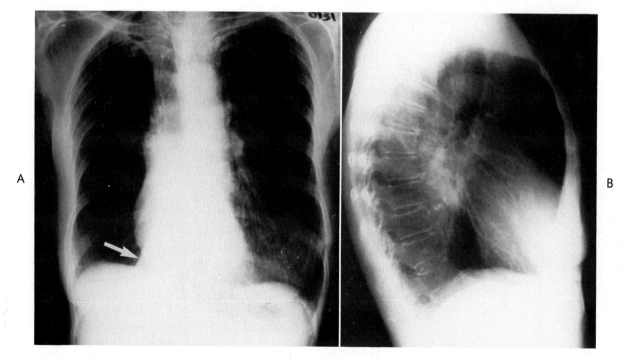

Fig. 10-39. Right lower lobe atelectasis. **A,** PA chest radiograph reveals what appears to be triangular widening of the right lower mediastinum *(arrow)*. **B,** Lateral chest radiograph reveals posterior density silhouetting and obscuring the posterior right diaphragm.

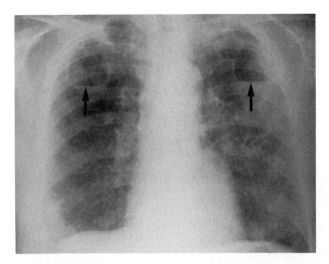

Fig. 10-40. Tuberculosis with cavities. Bilateral upper lung fibronodular changes are present. Thin-walled cavities are typical of tuberculosis. However, cavities with fluid levels *(arrows)* are unusual and often indicate superinfection, bleeding, or fluid from some other cause, such as congestive heart failure. Other granulomatous diseases such as a fungal infection may also manifest with thin-walled cavities.

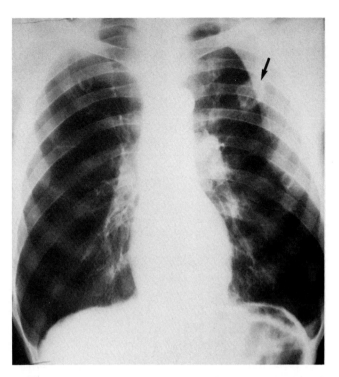

Fig. 10-41. Pulmonary cavitation from infection. There are cavities with irregular walls in the left upper lung *(arrow)*. These lesions can represent hematogenous spread of infection, although the upper lung location is somewhat unusual for hematogenous dissemination. *Pseudomonas aeruginosa* was found by culture.

lateral chest radiograph (see Fig. 10-45, *B*). As with lobar or segmental consolidation, the location of lobar atelectasis can often be ascertained by the presence of the "silhouette sign" with loss of definition of the heart border and hemidiaphragms. For instance, an atelectatic lower lobe projects through the heart border as a sharp, oblique, homogeneous density (Fig. 10-39), which is especially prominent on overpenetrated PA and oblique radiographs. Displacement of a major fissure inferoposteriorly on the lateral radiograph confirms the diagnosis of lower lobe atelectasis. Furthermore, visualization of a major fissure on a frontal radiograph often indicates lower lobe collapse.

Subsegmental atelectasis may appear as a linear plate-like or discoid density. Even small areas of atelectasis can cause increased shunt fractions and hypoxemia. When atelectasis is caused by multiple peripheral mucous plugs, the radiographic pattern may resemble consolidation rather than volume loss.[20]

Air-containing sacs and cavities

Bullae, blebs, and *cysts* are terms for thin-walled, air-containing sacs in the lung. If these structures become infected, the wall of the sac usually becomes thicker, and air-fluid levels may appear. Thin-walled, air-containing sacs may be caused by congenital conditions, emphysema, previous infection, or dilated, destroyed airways (e.g., as a result of cystic bronchiectasis).

The term *cavity* implies the destruction of the pulmonary parenchyma with necrosis and discharge of material into the bronchi. If an air-fluid level is present, the cavitary nature of the sac is supported. Common causes of cavities include infection, neoplasm, infarction, vasculitis,

and collagen vascular disease. Cavities caused by malignant disease tend to have nodular and irregular inner walls, although the outer walls may be sharply or poorly defined. Benign and inflammatory cavities usually have smooth inner walls (Fig. 10-40). In addition, the thicker the wall of the cavity (especially if the cavity diameter is greater than 2 cm), the greater the probability of malignancy. The exception to that rule is the cavity that has developed very rapidly over a few days, which is usually traumatic or infectious in origin (Fig. 10-41). A pneumatocele is a cystic space that may develop after lung injury, for example, in staphylococcal pneumonia in the young patient. Pneumatoceles usually resolve with therapy after several weeks.

Nodules and masses

Unless a lung lesion has detectable calcification or is stable in size for at least 2 years, biopsy and pathologic tissue diagnosis is usually necessary because the mass may be malignant. Any calcification is evidence of nonmalignancy although, rarely, calcification will be present adjacent to a neoplasm. Furthermore, metastases from osteogenic sarcoma or chondrosarcoma may occasionally exhibit calcification.[21] A central ("bull's eye") calcification or symmetric lamellar calcification strongly suggests the diagnosis of a benign granuloma.

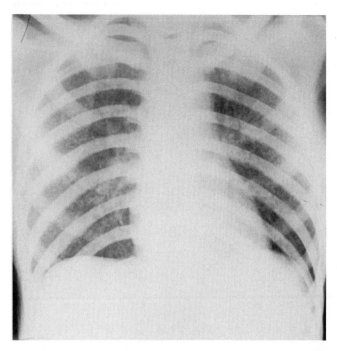

Fig. 10-42. Miliary tuberculosis. Hematogenous spread of tuberculosis is one of the more common causes of the miliary pattern. The pattern of uniform tiny nodules is called *miliary*, because it resembles seeds of the grain, millet.

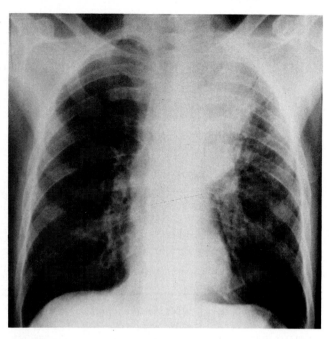

Fig. 10-44. Left upper lobe malignancy. There is a mass in the left upper hemithorax, silhouetting the mediastinum. Inflammatory disease rarely may present with this appearance.

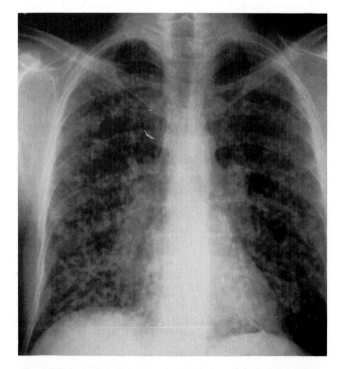

Fig. 10-43. Histoplasmosis. There are multiple parenchymal nodules resulting from inhalation of *Histoplasma capsulatum*, frequently found around bird droppings.

Common causes of diffuse, tiny (1 to 2 mm) nodules (miliary nodules) include granulomatous infection (such as the miliary pattern of tuberculosis or fungal infection), sarcoidosis, neoplasm, eosinophilic granuloma, and silicosis. These tiny, uniform, well-demarcated nodules nearly always represent nodular thickening of the pulmonary interstitium (Fig. 10-42). In general, multiple nonneoplastic granulomatous nodules tend to be of the same size (Fig. 10-43), whereas metastases are often of differing sizes. Multiple scattered nodules (0.5 to 3.0 cm in diameter) may be caused by neoplasm (especially metastasis), sarcoidosis, granulomatous infection, infarctions, silicosis, rheumatoid disease, vasculitis, septic emboli, and arteriovenous malformations. Large, ill-defined, fluffy, and unevenly distributed nodules generally have the same causes as alveolar consolidations.

Any of the causes of nodular lesions discussed previously may also present as a solitary nodule or mass. Most solitary nodules are due to primary or metastatic neoplasm, granuloma (tuberculous or fungal), hamartoma, abscess, or infarction. Less common causes include pneumonia, pulmonary sequestration, varices, and arteriovenous malformation.[2] If an isolated pulmonary nodule increases its diameter by 25% (doubles its volume) in less than 4 weeks or slowly over more than 2 years, it is most likely not malignant. Furthermore, lack of growth over a 2-year period usually excludes the diagnosis of malignancy. In general, malignant lesions double their volume in 1 to 6 months.[4]

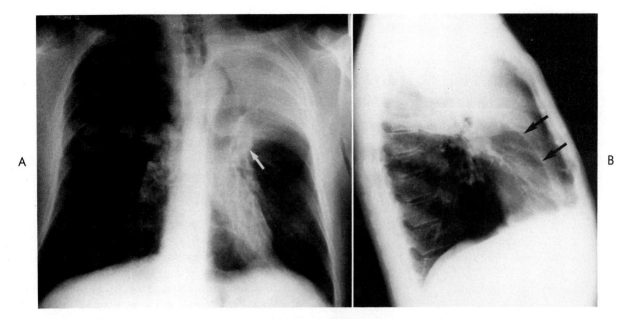

Fig. 10-45. Tumor with bronchial obstruction. PA **(A)** and lateral **(B)** chest radiographs reveal a left hilar mass obstructing the left upper lobe bronchus *(small arrow)* with left upper lobe and lingular atelectasis. PA radiograph reveals an increased density in the left upper hemithorax with partial silhouette loss of the left heart border. Lateral radiograph demonstrates anterior densities of left upper lobe and lingular atelectasis with anterior displacement of the left major fissure *(large arrows)*.

Neoplasm

Lung cancer is the most common malignancy (after skin cancer) in the United States. It is also the most common cause of death from cancer in men and (since 1985) in women. The best available data suggest that early diagnosis increases survival. Because initial symptoms of lung cancer are usually mild and nonspecific, the chest radiograph often provides the first major clue that lung cancer is present. The following radiographic findings may be detected individually or in combination in patients with lung cancer:[2]

- Mass (Fig. 10-44) or nodule.
- Enlarged, deformed, dense hilum or mediastinum.
- Segmental, lobar (Fig. 10-45), or total lung atelectasis.
- Segmental or lobar consolidation, particularly one that does not resolve or resolves incompletely.
- A persistent growing area of consolidation, which often represents alveolar cell cancer.
- A cavity, especially one with a thick, irregular, nodular wall.
- A poorly defined parenchymal density, particularly in the lung apex.
- Bone destruction, which can be due to metastatic disease or direct invasion of the chest wall.
- Septal lines, which can represent tumor spread or venous or lymphatic obstruction.
- Pleural effusion, which most often is due to tumor involvement of the pleura but may be caused by inflammatory disease or venous or lymphatic obstruction.

- A narrowed trachea or bronchus.
- An elevated hemidiaphragm, which may represent atelectasis or phrenic nerve paralysis.
- Hyperinflation of a lobe or segment caused by a ball-valve mechanism of an endobronchial tumor.
- Hyperlucency of a segment, lobe, or lung resulting from oligemia.
- Bronchocele, which is a collection of mucous secretions in a dilated bronchus distal to a neoplastic obstruction.
- Dilatation of the superior vena cava or azygous vein caused by mediastinal tumor spread.

Lung carcinoma can closely resemble pneumonia (Fig. 10-46), but air bronchograms do not occur except in alveolar cell carcinoma, giant cell carcinoma, or lymphoma of the lung. Incomplete resolution of atelectasis or consolidation with appropriate treatment should suggest that a neoplastic process is present. Therefore the patient with pneumonia should undergo serial radiographic studies until complete clearing occurs.

The edge of a peripheral malignant neoplasm is usually lobulated, notched, spiculated, or ill defined (Fig. 10-47). Because primary lung cancers do not calcify and because they generally have ill-defined borders, it is very unusual to radiographically identify a nodule caused by lung cancer until it is 1 cm or more in size. Occasionally, a lung tumor may engulf one or more pre-existing calcified granulomas to form eccentric calcifications. Squamous cell carcinomas can cavitate, whereas oat cell carcinomas almost never do.

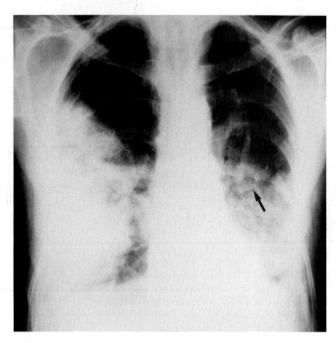

Fig. 10-46. Malignancy resembling alveolar consolidation. Several malignancies are manifested by a pattern of alveolar consolidation. This patient has alveolar cell carcinoma with air bronchograms *(arrow)*.

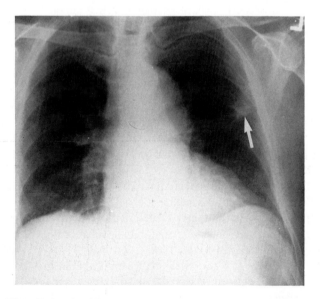

Fig. 10-47. Scarlike malignancy. Radiograph demonstrates an irregular density representing a primary neoplasm in the lateral left midlung *(arrow)*. This could also be a residual scar from inflammatory disease.

Unilateral or markedly asymmetric hilar enlargement may be caused by a primary lung carcinoma that has developed centrally or by hilar lymphadenopathy resulting from metastatic disease. Oat cell carcinoma often induces massive hilar and mediastinal adenopathy, along with either a small (less than 4 cm in diameter) mass or no primary tumor identifiable radiographically. However, atelectasis or pulmonary consolidation occurs frequently in association with a hilar mass in oat cell carcinoma. Diffuse or patchy calcification in hilar lymph nodes generally indicates previous granulomatous disease (infectious or noninfectious, such as silicosis), and further evaluation is usually unnecessary.[2]

The presence of bone destruction in the vicinity of a pulmonary shadow is virtually pathognomonic of primary lung carcinoma. Pulmonary infection (with the rare exception of actinomycosis) does not invade adjacent bone.[2]

Squamous cell carcinoma typically presents as a central or hilar mass. Adenocarcinoma often is identified as a shaggy or stellate, poorly defined peripheral nodule. Oat cell carcinoma typically presents with hilar and mediastinal lymph node involvement. Alveolar cell carcinoma often is a slowly growing, poorly defined peripheral infiltrate or mass that is initially misdiagnosed as pneumonia or parenchymal scarring. Bronchial adenoma, which is a carcinoid, is a very low-grade carcinoma usually manifested as a well-circumscribed hilar or perihilar round mass.

Malignant lymphoma, particularly Hodgkin disease of the lung, is usually accompanied by mediastinal adenopathy. Lymphoma may present radiographically as one or more areas of consolidation resembling pneumonia, masses simulating metastatic carcinoma, or reticulonodular shadowing resembling lymphangitic carcinomatosis. The diffuse lymphangitic form of neoplasm is common in non-Hodgkin lymphoma. The majority of mesotheliomas present as pleural effusions in patients with asbestosis. The Pancoast tumor, which involves the mediastinal aspect of the upper lobe, is often difficult to identify on a chest radiograph because of superimposed densities caused by normal mediastinal soft tissues and the bony thorax.

Pleural neoplasms are commonly due to metastatic disease or to direct extension from adjacent lung or breast carcinoma. Unlike parenchymal lesions, pleural masses typically taper toward the chest wall. Bony lesions are suggestive of adjacent extrapleural neoplasms.[2]

Additional radiographic studies may be indicated for further evaluation of lesions that are potentially neoplastic. For example, oblique chest radiographs, conventional tomograms, and fluoroscopic examinations can further define lung lesions. The CT scan is more sensitive than conventional methods for the detection of tiny lung nodules, and it can effectively document direct invasion of adjacent structures by neoplasm and mediastinal extension of malignancy (Fig. 10-48).

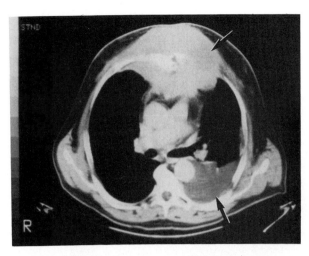

Fig. 10-48. CT scan through the midchest demonstrating sternal and rib destruction by a lymphoma. There is a mass in the anterior mediastinum as well as in the anterior thoracic wall *(upper arrow)*. A left pleural effusion is present *(lower arrow)*.

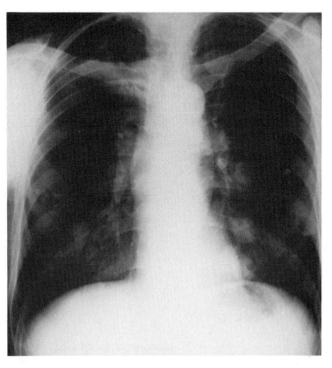

Fig. 10-49. Metastatic malignant pulmonary disease. Radiograph demonstrates multiple noncalcified pulmonary nodules of varying size, some of which are cavitating.

Causes of pleural effusion

Congestive heart failure
Infection
Neoplasm
Trauma
Pulmonary embolism
Hepatic disease
Renal disease
Pancreatitis
Collagen vascular disease
Inhalation injury
Hypoproteinemia
Ruptured esophagus
Obstruction of the great veins
Thoracic duct disruption
Subdiaphragmatic abscess
Iatrogenic origin
    Misplaced CVP catheter
    Post-abdominal surgery

Metastases and lymphomas

Metastatic disease may present as mediastinal or hilar lymphadenopathy or may cause pulmonary abnormalities. Hematogenous metastatic spread in the lung is generally characterized by small interstitial nodules that may grow rapidly (Fig. 10-49) and become more hazy, especially if they cause hemorrhage. The nodules are often subpleural and basilar because of the prevalence of small vessels and increased blood flow in these regions. Common causes of hematogenous metastatic disease include sarcomas, melanomas, trophoblastic malignancies, thyroid carcinomas, adenocarcinomas of the breast, colon, or pancreas, and squamous cell carcinomas, especially of the head and neck region. However, virtually any malignancy may cause these type of nodules.

Lymphangitic metastatic disease in the lungs appears as diffuse reticular interstitial infiltration with Kerley B lines that is most marked in the lower lung fields and especially near the hila. Nodularity may be present, but it is much more ill defined than in hematogenous metastatic disease and generally is distributed along with the bronchovascular structures. The appearance of lymphangitic spread resembles interstitial pulmonary edema, except for the absence of certain signs of LVF (especially enlargement of the upper lobe vessels) that are usually present with interstitial edema. Common causes of lymphangitic metastatic disease include carcinoma of the breast, stomach, lung, and lower genitourinary tract, including the prostate.[2]

Pleural effusion

A pleural effusion is a collection of fluid anywhere in the pleural space (see box at left). It may consist of water, blood, pus, chyle, and other exudates. On the upright chest radiograph, a volume of approximately 250 ml of effusion in the costophrenic angles is necessary before radiographic demonstration is possible. A lesser amount of fluid will first be visible in the posterior gutter angles on the lat-

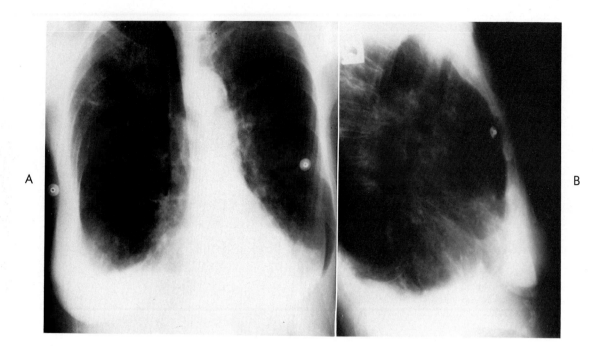

Fig. 10-50. Bilateral pleural effusions. PA (**A**) and lateral (**B**) chest radiographs reveal a loss of normal diaphragmatic curves with a meniscus at the costophrenic angles. Presence of free fluid can be further confirmed with a decubitus radiograph.

eral radiograph before effusion is detectable on the frontal (PA or AP) projection. A meniscus often occurs with pleural effusion because fluid has a tendency to layer higher laterally than centrally (Fig. 10-50). Large amounts of fluid can accumulate between the lung base and diaphragm; these subpulmonic pleural effusions can simulate an elevated hemidiaphragm. A clue to the presence of subpulmonic pleural fluid is that the apparent peak of the dome of the diaphragm shifts toward the lateral chest wall. In addition, a left-sided subpulmonic effusion may increase the distance between the gastric bubble and aerated lung (Fig. 10-51, *A*). Finally, subpulmonic effusions are usually associated with detectable fluid in the posterior gutter angles on the lateral radiograph (Fig. 10-51, *B*).

A lateral decubitus radiograph with the involved side down confirms the layering nature of a free pleural effusion (including a subpulmonic effusion). With slight Trendelenburg positioning, as little as 5 to 15 ml of fluid may be detected on a lateral decubitus radiograph.[2] The fluid floats into a dependent position that obscures the lateral chest wall and forms a fluid level (Fig. 10-51, *C*). With the involved side up, the fluid migrates into the mediastinal pleural space, and the nondependent costophrenic angle and lateral chest wall become sharply demarcated. Pleural thickening may blunt the costophrenic angle on the upright radiograph and may be indistinguishable from a small effusion. On the lateral decubitus radiograph, thickened pleura does not change in configuration as does free pleural fluid. However, a loculated pleural effusion may be difficult to differentiate from pleural thickening.

Free pleural effusion in the recumbent patient gravitates superiorly, laterally, and posteriorly and may not be discernible on the supine radiograph. However, the fluid can form an apical cap superiorly and can cause increased density in the hemithorax because of posterior layering. If the patient is too ill to lie on the side for a decubitus radiograph, a cross-table lateral radiograph may allow for detection of the posterior layering of a pleural effusion.[22] A totally opacified hemithorax may result from a pleural effusion.

Pleural fluid can extend up a major fissure and appear as a homogeneous density in the lower two thirds of the lung field on a frontal radiograph. Fluid can loculate in fissures ("fluid pseudotumor") or elsewhere in the pleural space. Fluid in a fissure (Fig. 10-52) is typically fusiform in shape (widest in the middle). Adhesions or anatomic variants, such as incomplete fissures, can cause fluid to loculate. Empyema or pus in the pleural space is often loculated or atypical in location. Empyema may also contain loculated air. If an air-fluid level develops in an area with pneumonia, a bronchopleural fistula (or infection with a gas-forming organism) may be present. Such a fistula allows air to enter the pleural space directly from a bronchus.

Some conditions cause pleural effusions that are bilateral (systemic lupus erythematosus, CHF, multiple pulmonary infarctions, hypoproteinemia), right-sided (secondary to ascites, as in Meigs syndrome, CHF, or liver abscess), or left-sided (pancreatitis, ruptured esophagus). "Spontaneous" esophageal rupture (Boerhaave syndrome) can be

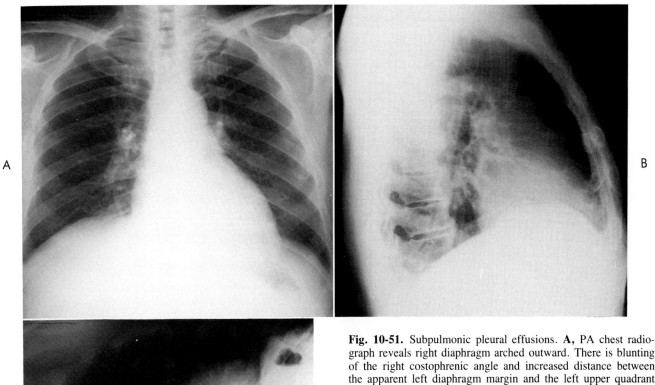

Fig. 10-51. Subpulmonic pleural effusions. **A,** PA chest radiograph reveals right diaphragm arched outward. There is blunting of the right costophrenic angle and increased distance between the apparent left diaphragm margin and the left upper quadrant gas-containing structures. **B,** Lateral chest radiograph reveals blunting of the posterior costophrenic angles. **C,** Right lateral decubitus radiograph confirms presence of right pleural effusion, separating the parietal from the visceral pleura. Left pleural effusion is also confirmed by the nonnormal distance between the left hemidiaphragm and the gastric bubble.

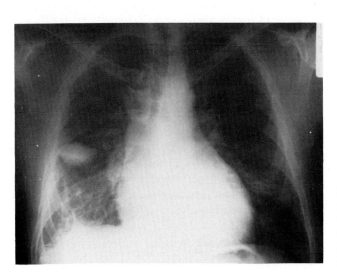

Fig. 10-52. "Pseudotumor" of pleural fluid loculated in the minor fissure. PA chest radiograph reveals indistinct pulmonary vascularity with a few Kerley B lines in the right costophrenic angle, representing congestive heart failure. Cardiomegaly is present. Elliptic density in the minor fissure is loculated pleural fluid.

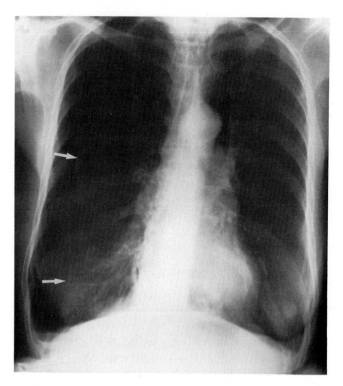

Fig. 10-53. Small-to-moderate pneumothorax. There is partial collapse of the right lung with air in the pleural space. Visceral pleural edge is clearly identified *(arrows)*. Patient was asthmatic.

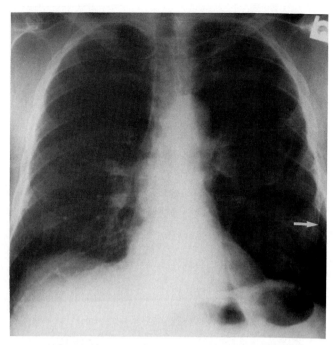

Fig. 10-54. Loculated pneumothorax. Postsurgical pleural scarring and adhesions confine this pneumothorax to the left lower pleura and costophrenic angle *(arrow)*.

associated with a left-sided pleural effusion because the site of rupture is typically the left posterolateral aspect of the distal portion of the esophagus, just proximal to the diaphragm.[3] Massive effusions are commonly due to malignant disease, especially metastases (lung, breast) but may also occur in CHF, cirrhosis, tuberculosis, empyema, trauma, and other conditions.[23]

Pneumothorax, pneumomediastinum, pneumopericardium

A pneumothorax is a collection of air between the visceral and parietal pleura. Spontaneous pneumothorax can occur after coughing or straining and is often associated with an underlying parenchymal abnormality, particularly apical blebs located immediately beneath the visceral pleura. Spontaneous pneumothorax occurs predominately in males between 20 and 40 years of age, is often recurrent, and may be associated with a small hemothorax. Penetrating or blunt trauma can cause a pneumothorax (see Chapter 5). Necrosis of the subpleural lung by infection can lead to a bronchopleural fistula and a loculated pneumothorax. Extension of air from a pneumomediastinum, ruptured alveoli, perforated esophagus, or tracheal tear can induce a pneumothorax. In addition, disorders such as asthma, staphylococcal pneumonia, metastatic disease, and pulmonary fibrosis are associated with pneumothorax

(Fig. 10-53). During placement of a subclavian or internal jugular venous catheter, a pneumothorax is a common complication; therefore, a chest radiograph should always be obtained after these procedures.

With a pneumothorax, the visceral pleura line can be visualized radiographically between the lung and pleural air space (Fig. 10-54) because air is less dense than the collapsed lung. Furthermore, no pulmonary bronchovascular markings can be identified in the areas of pleural air space. Faint vertical lines can represent skinfolds, and exclusion of a pneumothorax requires visualization of lung markings peripheral to these lines. Clinical comment on the size of a pneumothorax is based on the percentage of lung volume lost. For practical purposes, however, classification of a pneumothorax as marginal, moderate, massive (without tension), or tension is generally sufficient.[3]

Demonstration of a marginal pneumothorax may be enhanced on a PA upright radiograph exposed during expiration. The collapsed lung decreases in volume during expiration, whereas the pleural air-space volume remains constant. Therefore the lung draws away from the chest wall, rendering the pneumothorax more easily visible. If a patient who cannot assume the upright posture is placed in the decubitus position with the affected side up, air will accumulate in the uppermost pleural space and the weight of the heart will pull the lung away from the nondependent chest wall, rendering a marginal pneumothorax more detectable on the lateral decubitus radiograph. A pneumothorax may be impossible to detect on a supine radiograph if

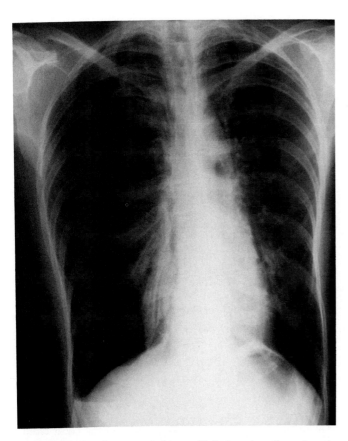

Fig. 10-55. Tension pneumothorax. Right lung is collapsed, and there is a slight shift of the mediastinum to the left.

air migrates into the anterior (uppermost) pleural space, while the lateral pleural surfaces remain in apposition. Therefore a negative supine chest radiograph does not exclude the diagnosis of pneumothorax.[3] However, pleural air space can often be visualized radiographically in the lateral costophrenic angles in the supine patient because these general areas may indeed be uppermost in the recumbent torso.

If a ball-valve effect occurs so that air continues to enter the pleural space during inspiration but cannot escape during expiration, a tension pneumothorax develops. This situation can be life-threatening because function of the involved lung, the heart and great vessels, and eventually the contralateral lung is compromised by the expanding pleural air-space mass and the increasing intrathoracic pressure. Venous return to the heart and cardiac output decrease. Immediate therapy (needle or chest tube decompression of the pneumothorax) may be required before chest radiographs are even obtained. The radiograph of a tension pneumothorax reveals a collapsed lung, mediastinal (aortic arch, right heart border) and tracheal shift away from the pneumothorax, depressed ipsilateral hemidiaphragm, and a relative increase in the size of rib inter-

spaces compared to the contralateral side (Fig. 10-55). If the lung is densely consolidated or if there are pleural adhesions, total lung collapse and mediastinal shift may be absent, in which case a depressed hemidiaphragm may be the only sign of a tension pneumothorax.[20]

Bronchospasm or inflammatory edema can cause a bronchiolar check-valve obstruction with air trapping, which leads to ruptured alveoli distally. Rupture of alveoli may also occur after a forceful valsalva maneuver (e.g., during vaginal delivery) or as a result of barotrauma in patients who require ventilatory support, especially if the lungs are poorly compliant as a result of inflammation or edema. Ruptured alveoli can release air into the interstitium, which may dissect medially along the peribronchial connective tissue sheaths to enter the hila and mediastinum to form a pneumomediastinum. This air can also extend into the pleural space to form a pneumothorax, into the pericardial sac through the perivenous spaces to form a pneumopericardium, inferiorly into the peritoneal cavity or retroperitoneum, and superiorly from the mediastinum through the fascial planes into the neck to form subcutaneous emphysema.

Pneumomediastinum is relatively common in infants and is unusual in adults. The most common cause in a nontraumatized patient is air leak during an acute asthma episode.[8] Other causes include trauma to the pharynx, esophagus, or tracheobronchial tree, rupture of the esophagus (Boerhaave syndrome), and gas entering the mediastinum from below the diaphragm after medical procedures during which air is introduced (see Chapter 5). The mediastinal pleura is displaced laterally and appears as a sharp, oblique, linear density that parallels the mediastinal border and is usually more apparent on the left side. Air translucency is often visible adjacent to the aortic knob, main pulmonary artery, and left hilum. On the lateral radiograph, the pneumomediastinum is characteristically visualized in the retrosternal space. Dissection of mediastinal air into the neck and chest wall is more common in adults than in children.[3] If the mediastinum is also widened, esophageal perforation with resulting mediastinal air and fluid accumulation must be considered.

Pneumopericardium may be difficult to distinguish radiographically from pneumomediastinum or a small pneumothorax. Air in the pericardial sac is confined to the anatomic distribution of the parietal pericardium, which terminates at the point of its reflection around the great vessels. Thus air that extends more cephalad than this level lies outside the pericardium. Furthermore, air in the mediastinum does not outline the heart border as accurately as a pneumopericardium.[3]

UPPER AIRWAY ABNORMALITIES

The radiographic evaluation of upper airway differential conditions (see box on pp. 279-280) is somewhat controversial; some clinicians prefer direct visualization. How-

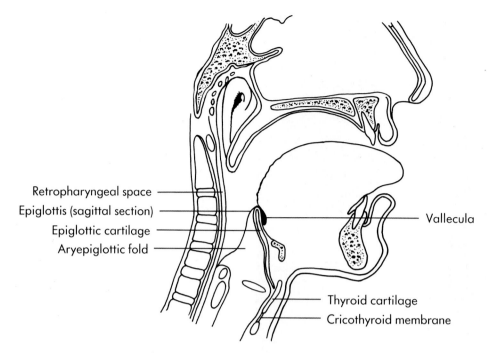

Fig. 10-56. Upper airway anatomy.

ever, the lateral neck radiograph may be valuable in the assessment of the airway and its relation to the mandible, tongue, palate, retropharyngeal soft tissues, and spine. The study allows for the assessment of the epiglottis, aryepiglottic folds, and subglottic trachea (Fig. 10-56).

The expiratory phase of respiration and flexion of the head and neck during lateral radiographic exposure can cause buckling and anterior displacement of the upper trachea and redundancy of the pharyngeal soft tissues, which can render radiographic interpretation of the neck quite difficult. The AP neck radiograph complements the lateral radiograph and allows for further assessment of the glottic and subglottic areas and the tracheal lumen. Tracheal buckling during expiration may simulate the radiographic appearance of tracheal deviation on the AP projection.

Croup

The most common cause of stridor in the febrile child is croup. Laryngotracheobronchitis, or croup, is a viral infection that causes inflammatory narrowing of the tracheobronchial tree. The most severe narrowing occurs in the subglottic trachea. A smooth concentric narrowing of this area is demonstrated on both AP and lateral neck radiographs in severe disease. The shape of the normal airway beneath the true vocal cords resembles a rounded archway. In croup, edema of the vocal cords and subglottic trachea produces an appearance that resembles a church steeple,[8] which is especially visible on the AP view (Fig. 10-57). However, most radiographic neck studies in children with croup are normal or may disclose only ballooning of the hypopharynx. Diffuse bilateral pulmonary hyperlucency caused by air trapping may be present on the chest radiograph.[24]

Epiglottitis

Epiglottitis or supraglottitis is an infectious inflammation of the glottic and supraglottic tissues that can produce life-threatening airway obstruction. The patient often presents with a fever of rapid onset, sore throat, drooling, and odynophagia. Dyspnea and sternal retractions may indicate the progression of airway edema. Radiography may be helpful in atypical or doubtful cases. If the diagnosis is obvious on clinical grounds, radiography is not needed and is contraindicated in the unstable child.

Only one view is required—the inspiratory, upright, lateral radiograph of the soft tissues of the neck. The tip of the normal epiglottis can appear slightly bulbous. In epiglottitis, edema of the epiglottis and the aryepiglottic folds can be identified radiographically. As a result of inflammatory swelling, the epiglottis becomes more vertically oriented and develops a convex contour of the anterior and posterior margins (Fig. 10-58). This radiographic appearance of the edematous epiglottis has been termed the *thumb sign*. In addition, the vallecula may appear constricted or obliterated on the neck radiograph. The subglottic trachea is usually not involved and appears normal radiographically.[1,24] The same radiographic criteria are used to evaluate the adult with possible epiglottitis.

Retropharyngeal abscess

Retropharyngeal abscess is an uncommon infection that generally occurs in children less than 4 years of age. The

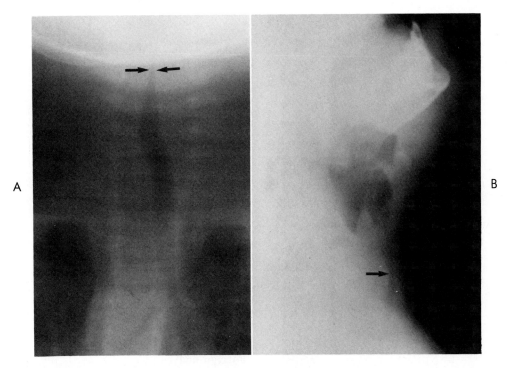

Fig. 10-57. Croup. AP (**A**) and lateral (**B**) chest radiographs demostrating laryngotracheobronchitis manifested by laryngeal edema with alteration of the normal vocal cord arch. There is a decrease in the size of the laryngeal lumen *(arrows)* on both views.

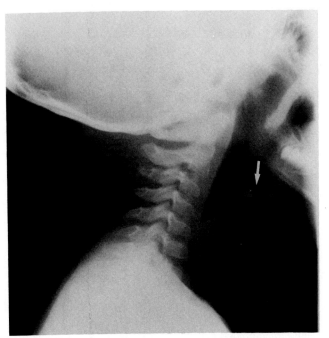

Fig. 10-58. Epiglottitis. Because of inflammation, the epiglottis is several times larger than normal *(arrow)*. Associated mucosal swelling has caused a decrease in caliber of the laryngeal lumen.

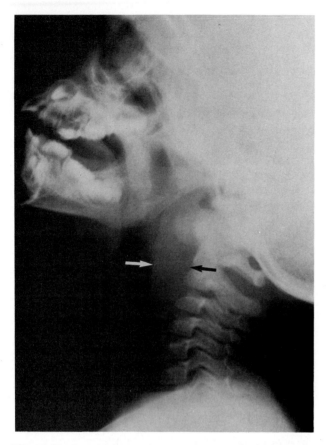

Fig. 10-59. Retropharyngeal abscess. There is a marked increase in the soft tissues anterior to the cervical spine *(between arrows)* consistent with cellulitis or abscess. Compare this radiograph with epiglottitis shown in Fig. 10-58.

abscess fills the potential space between the anterior border of the cervical vertebrae and the posterior wall of the esophagus. The child presents with a clinical picture resembling epiglottitis, but the onset of symptoms with retropharyngeal abscess is less abrupt. If the diagnosis is suspected, a lateral neck radiograph should be obtained. The radiograph reveals an increase in the width of the soft tissues anterior to the vertebrae (Fig. 10-59), often an acute cervical kyphosis, and occasionally an air-fluid level caused by gas in the abscess. The normal width of this retropharyngeal space is less than half that of the adjacent vertebral body. However, even limited flexion of the neck during exposure of the radiograph may cause a buckling of the retropharyngeal tissues that resembles a purulent collection. Therefore it is imperative that the neck radiograph be obtained during inspiration with the neck properly extended.

Bacterial tracheitis

Bacterial tracheitis is an unusual infection of childhood. Patients initially are diagnosed with severe viral croup or epiglottitis. The neck radiograph reveals tracheal narrowing, but the supraglottic area is normal.[24]

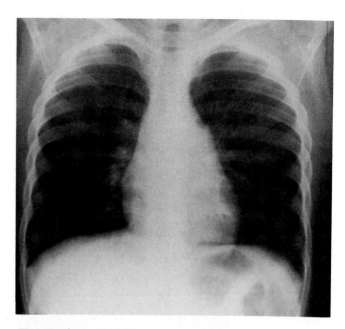

Fig. 10-60. Bronchiolitis. PA chest radiograph reveals generalized hyperinflation of the lungs. This may be the only radiographic finding in bronchiolitis.

Foreign body

For a discussion on the inhalation of foreign bodies, see Chapter 24.

PEDIATRIC LOWER AIRWAY ABNORMALITIES
Bronchiolitis

Bronchiolitis is an infection of the bronchioles that is characterized by wheezing; it is the most common lower respiratory infection in young children. Respiratory syncytial virus causes the majority of these infections. Most cases of bronchiolitis occur in the winter, and the majority of the children are between 2 and 8 months of age. The illness begins with cough and coryza; fever, tachypnea, wheezing, and signs of respiratory distress appear over a period of 2 to 5 days. The chest radiograph generally shows diffuse air trapping manifested by hyperinflation, low, flat hemidiaphragms, and an increased anteroposterior diameter of the chest (Fig. 10-60). Areas of atelectasis may occasionally be present. Streaky reticulonodular densities radiating from the hila are commonly visualized. Despite the often significant air trapping, pneumothorax and pneumomediastinum only rarely occur.[24]

Cystic fibrosis

Cystic fibrosis is a generalized disease of the exocrine and mucus-secreting glands. The mucus is abnormal and has increased viscosity. Currently, these patients often survive to adulthood because of improved therapy for respiratory complications. Hypersecretion of viscid mucus into the airways predisposes the patient to infection and may cause bronchial obstruction. Radiographic signs in the

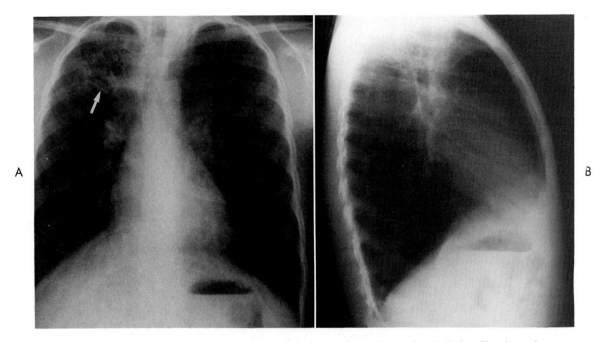

Fig. 10-61. Cystic fibrosis of the lung. **A,** PA chest radiograph reveals nodularity, fibrosis, and bronchiectasis, especially in the right upper lung. Bronchial wall thickening is evident *(arrow).* **B,** Lateral chest radiograph reveals lung hyperinflation with an increased AP diameter of the chest and an enlarged retrosternal space.

early stages of the disease are nonspecific and are caused by recurrent episodes of pneumonia. Persistent pulmonary hyperinflation may occur and is one of the earliest clues to the diagnosis of cystic fibrosis in children.

In the later stages of the disease, chest radiographs show generalized hyperinflation and diffuse interstitial shadowing in the lungs. Bronchial wall thickening produces a ring density when the end of the bronchus is visualized or parallel linear densities when the long axis of the bronchus is visible. Bronchiectasis is frequently present with an upper lung predominance and appears as cystlike ring shadows in the case of air-filled spaces or as circular densities if the spaces are fluid-filled (Fig. 10-61). Air-fluid levels may also be apparent in bronchiectatic areas. Segmental or lobar collapse and areas of bullous emphysema may develop. Lobar or segmental consolidations indicate acute pneumonia. Hilar adenopathy is frequent, and the development of pulmonary hypertension can cause concomitant enlargement of the pulmonary arteries. As cystic fibrosis progresses, cor pulmonale causes an increase in cardiac size. A pneumothorax may be a life-threatening complication in these patients, and hemoptysis can be severe.[1]

SUMMARY

Radiographic evaluation of the patient presenting with shortness of breath, either acutely or as an exacerbation of a chronic condition, is essential. Frequently, differential diagnostic considerations can be narrowed by initial assessment with imaging techniques, which often provide definitive diagnostic data.

REFERENCES

1. Alford BA, Keats TE: The infant and young child. In Grainger RG, Allison DJ, eds: *Diagnostic radiology; an Anglo-American textbook of imaging,* ed 1, vol 1, Edinburgh, 1986, Churchill-Livingstone.
2. Forrest JV, Feigin DS: *Essentials of chest radiology,* ed 1, Philadelphia, 1982, WB Saunders.
3. Harris JH Jr, Harris WH: *The radiology of emergency medicine,* ed 2, Baltimore, 1981, Williams & Wilkins.
4. Wilson AG: Interpreting the chest radiograph. In Grainger RG, Allison DJ, eds: *Diagnostic radiology: an Anglo-American textbook of imaging,* ed 1, Edinburgh, 1986, Churchill-Livingstone.
5. Felson B, Felson H: Localization of intrathoracic lesions by means of the postero-anterior roentgenogram, the silhouette sign, *Radiology* 55(3):363, 1950.
6. Breckenfeld JI, Stone AJ, and Victor LD: Cardiovascular disease. In Victor LD, ed: *An atlas of critical care chest roentgenography,* ed 1, Rockville, MD, 1985, Aspen Systems.
7. Wilson AG: Pulmonary infection. In Grainger RG, Allison DJ, eds: *Diagnostic radiology: an Anglo-American textbook of imaging,* ed 1, Edinburgh, 1986, Churchill-Livingstone.
8. Armstrong P: Chest. In Keats TE, ed: *Emergency radiology,* ed 2, Chicago, 1989, Year Book Medical Publishers.
9. Flower CDR: Diffuse pulmonary disease. In Grainger RG, Allison DJ, eds: *Diagnostic radiology: an Anglo-American textbook of imaging,* ed 1, Edinburgh, 1986, Churchill-Livingstone.
10. Weg JG: Chronic noninfectious parenchymal diseases. In Guenter CA, Welch MH: *Pulmonary medicine,* ed 2, Philadelphia, 1982, JB Lippincott.
11. Hublitz UF, Shapiro JH: Atypical pulmonary patterns of congestive heart failure in chronic lung disease, *Radiology* 93(5):995, 1969.
12. Flower CDR, Armstrong JD: Pulmonary oedema. In Grainger RG,

Allison DJ, eds: *Diagnostic radiolgoy: an Anglo-American textbook of imaging,* ed 1, Edinburgh, 1986, Churchill Livingstone.

13. Squire LF, Novelline RA: *Fundamentals of radiology,* ed 4, Cambridge, Mass, 1988, Harvard University Press.
14. Rubenstein E: Thromboembolism. In Rubenstein E, Federman DD, eds: *Scientific American medicine,* New York, 1989, Scientific American.
15. Pritchard JA, MacDonald PC, and Gant NF: *Williams' obstetrics,* ed 17, Norwalk, CT, 1985, Appleton-Century-Crofts.
16. Benedetti TJ: Obstetric hemorrhage. In Gabbe SG, Niebyl JR, Simpson JL, eds: *Obstetrics, normal and problem pregnancies,* ed 1, New York, 1986, Churchill-Livingstone.
17. Weinberger SE, Weiss ST: Pulmonary diseases. In Burrow GN, Ferris TF, eds: *Medical complications during pregnancy,* ed 3, Philadelphia, 1988, WB Saunders.
18. Wilson AG: Sarcoidosis. In Grainger RG, Allison DJ, eds: *Diagnostic radiology: an Anglo-American textbook of imaging,* ed 1, Edinburgh, 1986, Churchill-Livingstone.
19. Flower CDR: Asthma and emphysema. In Grainger RG, Allison DJ, eds: *Diagnostic radiology: an Anglo-American textbook of imaging,* ed 1, Edinburgh, 1986, Churchill-Livingstone.
20. Goodman LR: The postoperative and critically ill patient. In Grainger RG, Allison DJ, eds: *Diagnostic radiology: an Anglo-American textook of imaging,* ed 1, Edinburgh, 1986, Churchill-Livingstone.
21. Armstrong P: Pulmonary neoplasms. In Grainger RG, Allison DJ, eds: *Diagnostic radiology: an Anglo-American textbook of imaging,* ed 1, vol 1, Edinburgh, 1986, Churchill-Livingstone.
22. Victor LD, Yates D: Abnormal air and fluid. In Victor LD, ed: *An atlas of critical care chest roentgenography,* ed 1, Rockville, MD, 1985, Aspen Systems.
23. Wilson AG: The chest wall and pleura. In Grainger RG, Allison DJ, eds: *Diagnostic radiology: an Anglo-American textbook of imaging,* ed 1, Edinburgh, 1986, Churchill-Livingstone.
24. Fleisher GR: Infectious disease emergencies. In Fleisher GR, Ludwig S, eds: *Textbook of pediatric emergency medicine,* ed 2, Baltimore, 1988, Williams & Wilkins.

Aspiration

Brian R. Holroyd
Richard R. Lesperance

Aspiration has been described as "a diverse group of disorders that are linked by the common factor of soiling of the lower respiratory tract by foreign, nongaseous substances."[1] The potential for significant associated mortality (reported to be from 28%[2] to 62%[3] with gastric aspiration) and morbidity mandates careful emergency department consideration.

Several key principles must guide the clinical approach to this problem. First, every patient must be regarded as a potential victim of aspiration,[4] and those patients with characteristics that may increase this risk significantly must be recognized. Prevention must be considered a fundamental treatment.[5] Second, the type of substance aspirated dictates the clinical and radiographic presentation, the underlying pathophysiologic state, and the subsequent management of the patient. As the clinical presentation may be extremely varied, the possibility of aspiration must be considered in a wide variety of presenting complaints. The chest radiograph plays a significant role in the management process.[6]

ANATOMY

Several anatomic factors must be considered in the clinical and radiographic approach to aspiration. Gravity and the position of the patient at the time of aspiration deter-

mine the anatomic distribution of the aspirate.[7] The most dependent bronchopulmonary segments are at the greatest risk.[8]

The less acute angle of the right mainstem bronchus originating from the trachea, as compared with the left, accounts for the predominance of involvement of the right lung in aspiration.[1,3,8,9]

Clinical studies of aspiration[2,3] reveal that the most frequently affected lobe is the right lower lobe and the least frequently affected is the left upper lobe.

If a patient aspirates while in a supine position, the affected areas are usually the posterior segments of the upper lobes and the superior and posterior basal segments of either lower lobe [1,7,10] (Fig. 11-1). Involvement of the axillary subsegments of the right upper lobe may also suggest a diagnosis of aspiration.[10] If the patient is in an upright position at the time of aspiration, the basal segments of the lower lobes will be predominantly affected.[8,11] A large volume of aspirate may result in involvement of different lung segments or in diffuse bilateral involvement[1,9,10] (see Table 11-1). The radiographic silhouettes of bronchopulmonary segments commonly affected in aspiration are demonstrated in Fig. 11-2.

PREDISPOSING FACTORS

Since aspiration is a frequent problem seen in the emergency department and all patients must be considered at risk,[4] factors present that further increase the risk of aspiration warrant care for prevention and a heightened level of suspicion. These factors also indicate the need for clinical and radiographic examination. The presence of these risk factors must be determined by history and physical and radiographic examinations.

Aspiration is frequently an occult event. Several studies have clearly documented the presence of aspiration in patients who did not overtly manifest evidence of vomiting.[12,13]

The common denominator in significant aspiration is a disruption (either constant or intermittent) of the normal protective mechanisms, which allows oropharyngeal secre-

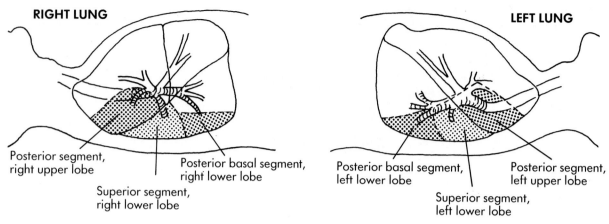

Fig. 11-1. Dependent bronchopulmonary segments with patient in supine position.

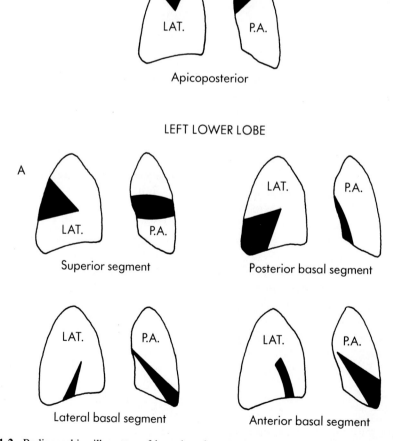

Fig. 11-2. Radiographic silhouettes of bronchopulmonary segments commonly involved in aspiration. **A,** Left lung. (Adapted from Healy JE Jr: *A synopsis of clinical anatomy,* Philadelphia, 1969, WB Saunders.)

tions, gastric contents, or exogenous liquids or solids to enter the tracheobronchial tree.[14]

Fishman[1] has classified risk factors into three major categories: mechanisms decreasing reflex protection, alterations in anatomy that predispose an individual to aspiration, and iatrogenic mechanisms (see box on p. 316).

Mechanisms decreasing reflex protection

The complex swallowing mechanism that projects ingested liquids and solids into the esophagus rather than into the tracheobronchial tree is essential in preventing aspiration. If this sequence of neuromuscular events is compromised or altered, an increased risk of aspiration results.[16,17] Additional protection is provided by the presence of the lower esophageal sphincter.[16]

Loss of reflex protection is present in many clinical situations seen in the emergency department. Patients with a decreased level of consciousness—including cardiopulmonary arrest,[18] trauma with altered mental status[4,19,20] (Fig. 11-3), and ingestion of central nervous system depres-

RIGHT LUNG

RIGHT UPPER LOBE

Posterior segment

RIGHT LOWER LOBE

Superior segment

Lateral basal segment

B

Posterior basal segment

Anterior basal segment

Medial basal segment

Fig. 11-2, cont'd. B, Right lung.

Predisposing factors and conditions for aspiration

Decreased reflex protection

Decreased level of consciousness
  Cardiopulmonary arrest
  Trauma
  Ingestion of CNS depressants
  Seizure disorder
  Coma
  General anesthesia
Central nervous system disorders (disruption of
  swallowing mechanism)
  Cerebrovascular accidents
  Bulbar neuropathy (myasthenia gravis; Guillain-Barré
    syndrome)
Use of depolarizing neuromuscular blocking agents
Impairment of protective body movements
  Neuromuscular paralysis or weakness
  Restrained patient
Chronic, debilitating illness

Anatomic alterations

Increased gastric volume or pressure
  Recent meal
  Excessive gastric secretions
  Delayed gastric emptying
  Gastric dilatation
  Intestinal obstruction
Tracheoesophageal fistula
  Congenital
  Traumatic
  Neoplastic
Esophageal pathologic conditions
  Achalasia
  Altered motility (i.e., scleroderma)
  Foreign body
  Strictures
Incompetent lower esophageal sphincter

Iatrogenic mechanisms

Nasogastric or feeding tubes
Tracheostomy
Endotracheal intubation
Esophageal tamponade (Sengstaken-Blakemore tube)
Esophageal obturator airway

From Fishman AP, ed: *Pulmonary diseases and disorders,* vol 2, ed 2, New York, 1988, McGraw-Hill.

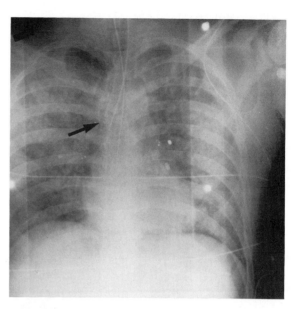

Fig. 11-3. Radiograph of 22-year-old male who sustained severe blunt head and chest trauma in a motor vehicle accident. The radiograph demonstrates wide-spread nonhomogeneous air-space consolidation consistent with pulmonary contusion. An endotracheal tube is in the right mainstem bronchus *(arrow).* Aspirated radio-opaque particulate material is in right upper lobe bronchus, right middle lobe bronchus, left upper lobe bronchus, and left lower lobe bronchus. Note, also, particulate radio-opaque matter in the esophagus and stomach.

sants, such as alcohol and narcotics[21]—are at significantly increased risk for aspiration.[1,9,14] In addition, during the process of endotracheal intubation, the patient is also at peril for aspiration.[5]

Various neurologic conditions may also compromise reflex airway protection. The patient with a seizure disorder may aspirate during a convulsion or during the post-ictal phase. Disruption of the swallowing mechanism may oc-

cur with a cerebrovascular accident[22] or in other neurologic disorders that produce bulbar neuropathy, including Guillain-Barré syndrome and myasthenia gravis.[1,9] Pharmacologic induction of a neuromuscular blockade inhibits any protective reflexes from preventing aspiration. Additionally, the increase in intragastric pressure that can occur with the administration of depolarizing neuromuscular blocking agents may allow regurgitation and subsequent aspiration.[23,24] The presence of neuromuscular paralysis (Fig. 11-4) or weakness impairs protective body movements, such as turning or bending in response to vomiting.[1] A restrained patient similarly is prevented from employing these protective movements. The presence of chronic, debilitating illness may also contribute to increased risk through decreased cough and gag reflexes,[25] decreased gastric emptying, and the use of feeding tubes.[9]

Alterations in anatomy predisposing individuals to aspiration

Alterations in the functional or structural anatomy of the oropharynx, larynx, or esophagus may predispose the patient to aspiration.

Factors contributing to increased gastric volume, such as a recent meal, gastric hypersecretion (e.g., secondary to stress or trauma), delayed gastric emptying (e.g., secondary to narcotic or anticholinergic drug use), and increased intragastric air[23] (e.g., from excessive mask ventilation) in-

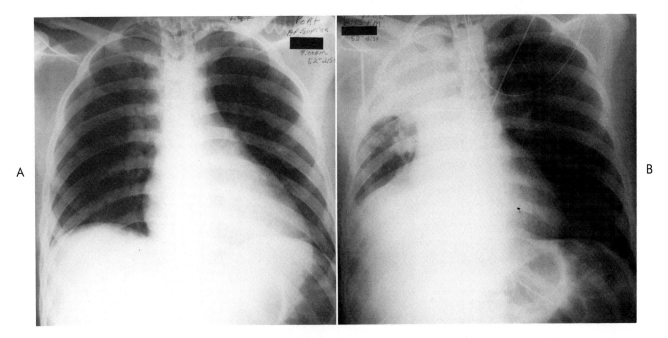

Fig. 11-4. Chest radiograph **(A)** of 19-year-old quadriplegic at 9 AM shows clear lungs. Radiograph **(B)** taken at 2:15 PM on same day shows marked atelectasis of right upper and lower lobes caused by acute aspiration. Only the right middle lobe remains inflated. There is a marked shift of the mediastinum to the right with elevation of the right hemidiaphragm.

crease the risk of subsequent aspiration.[16] Similarly, gastric dilatation, with ileus or mechanical bowel obstruction[26] or after trauma,[27] places the patient in jeopardy. Increased gastric pressure may overcome the mechanisms of the lower esophageal sphincter and allow aspiration to occur. The increased pressure is usually caused by increased gastric volume,[16] although occasionally mechanical factors may result in elevated intragastric pressure despite a normal volume (e.g., in a gravid uterus[28] or a markedly obese patient[16]). Any factor contributing to a reduction in lower esophageal sphincter tone may predispose the patient to aspiration.[16]

A tracheoesophageal fistula (TEF) may result from congenital, traumatic, or neoplastic causes. A TEF is characterized by spasms of coughing and dyspnea early or late after ingestion of solids or liquids, depending on the level of the fistula. Radiographic evidence of a TEF includes recurrent parenchymal infiltrates or outlining of the tracheobronchial tree when a barium swallow is performed.[1] Water-soluble contrast material should never be used if there is a risk of pulmonary aspiration of the contrast material, resulting in an induced pulmonary edema.

The presence of a Zenker diverticulum may predispose a patient, particularly in the recumbent position, to aspiration.[1] Soft tissue radiographs of the neck may also reveal an air-fluid level.[29] The definitive diagnosis can be made with a contrast-enhanced radiographic study of the pharyngoesophageal region.

The presence of esophageal pathologic states[30]—including achalasia[31] (Fig. 11-5), alterations in esophageal motility (i.e., scleroderma), esophageal foreign body,[32,33] or esophageal strictures—may impair esophageal emptying and thus increase the risk of aspiration. Early in the disorders, plain radiographs may not reveal any abnormalities, but they may suggest the diagnosis in more advanced cases. A dilated esophagus may be apparent on chest radiographs with an air-fluid level, the height of which reflects the severity of the obstruction.[34] In patients with achalasia, the gastric air bubble is frequently absent as a result of the underlying obstruction.[34] Patients with recurrent pulmonary complaints, such as dyspnea or wheezing (Fig. 11-5), or with recurrent radiographic infiltrates should be examined carefully to rule out the presence of significant esophageal pathologic conditions as the cause of their problem. Aspiration has been associated with gastroesophageal reflux in patients with chronic bronchial disease.[35]

Iatrogenic mechanisms

Various medical interventions can render a patient more prone to aspiration. The presence of a nasogastric tube may predispose the patient to aspiration through several mechanisms:[10,23,26,36]

- Physically rendering the esophageal sphincters incompetent.
- Stimulating increased gastric secretions.
- Giving the physician the possibly false reassurance that the patient's stomach is empty.
- Irritative effects causing gagging and regurgitation.

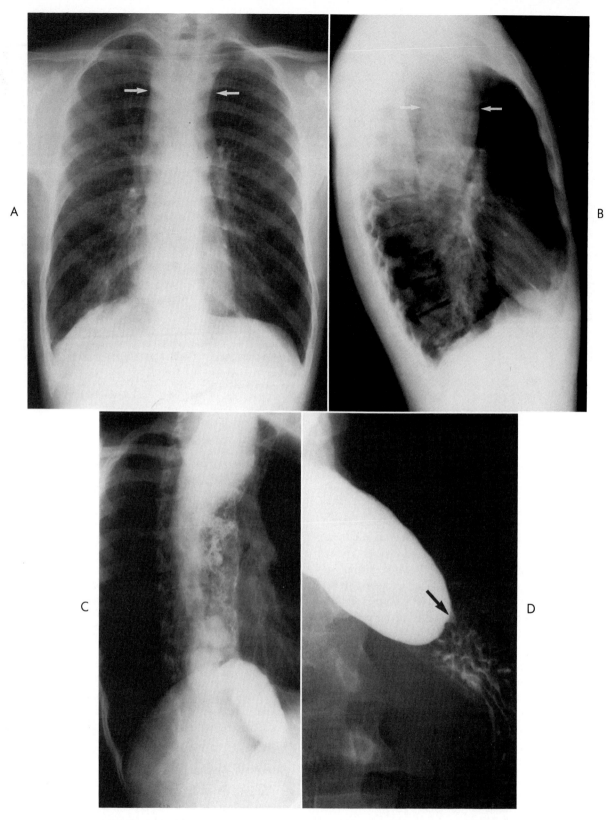

Fig. 11-5. Radiographs of 20-year-old male with multiple episodes of wheezing and broncho-spasm who was diagnosed as having asthma and was treated with bronchodilators. On presenta-tion with bronchospasm, a chest radiograph (**A**) was taken, revealing bilateral hyperinflation of lungs with some segmental consolidation, consistent with bronchopneumonia in the right lower lobe. There was also marked widening of the entire posterior mediastinum that is clearly caused by a radiograph markedly dilated esophagus *(arrows)*. Lateral radiograph (**B**) reveals esophagus *(arrows)* displacing tracheal air column anteriorly, as well as a right lower lobe bronchopneumo-nia superimposed on the distended lower esophagus. Barium esophagogram (**C**) shows classic changes of severe achalasia with a sigmoid esophagus containing barium intermixed with food material. Note the beaked appearance (**D**) of the distal esophagus *(arrow)* at the esophagogastric junction. This is one of the classic findings of achalasia.

A feeding tube may predispose the patient to aspiration when the rate of administration of nutrients is excessive or the patient is improperly positioned.[1,26] Nasogastric feedings have been noted to be aspirated in up to 38% of cases, despite the presence of endotracheal tubes or tracheostomies.[37]

A tracheostomy tube may contribute to aspiration through interference with the normal mechanism of glottic closure.[17,36] The incidence of aspiration with either a standard, uncuffed, metal tracheostomy tube or a small-volume, high-pressure cuff has been reported to be as high as 87% (whether or not the cuff was inflated).[36,38,39] This rate has been reduced to 15% with the use of high-volume, low-pressure cuffs.[36,39]

Endotracheal intubation also does not prevent aspiration (Fig. 11-6). The endotracheal tube abolishes epiglottic function and is not an effective replacement.[23] A 20% incidence of leakage around high-volume, low-pressure endotracheal tube cuffs and a 56% incidence of leakage around low-volume, high-pressure cuffs has been demonstrated.[40] Endotracheal intubation itself has been shown to disrupt reflex laryngeal function for hours after intubation, and thus the recently extubated patient may be predisposed to aspiration.[41]

Aspiration has been rated the most frequent major complication associated with the use of the Sengstaken-Blakemore tube for esophageal tamponade.[42,43] Use of a nasogastric tube or a modification of the standard Sengstaken-Blakemore tube with a provision to allow for removal of accumulated oral secretions from the esophagus, as well as strict avoidance of any oral intake, is essential to avoid aspiration in this circumstance.[43]

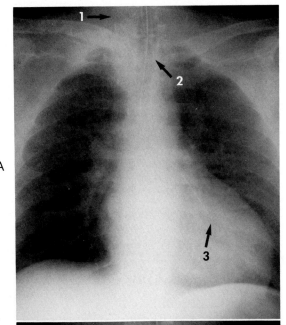

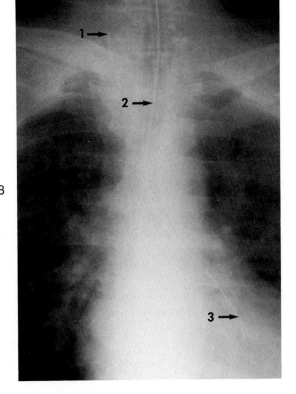

Fig. 11-6. Radiograph (**A**) and the coned-down view (**B**) demonstrate a right subclavian central venous pressure catheter *(arrow 1)* oriented cephalad with its tip in the right internal jugular vein. There is an endotracheal tube *(arrow 2)* with its tip in good position and a nasogastric tube *(arrow 3)* with its tip in the left lower lobe bronchus. Note that, despite the presence of the inflated endotracheal tube cuff, the nasogastric tube was easily placed in the tracheobroncheal tree. This illustrates that the inflated cuff of the endotracheal tube was no barrier to aspiration.

Table 11-1. Distribution of pulmonary aspiration

Pulmonary aspiration complex	Areas of distribution
Toxic liquid material (Mendelson syndrome)	Unilateral and bilateral involvement with almost equal frequency Lower lobe involvement more common than upper lobe involvement
Nontoxic liquid material	Bilateral involvement much more common than unilateral involvement Lower lobe involvement more common than upper lobe involvement
Foreign body or particulate material	Localization of aspirate in right main bronchus more frequently than in left main bronchus Localization of aspirate at tracheal bifurcation uncommon
Bacterial pneumonia or lung abscess	If patient recumbent, apical segments of right upper and lower lobes more common than those of left lobes If patient sitting, right lower lobe more common than left lower lobe

Adapted from Newman GE, Effman EL, and Putman CE: *Curr Probl Diagn Radiol* 1982.

Pulmonary aspiration complexes[11,14,15]

- Toxic liquid material
- Nontoxic liquid material
- Foreign body or particulate material
- Bacterial pneumonia or lung abscess

PULMONARY ASPIRATION MECHANISMS

An individual's response to aspiration depends on the nature, volume, frequency, and distribution of the aspirate.[26] Similarly, the patient's presentation (clinical and radiographic), clinical course, and appropriate therapy are dictated by characteristics of the material aspirated.[15] Bartlett's classification of pulmonary aspiration complexes,[11,14] as modified by Newman,[15] is based on the nature of the material aspirated (see box above). This classification lends itself well to the discussion of radiographic findings in the various types of aspiration (Tables 11-1 and 11-2).

Toxic liquid material

The classic example of aspiration of a toxic liquid is Mendelson syndrome[44]—the pulmonary aspiration of gastric acid. Various other aspirated substances—such as hypertonic contrast material,[15] hydrocarbons, bile,[45] alcohol, and animal fats[14]—are also in this category. The common denominator of these agents is their ability to initiate an inflammatory reaction independent of bacterial infection.[14]

Table 11-2. Summary of radiographic findings in pulmonary aspiration

Pulmonary aspiration complex	Radiographic findings
Toxic liquid material (Mendelson syndrome)	Alveolar infiltrate more common than mixed infiltrate or interstitial infiltrate Atelectasis noted, but effusions uncommon
Nontoxic liquid material	Mixed (alveolar or interstitial) parenchymal infiltrate much more common than alveolar infiltrate alone (interstitial infiltrate uncommon) Atelectasis and effusion occasionally noted
Foreign body or particulate material	If radio-opaque: primary localization If nonradio-opaque: secondary localization by air trapping, mediastinal shift, or lobar hyperinflation Possible inflammatory response with particulate matter (especially plant matter and nuts) or superimposed infection
Bacterial pneumonia or lung abscess	Consolidation of involved lobe Cavitation with or without air-fluid level within parenchymal consolidation

Adapted from Newman GE, Effman EL, and Putman CE: *Curr Probl Diagn Radiol* 1982.

In gastric acid aspiration both the volume and the pH (typically less than 2.4)[15] of the aspirate are of significance in determining the extent of pulmonary damage.[5] This discussion focuses on acute gastric acid aspiration and hydrocarbon aspiration because the other toxic aspirations are uncommon.

The onset of respiratory distress usually follows gastric content aspiration within a few minutes to less than 1 hour.[2,5] These clinical findings frequently include fever, tachycardia, diffuse rales, wheezes and rhonchi, and serious hypoxemia.[2,5] Cough, cyanosis, wheezing, and apnea are present in approximately one third of patients following gastric content aspiration.[2] The clinician must be aware that the predisposing factor for aspiration (e.g., altered mental status) may obscure these clinical findings.

The radiographic findings of acute gastric acid aspiration are variable, with no pathognomonic appearance[1,46,47] (Figs. 11-7 and 11-8). If a chest radiograph is obtained immediately after aspiration, the pulmonary parenchyma occasionally appears normal.[1,46] In studies of patients with gastric content aspiration, over 90% developed pulmonary infiltrates that were visible on the first radiograph.[2,46] Radiographic abnormalities related to aspiration alone rarely occur later than 24 to 36 hours after the aspiration event.[15]

The chest radiograph most commonly demonstrates al-

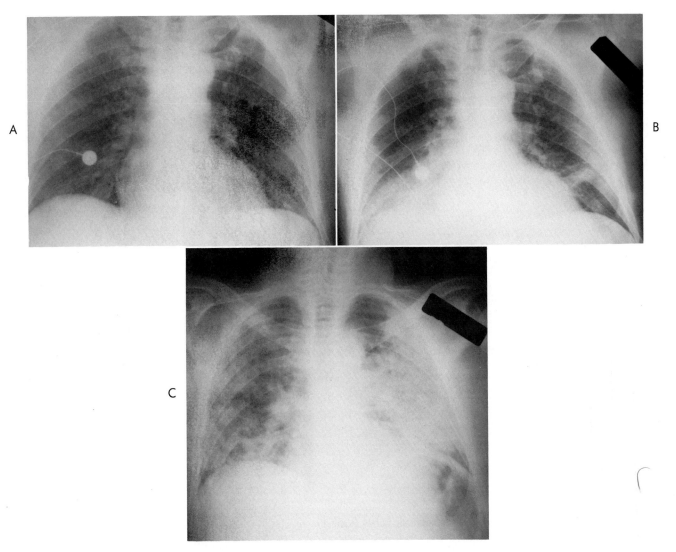

Fig. 11-7. Series of radiographs demonstrating radiographic progression following an acute aspiration. **A,** No significant abnormalities are noted on the initial chest radiograph. **B,** On a radiograph taken 3 days later, the patient has developed segmental and subsegmental atelectasis in the left lower lobe, as well as consolidation in the right lower lobe, representing a combination of atelectasis and aspiration pneumonia. **C,** Chest radiograph obtained 4 days after **B** shows wide-spread nonhomogeneous air-space consolidation. The pattern of noncardiogenic pulmonary edema and pneumonia (adult respiratory distress syndrome [ARDS]) is consistent.

veolar infiltrates in areas affected by the aspiration.[1,2,6,15,48] In a review of radiographic manifestations of aspiration of gastric contents, Landay[46] noted the presence of three major types of indicators for infiltrates: (1) confluent (densities homogeneous enough to outline an air bronchogram), (2) acinar (5 to 6 mm, poorly defined nodules), and (3) small irregular shadows, frequently including indistinct vascular markings. The most frequent indicator of an infiltrate were small irregular shadows. The acinar opacities are only seen at the periphery of a lesion because conflu-

ence occurs in more severely affected areas.[48] Although alveolar infiltrates were the most common in Kross' study[6] (45% of patients had aspirated gastric contents), mixed alveolar and interstitial infiltrates (21%) and interstitial infiltrates (9%) were also seen. If the aspiration is massive, a bilateral "white out" can occur on the chest radiograph[1] as a result of acute noncardiogenic pulmonary edema.

The distribution of infiltrates depends on multiple factors, including patient position, effect of gravity, airflow dynamics, and characteristics of the aspirate.[46] Most fre-

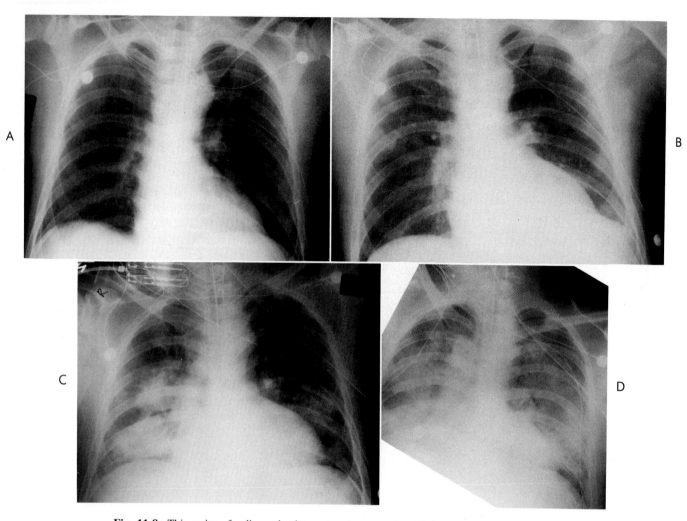

Fig. 11-8. This series of radiographs demonstrates progression of changes following an acute aspiration. **A,** Initial radiograph reveals clear lungs. **B,** Radiograph obtained later that day shows nonhomogeneous asymmetric consolidation in both lower lobes. Consolidation is more extensive on the right than the left. This is compatible with aspiration pneumonia. Patient has had an endotracheal tube placed. **C,** Radiograph obtained 2 days after **B** shows progression of aspiration pneumonia. Distribution of the disease remains unchanged. **D,** Radiograph obtained 1 day after **C** shows bilateral widespread air-space consolidation involving the central two thirds of the lungs, with sparing of the periphery. This pattern is consistent with noncardiogenic pulmonary edema and pneumonia (adult respiratory distress syndrome [ARDS]).

quently, the pattern of distribution is diffuse and bilateral.[2,6,15,46,48] The apices are frequently spared.[48] The most common pattern includes abnormalities in a radial distribution, diminishing with distance from the hilum, and infiltrates, increasing toward the lung bases.[46] Unilateral involvement has been noted in 26% to 45% of cases,[2,6,46] with a preference for the right lung.[6,46] If lateral radiographs are available, posterior and midlung infiltrates are seen most commonly.[46]

Atelectasis is an infrequent finding on initial radiographs; it was found in only 8% of patients in Bynum's study.[2] In Landay's study,[46] major atelectasis was not demonstrated on initial radiographs, although 5% of patients initially demonstrated segmental volume loss and

17% had small linear densities, probably representing minor degrees of platelike atelectasis.[46] Subsequently, 3% of patients developed lobar atelectasis and 17% developed significant segmental or subsegmental atelectasis during their hospitalization. The presence of atelectasis should raise the suspicion of aspiration of particulate matter.[49]

Pleural effusion is rare, occurring in less than 2% of initial chest radiographs.[2,46] Cavitation was not noted to occur from uncomplicated aspiration of gastric contents,[2,46] but, if present, it was suggestive of superimposed bacterial infection.[49]

The alveolar infiltrates associated with aspiration of gastric contents frequently resemble cardiogenic pulmonary edema.[1,6,15,48] The lack of cardiomegaly, the inabil-

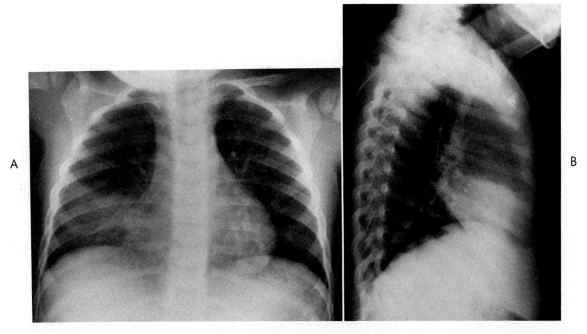

Fig. 11-9. Radiographs of 2-year-old child who ingested about 2 oz of gasoline while playing in the garage. Child subsequently became listless and febrile and was brought to emergency department the next day with respiratory distress. PA (**A**) and lateral (**B**), radiographs demonstrate right middle lobe infiltrate.

ity to demonstrate vascular congestion, and an asymmetric distribution of infiltrates may help to differentiate gastric acid aspiration from left ventricular failure.

Prognostication on the basis of the initial chest radiograph should be avoided.[47] No correlation was noted between the extent or type of initial radiographic abnormality and mortality or duration of illness.[2] Minimal radiographic changes should not be regarded as insignificant.[47]

If the gastric acid aspiration is uncomplicated, radiographic resolution of infiltrates occurs within 2 to 16 days, with a mean of 4½ days.[2] If radiographic clearing has not occurred in less than 7 days, the possibility of bacterial superinfection or chronic aspiration must be considered.[6]

Hydrocarbons. Although the toxicity of hydrocarbons may be manifest in several organ systems, aspiration of hydrocarbons into the lungs is the greatest cause of morbidity and mortality.[50] The chest radiograph is an essential component in the initial evaluation of a patient with hydrocarbon ingestion.

Radiographic changes in hydrocarbon aspiration may be present within 30 minutes after the event, and up to 98% of patients with pulmonary involvement manifest radiographic changes by 12 hours.[51] Radiographic abnormalities correlate poorly with the presence of clinical symptoms.[52] It is not unusual to find radiographic abnormalities in children who are completely asymptomatic and who have normal findings on physical examination[53] (Fig. 11-9).

The initial radiographic abnormalities are fine, punctate, mottled densities that appear in the perihilar region and midlung fields.[51-53] These mottled densities have a tendency to coalesce and to produce a picture of consolidation.[52-54] The radiographic changes most often occur bilaterally[52] and generally involve multiple lobes, although they are typically most severe in the lower lobes.[53,55] Evidence of obstructive emphysema, air trapping, and localized atelectasis may be present.[56] Subsequently, pleural effusions, pneumatoceles, and cysts may form.[56] Radiographic changes are at their maximum by 72 hours and, in the absence of complications, usually clear in 7 to 10 days.[56] Occasionally, a slower course may occur, peaking at 10 days and taking several weeks to resolve.

Nontoxic liquid material

Substances in the category of nontoxic liquid aspirates (nontoxic being a relative term) include water, tube feedings, blood, oropharyngeal secretions, or vomitus with a pH of greater than 3.[14,15] This type of aspiration tends to be more common and more benign than other forms.[15] The response to aspiration depends on the volume of the aspirate and its composition (especially its tonicity) and on the presence of large particles or irritating food material.[36]

The clinical manifestations of liquid nontoxic aspiration are widely variable, and the diagnosis may depend on the exclusion of other forms of aspiration (bacterial, foreign body, or toxic liquid material aspiration).[15] The final diagnosis of a nontoxic liquid aspiration often can be made only after a retrospective review of the patient's clinical and radiographic course.[15]

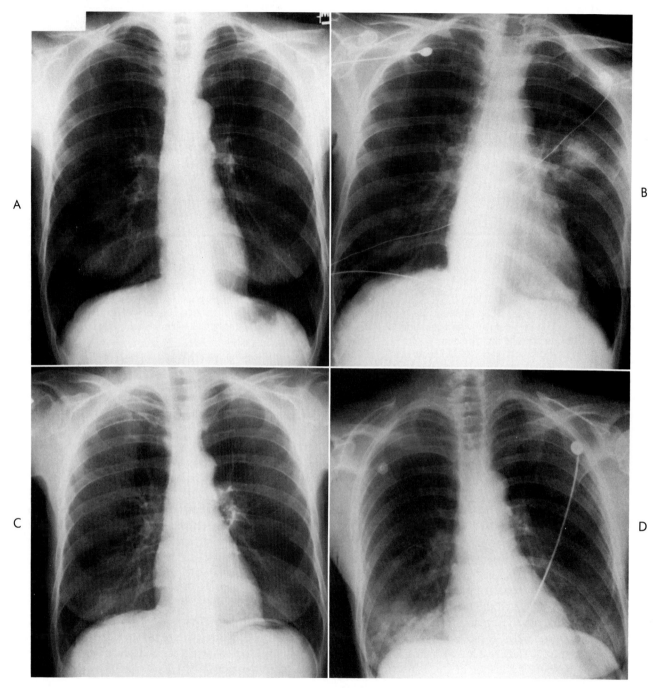

Fig. 11-10. A, Initial radiographic evaluation of a child with onset of repeated episodes of aspiration reveals no significant intrathoracic abnormalities. **B,** Chest radiograph obtained over 1 month later shows segmental consolidation of the superior segment and posterior basal segment of the left lower lobe. **C,** Chest radiograph obtained 4 days after **B** demonstrates resolution of this consolidation. **D,** Chest radiograph taken 1 month after **C** shows new segmental consolidation in the right lower lobe. **E,** Chest radiograph obtained 1 day after **D** shows considerable progression of the right lower lobe consolidation with development of new consolidation in the axillary region of the right upper lobe. There is also some new consolidation in the left lower lobe.

Chest radiographic findings are variable in nontoxic liquid aspiration—ranging from an essentially normal chest radiograph to an alveolar or interstitial pattern and atelectasis[15] (Fig. 11-10). In a study of aspiration of oropharyngeal secretions and food, the predominant radiographic feature was that of a mixed alveolar and interstitial infiltrate, which appeared most commonly in the lower lobes.[6] A shifting bilateral distribution occurred in 82% of these patients.[6] Atelectasis was present in 29% of cases.[6] Radiographic clearing was variable and depended on the chronicity of the aspiration.[6]

Chronic aspiration of nontoxic liquids may result in a superimposed pulmonary infection, with a potential for developing into complications of pulmonary fibrosis and bronchiectasis.[15]

Because nontoxic liquid aspirations frequently are re-

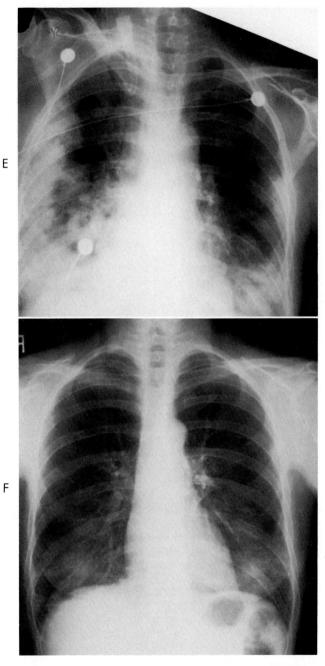

Fig. 11-10, cont'd. F, Chest radiograph obtained 3 days after **E** shows considerable clearing of the consolidation bilaterally, with only residual linear streaking and bronchial wall thickening in the lower lobes. This sequence of radiographic abnormalities is consistent with repeated bouts of aspiration. Note that, throughout the radiographic series, there are calcified left hilar nodes consistent with old granulomatous disease.

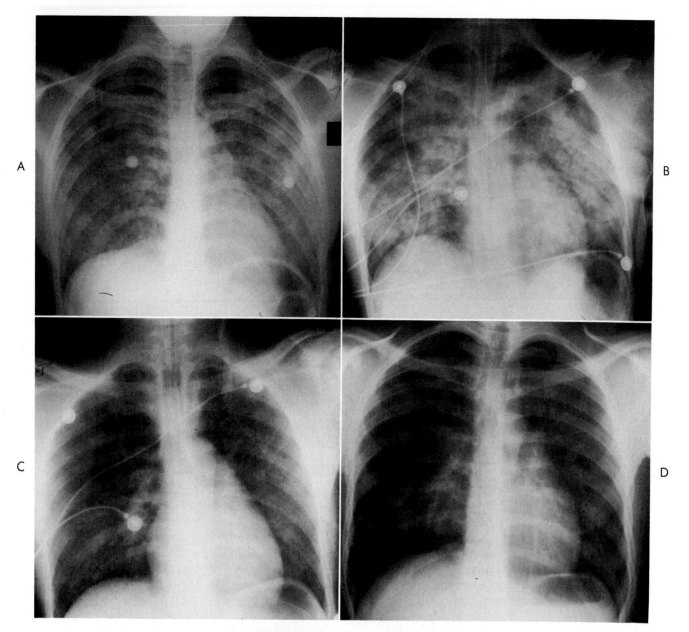

Fig. 11-11. A 22-year-old male presented after a near-drowning episode. **A,** Chest radiograph at 1:30 AM shows diffuse air-space consolidation throughout both lungs with air bronchograms. **B,** At 4 AM on the same day, consolidation has become more extensive and more confluent with relative sparing of the lung periphery. This pattern is characteristic of noncardiogenic pulmonary edema (in this case caused by the near-drowning incident). **C,** Radiograph obtained at 6:10 AM 1 day later shows marked clearing of pulmonary edema. **D,** Radiograph obtained 1 day after C shows some residual perihilar interstitial markings that may represent bronchopneumonia caused by aspiration.

current in nature (Fig. 11-10), consideration must be given to further evaluation, such as cineradiographic analysis of swallowing with neuromuscular disorders or barium esophagogram with esophageal disorders.[15]

In patients who have experienced near-drowning, the radiographic picture usually presents as one of several patterns. Occasionally, a victim of near-drowning may have no demonstrable abnormality on the initial chest radiograph.[57] The clinician must be very cautious in this circumstance because the lack of radiographic signs may be deceptive and by no means excludes significant pulmonary

pathologic states.[57] More commonly, the radiographic findings in near-drowning are those of pulmonary edema[47] (Fig. 11-11)—usually represented by a spectrum of two basic overlapping patterns.[57] In less severe cases, the chest radiograph may demonstrate partially confluent, coarse-to-fine alveolar infiltrates that are localized in the perihilar region with relative sparing of the bases, apices, and lateral lung fields.[57-59] The pattern is usually bilateral and, although often symmetric, may be more accentuated in either lung. This pattern tends to be the most frequent in cases of near-drowning.[57,58]

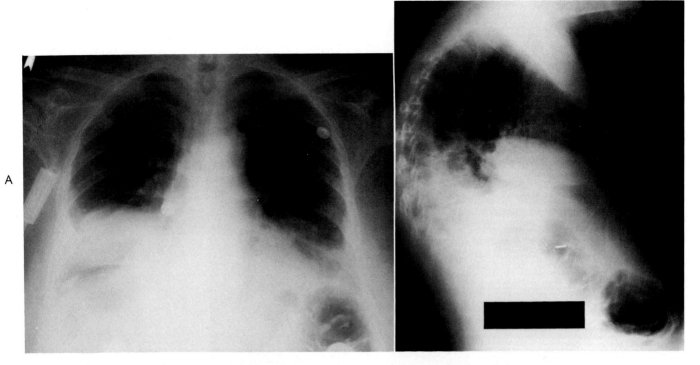

A

Fig. 11-12. PA **(A),** and lateral **(B),** chest radiographs of 69-year-old male demonstrate some confluent segmental consolidation in both lower lobes and in the right middle lobe where the lobe is partially atelectatic and has assumed a rounded contour, simulating a mass within the lobe. There is also a small right pleural effusion. Radiograph is characteristic of lipoid pneumonia from aspiration of mineral oil.

A second pattern is usually present in more severe cases and consists of a generally fine, confluent nodularity that blends into a homogeneous near total opacification of the entire lung field with little or no areas of relative sparing.[57,58]

Most survivors of near-drowning have significant clearing of the lung fields in 3 to 5 days, with complete radiographic resolution of infiltrates in 7 to 10 days.[57] If infiltrates persist for longer than 10 days, superimposed bacterial pneumonia must be considered.[57]

Lipoid pneumonia may result from the ingestion and subsequent inhalation of lipid materials (Fig. 11-12). Deposition of exogenous oil within the lung parenchyma produces varying degrees of tissue reaction, depending on the nature of the oily substance.[47] The majority of neutral vegetable oils are removed from the lung by mucociliary action and cough and result in little tissue reaction.[47] Animal fats, however, are rapidly hydrolyzed, and the resulting free fatty acids produce necrosis and subsequent fibrosis.[60] Mineral oil is the most common lipid aspirated by adults.[61]

Early in the course of lipoid pneumonia, the aspirated oil fills the small air spaces and produces an acinar or primary lobular pattern of air-space consolidation, appearing as small rosettes of no more than 6 mm in diameter on the radiograph.[62] If pulmonary involvement is more extensive, this pattern should be searched for at the margins of the process.[62] The oil is subsequently transported into the in-

terstitium by macrophages, which eventually break down, releasing the oil into the interstitium. This gradually results in the development of an interstitial radiographic pattern[61] with streaky and nodular infiltrates.[62] Fibrosis follows, with contraction and granuloma formation[62] producing a mass-like radiographic density[47] (Fig. 11-12). This process usually occurs in the lower lobes, and radiographic findings are out of proportion to the clinical manifestations of the process.[62,63] The end stage of lipoid pneumonia is frequently misdiagnosed as a bronchogenic carcinoma.[60,61] The diagnosis of lipoid pneumonia is confirmed by the finding of lipid-laden macrophages in the sputum.[62]

Computed tomography (CT scan) has been used to establish the diagnosis of lipoid pneumonia through detection of attenuation values of fat densities in pulmonary infiltrates.[64]

Foreign body or particulate material

The clinical manifestations of aspirated foreign material vary with the size of the aspirated substance. An object that is large enough to occlude the upper airway usually presents as an acute airway obstruction with signs of acute asphyxia.[14,15] Smaller objects are able to reach a more distal bronchus and may result in either complete or partial obstruction of the peripheral airway[5,14] (see Figs. 11-3 and 11-13). Patients who have aspirated foreign material tend

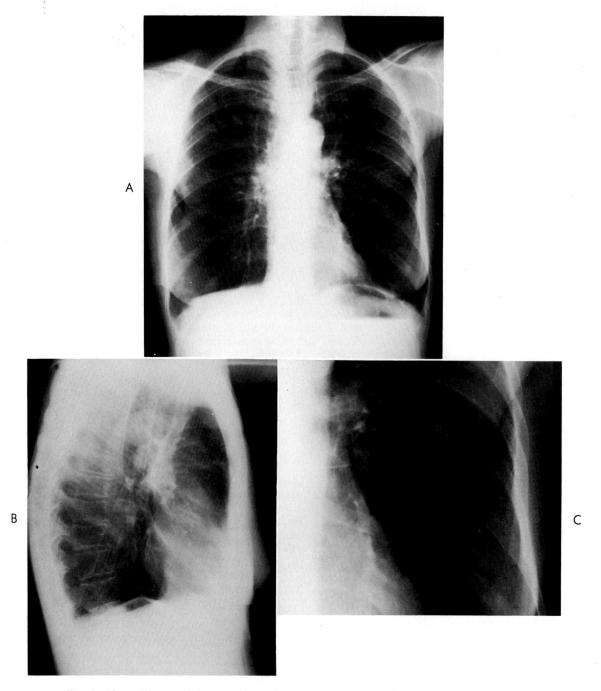

Fig. 11-13. A 63-year-old female with emphysema. Initial radiographs (**A** and **B**) with a coned-down view of the left hilar region (**C**) show patency of the central bronchi. Patient presented a month later after sustaining facial and dental trauma in an altercation.

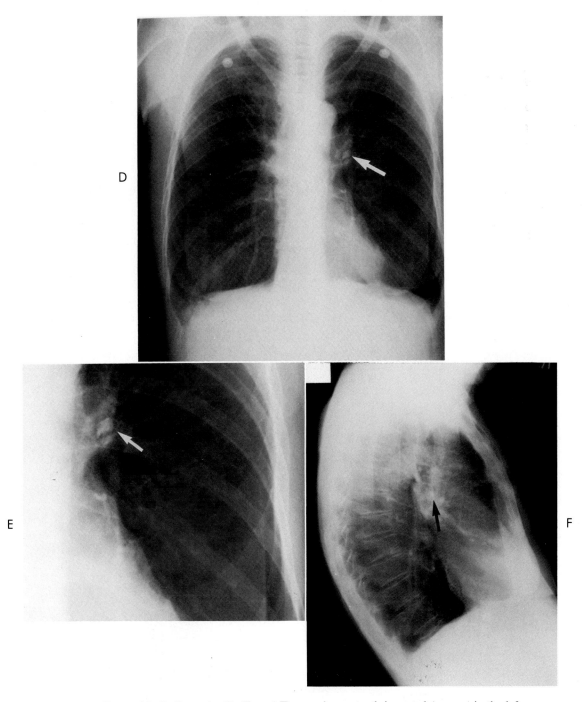

Fig. 11-13, cont'd. Radiographs (**D, E,** and **F**) now show a tooth impacted *(arrows)* in the left upper lobe bronchus.   *Continued.*

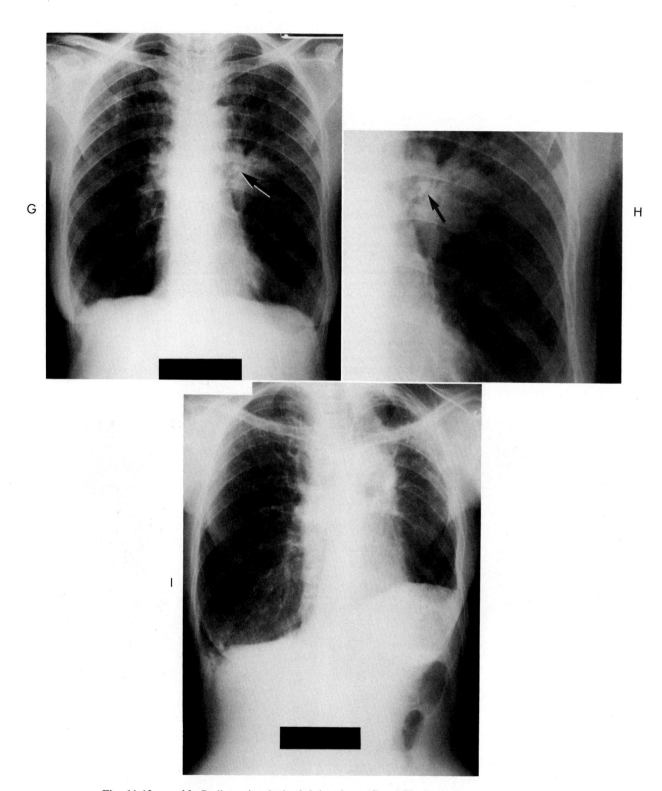

Fig. 11-13, cont'd. Radiographs obtained 6 days later (**G** and **H**) show obstructive pneumonitis secondary to impacted tooth *(arrows)* in the anterior segment of the left upper lobe. Radiograph obtained 4 months later (**I**) is a post-operative examination performed after left upper lobectomy.

to present in two distinct phases: (1) early, with evidence of airway obstruction or inflammation or (2) late, with bacterial complications caused by the foreign material.[14] A history documenting aspiration may be absent.[15] This type of aspiration is much more common in the pediatric than the adult population.[15] The most common material aspirated tends to be of organic origin (especially nuts and seeds), followed in frequency by a wide variety of inorganic material (such as needles, pins, tacks, can pull-tops, and plastic objects).[47]

The pulmonary reaction to aspirated material depends on several factors: its chemical composition; the size and shape of the particle; whether it can be removed by cough, phagocytosis, or disintegration[36,47]; and the presence and extent of injury directly produced to the mucous membrane.[65]

Vegetable particles tend to produce a much more rapid and intense response in the peripheral airway than do such inert materials as metal, teeth, and bone.[47] Commonly, the vegetable material produces prompt inflammatory changes, bronchial mucosal edema, and obstruction.[47] Aspirated vegetable particles have been noted to result in diffuse miliary nodules on chest radiographs, simulating other granulomatous disorders.[66]

Many authors note a predilection for foreign bodies to lodge in the right bronchial tree.[67-70] Several pediatric studies have noted a similar frequency in the distribution of foreign bodies between the right and left bronchial tree.[71,72]

Most radio-opaque foreign bodies are readily apparent on a standard chest radiograph[15,70] (see Figs. 11-3 and 11-13). Unfortunately, most foreign material aspirated is of tissue density (isodense) and is neither radio-opaque nor radiolucent.[67,72] In the case of such a foreign body, indirect evidence of its presence must be sought.[15]

The most common radiographic finding is that of hyperinflation that is distal to the partially obstructing foreign body and is produced by air trapping[67,70-72] (Fig. 11-14). This is manifested on the chest radiograph as a highly radiolucent zone of lung, whereas the remaining lung is relatively more radio-opaque.[8] A chest radiograph taken during expiration demonstrates the residual volume of the lungs.[8] In the presence of hyperinflation, resulting from partial bronchial obstruction by foreign material, the expiratory radiograph demonstrates a greater contrast between the radiolucent hyperinflated area and the remainder of the lung, a flattened hemidiaphragm on the affected side, and possibly a mediastinal shift away from the affected side[8]—all of which are signs of air trapping.

In children, hyperinflation may be a subtle finding[70] and timing of an expiratory radiograph may be difficult. Bilateral decubitus chest radiographs can be obtained to facilitate demonstration of hyperinflation. In a normal chest radiograph taken with the patient in the decubitus position,

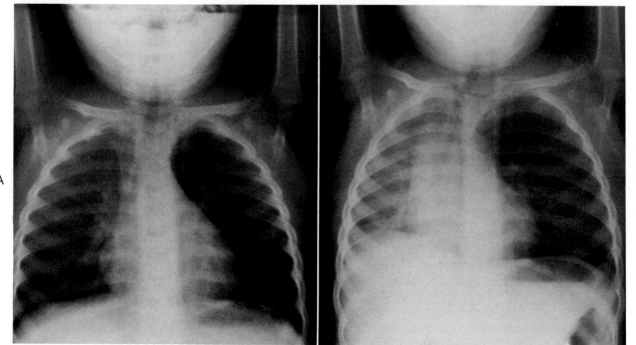

Fig. 11-14. Pediatric patient who aspirated a peanut within the left mainstem bronchus demonstrates classic air trapping on the inspiratory (**A**) and expiratory (**B**) chest radiographs, with hyperinflation of the left lung field exaggerated on expiration.

the dependent lung will have a loss of volume, as compared with the overlying lung.[70] When a partially obstructing foreign body is present on the dependent side, air trapping is demonstrated by the absence of volume loss in the dependent lung on the radiograph.[70]

At fluoroscopy during expiration, this air trapping may be manifested by a mediastinal shift to the opposite side, with immobility or flattening of the hemidiaphragm on the affected side.[65,73]

If the foreign material completely obstructs the bronchial lumen, volume loss will result[65,70] (see Fig. 11-4). Atelectasis is less common than the obstructive emphysema pattern that results from partial obstruction by a foreign body.[67,71,72] With complete atelectasis, there is decreased expansion of the involved hemithorax (see Fig. 11-4), and radiographs may show a shift of the mediastinum toward the involved side (constant on inspiration and expiration),[67] with elevation or depression of the hilum, elevation of the hemidiaphragm,[67] closer approximation of the ribs, and a smaller hemithorax.

Pulmonary infiltrates may occur distal to a foreign body[68,71,73] (see Fig. 11-13). There is nothing specific about pulmonary consolidation that occurs as a result of foreign body obstruction to distinguish it from some other cause.[73] Migratory pulmonary infiltrates have been caused by aspirated foreign bodies.[74]

The chest radiograph may appear normal in at least 20% of cases of endobronchial foreign body aspiration in children.[73] Factors associated with a normal appearance of the chest radiograph include small-sized and nonradioopaque particles.[15] A normal chest radiograph is significantly more common in upper airway enlodgement (above the carina), as compared with lower airway foreign body aspiration.[68] If the foreign body is not removed, complications, including pneumonia (often recurrent), bronchiectasis, lung abscess, empyema, and bronchial stenosis, can occur.[14,67]

Additional radiographs for aspirated foreign body have been suggested. Radionuclide perfusion lung scans may demonstrate diminished uptake in the involved lung,[75] but the finding is not specific.[73] Conventional tomography may be useful.[65] A CT scan, although not recommended routinely in the diagnosis of aspirated foreign body, may be of value in more difficult cases.[76]

Bacterial pneumonia or lung abscess

Two distinct patterns of bacterial infection are seen in individuals who aspirate.[36] In a patient who exhibits signifi-

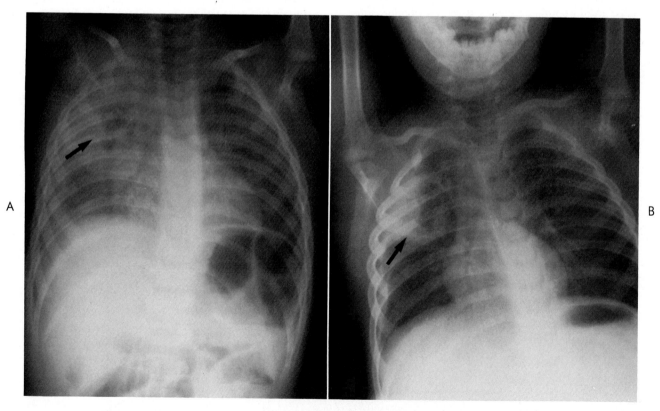

Fig. 11-15. Serial development of lung abscess from a necrotizing pneumonitis secondary to aspiration in a pediatric patient. **A,** Initial chest radiograph demonstrates a diffuse alveolar infiltrate and pleural effusion involving the right lung field with an area of necrotizing pneumonitis in the posterior segment of the right upper lobe *(arrow).* **B,** Chest radiograph 5 days later demonstrates considerable clearing of the pneumonitis and pleural effusion as well as development of a distinct thick-walled abscess cavity *(arrow).*

cant aspiration (usually of gastric contents), the damage done to the lung by the aspirate renders it susceptible to secondary infection. Infection does not play a significant role in the initial stages after gastric content aspiration. The predominant organisms in this type of infection tend to be aerobic rather than anaerobic, with gram-negative organisms such as *Pseudomonas aeruginosa* and gram-positive organisms such as staphylococci being frequent isolates.[2,9,36]

The second pattern of infection is associated with aspiration of a small, heavily infected inoculum such as an oropharyngeal secretion.[15,36] The event may not be evident until signs of infection develop.[36] This type of aspiration is probably the initial focus of infection in patients who develop nonspecific lung abscess, necrotizing pneumonia, or empyema after aspiration.[14,36] Patients with bacterial aspiration may present with an acute bacterial pneumonia with productive cough, fever, or pleuritic chest pain or with a more chronic course of weight loss and anemia.[15] In nonhospitalized patients, anaerobic organisms predominate,[36] whereas in hospitalized patients, facultative anaerobic and aerobic organisms are more common.[36,77] Aspirates grossly contaminated with bacteria (as may occur in bowel obstruction) have been noted to be uniformly fatal.[36,78,79]

The usual anatomic sites for infection are those subject to gravitational flow[14]—the posterior segments of the upper lobes and superior segments of the lower lobes in a recumbent position (see Fig. 11-1) and the basal segments of the lower lobes in an upright position.

Pleuropulmonary infection after aspiration may present with any combination of pneumonia, lung abscess, necrotizing pneumonia, and empyema.[1]

The radiographic appearance of bronchopneumonia—a patchy, confluent alveolar infiltrate—may be difficult to differentiate from the inflammatory changes resulting from gastric acid aspiration.[80] Fever, leukocystosis, and pulmonary infiltrates are common after gastric content aspiration and are not useful in differentiating infection.[10] Clinical parameters that may help differentiate the presence of bacterial pleuropulmonary infection in the setting of aspiration include:[7,10]

- Increasing temperature.
- New or extending pulmonary infiltrates occurring 36 to 48 hours after aspiration.
- Increasing leukocytosis.
- Purulent sputum.
- Confirmatory Gram stain and culture results.
- Unexplained clinical deterioration.

Necrotizing pneumonia usually manifests itself radiographically in a segmental or lobar distribution.[80] Dense pulmonary consolidation may surround multiple cystic areas with fluid levels,[80] indicating the occurrence of lung necrosis. Pleural effusions or empyema commonly accompany necrotizing pneumonia.[80]

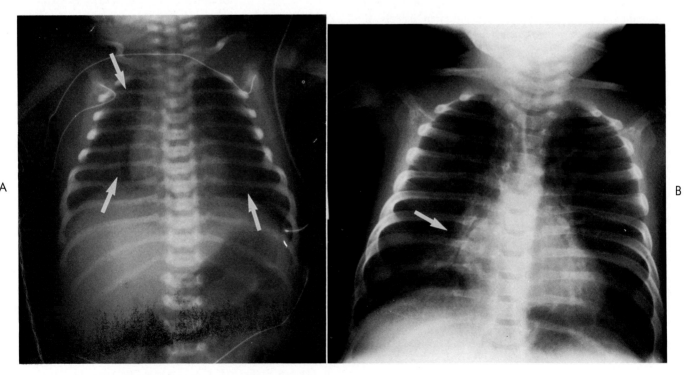

Fig. 11-16. Meconium aspiration in the newborn. **A,** Initial chest radiograph demonstrates patchy infiltrates in the right upper lung field and in both lower lung fields with atelectasia and peripheral hyperinflation *(arrows)*. The patient required high concentrations of oxygen therapy to maintain normal pulmonary function. **B,** Chest radiograph 3 months later demonstrates generalized peripheral hyperinflation and an interstitial infiltrate *(arrow)* in the right middle lobe, indicative of bronchopulmonary dysplasia secondary to oxygen toxicity. (Courtesy Antigoni Kencos, MD.)

The radiographic picture of a lung abscess is that of a thick-walled cavity in a dependent portion of the lung.[80] The outer edge of the abscess may have indistinct margins caused by the inflammation surrounding the cavity.[80] An air-fluid level may be present if the bronchus leading to the cavity is patent and some of the liquid contents of the cavity have been expectorated[15,80] (Fig. 11-15).

PEDIATRIC CONSIDERATIONS

The aspiration of hydrocarbons and foreign bodies in pediatric patients has been discussed previously.

The radiographic changes found in meconium aspiration (Fig. 11-16) in a newborn consist of a moderate-to-marked degree of patchy and or confluent infiltrate.[47] Evidence of air trapping (i.e., depressed diaphragms, intercostal bulging of pulmonary parenchyma, and reduced cardiothoracic ratio) may be seen in more severe cases,[47] but these are not consistently present.[81] Pneumothorax or pneumomediastinum may develop.[47,81] Pleural effusion has been noted in up to 27% of infants, with manifestations of pulmonary consolidation.[81]

SUMMARY

The physician must constantly be aware of the possibility of aspiration, from the viewpoint of prevention, especially in the patient with significant risk factors, and in the differential diagnosis of the multitude of presenting complaints that may have aspiration as a cause. The clinical and radiographic presentations, in addition to aspects of subsequent patient management, are determined by the type of material aspirated. The clinician must recognize the dependent bronchopulmonary segments in various patient body positions and thus the predisposition to development of disease processes resulting from aspiration in these segments.

The authors wish to express their gratitude to Marjorie Glines for preparation of the manuscript and to the Medical Media Service at Veteran's Administration Medical Center, Fresno, California, for their assistance in preparation of the graphics and photographs.

REFERENCES

1. Epstein PE: Aspiration diseases of the lungs. In Fishman AP, ed: *Pulmonary diseases and disorders*, vol 2, ed 2, New York, 1988, McGraw-Hill.
2. Bynum LJ, Pierce AK: Pulmonary aspiration of gastric contents, *Am Rev Respir Dis* 114:1129, 1976.
3. Cameron JL, Mitchell WH, and Zuidema GD: Aspiration pneumonia: clinical outcome following documented aspiration, *Arch Surg* 106:49, 1973.
4. Cameron JL, Zuidema GD: Aspiration pneumonia: magnitude and frequency of the problem, *JAMA* 219:1194, 1972.
5. Jayne HA: Aspiration pneumonia, *Top Emerg Med* 2(2):45, 1980.
6. Kross DE, Effmann EL, and Putman CE: Adult aspiration pneumonia, *Am Fam Physician* 22(1):73, 1980.
7. Murray HW: Pulmonary infection following aspiration, *Emerg Decis* 4(6):10, 1988.
8. Meschan I, Farrer-Meschan RM, ed: Roentgen signs in diagnostic imaging. In *The chest*, ed 2, vol 4, Philadelphia, 1987, WB Saunders.
9. Arms RA, Dines DE, and Tinstman TC: Aspiration pneumonia, *Chest* 65(2):136, 1974.
10. Kirsch CM, Saunders A: Aspiration pneumonia: medical management, *Otolaryngol Clin North Am* 21(4):677, 1988.
11. Bartlett JG: Aspiration pneumonia, *Clin Notes Resp Dis* 18:3, 1980.
12. Gardner AMN: Aspiration of food and vomit, *Q J Med* 27:227, 1958.
13. Amberson JB Jr: Aspiration bronchopneumonia, *Int Clin* 22:126, 1937.
14. Bartlett JG, Gorbach SL: The triple threat of aspiration pneumonia, *Chest* 68(4):560, 1975.
15. Newman GE, Effman EL, and Putman CE: Pulmonary aspiration complexes in adults, *Curr Probl Diagn Radiol* 11(4):1, 1982.
16. Kinni ME, Stout MM: Aspiration pneumonitis: predisposing conditions and prevention, *J Oral Maxillofac Surg* 44(5):378, 1986.
17. Blitzer A: Evaluation and management of chronic aspiration, *NY State J Med* 87(3)154, 1987.
18. Lawes EG, Baskett PJF: Pulmonary aspiration during unsuccessful cardiopulmonary resuscitation, *Intensive Care Med* 13(6):379, 1987.
19. Broe PJ, Toung TJK, and Cameron JL: Aspiration pneumonia, *Surg Clin North Am* 60(6):1551, 1980.
20. Volpe BT, Bradstetter RD: Delayed pneumonia after aspiration of a dashboard fragment, *J Trauma* 25(12):1173, 1985.
21. Aldrich T, Morrison J, and Cesario T: Aspiration after overdose of sedative or hypnotic drugs, *South Med J* 73(4):456, 1980.
22. Horner J et al: Aspiration following stroke: clinical correlates and outcome, *Neurology* 38(9):1359, 1988.
23. Hupp JR, Peterson LJ: Aspiration pneumonitis: etiology, therapy and prevention, *J Oral Surg* 39(6):430, 1981.
24. Andersen N: Changes in intragastric pressure following the administration of suxamethonium, *Br J Anaesth* 34(6):363, 1962.
25. Pontoppidan H, Beecher HK: Progressive loss of protective reflexes in the airway with the advance of age, *JAMA* 174(18):77, 1960.
26. Stewardson RH, Nyhus LM: Pulmonary aspiration, *Arch Surg* 112:1192, 1977.
27. Cogbill TH et al: Acute gastric dilatation after trauma, *J Trauma* 27(10):1113, 1987.
28. Ruggera G, Taylor G: Pulmonary aspiration in anesthesia, *West J Med* 125:411, 1976.
29. Jones B, Gayler BW, and Donner MW: Pharynx and cervical esophagus. In Levine MS, ed: *Radiology of the esophagus*, Philadelphia, 1989, WB Saunders.
30. Barrett NR: Association of esophageal and pulmonary diseases, *Postgrad Med* 36:470, 1964.
31. Anderson HA, Holman CB, and Olsen AM: Pulmonary complications of cardiospasm, *JAMA* 151(8):608, 1953.
32. Newman DE: The radiolucent esophageal foreign body: an often-forgotten cause of respiratory symptoms, *J Pediatr* 92(1):60, 1978.
33. Smith PC, Swischuk LE, and Fagan CJ: An elusive and often unsuspected cause of stridor or pneumonia (the esophageal foreign body), *AJR* 122(1):80, 1974.
34. Laufer I: Motor disorders of the esophagus. In Levine MS, ed: *Radiology of the esophagus*, Philadelphia, 1989, WB Saunders.
35. Crausaz FM, Favez G: Aspiration of solid food particles into lungs of patients with gastroesophageal reflux and chronic bronchial disease, *Chest* 93(2):376, 1988.
36. Wynne JW, Modell JH: Respiratory aspiration of stomach contents, *Ann Intern Med* 87(4):466, 1977.
37. Winterbauer RH et al: Aspirated nasogastric feeding solution detected by glucose strips, *Ann Intern Med* 95(1):67, 1981.
38. Cameron JL, Reynolds J, and Zuidema GD: Aspiration in patients with tracheostomies, *Surg Gynecol Obstet* 136:68, 1973.
39. Bone DK et al: Aspiration pneumonia: prevention of aspiration in patients with tracheostomies, *Ann Thorac Surg* 18(1):30, 1974.
40. Spray SB, Zuidema GD, and Cameron JL: Aspiration pneumonia incidence of aspiration with endotracheal tubes, *Am J Surg* 131(6):701, 1976.

41. Burgess GE III et al: Laryngeal competence after tracheal extubation, *Anesthesiology* 51(1):73, 1979.
42. Conn HO: Hazards attending the use of esophageal tamponade, *N Engl J Med* 259(15):701, 1958.
43. Glauser JM: Balloon tamponade of gastroesophageal varices. in Roberts JR, Hedges JR, eds: *Clinical procedures in emergency medicine,* Philadelphia, 1985, WB Saunders.
44. Mendelson CL: The aspiration of stomach contents into the lungs during obstetric anesthesia, *Am J Obstet Gynelol* 52:191, 1946.
45. Chokshi SK, Asper RF, and Khandheria BK: Aspiration pneumonia: a review, *Am Fam Physician* 33(3):195, 1986.
46. Landay MJ, Christensen EE, and Bynum LJ: Pulmonary manifestations of acute aspiration of gastric contents, *AJR* 131:587, 1978.
47. Berkmen YM: Aspiration and inhalation pneumonias, *Semin Roentgenol* 15(1):73, 1980.
48. Wilkins RA et al: Radiology in Mendelson's syndrome, *Clin Radiol* 27:81, 1976.
49. Woodring JH et al: Pulmonary aspiration of gastric contents, *J Ky Med Assoc* 83(6):299, 1985.
50. Karlson KH Jr: Hydrocarbon poisoning in children, *South Med J* 75(7):839, 1982.
51. Daeschner CW, Blattner RJ, and Collins VP: Hydrocarbon pneumonitis, *Pediatr Clin North Am* 4:243, 1957.
52. Eade NR, Taussig LM, and Marks MI: Hydrocarbon pneumonitis, *Pediatrics* 54(3):351, 1974.
53. Klein BL, Simon JE: Hydrocarbon poisoning, *Pediatr Clin North Am* 33(2):411, 1986.
54. Foley JC et al: Kerosene poisoning in young children, *Radiology* 62(6):817, 1954.
55. Olstad RB, Lord RM: Kerosene intoxication, *Am J Dis Child* 83(4):446, 1952.
56. Victoria MS, Nangia BS: Hydrocarbon poisoning: a review, *Pediatr Emerg Care* 3(3):184, 1987.
57. Hunter TB, Whitehouse WM: Fresh water near-drowning: radiological aspects, *Radiology* 112:51, 1974.
58. Rosenbaum HT, Thompson WL, and Fuller RH: Radiographic pulmonary changes in near-drowning, *Radiology* 83:306, 1964.
59. Putman CE et al: Drowning: another plunge, *AJR* 125(3):543, 1975.
60. Rachappa B, Murthy HSN, and Rogers WF: A case of lipoid pneumonia, *Practitioner* 228(1391):519, 1984.
61. Lipinski JK, Weisbrod GL, and Sanders DE: Exogenous lipoid pneumonitis: pulmonary patterns, *AJR* 136(5):931, 1981.
62. Weill H et al: Early lipoid pneumonia: roentgenologic, anatomic and physiologic characteristics, *Am J Med* 36:370, 1964.
63. Kennedy JD et al: Exogenous lipoid pneumonia, *AJR* 136(6):1145, 1981.
64. Joshi RR, Cholankeril JU: Computed tomography in lipoid pneumonia, *J Comput Assist Tomogr* 9(1):211, 1985.
65. Ribaudo CA, Grace WJ: Pulmonary aspiration, *Am J Med* 50:510, 1971.
66. Kaplan SL et al: Miliary pulmonary nodules due to aspirated vegetable particles, *J Pediatr* 92(3):448, 1978.
67. Aytac A et al: Inhalation of foreign bodies in children: report of 500 cases, *J Thorac Cardiovasc Surg* 74(1):145, 1977.
68. Laks Y, Barzilay Z: Foreign body aspiration in childhood, *Pediatr Emerg Care* 4(2):102, 1988.
69. Bose P, Mikatti NE: Foreign bodies in the respiratory tract: a review of forty-one cases, *Ann R Coll Surg Engl* 63:129, 1981.
70. Salzberg AM, Krummel T: Respiratory foreign bodies, *Top Emerg Med* 4:8, 1982.
71. Keith FM et al: Inhalation of foreign bodies by children: a continuing challenge in management, *Can Med Assoc J* 122:52, 1980.
72. Moazam F, Talbert JL, and Rodgers BM: Foreign bodies in the pediatric tracheobronchial tree, *Clin Pediatr* 22:148, 1983.
73. Reed M: Radiology of airway foreign bodies in children, *J Can Assoc Radiol* 28:111, 1977.
74. Hargis JL, Hiller FC, and Bone RC: Migratory pulmonary infiltrates secondary to aspirated foreign body, *JAMA* 240(22):2469, 1978.
75. Rudavsky AZ, Leonidas JC, and Abramson AL: Lung scanning for the detection of endobronchial foreign bodies in infants and children, *Radiology* 108:629, 1973.
76. Berger PE, Kuhn JP, and Kuhns LR: Computed tomography and the occult tracheobronchial foreign body, *Radiology* 134:133, 1980.
77. Lorber B, Swenson RM: Bacteriology of aspiration pneumonia: a prospective study of community and hospital acquired cases, *Ann Intern Med* 81:329, 1974.
78. Hamelberg W, Bosomworth PP: Aspiration pneumonitis: experimental studies and clinical observations, *Anesth Analg (Cleve)* 43:669, 1964.
79. Vilinskas J, Schweizer RT, and Foster JH: Experimental studies on aspiration of contents of obstructed intestine, *Surg Gynecol Obstet* 135:568, 1972.
80. Epstein PE: Aspiration diseases of the lungs. In Fishman AP, ed: *Pulmonary diseases and disorders,* ed 1, vol 2, New York, 1980, McGraw-Hill.
81. Gooding CA, Gregory GA: Roentgenographic analysis of meconium aspiration of the newborn, *Radiology* 100:131, 1971.

CHAPTER 12

Chest Pain

Richard V. Aghababian
Cynthia B. Umali

Chest pain is a symptom that evokes trepidation in patients and emergency care providers alike. Not surprisingly, chest pain frequently prompts emergency department visits. Since chest pain may be an indicator of an acute and potentially fatal cardiovascular condition, such patients must be given high priority when accessing emergency medical services.

Prehospital care protocols facilitate early intervention. Paramedics start intravenous lines, administer pain medication, and initiate monitoring devices. In the current era of thrombolytic therapy, patients with chest pain are triaged directly to the critical care area of the emergency department while their vital functions are being monitored. Rapid intervention may be life-saving for such patients and, if they survive, may have a profound impact on the quality of their lives. Patients with a clinical history, physical examination, and ECG consistent with life-threatening cardiac or pulmonary disease require emergent radiographic evaluation to narrow down the diagnostic options; concurrent conditions such as thoracic aneurysm may limit subsequent therapeutic alternatives, such as initiating thrombolytic agents.

Many disease processes producing chest pain are not life threatening. These generally involve inflammation of intrathoracic structures or the chest wall. No single piece of data from the patient's history, physical examination, or ancillary testing (ECG) clearly identifies the underlying disease process.[7] In many cases, the objective data available to the clinician are relatively nonspecific, leading to a host of differential considerations. Esophageal reflux may produce a burning or dull substernal discomfort with radiation to the throat that may be indistinguishable from the pain of acute myocardial ischemia.[1,2] Response to trials of antacids or nitroglycerin may be useful but are certainly not diagnostic. Furthermore, both disease processes may co-exist, so responses to therapeutic trials are usually not specific or sensitive sufficiently to confirm a single diagnosis.[8]

In the emergency department, the physician must arrive at a provisional diagnosis of the patient's condition that allows for conservative management while minimizing diagnostic and therapeutic errors. Indeed, some patients may be discharged with life-threatening disease while others with stable conditions will be hospitalized. Errors in diagnosis for patients with chest pain have enormous implications in terms of morbidity and mortality. Consequently, only one third of patients admitted to intensive care units with suspected acute myocardial infarctions are subsequently "ruled-in" by serial ECGs and enzyme determinations.

Retrospective evaluations have demonstrated that a small percentage of patients presenting to the emergency department with chest pain and discharged home actually are experiencing an acute myocardial infarction. Analysis of this latter group of patients reveals that they tend to be younger than typical patients experiencing an acute myocardial infarction, have less typical chest pain, and lack diagnostic findings on the ECG.[3-5]

Each encounter with a patient experiencing chest pain requires diagnostic acumen to acquire and synthesize appropriate historic and physical data before intervention. Radiographic tests often provide critical pieces of data that can influence the clinician's decision.

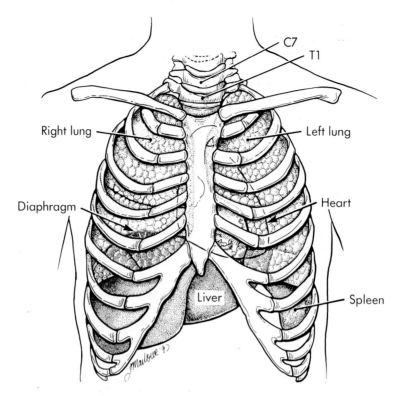

Fig. 12-1. Thoracic cavity and anatomic relationships.

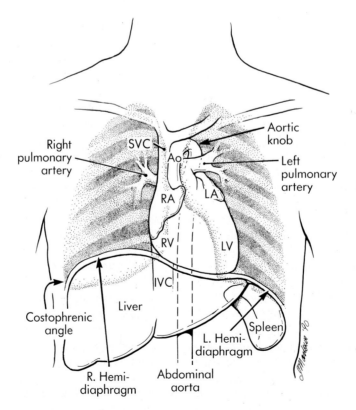

Fig. 12-2. Anatomic outline of radiographic findings. *SVC*, superior vena cava; *Ao*, aorta; *RA*, right auricle; *LA*, left auricle; *RV*, right ventricle; *LV*, left ventricle; *IVC*, inferior vena cava.

ANATOMY

The normal anatomy of the cardiopulmonary system is clearly delineated on chest radiographs. The location of the heart within the thorax can be seen as well as the outline of the chambers of the heart (Figs. 12-1 to 12-3). Abnormalities of pulmonary parenchyma should be evident. In the child, the thymus may be particularly evident, often appearing as a widening of the superior mediastinum, or the "sail sign" (Figs. 12-4 and 12-5).

PATHOPHYSIOLOGY

To understand the nature of pain in the chest and related organs, it helps to understand the nature of the underlying organs and their sensory innervation.

Pulmonary function

Ventilation requires the contraction of the intercostal muscles to allow the chest to expand in diameter and thereby in volume, propelling air into the bronchial tree and ultimately the alveoli. Relaxation of the intercostal muscles permits recoil of the elastic connective tissues in the chest wall and pulmonary tree, resulting in exhalation of air from the alveoli and bronchi. The thoracic volume may be increased by employing the accessory muscles, which can be used to increase the speed of change in thoracic volume.

Oxygen diffuses from the alveoli into pulmonary capillary hemoglobin while CO_2 diffuses in the opposite direction. Since the distance between the alveoli and pulmonary capillaries is small and capillary flow is slow, sufficient

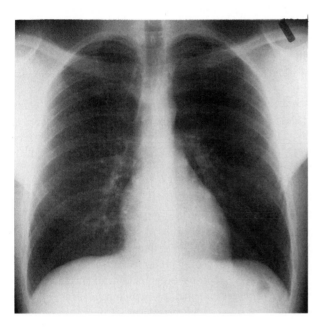

Fig. 12-3. Normal chest radiograph.

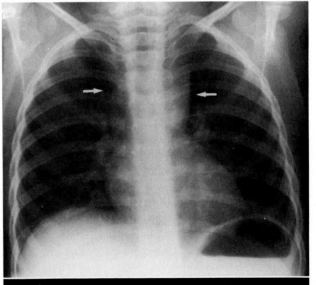

A

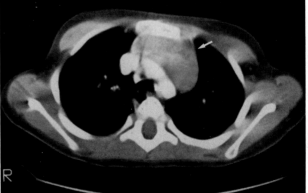

B

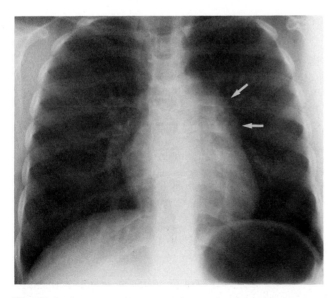

Fig. 12-4. Anterosuperior mediastinal mass secondary to normal thymus in a child. Note lobulated contour of the thymus *(arrows)*.

Fig. 12-5. A, Widened superior mediastinum secondary to thymus tissue *(arrows)*. **B,** CT scan of patient demonstrating normal thymus tissue *(arrow)*.

time is normally available to allow O_2 and CO_2 diffusion to occur.

Pathologic conditions may impair ventilation. Inflammatory processes may involve pulmonary or pleural tissue and produce infiltrates in pulmonary segments or at the lung base resting on the diaphragm. Pulmonary infection can lead to localized consolidation with alveolar damage and destruction. Increased pressure in the pulmonary capillary bed as a result of altered pulmonary flow may lead to pleural effusions and increased interstitial fluid (see Chapter 10).

Cardiac function

Cardiac function supports circulation. The low-pressure right side maintains pulmonary blood flow for gas exchange, propelling blood returning from the venous system. The left-sided high-pressure output provides support for tissue perfusion of organs of the body via the aorta, which loops in the upper thorax before descending through the diaphragm. When the myocardium is damaged by coronary occlusion, perfusion is impaired diffusely with concurrent enlargement of the heart due to muscle injury. Subsequently, poor coronary output leads to increased pulmonary arterial pressure and leakage of plasma into the interstitial and pleural spaces and, potentially, into the alveoli. Organ ischemia, injury, or sudden dilatation may cause chest pain.

Cardiac dilatation or aneurysm formation in the thoracic aorta produce characteristic radiographic changes.

Esophageal function

The esophagus lies behind the trachea in the upper thorax and descends posteriorly in the upper thorax and posteriorly through the diaphragm to the stomach. The lower esophageal sphincter muscle normally controls the direction of food into the stomach and inhibits regurgitation. If the sphincter is dysfunctional, acid gastric contents may reflux into the esophagus producing inflammation; spasm or stricture may result. This may produce blockage of food and esophageal inflammation.

Esophageal inflammation or spasm may cause chest pain. Additionally, pressure of the gastric fundus on the diaphragm may produce discomfort.[1,2]

Sensory innervation

Sensory innervation of the chest helps to explain the nature of some clinical presentations. Pain in the thoracic dermatomes is perceived by afferent sensory fibers of the T1 to T6 posterior spinal roots that form part of the intercostal nerves. The afferent sensory fibers of the T1 to T4 posterior roots are perceived in the T1 and T4 dermatomes. Since the afferent sensory fibers communicate with adjacent fibers from above and below the dermatomes, painful stimuli may be perceived over two to three dermatomes. Fibers from the T5 and T6 and lower thoracic intercostal posterior nerve roots carry afferent sensory information from the lower thoracic wall, diaphrag-

matic pleura, and peripheral portions of the diaphragm (as well as liver, gallbladder, pancreas, duodenum, and stomach). Irritation of the lower pleura may be referred to the lower thorax, lumbar area, and upper abdominal region.

The parietal pleura is supplied with sensory nerves from the intercostal nerves and diaphragm. Inflammation and stretching of the pleura may cause stimulation. Pleural pain often diminishes during expiration or breath-holding and is usually not exacerbated by chest wall pressure.

The presence of inflammatory stimuli and irritation of the visceral organs of the mediastinum contained within the thorax (myocardium, pericardium, aortic and pulmonary vessels, esophagus, lymph nodes, and mediastinal structures) may produce indistinguishable chest pain that will seem similar in quality, located retrosternally, or be poorly localized regardless of the source. The pain may seem to originate in the lower chest and epigastrium.

Afferent fibers from the phrenic nerve, which innervates the central portion of the diaphragm, also receive afferent innervation from the supraclavicular fossa area between the neck and shoulder. The sensory afferents of the phrenic nerve enter the cervical cord primarily at the C3 and C4 posterior nerve roots. Irritation of the central portion of the diaphragm, therefore, can produce poorly localized pain involving the lower thorax, neck, and shoulder simultaneously. Inflammation of organs adjacent to the diaphragm may produce similar pain as well as accumulation of body fluids over the diaphragm.

The pain produced by inflammation of the thoracic organs may be accentuated by coughing, sneezing, deep breathing, or other rapid movements. Chest pain produced by components of the chest wall may occasionally be localized and then reproduced with a cough or deep breath over the chest surface. Visceral pain cannot usually be localized in a similar manner.

CLINICAL EVALUATION

In differentiating pathologic conditions, a systematic approach to data collection must first emphasize a careful history and physical examination and then focus on analysis of ancillary data. Radiographic assessment is often central in patient evaluation.

Patient history

The patient's history should focus on identification of pre-existing conditions, pertinent medical background, and a detailed description of the pain. The latter is probably the most important aspect of assessment. The description of the pain should include:

- Pattern of onset of pain with respect to rapidity and progression; focus on the time from onset to maximum intensity.
- Nature and severity of the pain; sharp, dull, crushing, lancing; relative assessment of severity.
- Consistency of pain: constant or intermittent.
- Reproducibility of pain with deep breathing, movement, pressure, laughing, sneezing, position, meals.

- Exacerbation of pain with motion, coughing, breathing, or sneezing.

Associated findings should be defined, including tachycardia, tachypnea, cyanosis, orthostatic hypotension, palpitations, cough, syncope or near-syncope, dysphagia, hematemesis, melena, recent stress, weight loss, and recurrence of pain.

The patient's past medical history should focus on considerations such as recent physical exertion, known cardiovascular or other systemic disease, ulcer, and cancer. Cardiovascular risk factors, including diabetes mellitus, hyperlipidemia, smoking, family history, obesity, and lack of exercise, should be defined. Current medications and exposures should be noted.

Physical examination

The physical examination provides important clues to the need for immediate stabilization and intervention. Vital signs must be ascertained, assessing for tachycardia, tachypnea, hypotension, abnormal rhythm, differential blood pressure, and jugular venous distention. Cyanosis, pallor, sweating, and capillary perfusion should be assessed while mental status is monitored.

Cardiac evaluation should include notation of jugular venous distention and auscultation for heart sounds, clicks, murmurs, rubs, and gallops. Pulmonary examination should assess breath sounds, with attention to wheezing, rhonchi, rales, asymmetry of breath sounds, crepitus, retractions, asymmetry of the trachea, and distress. The chest should be palpated for areas of focal tenderness. Percussion may be useful in detecting dullness resulting from fluid accumulation.

Abdominal evaluation should look for tenderness, masses, guarding, rebound, hematest positive stool, and specific epigastric discomfort. Peripheral edema, pulses, rashes, and phlebitis should be noted.[6]

Ancillary data may include ECG, electrolytes, cardiac enzymes, liver function tests, amylase, and other relevant studies. Serial ECG and CK-MB isoenzyme determinations are essential in confirming the diagnosis of acute myocardial infarction.

Radiographic assessment is essential. The chest radiograph remains the primary modality; ventilation/perfusion scans, ultrasonography, CT scan, and MRI may be additional techniques that are ancillary in the complete evaluation.

Chest radiograph analysis

A systematic approach to the evaluation of a chest radiograph is essential to avoid missing important findings (see Chapter 10 for a more in-depth discussion of specific entities). Obviously, the radiograph must be technically adequate from the perspective of exposure, symmetry and content, and the inspiratory/expiratory phase.

The emergency physician should systematically evaluate outside structures on the radiograph and then proceed centrally. The radiograph should be evaluated from top to bottom and right to left. Soft tissues of the thorax should be examined for masses, air, calcification, and absence of a structure.

Bones should be assessed for their density. Osteopenia as well as lytic, lucent, blastic, and sclerotic lesions should be sought. There should be evaluation for fractures or dislocations.

The pleura is not generally seen unless it is abnormally thickened, calcified, or outlined by a pneumothorax. Costophrenic angles should remain sharp unless there is an effusion. Decubitus views may be helpful in clarifying the nature of suspected effusions.

The lungs should be symmetrically lucent with increasing lucency from top to bottom. There should be no opacities or densities suggesting a mass, pneumonia, or atelectasis. Air-fluid levels may be present in cavities. Calcifications should be noted.

The vessels of the pulmonary vasculature should be normal in size and without unusual convexities that suggest a mass. There should be a 2:3 ratio in the relative caliber of upper and lower lobe vessels. The arborization or division of the vessels should be smooth. Side-by-side vessels and bronchus on-end should be of equal size. Vessels should not be attenuated; hypovascularity should not be present.

The airway from the nasopharynx (if included) should be patent to the distally visible bronchi. Narrowing may be observed near the glottis and at the point of impression of the aortic knob.

Mediastinal and cardiac silhouettes should be observed for contour, relationships, and size. The anterior mediastinum seen on the lateral view behind the sternum should be lucent and clear. The great vessels and trachea should not be displaced. The area behind the heart and anterior to the vertebrae should not have a mass density. Junction lines and those of the pleural reflection should not be deviated. No air should outline the edges of the mediastinum nor be within the cardiac silhouette.

The diaphragm should be smooth. Although often of equal height, it is not uncommon for the right side to be slightly elevated.

A systematic approach to the evaluation makes identification of abnormalities and differentiation from normal variables easier. Approaching chest pain by diagnostic imaging is outlined in Fig. 12-6. Specific entities referenced in the box on p. 344 are discussed in greater depth in Chapters 5, 10, 11, 24, and 26.

DIFFERENTIAL CONSIDERATIONS

The differential considerations in the patient with chest pain include a host of diagnostic entities that may generally be distinguished using diagnostic imaging techniques. Although the chest radiograph forms the initial basis for decision-making, additional studies may be useful in further clarifying underlying or contributing conditions (see Fig. 12-6).

The box on p. 344 outlines etiologic considerations that must be excluded in evaluating the patient with chest pain.

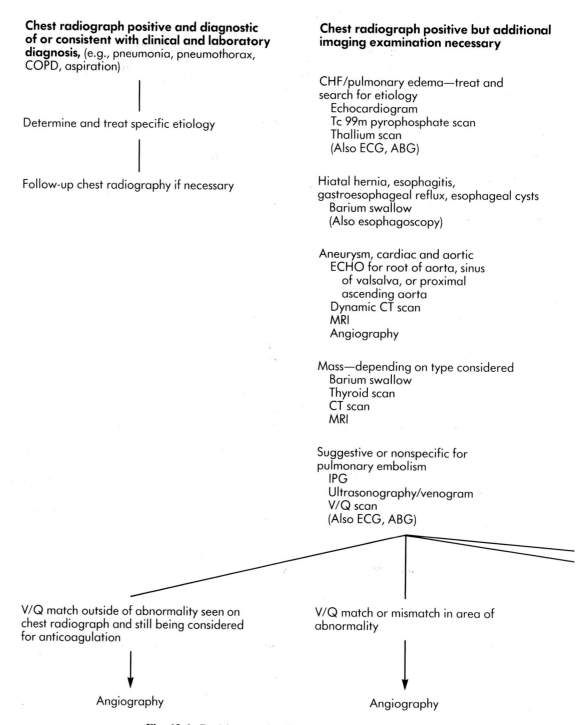

Chest radiograph positive and diagnostic of or consistent with clinical and laboratory diagnosis, (e.g., pneumonia, pneumothorax, COPD, aspiration)

Determine and treat specific etiology

Follow-up chest radiography if necessary

Chest radiograph positive but additional imaging examination necessary

CHF/pulmonary edema—treat and
search for etiology
    Echocardiogram
    Tc 99m pyrophosphate scan
    Thallium scan
    (Also ECG, ABG)

Hiatal hernia, esophagitis,
gastroesophageal reflux, esophageal cysts
    Barium swallow
    (Also esophagoscopy)

Aneurysm, cardiac and aortic
    ECHO for root of aorta, sinus
        of valsalva, or proximal
        ascending aorta
    Dynamic CT scan
    MRI
    Angiography

Mass—depending on type considered
    Barium swallow
    Thyroid scan
    CT scan
    MRI

Suggestive or nonspecific for
pulmonary embolism
    IPG
    Ultrasonography/venogram
    V/Q scan
    (Also ECG, ABG)

V/Q match outside of abnormality seen on chest radiograph and still being considered for anticoagulation

V/Q match or mismatch in area of abnormality

Angiography

Angiography

Fig. 12-6. Decision tree for diagnostic imaging of chest pain.

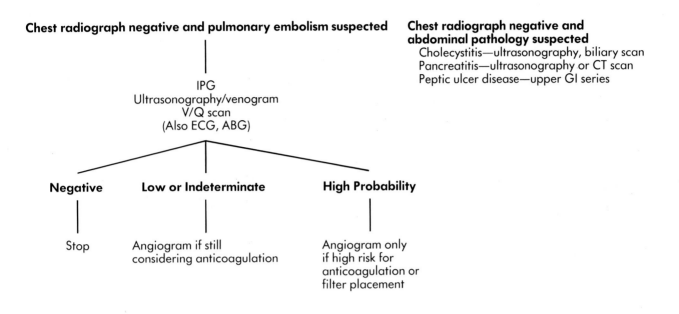

Chest radiograph negative and pulmonary embolism suspected

IPG
Ultrasonography/venogram
V/Q scan
(Also ECG, ABG)

Negative

Stop

Low or Indeterminate

Angiogram if still
considering anticoagulation

High Probability

Angiogram only
if high risk for
anticoagulation or
filter placement

**Chest radiograph negative and
abdominal pathology suspected**
Cholecystitis—ultrasonography, biliary scan
Pancreatitis—ultrasonography or CT scan
Peptic ulcer disease—upper GI series

V/Q mismatch outside area of radiographic
abnormality and high risk for anticoagulation or
candidate for filters, venous occlusion, or embolectomy

Angiography regardless of
V/Q findings

Diffuse abnormality such
as COPD, CHF, pneumonia

Angiography

Fig. 12-6, cont'd.

Chest pain: etiologic considerations

Infectious disease

Pneumonia (Figs. 12-7 to 12-11)
  Etiology
    Bacterial
    Viral
    Fungal: coccidiomycosis, histoplasmosis
    Parasitic: toxoplasmosis, pneumocystis
    Tuberculosis
  Lobar involvement: lobar, segmental, retrocardiac
Abscess (Fig. 12-12)
Aspiration (Fig. 12-13)

Congenital lesions

Deformity of thoracic spine (Fig. 12-14)
Deformity of chest wall
Congenital cyst
Marfan syndrome (rib notching)
Congenital heart lesions
Cystic fibrosis (Fig. 12-15)

Cardiovascular disease

Acute myocardial infarction
Congestive heart failure
Pulmonary edema (cardiac or noncardiac) (Figs. 12-16 and 12-17)
Pulmonary emboli and infarction (Figs. 12-18 and 12-19)
Pericardial tamponade and effusion (Fig. 12-20)
Thoracic aortic dissection and aneurysm (Fig. 12-21)

Pulmonary disease

Chronic obstructive pulmonary disease (COPD) (Figs. 12-22 and 12-23)
Emphysema, asthma, and bronchiectasis
Allergic disease (inflammatory, infiltrate, hypersensitivity)
Pleural effusion (infectious, infarction, reactive) (Fig. 12-24)
Pleuritis
Chronic inflammation and fibrosis

Malignancy

Primary lung, pleura, and mediastinum (Figs. 12-25 to 12-29)
Metastatic (Fig. 12-30)

Collagen/vascular disease

Systemic lupus erythematosus
Ankylosing spondylitis
Rheumatoid arthritis
Myositis
Sarcoidosis

Adult respiratory distress syndrome (ARDS)

Near-drowning (Fig. 12-31)
Prolonged shock state

Gastrointestinal disease

Esophagitis and esophageal reflux (Fig. 12-32)
Hiatal hernia

Miscellaneous

Spontaneous pneumothorax (Figs. 12-31, 12-33, and 12-34)
Osteopenia
Post-operative changes
Foreign bodies: tubes, wires, central lines, pacemakers, prosthetic valves, ingestions

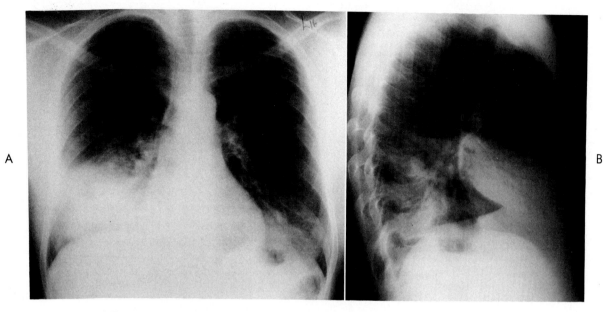

A

B

Fig. 12-7. A, Right middle and left lower lobe posterior segmental pneumonia. **B,** Lateral view. Note air bronchograms in these areas of consolidation.

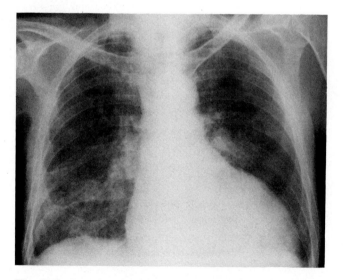

Fig. 12-8. Bronchopneumonia producing linear and patchy densities in the right lower lobe.

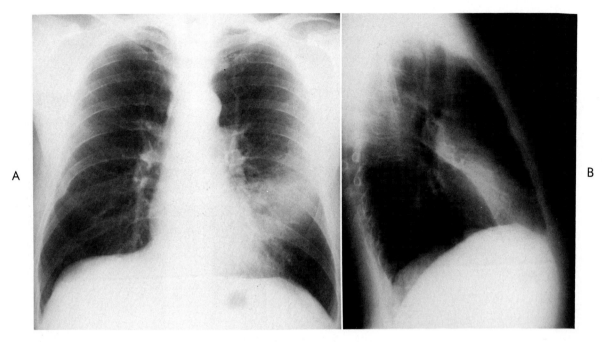

Fig. 12-9. A, Pneumococcal pneumonia involving the lingula. Increased density obliterating a portion of the left heart border. **B,** Lateral view confirms finding with increase in the density of the lingula.

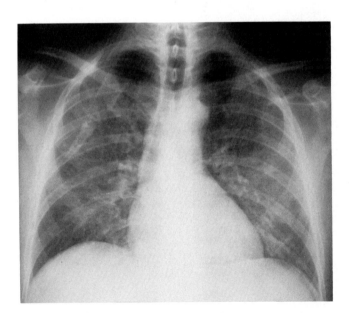

Fig. 12-10. Diffuse, bilateral interstitial infiltrates from *Pneumocystis carinii* pneumonia.

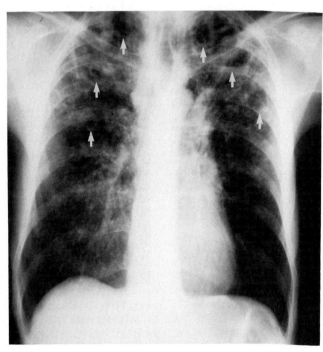

Fig. 12-11. Bilaterally, predominantly upper lobe densities from *Mycobacterium tuberculosis* with cavitation *(arrows)*.

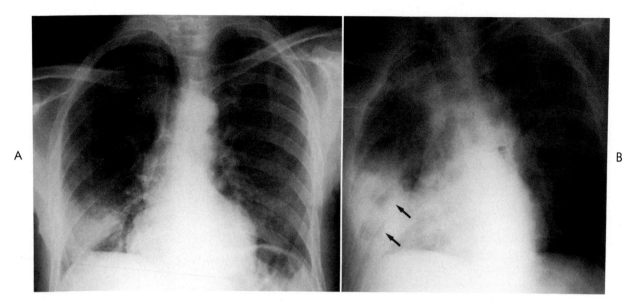

Fig. 12-12. A, Abscess noted by somewhat rounded density in right middle lobe. **B,** Cavitation of abscess demonstrating lucent areas *(arrows)* on follow-up radiograph 3 weeks later.

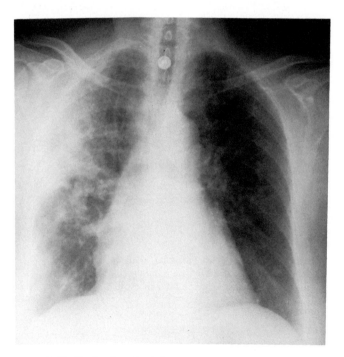

Fig. 12-13. Predominantly right upper lobe densities from aspiration pneumonia.

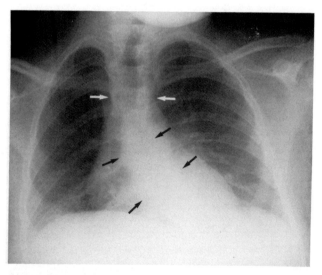

Fig. 12-14. Scoliosis of the dorsal spine *(arrows)* can cause chest pain.

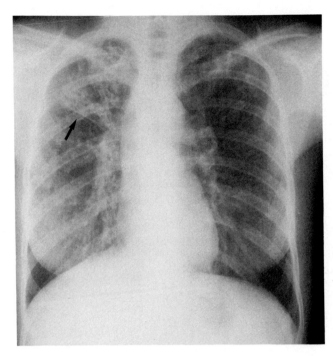

Fig. 12-15. Bilateral interstitial linear cystic and nodular densities accompanying cystic fibrosis. Volume loss is also noted in the right upper lobe with a shift of the minor fissure *(arrow).*

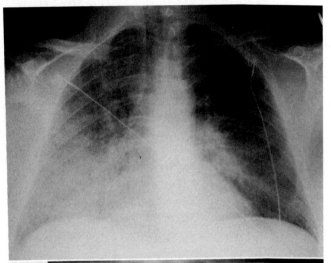

A

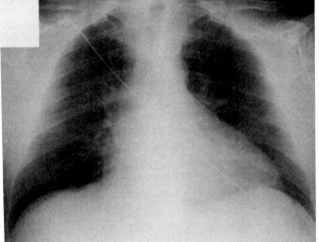

B

Fig. 12-16. A, Bilateral alveolar densities from pulmonary edema, more marked on the right side of the chest. **B,** Clearing of pulmonary edema 12 hours after therapy.

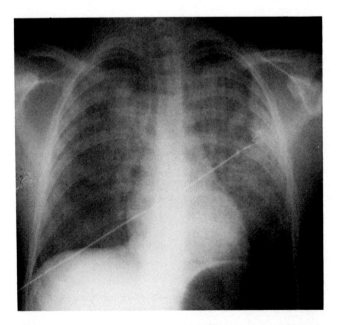

Fig. 12-17. Diffuse bilateral alveolar infiltrates representing pulmonary edema. Normal cardiac size suggests either noncardiac origin or sudden massive myocardial infarction, rupture of papillary muscle, or early adult respiratory distress syndrome (ARDS).

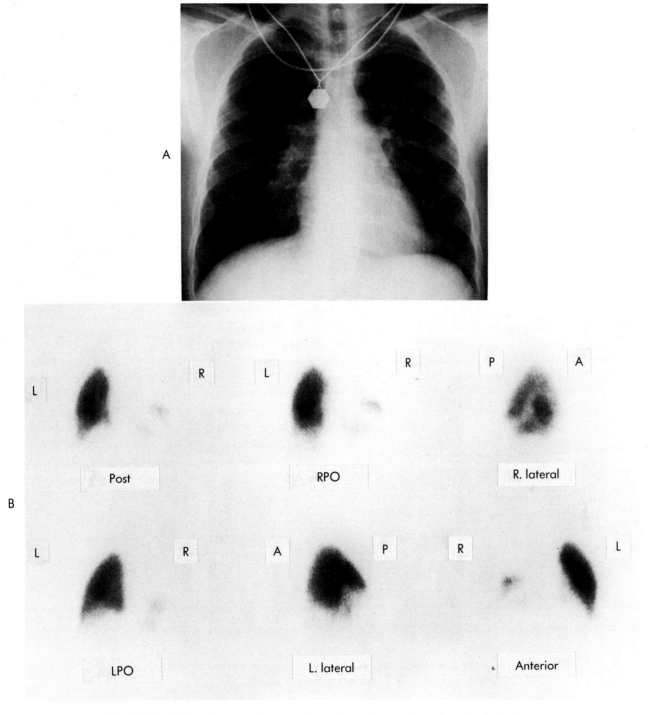

Fig. 12-18. A, Normal chest radiograph in a patient with pleuritic chest pain. **B,** Perfusion scan shows complete absence of perfusion to the right lung resulting from a pulmonary embolism.

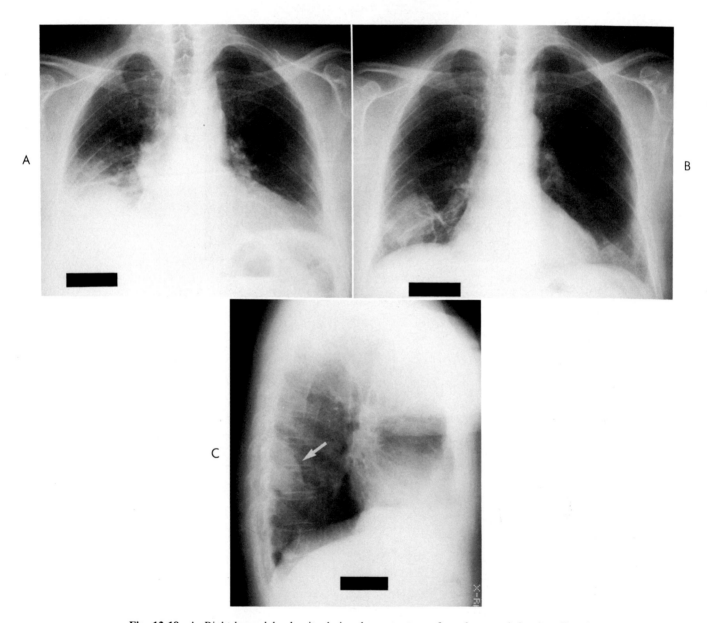

Fig. 12-19. A, Right lower lobe density during the acute stage of a pulmonary infarction. **B** and **C,** Area of infarction *(arrow)* of the right lower lobe 10 days later.

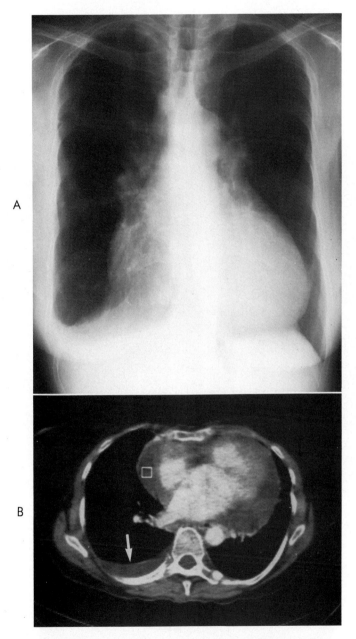

Fig. 12-20. A, Enlargement of cardiac silhouette from pericardial effusion. Note blunted right costophrenic angle. **B,** CT scan shows pericardial effusion *(cursor)* and right effusion *(arrow)*.

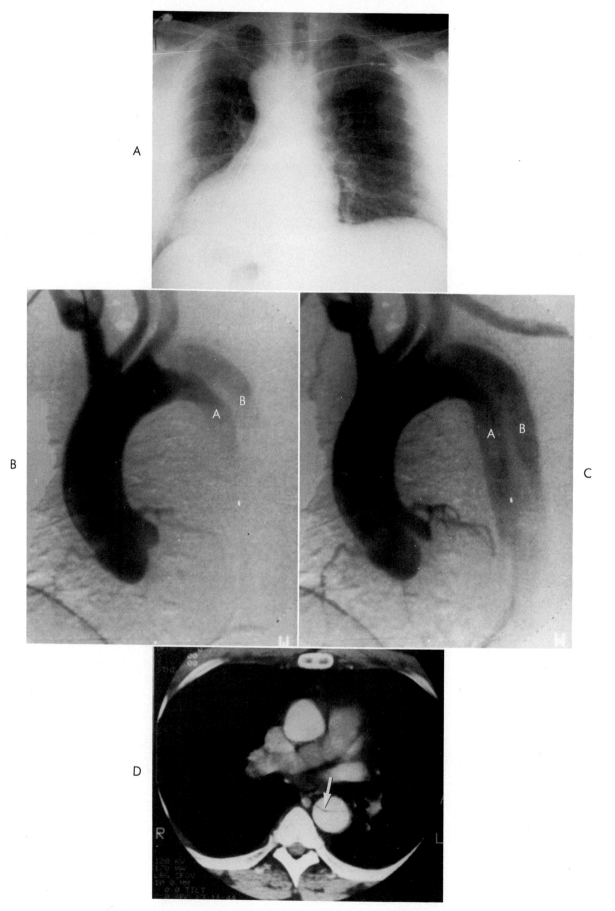

Fig. 12-21. A, PA chest radiograph shows a widened superior mediastinum and slightly prominent aortic knob consistent with a dissecting aortic aneurysm. **B** and **C,** Angiogram shows the true *(A)* and false *(B)* lumen of the dissecting aneurysm. **D,** CT scan shows the flap *(arrow)* between the true and false lumen of the aorta.

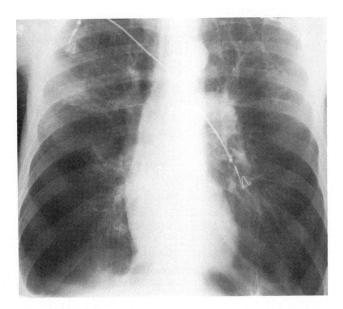

Fig. 12-22. Hyperexpanded lower lobes, crowded bilateral upper lobe vessels, and flattened hemidiaphragms in a patient with chronic obstructive pulmonary disease (COPD).

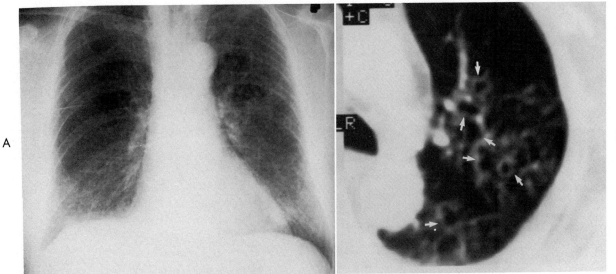

A

B

Fig. 12-23. A, Bilateral basal linear densities, more marked on the left base from bronchiectasis. **B,** CT scan shows the ectatic bronchi *(arrows)* in the left lower lobe.

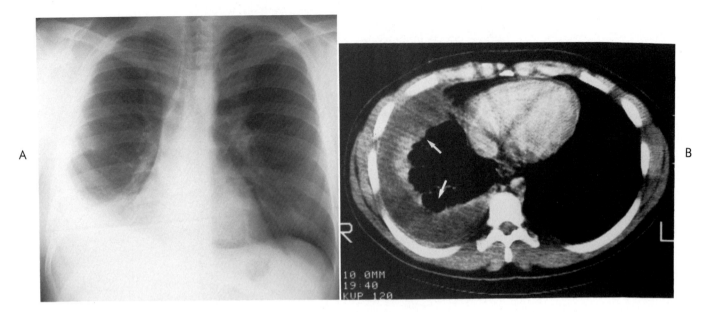

Fig. 12-24. **A,** Blunted right costophrenic angle secondary to pleural effusion. **B,** CT scan showing the right pleural effusion *(arrows)*.

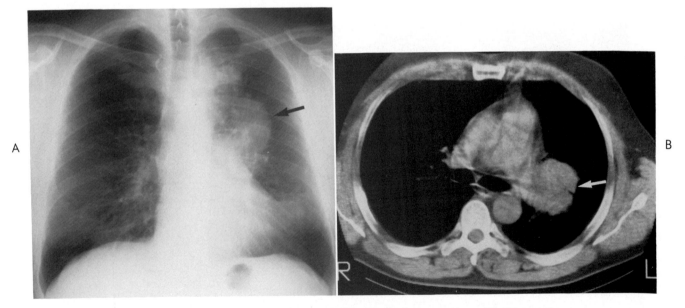

Fig. 12-25. **A,** Left hilar mass *(arrow)* representing bronchogenic carcinoma. **B,** CT scan showing same mass *(arrow)*.

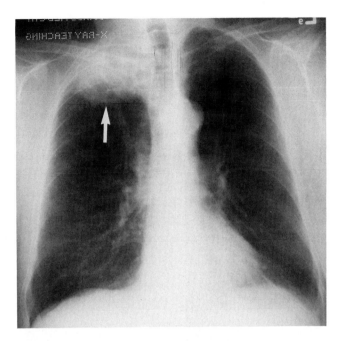

Fig. 12-26. Pancoast tumor *(arrow)* (bronchogenic carcinoma in the right superior sulcus) producing pain.

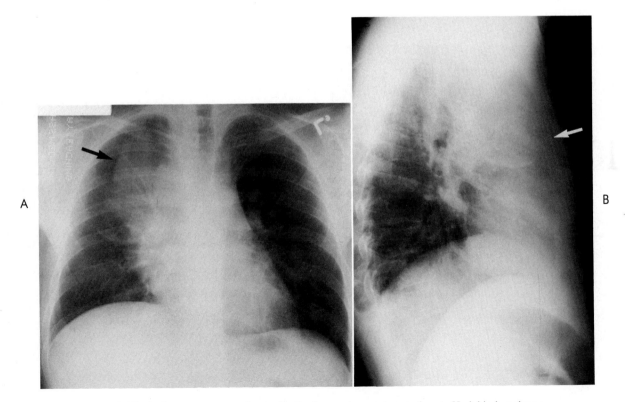

Fig. 12-27. A, Large anterosuperior mediastinal mass *(arrows)* secondary to Hodgkin lymphoma. **B,** Lateral radiograph showing the absence of a normal retrosternal clear space and the presence of a soft tissue density in this area *(arrow).*

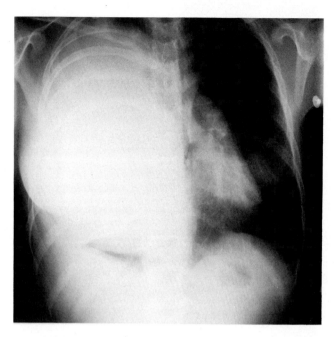

Fig. 12-28. Large mass (Ewing's sarcoma) in the right hemithorax causing splaying and destruction of the ribs.

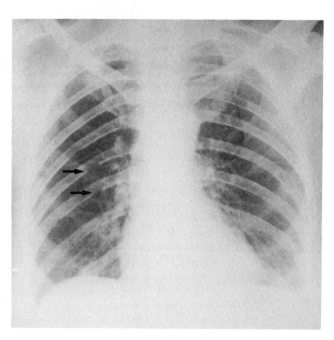

Fig. 12-30. Lytic lesions *(arrows)* secondary to multiple myeloma, causing chest pain.

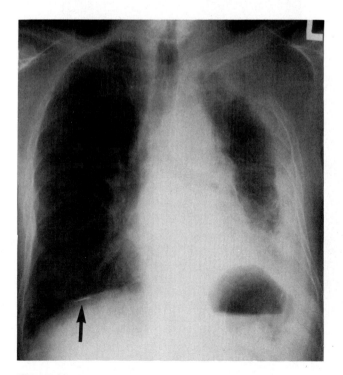

Fig. 12-29. Pleural mesothelioma involving the left side in a patient with asbestos exposure. Note the calcified diaphragmatic plaque on the right *(arrow)*.

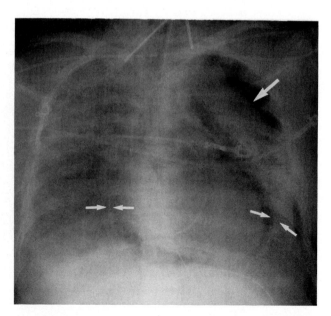

Fig. 12-31. Patient with pneumopericardium. Note pericardium *(small arrows)*, left pneumothorax *(large arrow)*, and parenchymal findings consistent with adult respiratory distress syndrome (ARDS).

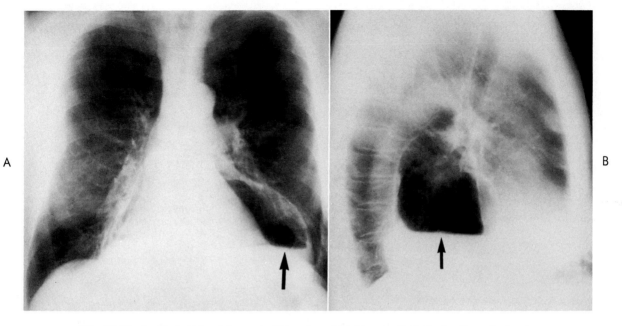

Fig. 12-32. A, Air-fluid level *(arrow)* within a large hiatal hernia. **B,** Lateral radiograph showing the hernia and air-fluid level *(arrow)*.

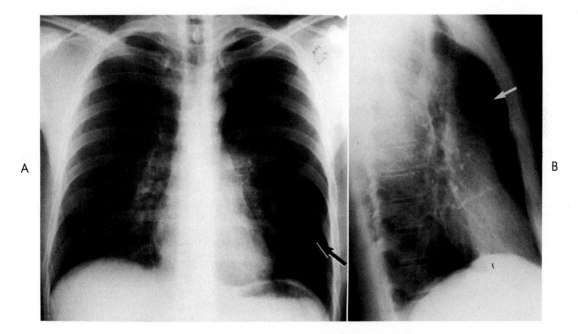

Fig. 12-33. A, More lucent left hemithorax, absence of vascular markings in the upper lung field, and visceral pleura outlined by air on both sides *(arrow)* in the left lung base of a patient with spontaneous pneumothorax. **B,** Lateral radiograph showing visceral pleura outlined by air on both sides *(arrow)*.

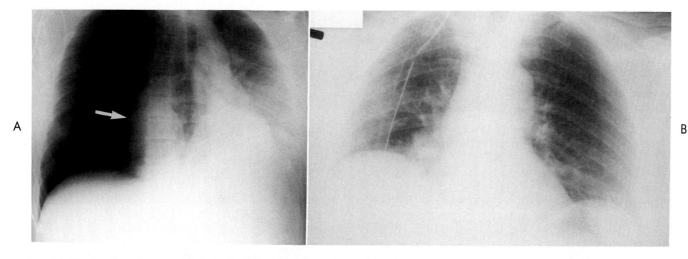

Fig. 12-34. A, Absent lung markings on the right side and a shift of the mediastinum to the opposite side with a collapsed right lung *(arrow)* in a patient with tension pneumothorax. **B,** Complete evacuation of the pneumothorax after placement of a chest tube.

SUMMARY

Chest radiographs in the patient presenting with chest pain are an essential component of patient evaluation. Additional imaging modalities may provide further diagnostic information that can confirm the etiology.

REFERENCES

1. Davies HA, Jones DB, and Rhodes J: Esophageal angina as the cause of chest pain, *JAMA* 248:2274, 1982.
2. Richter JE, Castell DO: Gastroesophageal reflux, *Ann Intern Med* 97:93, 1982.
3. Goldman L et al: A computer-derived protocol to aid in the diagnosis of emergency room patients with acute chest pain, *New Engl J Med* 307:588, 1982.
4. Lee TH, Rown GW, Weisberg MC et al: Clinical characteristics and natural history of patients with acute myocardial infarction sent home from the emergency room, *Am J Cardiol* 60;219, 1987
5. Lee TH et al: Sensitivity of routine clinical criteria for diagnosing myocardial infarction within 24 hours of hospitalization, *Ann Intern Med* 106:181, 1987.
6. DeGowan EL, DeGowan RL: *Diagnostic examination,* ed 2, New York, 1971, MacMillan.
7. Lee TH, Cook F, Weisberg M et al: Acute chest pain in the emergency room: identification and examination of low-risk patients, *Arch Intern Med* 145:65, 1985.
8. Levin HJ: Difficult problems in the diagnosis of chest pain, *Am Heart J* 100:108, 1980.

C H A P T E R *13*

Acute Abdominal Pain

George L. Sternbach
Suzanne Z. Barkin

Plain Radiographs
    Acute appendicitis
    Intestinal obstruction
    Acute cholecystitis
    Pneumoperitoneum
    Pancreatitis
    Ureterolithiasis
    Mesenteric infarction
    Foreign body
    Intussusception
Positional Radiographs
    Pneumoperitoneum
    Intestinal obstruction
    Aortic aneurysm
Ultrasonography
    Aortic aneurysm
    Ectopic pregnancy
    Biliary tract disease
    Urinary obstruction
Radionuclide Scanning
    Hepatobiliary scanning
    Other entities
Computed Tomography
    Aortic aneurysm
    Retroperitoneal hemorrhage
    Mesenteric infarction
    Appendicitis
    Diverticulitis
    Pancreatitis
Barium Enema
    Intussusception
    Appendicitis
    Colonic obstruction
Intravenous Urography
Angiography
    Gastrointestinal bleeding
    Mesenteric infarction
Summary

By far the most important element in the evaluation of the patient with acute abdominal pain or associated dysfunction (e.g., vomiting, abdominal distention) is clinical assessment. History and physical examination will generally provide the most important information regarding severity and likely diagnosis. Although diagnostic radiographic techniques are frequently applied to such cases, they rarely identify the causative problem unless the clinician already possesses a strong notion of the likely diagnosis. It is usually unproductive to order studies in shotgun fashion if nonspecific information has been garnered from the physician's encounter with the patient. The suggested use of plain radiographs and special studies in common acute abdominal problems is presented in Table 13-1.

PLAIN RADIOGRAPHS

Although plain radiographs are frequently ordered in the diagnostic evaluation of the patient with acute abdominal complaints, there are limitations to the information provided by the plain supine and the upright radiograph. Although many clinical entities that cause acute abdominal pain do produce findings that are radiographically discernible, many of these findings are subtle and nonspecific. The radiographic signs indicative of free intraperitoneal fluid are a case in point. Radiographs are not particularly sensitive to small amounts of intraperitoneal hemorrhage. Conversely, when a large enough quantity of intraperitoneal blood is present to produce clear radiographic signs, this information can probably be ascertained by the clinical appearance of the patient.

A diagnosis may, therefore, be supported by radiographic findings, but the clinical evaluation of the patient is often far more important in identifying the cause of abdominal symptoms. Furthermore, radiographic findings may not accurately reflect a disease process, particularly if the study is obtained a relatively short time after the onset of symptoms.

The supine abdominal radiograph studies the area of the abdomen from the diaphragm to the pelvis. The spine,

Table 13-1. Use of plain radiographs and special studies in evaluation of acute abdominal problems

Clinical entity	Supine abdominal radiograph	Postional radiograph	Additional radiographic studies
Leaking abdominal aortic aneurysm	Not routinely indicated	Lateral abdomen (stability permitting)	CT scan or ultrasonography (stability permitting)
Appendicitis	Not routinely indicated	Not indicated	Barium enema in select cases
Cecal volvulus	Frequently diagnostic	Not indicated	Barium enema in select cases
Cholecystitis	Not routinely indicated	Not indicated	Gallbladder ultrasonography
Colonic obstruction	Frequently diagnostic	Upright abdomen	Barium enema
Ectopic pregnancy	Not routinely indicated	Not indicated	Pelvic ultrasonography
Foreign body	Frequently diagnostic	Lateral abdomen in select cases	Not indicated
Intussusception	May suggest diagnosis	Not indicated	Barium enema
Mesenteric infarction	May suggest diagnosis	Not indicated	CT scan
Pancreatitis	Not routinely indicated	Not indicated	CT scan or ultrasonography in select cases
Pneumoperitoneum	Frequently normal	Upright chest or lateral decubitus	Gastrograffin swallow or CT scan in select cases
Retroperitoneal hemorrhage	Not indicated	Not indicated	Abdominal CT scan
Small bowel obstruction	May be diagnostic	Upright or lateral decubitus	Barium small bowel series in select cases
Sigmoid volvulus	Frequently diagnostic	Not indicated	Barium enema in select cases
Ureterolithiasis	May suggest diagnosis	Not indicated	IVP or renal ultrasonography

lower ribs, and portions of the bony pelvis are visible as are the borders of the kidneys, the psoas muscles (Fig. 13-1), and the posterior margins of the liver and spleen (although the spleen cannot be visualized in about one half of the cases). The pattern of intraluminal gastrointestinal gas is always of interest. There is normally a small amount of gas in the stomach and a variable quantity in the colon. The presence of a small amount of gas irregularly distributed in the small bowel is a normal finding. Of particular importance in evaluating the gas pattern is identification of a sentinel loop. Although nonspecific, this may be indicative of a localized reflex ileus involving a single loop (or several loops) of small bowel affected by a focal inflammatory process, such as appendicitis, cholecystitis, or pancreatitis (Fig. 13-2).

Acute appendicitis

Appendicitis is a clinical diagnosis, and plain radiographic findings are subtle and so rarely diagnostic that abdominal studies should not be routinely performed. Surgical consultation should be obtained for the patient who is suspected on clinical grounds of having acute appendicitis. Radiography of the abdomen is not necessary in such cases.

However, some findings of acute appendicitis may appear on the plain radiograph. There is frequently a paucity of gas noted in the gastrointestinal tract, the consequence of anorexia, vomiting, and diarrhea. A sentinel loop may be seen in the right lower quadrant. Other plain radiographic findings include lumbar scoliosis with concavity to the right (representing splinting of the psoas and paraspinal muscles), indistinctness of the right psoas margin, air in the appendix, and the presence of a calcified appendicolith in the right lower quadrant or in the pelvis (Fig. 13-3). The presence of an appendicolith virtually confirms the diagnosis of acute appendicitis, but it appears in only 13% of cases and is often preceded or accompanied by diagnostic physical signs.[1]

Intestinal obstruction

Plain radiographs of the abdomen are key to the diagnosis of intestinal obstruction. Although findings diagnostic of this entity can sometimes be identified on the supine radiograph, obtaining an upright view is recommended. If the patient is too ill to tolerate the upright position, a lateral decubitus view should be obtained. Findings of intestinal obstruction are discussed in the section on positional radiographs.

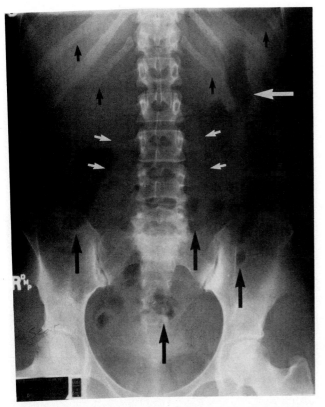

Fig. 13-1. Normal KUB demonstrates a nonspecific bowel gas pattern with gas in the ascending, transverse, and descending colon and in the rectum *(large vertical arrows)* as well as in the stomach *(large horizontal arrow)*. The liver, the spleen, and the kidney shadows *(small vertical arrows)*, the psoas shadows *(small paired arrows)*, and the lower ribs, the lumbar spine, and the bony pelvis are also visualized. (Courtesy Garry Malnar, DO.)

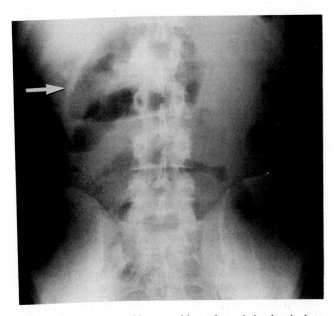

Fig. 13-2. A 38-year old man with perforated duodenal ulcer. Focal ileus (sentinel loop) *(arrow)* is demonstrated.

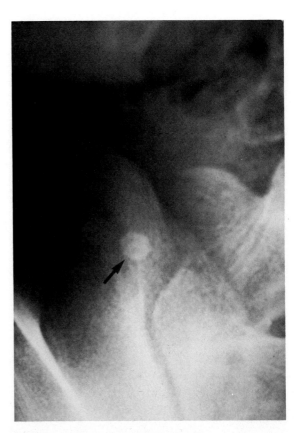

Fig. 13-3. Calcified appendicolith *(arrow)* overlying the pelvis in a patient with acute appendicitis.

Acute cholecystitis

The plain radiograph is normal in most cases of cholecystitis. The most common abnormal finding is the presence of a sentinel loop in the right upper quadrant. Scoliosis with concavity to the right may also be seen. If calcified gallstones are present (Fig. 13-4), these can be identified, but only 15% to 20% of gallstones contain enough calcium to be visible on plain radiographs.[2] Other findings suggestive of acute cholecystitis include an enlarged gallbladder shadow, gallbladder wall calcification, air in the wall of the gallbladder (in emphysematous cholecystitis) or in the biliary tree (with cholecystoenteric fistula).[3]

If acute cholecystitis is suspected, obtaining a plain radiograph of the abdomen will add little to the diagnostic progression of the case. To confirm the diagnosis, either abdominal ultrasonography or hepatobiliary scanning are the imaging studies of choice (see later discussion).

Pneumoperitoneum

Free air within the abdominal cavity is most commonly the result of perforation of the gastrointestinal tract, usually by a gastric or duodenal ulcer. Although pneumoperitoneum produces findings on supine abdominal radio-

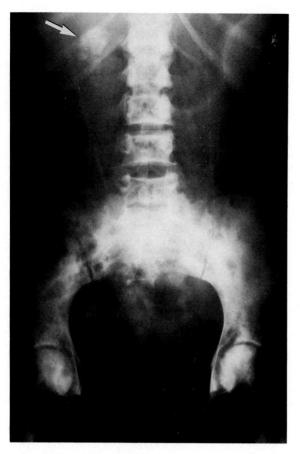

Fig. 13-4. Gallstones *(arrow)* in the right upper quadrant in a patient with sickle cell disease.

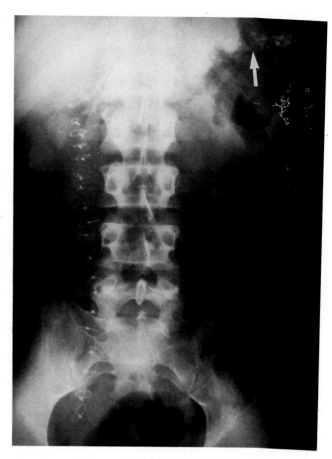

Fig. 13-5. Pancreatic calcifications *(arrow)* visible in the left upper quadrant in a patient with chronic pancreatitis.

graphs, the most expeditious method of identifying free air is by means of positional radiographs (see later discussion).

Pancreatitis

There are a multitude of radiographic findings (Fig. 13-5) associated with acute pancreatitis (sentinel loops, colon cut-off sign, loss of the left psoas margin, left pleural effusion), but these are relatively nonspecific and unlikely to distinguish pancreatitis from other causes of an acute abdomen. The diagnosis is most frequently established by identifying an elevated serum amylase or lipase level in the patient with a compatible clinical picture.

Ureterolithiasis

Most ureteral calculi are radio-opaque, but many are small and may be difficult to identify or to distinguish with certainty from phleboliths, radiodense bowel content, and other calcifications.[4] Although plain radiographs are frequently performed on patients with suspected ureterolithiasis, they usually precede a more definitive study rather than being diagnostic (Fig. 13-6).

Mesenteric infarction

Both the clinical and radiographic pictures of this serious condition are frequently subtle and nonspecific. A normal plain radiograph of the abdomen does not exclude acute mesenteric ischemia. Slightly dilated gas-filled or fluid-filled loops of small bowel are the most common radiographic findings. Early in the course, a paucity of bowel gas may be present. "Thumbprinting" of the intestine, an irregular intestinal contour due to submucosal hemorrhage and edema, is the best known finding but may also be seen in malignancy and a variety of inflammatory diseases. When intestinal necrosis occurs, gas may dissect into the bowel wall or appear in the portal venous system (Fig. 13-7). A CT scan may be done if mesenteric infarction is suspected, and plain radiographs are not diagnostic (see later discussion).

Foreign body

Radio-opaque intraluminal gastrointestinal foreign bodies are often readily apparent on plain radiographs, their configuration varying, depending on the object involved (Fig. 13-8) (see Chapter 24).

Fig. 13-6. A, Scout radiograph of excretory urogram demonstrates right ureteric calculus *(arrow)* at ureterovesical junction. **B,** Radiograph of same patient 2 hours after injection of intravenous contrast material shows partial obstruction of right upper tract and edema around ureteral calculus *(arrow)*.

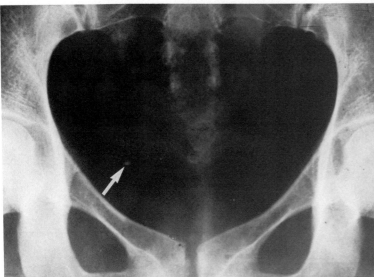

A

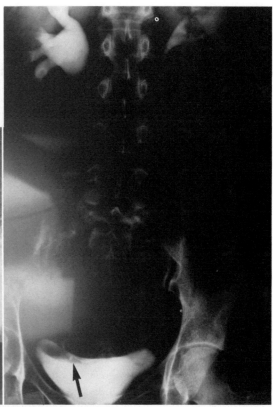

B

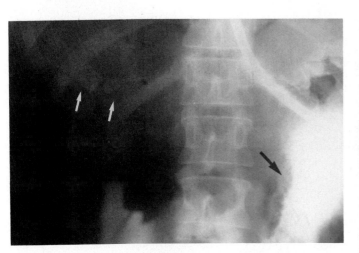

Fig. 13-7. Gas is seen in portal veins *(curved arrows)* and in stomach wall *(single arrow)* of 44-year old man with phlegmanous gastritis (secondary to acid ingestion).

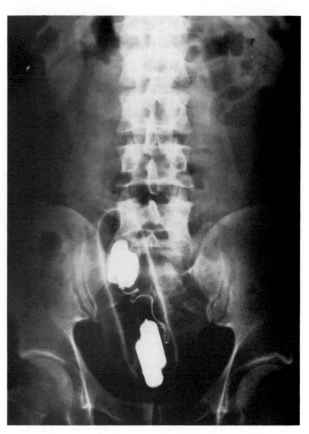

Fig. 13-8. Rectal foreign body.

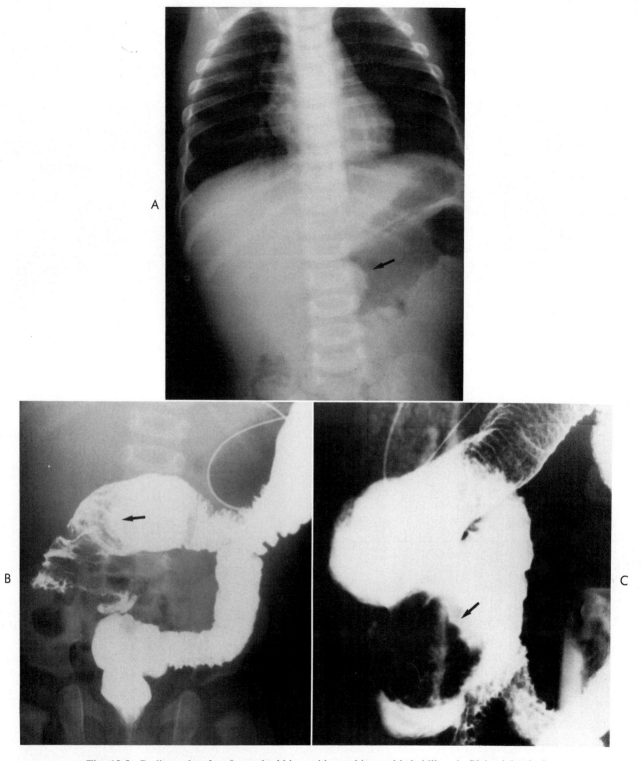

Fig. 13-9. Radiographs of an 8-month old boy with vomiting and irritability. **A,** Plain abdominal radiograph shows a soft tissue density *(arrow)* in the midtransverse colon. An intussusception was noted at surgery. **B,** Same patient. Barium enema shows filling defect in the region of the hepatic flexure *(arrow).* **C,** Barium enema spot radiograph shows filling defect in region of cecum *(arrow).*

Intussusception

Intussusception classically occurs in children 6 months to 2 years of age. Early in the course of intussusception, a normal gas pattern is present on the plain radiograph, although there may be a paucity of gas in the area of the intussusception. Occasionally, the suggestion of a soft tissue mass is identified in the upper or lower right quadrant. When intussusception is present for a prolonged period, the radiographic picture of obstruction is produced. When intussusception is suspected, one should proceed to confirm the diagnosis and simultaneously attempt hydrostatic reduction with a barium enema (Fig. 13-9).

POSITIONAL RADIOGRAPHS

Plain film radiographic demonstration of an abnormal distribution of intraluminal and extraluminal gas or fluid within the abdominal cavity or the presence of intravascular calcification may be extremely useful in defining the cause of abdominal symptoms. Because positional radiographs best demonstrate these findings, their appropriate use is imperative.

Pneumoperitoneum

The upright chest radiograph is the best study for demonstration of pneumoperitoneum and may demonstrate as little as 1 milliliter of air.[5] The upright chest radiograph is

superior to the upright abdominal study because on the upright chest radiograph, the diaphragmatic domes are penetrated tangentially by the x-rays, and the exposure is optimal for depicting small amounts of free intraperitoneal air (Figs. 13-10 and 13-11). Placing the patient in the left lateral decubitus position for a few minutes before the up-

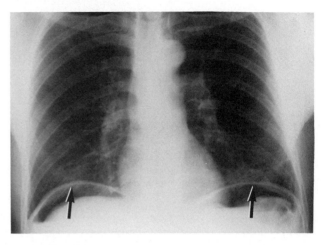

Fig. 13-10. Upright chest radiograph in a patient with a perforated duodenal ulcer (same patient as Fig. 13-2). Free air underlies both hemidiaphragms *(arrows).*

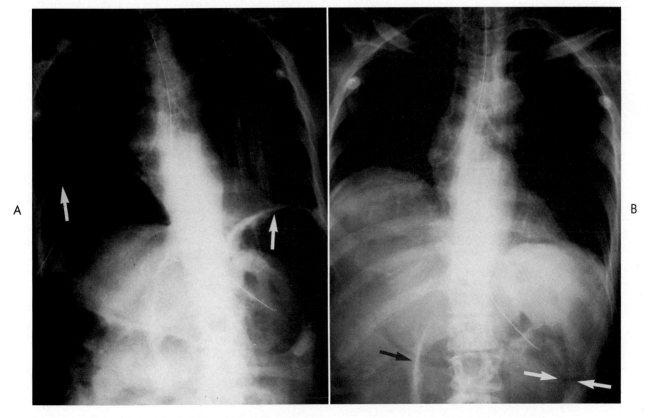

Fig. 13-11. A, Colonic perforation producing massive amount of free air underlying both hemidiaphragms *(arrows).* The study was performed in the upright position. **B,** Same patient with the chest radiograph performed in the supine position. Falciform ligament *(arrow)* is outlined by free air, and the "football sign" of pneumoperitonium is demonstrated *(paired arrows).*

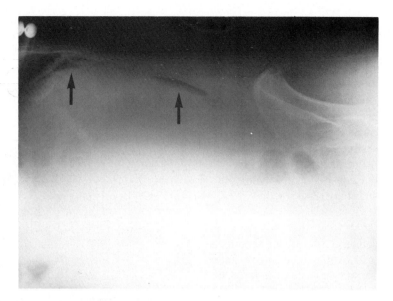

Fig. 13-12. Lateral decubitus radiograph of the abdomen reveals free intraperitoneal air *(arrows)* due to rupture of a colonic diverticulum.

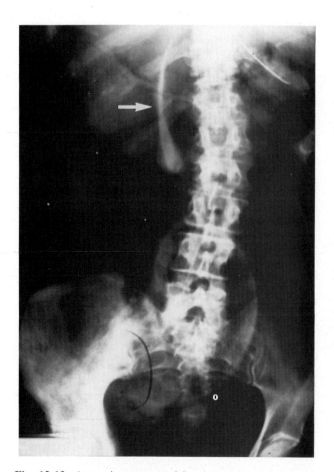

Fig. 13-13. A massive amount of free intraperitoneal air outlining the falciform ligament *(arrow)* of the liver.

right position is assumed permits visualization of the most minute quantities of free intraperitoneal air.[5]

In patients who are too ill to stand, a left lateral decubitus abdominal radiograph may be performed. This will demonstrate free air trapped between the edge of the liver and the lateral abdominal wall (Fig. 13-12). Because it frequently takes as long as 10 minutes for free air to rise to the highest point in the abdomen, patients should optimally be in this position for at least this length of time before the exposure is made.[6]

The presence of free air can sometimes be identified on supine radiographs, but substantially more air must be present than that which can be identified on the upright chest radiograph. Visualization of the outer as well as the inner wall of a loop of bowel (Rigler's sign) is an indication that extraluminal gas is present. Peritoneal reflections on the inner surface of the anterior abdominal wall are normally not seen but may be oulined by the presence of large amounts of free air. The falciform ligament of the liver, the urachus, and the umbilical ligaments can be outlined in this fashion (Fig. 13-13).

Intestinal obstruction

The hallmarks of any intestinal obstruction are the accumulation of gas and fluid above the site of obstruction. Gas-filled loops of bowel are typically dilated and can often readily be seen on the supine radiograph, but air-fluid levels are best visualized on upright or lateral decubitus radiographs (Fig. 13-14).

Distended loops of small bowel can usually be recognized 3 to 5 hours after the onset of small bowel obstruction.[4] Air-fluid levels are characteristically located at different heights in a single loop of small bowel. The location

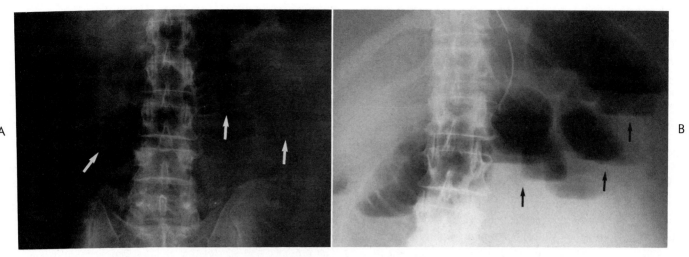

Fig. 13-14. A, Supine radiograph reveals dilated loops of small bowel *(arrows)* secondary to adhesions in 54-year-old man with a small bowel obstruction. **B,** Upright abdominal radiograph shows air-fluid levels *(arrows)* in same patient.

of these loops is generally in the central portion of the abdomen rather than around the periphery. When obstruction is complete, little or no gas will be found in the colon.

When a number of distended loops are present, they tend to lie one above the other in a transverse ladder-like pattern. The outlines of the valvulae conniventes, which completely traverse the diameter of the small bowel, are visible. Small amounts of gas may be caught between the valvulae conniventes to produce a "string of beads" appearance on the supine or upright radiograph.

The radiographic picture of colonic obstruction involves distention of the colon and sometimes the small intestine as well (although the ileocecal valve is usually competent). The colon is typically distended with gas to the level of the obstruction with a paucity of gas distal to this point. The presence of gas in the small bowel depends on the competence of the ileocecal valve. If the valve is competent, little or no gas will be present in the small bowel. In the presence of valvular competence, the cecum may dilate and rupture of the cecum, the weakest portion of the colon, is a hazard. A cecum greater than 9 cm in diameter is considered in danger of imminent perforation.

Volvulus of the sigmoid colon is a form of colonic obstruction in which a redundant loop of colon twists on its mesenteric axis. This appears radiographically as a massively distended loop of bowel emerging from the pelvis, which may reach to the diaphragm and have a "bent inner tube" or beak-like appearance. Fluid levels may be present in this loop on an upright or lateral decubitus radiograph.

In cecal volvulus, the dilated loop is generally located in the epigastrium or the left upper quadrant and has a "kidney bean" shape. Although there is typically little gas in the left colon, there are frequently gas-filled loops of small bowel, which may even obscure the presence of the volvulus itself (Fig. 13-15).

Intestinal obstruction must frequently be distinguished

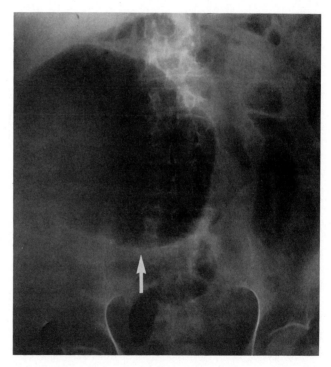

Fig. 13-15. Supine radiograph demonstrates cecal volvulus *(arrow)* in a 66-year-old man.

from adynamic ileus, also known as paralytic ileus. This condition occurs when intestinal peristalsis ceases and accumulation of gas and fluid in the bowel results. Adynamic ileus may be the consequence of an intra-abdominal inflammatory process, such as appendicitis or pancreatitis, trauma, electrolyte imbalance, or a number of other disorders.

The radiographic picture of adynamic ileus is one of generalized distention of the small bowel and colon with gas and fluid. The colon typically displays more distention than the small bowel. Although fluid levels may be seen, they are not as prominent a feature as in mechanical obstruction. An entity known as pseudo-obstruction produces radiographic findings similar to colonic obstruction but without a mechanical cause. Most commonly found in elderly patients with chronic medical illness (such as congestive heart failure, myxedema, or chronic renal failure), pseudo-obstruction may require differentiation from mechanical colonic obstruction by means of a barium enema.

Aortic aneurysm

A frequently used diagnostic technique for the determination of aortic aneurysm is the plain lateral abdominal radiograph. Before the availability of more sophisticated imaging studies, such as ultrasonography and computed tomography (CT scan), the plain radiograph was the initial test of choice for confirming the presence of an aortic aneurysm. Mural aortic calcification outlining the aneurysm may be seen on this radiograph and is sometimes evident on the supine radiograph as well. However, this finding may be absent, subtle, or obscured by the presence of other densities. Twenty percent to 45% of cases fail to demonstrate any diagnostic plain film findings.[7]

When classic physical findings of acute abdominal aortic rupture are present, the diagnosis is evident on clinical grounds and no further diagnostic evaluation is indicated. In such circumstances, consultation should be obtained with a vascular surgeon, and the patient should be stabilized and readied for immediate emergency surgery. Any actions that delay surgical intervention are deleterious and may even prove fatal. If the presentation is atypical and the diagnosis uncertain, steps should be taken to obtain an abdominal ultrasonogram or a CT scan to confirm the diagnosis. A portable lateral abdominal radiograph may be obtained while one of these studies is readied, and, if an aneurysm is identified, the patient should proceed to surgery. If the plain radiograph is negative, the patient should proceed to the more sophisticated diagnostic evaluation. An acute leaking aneurysm should generally be diagnosed by an enhanced CT scan (see discussion following) rather than by angiography, which has little role in the acute setting.[13]

ULTRASONOGRAPHY

Abdominal and pelvic ultrasonography offer many diagnostic applications in the evaluation of selected emergency department patients. There are a number of advantages to ultrasonography: it is noninvasive, does not require use of radiographic contrast material, may be performed as a portable examination in the unstable patient, and there are no contraindications to the performance of ultrasonography in pregnant women, which may be particularly important for the emergency patient in whom the possibility of an early pregnancy may have been overlooked.

There are, however, a number of limitations to the emergency use of ultrasonography. Interpretation may be hindered by technical factors such as patient obesity or the presence of bowel gas. Most emergency physicians are not trained in ultrasonography and consultation with a trained radiologist must be obtained.

Aortic aneurysm

Although the diagnosis of aortic aneurysm may be obvious when classic physical findings of aortic rupture are present, aneurysm as an entity has a quite variable clinical presentation. In instances in which the diagnosis is uncertain, emergency ultrasonography may be of benefit in defining an aneurysm but may not be diagnostic of a leak. Ultrasonography is frequently an integral part of the non-emergency evaluation of the patient with aortic aneurysm. The presence and size of the aneurysm may be delineated ultrasonographically (Fig. 13-16). Adjacent soft tissue fluid collection suggests aneurysmal leakage.

The abdominal CT scan has a number of advantages over ultrasonography in dealing with aneurysm, including the ability to reveal the relationship of the aneurysm to the renal vessels. As a diagnostic entity, the CT scan is superior to ultrasonography in providing information about aortic aneurysm leakage (see discussion following); however, the patient must be removed from the emergency department in order for a CT scan to be performed. This represents a marked disadvantage for patients who are at risk for abrupt clinical deterioration.

Ectopic pregnancy

Pelvic ultrasonography, especially when used in conjunction with sensitive serum pregnancy tests, has markedly altered the diagnostic process for confirming suspected ectopic pregnancy (see Chapter 21). Ultrasonography is indicated in any patient in whom ectopic pregnancy is suspected as a result of clinical evaluation and a positive β-subunit human chorionic gonadotropin (hCG) pregnancy test.

Despite the effectiveness of the combined use of an hCG test and ultrasonography in identifying ectopic pregnancy, some enthusiasm remains for culdocentesis as an initial diagnostic test for ruptured ectopic pregnancy. However, although aspiration of defibrinated blood from the cul-de-sac is suggestive of ruptured ectopic pregnancy, such blood may be from another source. In addition, a dry tap or even a negative aspiration must be considered with caution, as culdocentesis will yield blood in only 65% of cases of unruptured ectopic pregnancy.[8]

Biliary tract disease

Ultrasonography is a valuable diagnostic procedure in evaluating the patient with right upper quadrant abdominal pain. It has become the method of choice for identifying cholelithiasis and has been recommended as the study of choice for cholecystitis when an immediate diagnosis is needed.[9]

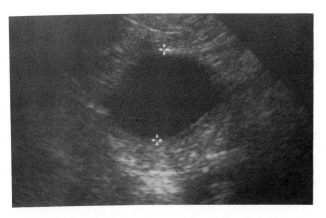

Fig. 13-16. Transverse ultrasonogram of the abdominal aorta just above the umbilicus shows an abdominal aortic aneurysm measuring 6 cm in 85-year-old man presenting with a syncopal episode.

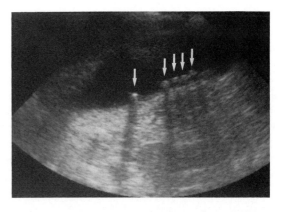

Fig. 13-17. Longitudinal ultrasonogram shows a fluid-filled gallbladder with multiple gallstones *(arrows)* exhibiting acoustic shadowing in 38-year old woman presenting with abdominal pain.

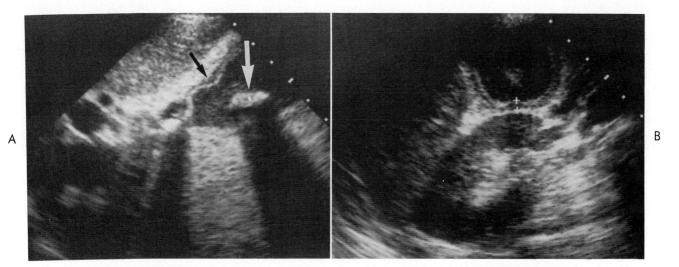

Fig. 13-18. A, Longitudinal ultrasonogram shows a gallstone *(large arrow)* exhibiting acoustic shadowing and a small amount of pericholecystic fluid *(small arrow)* in a 36-year old man with AIDS and abdominal pain. **B,** Transverse ultrasonogram of the same patient reveals a thickened gallbladder wall. The distance between the crosses is 4 mm. Normal is less than or equal to 3 mm.

Ultrasonography is nearly 100% accurate in detecting gallbladder calculi[3] (Fig. 13-17). However, the mere presence of cholelithiasis is not diagnostic of acute cholecystitis, and this is of diagnostic concern for the emergency physician in cases of right upper quadrant abdominal pain. Additional ultrasonographic findings suggestive of cholecystitis are the presence of pericholecystic fluid, wall thickening, distention, and a rounded rather than an oval shape (Fig. 13-18) as well as focal tenderness when the transducer is applied directly over the gallbladder. Although all these findings suggest cholecystitis, none are pathognomonic. Their presence has, however, been shown to demonstrate a pathologic correlation with acute cholecystitis.[10]

Because of the limitations of ultrasonography in diagnosing cholecystitis, scanning with technetium 99m HIDA (hyoponic iminodiacetic acid) has been preferred by some physicians as the initial screening technique for acute cholecystitis. Unlike radionuclide imaging, however, ultrasonography can visualize other structures in the region, such as the liver, pancreas and kidneys, any of which may be the source of abdominal pain. Ultrasonography may be performed at the bedside and is safe for use in pregnancy because the patient is not exposed to ionizing radiation.

Ultrasonography is independent of hepatic function. However, it is highly dependent on the diagnostic skills of the ultrasonographer and radiologist.

Urinary obstruction

Ultrasonography has been shown to be effective in the diagnosis of urinary obstruction due to ureterolithiasis.[11] However, its use in diagnosing this entity remains highly individual, and many clinicians prefer to perform an intravenous pyelogram (IVP). Obstruction is demonstrated ultrasonographically by dilatation of the urinary collecting system (Fig. 13-19). However, such dilatation can occur as a result of causes other than calculous obstruction. Diagnosis of ureterolithiasis on the basis of hydronephrosis is somewhat treacherous; calculi can sometimes be visualized ultrasonographically but this is the exception.

The principal advantage of ultrasonography over intravenous pyelography is that radiographic contrast material need not be used, and adverse contrast reactions can thereby be avoided. Although false positive tests may occur, a normal ultrasonogram virtually excludes the diagnosis of significant urinary tract obstruction.[12]

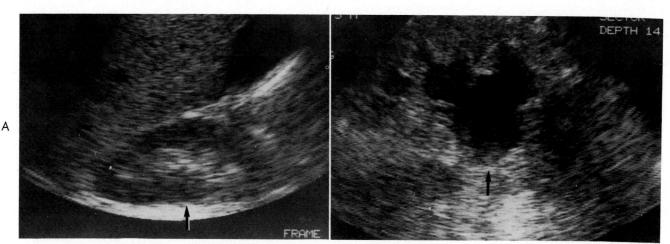

Fig. 13-19. A, Longitudinal ultrasonogram of the right kidney *(arrow)* shows no evidence of hydronephrosis in 75-year-old man. **B,** Longitudinal ultrasonogram of left kidney in same patient demonstrates moderate hydronephrosis *(arrow).*

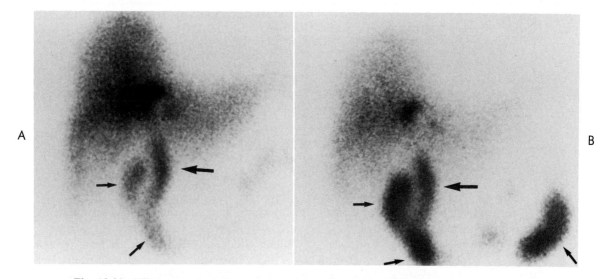

Fig. 13-20. HIDA scan. **A,** At 25 minutes, activity of the radionuclide is seen in the biliary system *(large arrow)* and small bowel *(small arrows).* No activity is seen in the gallbladder. **B,** At 60 minutes, activity of radionuclide is more clearly seen in the common bile duct and small bowel *(arrows).* There is still no activity in the gallbladder. At surgery, acute cholecystitis was found.

RADIONUCLIDE SCANNING
Hepatobiliary scanning

Hepatobiliary scanning involves a study of gallbladder function and has nearly 100% accuracy in identifying acute cholecystitis. Technetium 99m HIDA is taken up in the liver and excreted in the bile. Visualization of the liver, gallbladder, and biliary tree is thereby accomplished. If visualization of the gallbladder within an hour of administration of the radionuclide is accomplished, a diagnosis of acute cholecystitis is virtually excluded, even in acalculous disease.[3] Hepatobiliary scanning has been demonstrated to be 95% to 100% specific and sensitive in diagnosing acute cholecystitis (Fig. 13-20).

Those who favor this diagnostic technique as the initial method of choice point out its simplicity, lack of need for abdominal manipulation, and operator independence of the study. However, radionuclide scanning involves the administration of ionizing radiation, and the study requires from 1 to 4 hours for completion. Utility is limited in the patient with significant pre-existing hepatic dysfunction.

There is considerable controversy regarding whether ultrasonography or radionuclide scanning is the screening procedure of choice in the patient with right upper quadrant pain. The time requirements mitigate strongly against radionuclide scanning as the preferred procedure in the emergency department. Ultrasonography also provides more information about contiguous abdominal organs. Although radionuclide scanning is the more accurate test, the logistics of its application render it less practical for use in the emergency patient. It should be obtained following ultrasonography if the ultrasonogram is nondiagnostic, and there is continued concern about the presence of cholecystitis.

Other entities

Radionuclide scanning is not commonly used in the emergency department for evaluation of other acute abdominal conditions. Although scanning techniques with technetium 99m sulfur colloid and technetium 99m–labelled red blood cells are widely available for localizing gastrointestinal hemorrhage (Fig. 13-21), these studies are generally not the first diagnostic procedures carried out in the emergency department. Scanning with the radionuclides technetium 99m pertechnetate for Meckel diverticulum and indium-111–labelled leukocytes for intra-abdominal abscess are likewise seldom carried out in the emergency department setting (see Chapter 14).

COMPUTED TOMOGRAPHY

The CT scan has gained greater use in the emergency evaluation of patients with certain acute abdominal disorders because of the range of organs that can be visualized with the scan, eliminating the need for more invasive techniques.

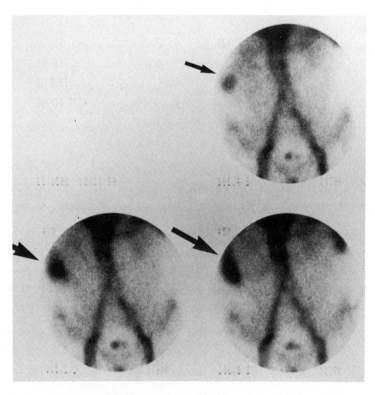

Fig. 13-21. Technetium 99m red blood cell scan demonstrates a focus of active bleeding beginning in the cecum *(small arrow)* and proceeding distally on subsequent scans into the ascending colon *(larger arrows)* in 46-year-old man with melena.

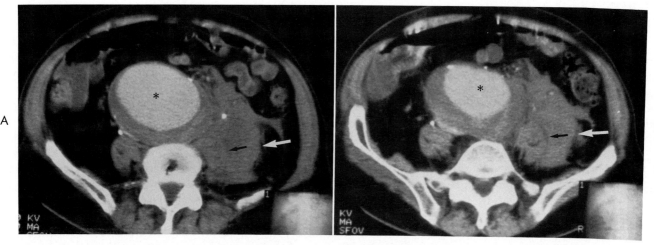

Fig. 13-22. A, CT scan of same patient as in Fig. 13-16. Contrast material is seen in an abdominal aortic aneurysm *(asterisk)*. The soft tissue density to the left *(large arrow)* represents leakage into the retroperitoneum. The left psoas muscle *(small arrow)* can be distinguished from the retroperitoneal hemorrhage. **B,** Same patient, CT scan at a more caudal level.

Aortic aneurysm

The CT scan is highly accurate in defining the presence and size of an abdominal aortic aneurysm. Because it can detect retroperitoneal and perianeurysmal hemorrhage, it is the method of choice for the hemodynamically stable patient with suspected aneurysmal leakage[13] (Fig. 13-22).

Retroperitoneal hemorrhage

The CT scan is probably the diagnostic study of choice when retroperitoneal hemorrhage is being considered. It depicts the presence and extent of hemorrhage occuring in patients with excessive anticoagulation, a bleeding diathesis, or as a consequence of various retroperitoneal tumors.[16]

Mesenteric infarction

The CT scan may be extemely useful in the diagnosis of bowel infarction.[14] The findings on the CT scan indicative of bowel infarction are analogous to those seen on plain radiographs. However, the CT scan is superior to plain radiographs in detecting and localizing abnormal collections of air in the abdomen (portal vein, mesenteric veins, or in the bowel wall), which are the most useful indication of intestinal infarction. Bowel wall thickening, sometimes called "thumbprinting," may also be more readily apparent on the CT scan than on plain radiographs (Fig. 13-23).

Appendicitis

The CT scan findings in acute appendicitis include appendiceal wall thickening, edema of the mesentery, and a pericecal mass. The normal appendix itself may occasionally be visualized.[15] Complications of appendicitis, such as periappendiceal abscess, can be diagnosed by CT scan (Fig. 13-24). Although the CT scan is not indicated in most instances in which appendicitis is being considered, it may be useful in atypical cases.

Diverticulitis

CT scan may be very helpful in confirming diverticulitis. Thickening of the bowel wall and the presence of pericolic inflammation are primary findings.[16] The CT scan may also detect contiguous abscess formation (Fig. 13-25).

Pancreatitis

Pancreatitis is usually diagnosed clinically and biochemically. The CT scan may be useful to show the extent of the disease or to demonstrate complications such as abscess or pseudocyst formation in a patient with a protracted course (Fig. 13-26).

BARIUM ENEMA

Barium enema is rarely used in the emergency evaluation of the patient with abdominal pain, but indications do exist for specific entities.

Intussusception

Barium enema is not only the preferred diagnostic procedure in intussusception (see Fig. 13-9, *B* and *C*) but frequently also is a therapeutic one. A first episode of intussusception can usually be hydrostatically reduced by barium enema, and a first recurrence should likewise be treated.[18] Subsequent recurrences of intussusception may require surgical intervention. Barium enema should be performed early in the course of a suspected case since the longer an intussusception remains untreated, the more difficult a hydrostatic reduction is likely to become. Contraindications to barium enema include the presence of free intraperitoneal air and findings of generalized peritonitis; these indicate that intestinal perforation has occurred. Water-soluble contrast material should be used in infants less than 3 months old and in patients in whom there is increased risk of intestinal perforation (e.g., plain film radiographic evidence of intestinal obstruction).[18]

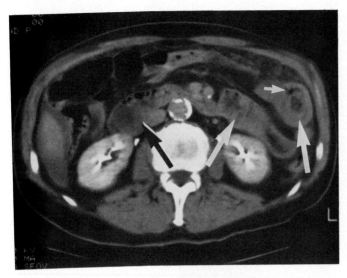

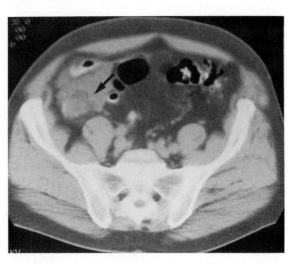

Fig. 13-23. CT scan of mesenteric infarction demonstrates dilated loops of small bowel with markedly thickened walls secondary to submucosal hemorrhage and edema *(large arrow)*. Also note intramural gas within necrotic bowel wall *(small arrows)*. (Courtesy Marylyn Rosencranz, DO.)

Fig. 13-24. CT scan demonstrates pericecal fluid *(arrow)* in 61-year-old man. A periappendiceal abscess was identified at surgery.

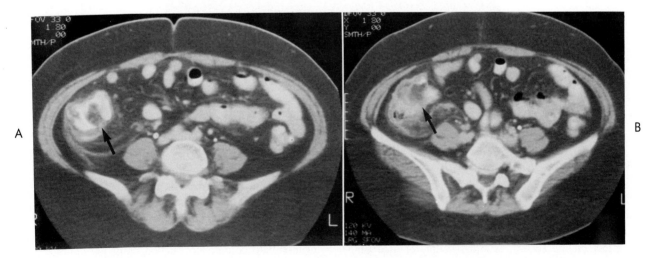

Fig. 13-25. A, CT scan of a 50-year-old woman with blood in the stool, showing a fluid collection in the region of the cecum *(arrow)*. A diverticulum with associated abscess was found at surgery. **B,** CT scan at a more caudal level demonstrates fluid collection in the region of the cecum *(arrow)*.

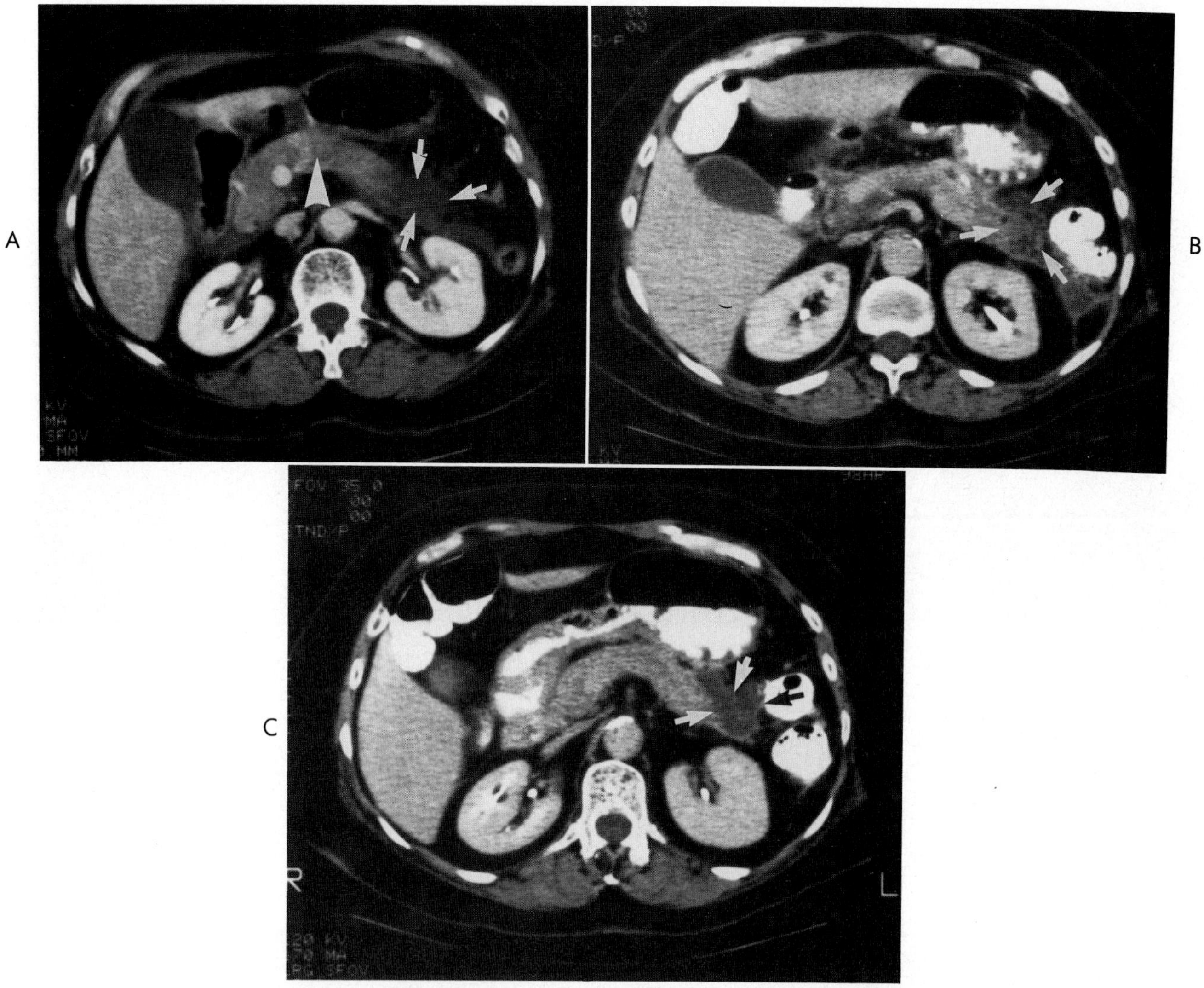

Fig. 13-26. CT scan of acute pancreatitis with complications. **A,** Initial CT scan demonstrates a diffusely enlarged and edematous pancreas *(large arrowhead)* with peripancreatic fluid obscuring the tail of the pancreas *(small arrows)*. **B,** Follow-up CT scan demonstrates a collection of air and fluid in the region of the tail of the pancreas *(small arrows)* consistent with necrotizing hemorrhagic pancreatitis. **C,** CT scan demonstrates the subsequent development of a pseudocyst within the tail of the pancreas *(small arrows)*. (Courtesy Marian P Demus, MD.)

Appendicitis

Barium enema may be used in the evaluation of the patient with suspected appendicitis. Findings suggestive of appendicitis on barium enema are the failure of the appendix to fill with barium and the presence of an extrinsic mass effect on the cecum, terminal ileum, or ascending colon (Fig. 13-27). However, these findings are not specific for acute appendicitis, and they may be seen in a number of other entities, including pelvic inflammatory disease, endometriosis, regional enteritis, and ileocecal infection with *Yersinia enterocolitica*.[17]

Patients in whom barium enema is likely to prove useful are those who have atypical presentations and those in whom there is underlying illness that renders them high-risk surgical candidates.[18]

Colonic obstruction

A barium enema may be required in instances of suspected colonic obstruction to verify the diagnosis, identify the site and cause of the obstruction, and plan a surgical procedure. It may be necessary to use a barium enema to differentiate colonic obstruction from pseudo-obstruction (see previous discussion) (Fig. 13-28).

INTRAVENOUS UROGRAPHY

In the emergency department, the intravenous pyelogram (IVP) is most commonly obtained in the evaluation of calculous obstruction of the urinary tract. Although ultrasonography may also be a useful tool in the assessment of this entity (see previous discussion), the IVP provides the most detailed depiction of the urinary tract. This study

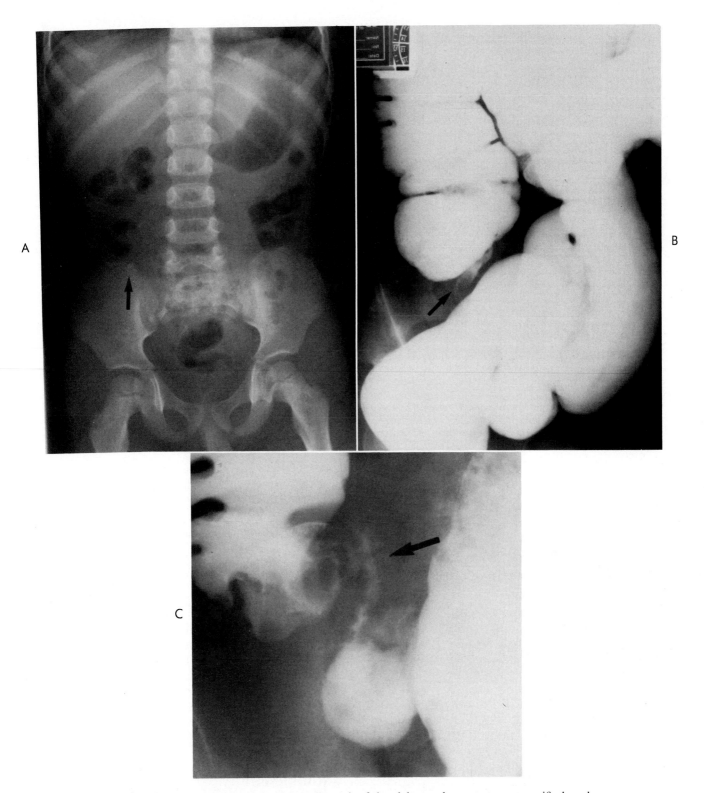

Fig. 13-27. Appendicitis. **A,** Plain radiograph of the abdomen demonstrates nonspecific bowel gas pattern and a calcification suspicious for an appendiceal fecolith *(arrow).* **B,** Barium enema demonstrates an incompletely filled appendix, outlining the fecolith *(arrow).* **C,** Barium enema in another patient visualizes the more classic findings of appendicitis: nonfilling of the appendix, cecal spasm, and mass effect on the cecum. Barium has refluxed into the terminal ileum *(arrow).*

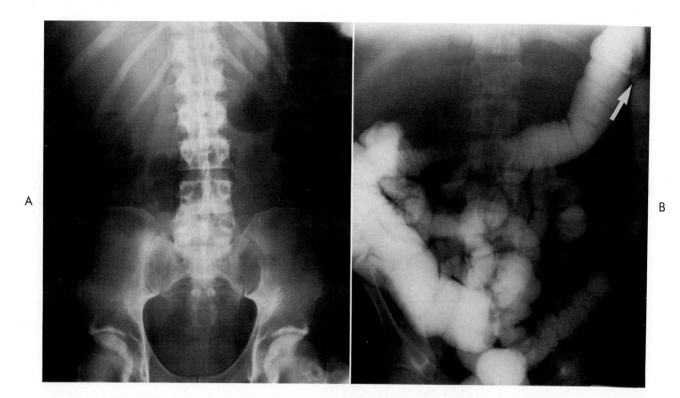

Fig. 13-28. Barium enema differentiating colonic pseudo-obstruction (acute pancreatitis) from colonic obstruction. **A,** Plain radiograph of the abdomen demonstrates a gas-filled transverse colon and splenic flexure with the absence of gas in the left colon. **B,** Barium enema visualizes no obstruction to the retrograde flow of barium. Spasm is demonstrated at the distal splenic flexure *(arrow).*

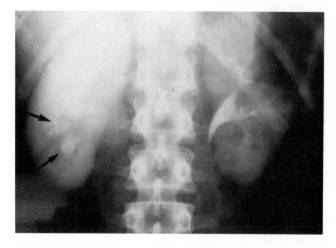

Fig. 13-29. Right ureterovesical calculus causing a prolonged nephrogram phase. This radiograph, taken 60 minutes after injection of intravenous contrast material, shows contrast material in the right calyceal system *(arrows).*

can precisely document the presence and location of calculi, demonstrate the remainder of the urinary tract, and most reliably confirm or exclude this system as the site of origin of abdominal symptoms (Fig. 13-29).

The major limitation with IVP is that radiographic contrast material must be used, which produces the risk of adverse contrast reactions (see Appendix). The major catego-

ries of serious reactions are allergy and nephrotoxicity. Contrast material allergy can occur in any study in which contrast is used. Contrast material–induced renal failure results in elevation of serum creatinine and oliguria. These effects are usually transient and self-limiting although serious renal failure may result. Factors that predispose to renal failure include renal insufficiency (serum creatinine >1.6 mg/dl), advanced age, dehydration, diabetes, hyperuricemia, multiple myeloma, and multiple exposures to contrast material within 24 hours. Pre-existing renal insufficiency is probably the most important of these factors.[19] In other than previously healthy young adults with acute renolithiasis, BUN and serum creatinine levels should be ascertained before performance of the IVP in order to identify the patient with subclinical renal insufficiency. Although the incidence of this complication is extremely low, consideration should be given to the use of ultrasonography as an alternative diagnostic study in high-risk patients.

ANGIOGRAPHY

For many clinical entities in which emergency abdominal angiography was previously indicated, the studies of choice have become noninvasive ones, particularly the CT scan and ultrasonography. Consequently, abdominal angiography is rarely used in the emergency department setting, and the need for its use should be determined in conjunction with consultants.

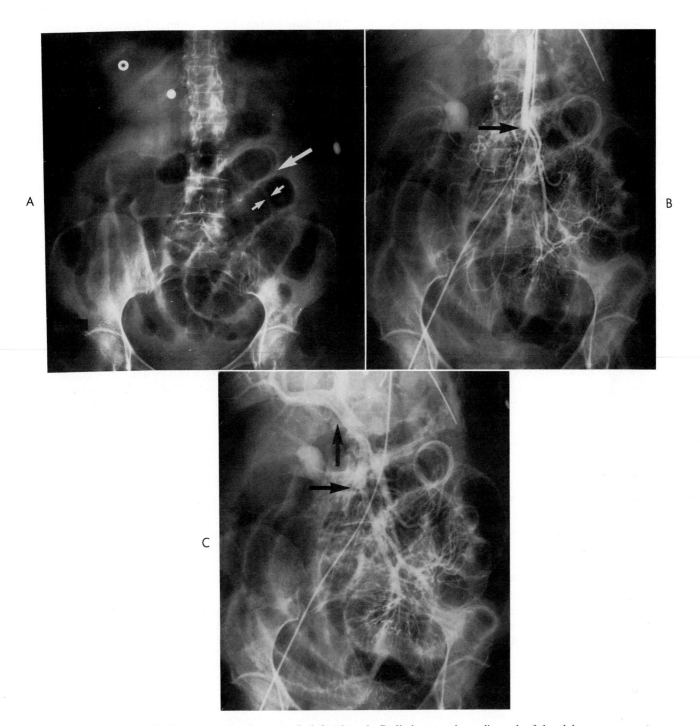

Fig. 13-30. Angiogram of mesenteric infarction. **A,** Preliminary supine radiograph of the abdomen demonstrates markedly dilated loops of small bowel with edematous bowel wall *(large arrow)* and valvulae conniventes *(opposing paired arrows)*. **B,** Superior mesenteric angiogram, in the arterial phase, demonstrates occlusion of the superior mesenteric artery *(arrow)* with opacification of two intestinal arterial branches proximal to the site of occlusion. **C,** Superior mesenteric angiogram, in the venous phase, demonstrates nonfilling of the major branches of the superior mesenteric vein *(horizontal arrow)* with the portal vein *(vertical arrow)* well opacified. (Courtesy Tony KY Chan, MD.)

Gastrointestinal bleeding

For a discussion of angiography in evaluating bleeding from the gastrointesinal tract, see Chapter 14.

Mesenteric infarction

Emergency angiography is frequently essential in diagnosing and defining the nature of mesenteric infarction or ischemia (Fig. 13-30). Embolism, thrombosis, and mesenteric vasoconstriction can be diagnosed and the adequacy of the splanchnic circulation evaluated. The instillation of intra-arterial vasodilators can also be performed via the angiographic catheter.

SUMMARY

Although many causes of acute abdominal pain produce findings that are discernible on plain radiographs, many of these findings are subtle and nonspecific. Therefore clinical evaluation generally provides the most information regarding a likely diagnosis and directs further studies. The supine abdominal radiograph may be expected to suggest the correct diagnosis in cases of small bowel or colonic obstruction and sigmoid or cecal volvulus. Positional radiographs will delineate intravascular calcification or the abnormal distribution of intraluminal and extraluminal gas or fluid within the abdominal cavity. The appropriate use of positional radiographs may lead to the diagnosis of pneumoperitoneum, intestinal obstruction, and aortic aneurysm.

Abdominal and pelvic ultrasonography have great application in selected patients. Among the clinical entities in which ultrasonography is likely to be diagnostic are leaking aortic aneurysm, ectopic pregnancy, biliary disease, and urinary tract obstruction. Hepatobiliary radionuclide scanning is an alternative diagnostic method to ultrasonography that has nearly 100% accuracy in identifying acute cholecystitis.

The CT scan has gained greater use in the emergency department and replaces various invasive techniques as the diagnostic method of choice because of the range of organs visualized and the pathologic entities elucidated. Among these entities are leaking aortic aneurysm, retroperitoneal hemorrhage, mesenteric infarction, appendicitis, diverticulitis, and pancreatitis. Other diagnostic radiographic techniques useful in various cases of acute abdominal pain include barium enema, intravenous urography, and angiography.

REFERENCES

1. Graham AD, Johnson HF: The incidence of radiographic findings in acute appendicitis compared to 200 normal abdomens, *Military Med* 131:272, 1966.
2. Cox GR, Browne BJ: Acute cholecystitis in the emergency department, *J Emerg Med* 7:501, 1989.
3. Laing FC: Diagnostic evaluation of patients with suspected acute cholecystitis, *Radiol Clin North Am* 21:477, 1983.
4. Field S: Plain films: the acute abdomen, *Clin Gastroenterol* 13:3, 1984.
5. Miller RE, Nelson SW: The roentgenologic demonstration of tiny amounts of free intraperitoneal gas: experimental and clinical studies, *AJR* 112:574, 1971.
6. Bryant LR, Wiot JF, and Kloecker RJ: A study of the factors affecting the incidence and duration of postoperative pneumoperitoneum, *Surg Gynecol Obstet* 117:145, 1963.
7. Gomes MN, Schellinger, and Hurnagel CA: Abdominal aortic aneurysms: diagnostic review and new technique, *Ann Thorac Surg* 27:480, 1979.
8. DeCherney AH, Jones EE: Ectopic pregnancy, *Clin Obstet Gynecol* 28:305, 1986.
9. Bartrum RJ, Crow HC, and Foote SR: Ultrasonic and radiographic cholecystography, *N Engl J Med* 296:538, 1977.
10. Lim JH, Ko YT, and Kim SY: Ultrasound changes of the gallbladder wall in cholecystitis: a sonographic-pathological correlation, *Clin Radiol* 38:389, 1987.
11. Ellenbogen PH, Scheible FW, Talner LB et al: Sensitivity of gray scale ultrasound in detecting urinary tract obstruction, *AJR* 130:731, 1978.
12. Jeffrey RB, Federle MP: CT and ultrasonography of acute renal abnormalities, *Radiol Clin North Am* 21:515, 1983.
13. Bandyk DF: Preoperative imaging of aortic aneurysms, *Surg Clin North Am* 69:721, 1989.
14. Federle MP, Chun G, Jeffery RB et al: Computed tomography findings of bowel infarction, *AJR* 142:91, 1984.
15. Shapiro MP, Gale ME, and Gerzof SG: CT of appendicitis, *Radiol Clin North Am* 27:753, 1989.
16. Shaff MI, Tarr RW, Partain CL et al: Computed tomography and magnetic resonance imaging of the acute abdomen, *Surg Clin North Am* 68:233, 1988.
17. Fedyshin P, Kelvin FM, and Rice RP: Nonspecificity of barium enema findings in acute appendicitis, *AJR* 143:99, 1984.
18. Merten DF: The acute abdomen in childhood, *Curr Probl Diagn Radiol* 15:335, 1986.
19. Byrd L, Sherman RL: Radiocontrast induced renal failure—a clinical and pathophysiologic review, *Medicine* 58:270, 1979.

Gastrointestinal Hemorrhage

Peter Rosen

Suzanne Z. Barkin

There are few instances in the practices of emergency medicine and radiology where diagnosis and therapy are so closely related as in treating emergency cases of gastrointestinal hemorrhage. The patient with uncontrollable gastrointestinal bleeding is one of the few exceptions to the rule that stabilization and therapy take precedence over diagnosis since often they will be one and the same.[1,2] For example, it may well be that during the same procedure a diagnosis and definitive treatment are achieved, as in angiography and embolization of the patient with exsanguinating hemorrhage from the colon.[3,4]

Nevertheless, for most patients, radiographic determination of the cause of hemorrhage will not be obtained in the emergency department but only after the patient has achieved stability and probably after the hemorrhage has been controlled.[2,5]

The radiographic approach to upper gastrointestinal bleeding reflects the specific part of the gastrointestinal tract involved: nasopharynx, esophagus, stomach, and duodenum. Causes of lower gastrointestinal bleeding involve the small bowel (distal to the ligament of Treitz) and the colon.

NASOPHARYNX

Nasopharyngeal bleeding is often produced by trauma, and in these instances the hemorrhage is usually not subtle. The cause of the bleeding is often determined by direct inspection. Bleeding in the posterior pharynx, or the posterior nose, may be identified by inference rather than direct inspection and controlled by blind pressure (e.g., the posterior nasal pack).[6] Radiology has little to offer in determining the cause of direct hemorrhage, but plain radiographs of the facial bones or a CT scan will provide information about any fractures that are present and may provide useful information to the plastic or oral surgeon or otolaryngologist in defining the type of repair that will provide optimal benefit to the patient (see Chapter 4). In most of these patients, the bleeding is either self-limited or can be controlled by treatment before diagnosis.

There are, however, a group of patients whose source of hemorrhage is more obscure; they may present with the vomiting of coffee ground material or bright red blood from an unsuspected tumor of the nasopharynx. The patient is not aware of having swallowed the blood until it causes vomiting. While these tumors are often inspected directly with endoscopy to obtain a biopsy for tissue identification, a CT scan may be helpful in demonstrating the extent of surrounding invasion or to actually provide the first clue to the presence of tumor.[7]

While most traumatic causes of nasopharyngeal hemorrhage are self-limited, the occasional patient will bleed so vigorously that some form of operative intervention may be necessary. Usually this involves the surgical repair of a traumatic lesion. However, unresponsive pure nasal hemorrhage may require angiographic embolization of the nasal and maxillary branches of the external carotid artery before the otolaryngologist surgically ligates the external carotid artery [7] (Table 14-1).

ESOPHAGUS

The esophagus can be the source of both minor and major hemorrhage. In the face of relatively minor bleeding, radiographic diagnosis can be very helpful in the elucidation of the exact cause. As a first principle, the patient must be stable before undergoing radiographic investigation. This usually means that the patient should be admitted and treated for upper gastrointestinal bleeding before being investigated.

While endoscopy is usually the means of identifying the cause of bleeding, there are some pathologies for which

Table 14-1. Approaches to the patient with bleeding from the nasopharynx and esophagus

Site	Emergency medicine	Radiology
Nose	Attempt to determine site of hemorrhage by direct inspection Control hemorrhage with direct pressure or indirect packing Admit patient to otolaryngologist for persistent bleeding or after posterior or bilateral anterior nasal packing	CT scan for suspected tumors of posterior nasopharynx Selected angiography of the external carotid artery for embolization of persistent hemorrhage
Pharynx	Perform direct inspection to determine site of hemorrhage Use direct pressure for control For deeper bleeding, obtain endoscopy to locate the site of bleeding Admit to otolaryngologist, general surgeon, or thoracic surgeon for surgical control of persistent hemorrhage Admit to gastroenterologist for diagnosis of controlled bleeding	CT scan for bulky tumors or to determine extent
Esophagus	Stabilize patient as for any upper GI hemorrhage If bleeding is bright red, persistent, and massive, treat for bleeding varices and use Sengstaken tube for persistent hemorrhage Obtain early endoscopy for diagnosis Consider radiographic studies for recurrent bleeding in stable patients only	Barium swallow to elucidate diverticulae Barium swallow to electively demonstrate varices, stricture, or hiatal hernia CT scan for tumor Radionuclide scan for active bleeding site Angiography for demonstration of portal and splenic venous anatomy

radiographic techniques are superior. For example, in the case of a Zenker diverticulum, it is easy to miss the orifice of the diverticulum with endoscopy, but it will be well demonstrated by barium swallow (Fig. 14-1).

Tumors of the esophagus also require a combination of endoscopy and radiographic techniques. Both a barium swallow and a CT scan may be useful; the CT scan can establish the extent of tumor.

Schatzki ring and hiatal hernia are well demonstrated with a barium swallow (Figs. 14-2 and 14-3), but it requires endoscopy to determine the source and location of the hemorrhage. Radiographic studies will probably be done only after the hemorrhage has been controlled and endoscopy performed.

Esophageal variceal bleeding is the source of the most severe major upper gastrointestinal hemorrhage. The cause is often suspected from the clinical appearance of the patient who frequently has all the physical stigmata of cirrhosis (spider aneurysms, beefy tongue and palms, ascites, jaundice, hemorrhoids, caput medusa, and splenomegaly). Since cirrhosis is also associated with a high incidence of duodenal ulceration as well as gastric or duodenal varices, the patient will most likely have the source of hemorrhage determined by endoscopy.[8-10]

Esophageal varices are easily demonstrated on a barium swallow (Fig. 14-4), but this will not show whether the varix is bleeding. A radionuclide study can show the site of hemorrhage, but most actively bleeding patients are too unstable for this procedure. Some gastroenterologists will obtain this study to assist in the guidance of sclerosing therapy.

Splenoportography is also a useful radiographic study, especially for the patient with recurrent bleeding after a splenorenal shunt. While these studies are most likely to be obtained during hospitalization or during surgery for shunting, they are occasionally performed during emergency department evaluation of recurrent bleeding (see Table 14-1).

STOMACH AND DUODENUM

The vast majority of cases of upper gastrointestinal hemorrhage are caused by lesions in the stomach and duodenum. One can often obtain a clue to their location by a history of ingestion of a medication or substance that penetrates the mucosal barrier, such as aspirin, ibuprofen, or some other nonsteroidal or steroidal medication. Alcohol is probably the most commonly abused substance that produces gastrointestinal bleeding. Coffee-ground material, hematemesis, or the passage of melena are clues to hemorrhage. Gastric lesions are more likely to produce hematemesis than duodenal lesions, but if the bleeding is brisk enough, even distal duodenal lesions are capable of producing bright red hematemesis.

Early diagnosis of lesions in this part of the gut depends on the endoscopist although, if the patient presents with a history or evidence of bleeding (such as anemia with hemoccult positive stools), the initial workup may be a barium swallow rather than endoscopy. Certainly duodenal and gastric ulcerations are well demonstrated on barium swallow (Figs. 14-5 and 14-6). Although gastritis is not consistently seen on barium swallow, proximal duodenal lesions are sometimes missed on endoscopy and may be better demonstrated by radiographic technique. Endoscopy is very useful in revealing Mallory-Weiss tears that are not easily seen on barium swallow or a CT scan.

The diagnosis of pseudo-aneurysm of the aorta requires

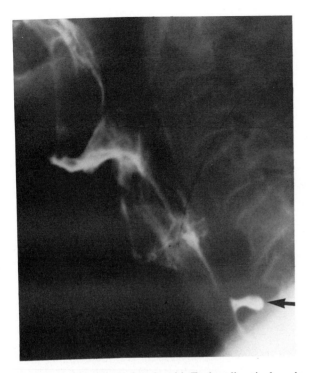

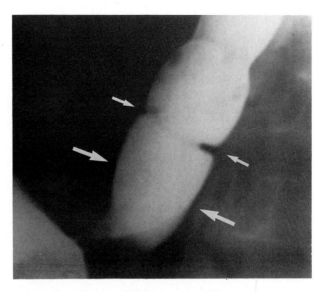

Fig. 14-3. A 67-year-old female with hiatal hernia *(large arrows)* and Schatzki ring *(small arrows)*.

Fig. 14-1. A 73-year-old female with Zenker diverticulum demonstrated on barium swallow *(arrow)*.

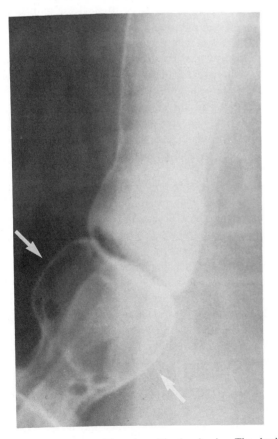

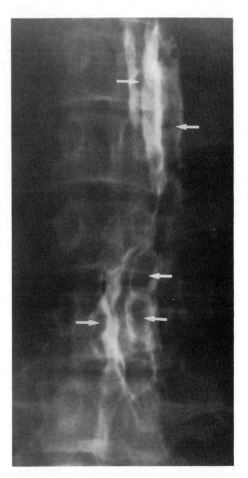

Fig. 14-2. A 77-year-old male with dysphagia. The barium swallow demonstrates a hiatal hernia *(arrows)*.

Fig. 14-4. A 42-year-old male with a history of alcohol abuse, presenting with hematemesis. The barium swallow demonstrates varices of the distal esophagus *(arrows)*.

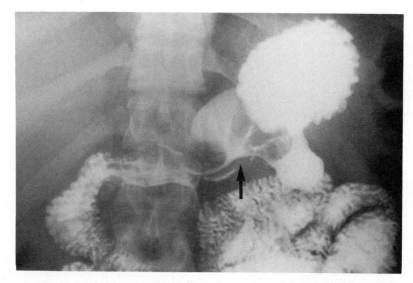

Fig. 14-5. A 30-year-old female presenting with hematemesis. The barium swallow demonstrates a giant gastric ulcer on the greater curvature *(arrow)*.

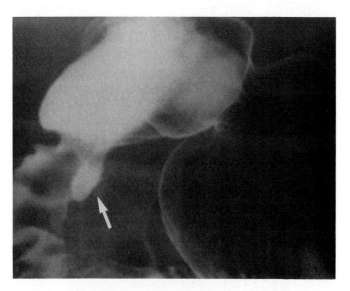

Fig. 14-6. A 37-year-old male with melena. A post-bulbar ulcer *(arrow)* is seen on the barium swallow.

early intervention. If the aortic enteric fistula is primary, it will often be missed until the patient has obvious clinical evidence of rupture. Clues to diagnosis may be detected on physical examination of the aorta or by observing calcification of the aortic wall on a lateral abdominal radiograph. Unfortunately, it is not helpful to do routine radiographs of the abdomen during the management of patients with upper gastrointestinal bleeding. Unless the emergency physician palpates an aneurysm, it is probable that the aneurysmal cause of the bleeding will be missed. It may be suggested if endoscopy reveals an ulceration in the third portion of the duodenum.

The possibility of aneurysmal bleeding is much more likely to be considered if an aneurysm has already been re-paired. In this case, any gastrointestinal bleeding must be related to the vascular disease the patient has already been proved to have. The lesion can be shown by a CT scan or by ultrasonography, especially if there is an abscess at the suture line. The choice of the procedure will depend on the availability of each modality. The most likely available procedure will be a CT scan. Endoscopy is less useful; however, if one sees an area of ulceration in the third portion of the duodenum that overlies an aortic bypass graft, one must prove that no aortoenteric fistula exists. Angiography might reveal the lesion if there is active bleeding but is likely to be unhelpful if the bleeding has stopped.[12-14]

Ulcerations of the third portion of the duodenum or other unusually located duodenal ulcerations are indications for a CT scan since these are often the sites of carcinoid or other unusual tumors.

Other rare causes of upper gastrointestinal bleeding will also require special radiographic investigation, and, unless the patient is actively bleeding, a CT scan will be the optimal modality. A CT scan also may be suggested when there is bleeding from the common bile duct or when there is a history of pancreatitis.

During active bleeding, a radionuclide scan may demonstrate the site of bleeding (Fig. 14-7) as well as an angiogram.[15] The advantage of the latter procedure is that if the bleeding vessel is identified, an embolization procedure can be considered.

While a barium swallow is useful to demonstrate gastric or duodenal ulceration, it is less likely to predict the subsequent course of the patient's recovery than is endoscopy. Therefore the greatest number of patients will benefit from early endoscopy, and radiographic evaluation is reserved for follow-up of the patient after the initial episode of bleeding is controlled.

For recurrent episodes of bleeding, especially if no

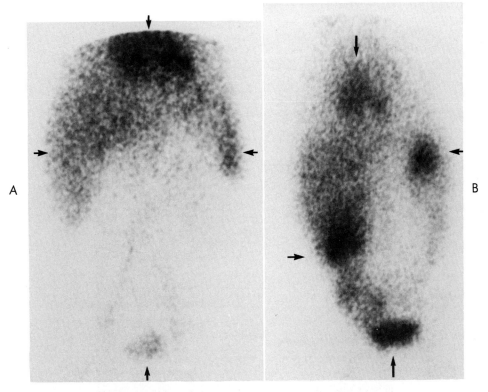

Fig. 14-7. A 19-month-old male infant with abdominal pain and hematest positive stool investigated by radionuclide red blood cell–tagged scan. **A,** At 25 minutes, the study appears normal. Note bladder, liver, spleen, and cardiac activity *(arrows)*. **B,** Four-hour delayed scan shows focal areas of radionuclide uptake in the hepatic and splenic flexures *(long arrows)* consistent with a gastrointestinal hemorrhage.

Table 14-2. Approaches to the patient with bleeding from the stomach and duodenum

Site	Emergency medicine	Radiology
Stomach and duodenum	Stabilize the patient Obtain early endoscopy Admit the patient to ICU if there is active bleeding, the patient is older than 60, or the patient is unstable	Barium swallow for location of gastric or duodenal lesions CT scan for possible aortoenteric fistula and for the location of hemorrhage that cannot be located with barium swallow or with endoscopy CT scan for patients with unusually located ulcers Radionuclide studies or angiography with embolization (if appropriate) for patients whose bleeding continues or who are not surgical candidates

cause for the patient's bleeding has been identified on endoscopy or with the barium swallow, it may be helpful to initiate a work-up with radionuclide studies or angiography.

Since these patients are well managed surgically, embolization procedures are reserved for patients who have not been found to have a source for their bleeding, who are thought to be in too poor condition for surgical therapy, or whose bleeding source is in an anatomically inaccessible location (such as an intra-hepatic lesion).

A CT scan may also be helpful in identifying recurrent bleeding after surgical therapy as well as in elaborating the details of rare causes of bleeding such as diaphragmatic hernia or pancreatitis.[16] Potential sources of bleeding in acute pancreatitis include varices, gastritis, and stress ulcers; inflammatory erosions of the duodenum and transverse colon; and leaking pseudo-aneurysms of the splenic, gastroduodenal, left gastric, and pancreaticoduodenal or hepatic arteries (Table 14-2).

SMALL BOWEL

Primary ulcerations rarely occur in the small bowel distal to the ligament of Treitz. There are, however, a number of congenital problems as well as post-traumatic le-

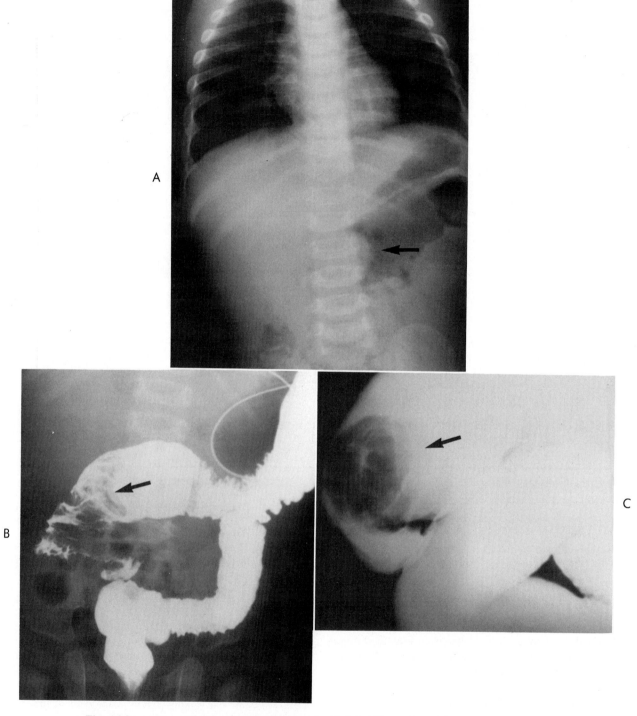

Fig. 14-8. An 8-month-old male infant presented with irritability and vomiting. **A,** Plain abdominal radiograph shows soft tissue density *(arrow)* in the midtransverse colon. **B** and **C,** Barium enema demonstrates filling defect in hepatic flexure *(arrow)*. At surgery, an intussusception was found that was reduced manually.

Table 14-3. Approaches to the patient with bleeding from the small bowel

Site	Emergency medicine	Radiology
Small bowel	Stabilize the patient with nasogastric suction, intravenous fluids, and blood as needed Look for physical stigmata of congenital disease Admit to ICU depending on rate of bleeding and overall condition of the patient	For most lesions of the small bowel, an enhanced CT scan is most useful Barium small bowel series for congenital lesions and suspected inflammatory bowel disease Angiography to identify mesenteric arterial disease or for embolization of diffuse angiomata Barium enema is most useful for intussusception; however, intussusception has also been demonstrated on CT scans

sions that may be the source of significant hemorrhage. Since lesions distal to the ligament of Treitz rarely if ever produce melena, the clinical presentation is usually bright red bleeding from the rectum. The age of the patient (usually below the fifth decade) provides a useful clue that the bleeding arises from above the colon. Physical stigmata of vascular disease may suggest Peutz-Jeghers syndrome, which includes multiple hamartomas of the small bowel and vascular abnormalities of the oral mucosa. Similarly, girls with Turner syndrome (ovarian agenesis), who are recognizable by their small stature, webbed neck, and shortened little fingers, may have multiple vascular angiomata of the small bowel that give rise to severe hemorrhage. These lesions may be demonstrated on an enhanced CT scan, which should be obtained after the patient has become stable. Angiography may also reveal the source of the bleeding, and embolization of the superior mesenteric artery may be necessary for control of the hemorrhage.[17] Surgery is often frustrating and futile in patients with these syndromes since there are so many lesions that the exact site of the hemorrhage cannot be determined, and there is too diffuse a presence of angiomata to allow surgical resection.

Blunt trauma may be the cause of the formation of stricture formation of the small bowel, and this may be the site of hemorrhage although small bowel obstruction is a more frequent presentation.

Congenital duplications of the small bowel can be a site of hemorrhage, and these will most likely be identified on the barium small bowel series.

Another cause of bleeding from the small bowel is a Meckel diverticulum. The diagnosis of symptomatic Meckel diverticulum is best made with angiography.[18]

Intussusception causes bleeding with currant jelly stools but more often presents with severe abdominal pain or with a child who appears "wiped out." On occasion, however, the parents may not have observed the severe "colic" that occurred in the middle of the night. The intussusception may have partially relieved itself no longer causing pain. These children should have a barium enema if they are stable (after consultation with a surgeon since there may be a persistent invagination of the small bowel that

will respond to the enema (Fig. 14-8) (see also Chapter 13).

Inflammatory disease of the small bowel rarely produces isolated bleeding although regional enteritis can present in this fashion. Barium small bowel series may demonstrate lesions characteristic of regional enteritis, but angiography may be necessary to identify the segment that is bleeding.[19]

Tumors of the small bowel are more common than is generally realized and are often benign. An enhanced CT scan is helpful in elaborating this cause of bleeding. The more malignant variety of small bowel tumor may give some chemical evidence of its presence, but the CT scan is useful not only in identifying the primary tumor but possibly metastatic sites as well.

In the patient with severe arteriosclerotic cardiovascular disease, superior mesenteric arterial stenosis is a rare cause of gastrointestinal hemorrhage; however, it is difficult to identify. There are no classic clinical presentations, and often the stenosis is only diagnosed when an angiogram is obtained to evaluate an elderly patient with abdominal pain who has signs of vascular disease and for whom no specific cause of the pain can be found. It is sometimes possible to obtain a history of intestinal angina after eating, but often the patient enters the emergency department with nonspecific abdominal pain. At times this is unrelenting, but, unfortunately, many patients seem to tolerate the pain without much complaint. Unexplained metabolic acidosis may be caused by poor perfusion of the small bowel. Since the cause of bleeding is usually necrosis of the bowel, these patients are often moribund and not ideal candidates for either a diagnostic procedure or surgery. The ideal diagnostic modality is angiography (Table 14-3).[20]

COLON

The colon is the site of many pathologies that may produce significant hemorrhage. The most common cause of lower gastrointestinal bleeding is anal fissure in infants and hemorrhoids in adults. Since these are easily identified on physical examination, they will not be discussed further.

The next most common cause of significant hemorrhage

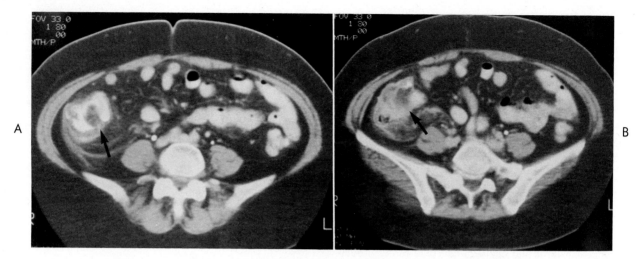

Fig. 14-9. A 50-year-old female presenting with melena. **A,** CT scan demonstrates a fluid collection in the region of the cecum *(arrow)*. At surgery, a diverticulum with associated hemorrhage and abscess was found. **B,** CT scan, at a more caudal level, again demonstrates fluid collection in the region of the cecum *(arrow)*.

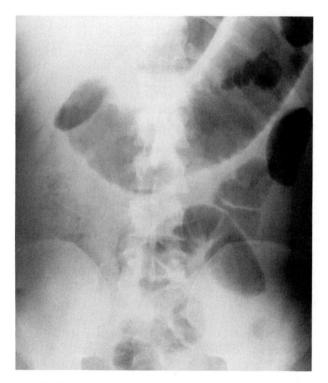

Fig. 14-10. A 36-year-old male with known ulcerative colitis complained of abdominal pain and blood from the rectum. Plain abdominal radiograph shows dilatation of the transverse colon, loss of haustral markings, and an irregular, nodular appearance of the bowel wall. Findings suggest toxic megacolon.

in the adult is diverticulosis. While diverticulae are readily diagnosed with barium enema, the enhanced CT scan has become more useful in the diagnosis of this problem and may well indicate the location of the hemorrhage (Fig. 14-9). The CT scan can be a useful guide to surgery should bleeding persist, or it can assist in localizing the appropriate vessel for successful embolization.

Should the CT scan not be available, barium enema can still be used to suggest the diagnosis; it has also been considered therapeutic by controlling bleeding in some patients.

Polyps and tumors are likely to be seen on physical examination or with endoscopy, which has the added advantage of providing a tissue diagnosis with biopsy and perhaps removal of the polyp. If bleeding is very vigorous, it may preclude endoscopy and may require angiography, both to provide diagnosis of the site of hemorrhage as well as possible treatment by embolization.

Inflammatory disease of the colon can often cause significant hemorrhage, but radiography is rarely required to identify this disease since it is more easily recognized at sigmoidoscopy. Because of the risk of perforation, the diagnosis of toxic megacolon should be made with plain radiographs for patients with known ulcerative colitis who present with acute hemorrhage (Fig. 14-10). Such hemorrhage is an indication for early surgery in patients who might otherwise be treated medically.

Barium enema is not often used for diagnosis of other sources of acute bleeding in the colon but is useful in conjunction with colonoscopy in right colon lesions that present as anemia, or intermittent bleeding.

An enhanced CT scan is also useful for elaboration of possible metastatic disease in patients with demonstrated tumors as the source of bleeding.

Table 14-4. Approaches to the patient with lower gastrointestinal hemorrhage

Site	Emergency medicine	Radiology
Colon	Stabilize the patient with intravenous fluids and blood as indicated Admit the patient to ICU depending on stability, age of the patient, and activity of bleeding Obtain early endoscopy if the source of the bleeding is not obvious from physical examination	Enhanced CT scan once the patient has been stabilized If CT scan is not available, barium enema to both diagnose and attempt to control bleeding Angiography for both diagnosis as to site and for embolization therapy for persistent bleeding For patient with known ulcerative colitis, plain abdominal radiograph to exclude the presence of toxic megacolon For patient with unknown source of anemia or in whom active bleeding has ceased, enhanced CT scan and barium enema in conjunction with colonoscopy

Vascular disease of the colon is uncommon but may occur as a complication of aortic aneurysm surgery. Endoscopy is probably more useful than radiographic diagnosis in patients who develop this complication since the bleeding is most often caused by necrosis of the colon, which can be visualized at sigmoidoscopy (Table 14-4).

SUMMARY

Radiology plays a significant role in the diagnosis and management of gastrointestinal hemorrhage. Attempts to stabilize the patient before diagnosis are warranted, as with all critical patients, but there will be conditions that warrant radiographic interventions for therapy as well.

REFERENCES

1. Eckstein MR, Athanasoulis CA: Gastrointestinal bleeding: an angiographic perspective, *Surg Clin North Am* 64:37, 1984.
2. Schlup M, Barbezat GO, and Maclaurin BP: Prospective evaluation of patients with upper gastrointestinal haemorrhage, *N Z Med J* 97:511, 1984.
3. Browder W, Cerise EJ, and Litwin MS: Impact of emergency angiography in massive lower gastrointestinal bleeding, *Ann Surg* 204:530, 1986.
4. Waye JD: A diagnostic approach to colon bleeding, *Mt Sinai J Med (NY)* 51:491, 1984.
5. Meyerovitz MF, Fellows KE: Angiography in gastrointestinal bleeding in children, *AJR* 143:837, 1984.
6. Cantrill SV, McGill J, and Kulig K: Facial trauma and epistaxis. In Rosen P, Baker FJ II, Barkin RM et al, eds: *Emergency medicine: concepts and clinical practice*, vol 1, ed 2, St Louis, 1988, CV Mosby.
7. Mulvaney TJ, Partlow RC Jr, and Weymuller EA Jr: Emergencies of the ear, facial structures and upper airway. In Wilkins EW Jr, ed: *Emergency medicine: scientific foundations and current practice*, ed 3, Baltimore, 1989, Williams & Wilkins.
8. Agha FP: The esophagus after endoscopic injection sclerotherapy: acute and chronic changes, *Radiology* 153:37, 1984.
9. Valla D, Huet PM, LaFortune M et al: Vasopressin perfusion of esophageal varices in cirrhotic patients: cineangiographic study, *Radiology* 152:45, 1984.
10. Widrich WC, Srinivasan M, Semine MC et al: Collateral pathways of the left gastric vein in portal hypertension, *AJR* 142:375, 1984.
11. Winn M, Weissmann HS, Sprayregen S et al: The radionuclide detection of lower gastrointestinal bleeding sites, *Clin Nucl Med* 8:389, 1983.
12. Athow AC, Sheppard L, and Sibson DE: Selective visceral angiography for unexplained acute gastrointestinal bleeding in a district general hospital, *Br J Surg* 72:120, 1985.
13. Hietala SO, Ghahremani GG, Crampton AR et al: Arteriographic evaluation of postsurgical stomach, *Gastrointest Radiol* 10:31, 1985.
14. Myllyla V, Paivansalo M, and Leinonen A: Angiographic diagnosis at gastrointestinal hemorrhage, *Diagn Imaging Clin Med* 53:135, 1984.
15. Mark AS, Moss AA, McCarthy S et al: CT of aortoenteric fistulas, *Invest Radiol* 20:272, 1985.
16. Schroder T, Kivisaari L, Somer K et al: Significance of extrapancreatic findings in computer tomography (CT) of acute pancreatitis, *Eur J Radiol* 5:273, 1985.
17. van der Vliet AH, Kalff V, Sacharias N et al: The role of contrast angiography in gastrointestinal bleeding with the advent of technetium labelled red blood cell scans, *Australas Radiol* 29:29, 1985.
18. Geelhoed GW, Druy EM, and Steinberg WM: Recurrent bleeding from Meckel's diverticulum in an adult: angiographic demonstration after normal scans, *South Med J* 79:65, 1986.
19. Asakura H, Takagi T, Kobayashi K et al: Microangiographic findings of massive intestinal bleeding in a patient with Crohn's disease: a case report, *Angiology* 36:802, 1985.
20. Athanasoulis CA, Waltman AC, and Geller SC: Angiography: a diagnostic and therapeutic aid in emergencies. In Wilkins EW Jr, ed: *Emergency medicine: scientific foundation and current practice*, ed 3, Baltimore, 1989, Williams & Wilkins.

C H A P T E R *15*

Altered Consciousness and Syncope

DePriest Whye, Jr.

Jeremy Young

Robert A. Barish

ALTERED CONSCIOUSNESS

Technologic developments within the field of radiology have tremendously advanced the accuracy and rapidity with which major neurologic disorders are evaluated (see later discussion on syncope and Chapter 17). Computed tomography (CT scan) has increased the understanding of neuropathologic processes and has allowed identification of intracranial lesions that before were detectable only by invasive means.[1] Serious intracranial lesions such as neoplasms, hemorrhages, and infections now have a greater potential for immediate recognition and therapy. The widespread availability of the CT scan has greatly benefited the management of a variety of neurologic emergencies.

The CT scan as a diagnostic tool in evaluating altered consciousness enables rapid determination of etiology and immediate therapeutic intervention, thereby reducing morbidity and mortality associated with lesions such as subdural hematoma and epidural hematoma.[1-3] However, in some situations in which surgical or medical intervention is limited, such as in intracerebral hematomas, brain stem hemorrhage, and intracranial neoplasms, the outcome has not changed appreciably.[1,4] The presence of coma implies profound brain dysfunction with seriously limited potential for reversal.

When treating brain insults and injuries, diagnosis is of paramount importance in the prevention of irreversible brain damage and in the preservation of brain function. The major determinants of patient outcome are the institution of proper resuscitation procedures and the rapid identification of reversible brain pathology. Recognition of the neuropathologic lesions that contribute to the development of altered states of consciousness has been considered crucial to the establishment of a definitive patient management plan. Such a plan, if instituted early, may reverse a fulminant intracerebral pathologic process.

The CT scan is an invaluable tool and has been demonstrated to be sensitive, safe, and reliable.[5] Continued development and upgrading of the technology has delivered more rapid and sophisticated scanners capable of producing better image quality. Skull radiographs and radionuclide brain scans have been virtually supplanted, and the CT scan has become the mainstay diagnostic procedure. Therefore a fundamental understanding of the basic technology is indispensable, including the type and quality of scanners, indications for scanning, indications for enhancement, and the logistics involved in scanning techniques; this assures appropriate application in solving diagnostic problems (see the Appendix).

The discussion that follows highlights the important features of radiographic intervention in the management of altered consciousness. Comprehension of the role of radiographic diagnostic procedures in the era of the CT scan is essential in facilitating this process.

Definitions

Consciousness and behavior can be thought of in terms of awareness, content, and arousal; the precise functions depend on normal brain integrity and activity. *Consciousness* is a state of awareness of self and environment and implies a functional cerebral cortex capable of providing goal-directed or purposeful behavior. Conscious behavior consists of two distinct physiologic components, content and arousal. The cerebral cortex provides the structural basis for the content of consciousness, whereas neural structures within the brain stem produce arousal. The content of consciousness encompasses cognitive and affective functions. Any significant impairment of the cerebral cortex may disrupt normal cognitive and behavioral function, potentially rendering the patient with a diminished content of consciousness.

Cognitive function, however, cannot occur without a stimulus to sustain an alert state. Arousal denotes a state of wakefulness that depends on an intact cortex, but more importantly, on normal brain stem function. The ascending reticular activating system (ARAS) is responsible for arousal and, when stimulated, causes wakefulness and alert behavior. The ARAS originates just ventral to the fourth ventricle and travels through the brain stem, pons, midbrain, and thalamus, receiving collaterals from sensory systems at every level. Spinothalamic input is particularly abundant and potentially explains why painful stimuli incite arousal. The ARAS projects diffusely to the cortex from the thalamus, maintaining a normal alert state and wakefulness. Given this anatomic and physiologic relationship, it is clear that altered consciousness may occur if either content or arousal is affected.

Altered conciousness includes neurologic states ranging from delirium to coma, each suggesting varying degrees of cortical or brain stem dysfunction. *Delirium* is a clouding of consciousness with reduced awareness of the environment. This condition is distinguished by disorientation, fear, irritability, misperception of visual stimuli, and visual hallucinations. Aberrations of arousal and attention may alternate between hyperactivity and somnolence. *Coma* is an altered state of consciousness in which the organism is totally unresponsive to external stimuli and is completely unaware of self or surrounding environment.[6,7]

Pathophysiology

The alteration of consciousness known as coma occurs when various pathologic conditions exert a deleterious effect at the cortical level or the level of the brain stem. The alterations in consciousness may be due to diffuse cortical dysfunction or disruption of brain stem function. Pathologic conditions or agents may cause a direct injury to the brain stem matter or an indirect effect as a consequence of intracranial hypertension and an accompanying brain herniation. Because of space-occupying effects, intra-axial (intracerebral) or extra-axial (extracerebral) masses may result in several well known brain herniation syndromes. Cerebral edema alone, or in association with a mass lesion, can also contribute to increased intracranial pressure (ICP).[6]

Coma can be attributed to several pathophysiologic mechanisms involving specific regions of the brain. *Supratentorial lesions, infratentorial lesions,* and *metabolic encephalopathy* are the general pathophysiologic categories under which coma is classified, and each category has a characteristic clinical evolution depending on the territory of the brain involved and the associated herniation syndrome.

Supratentorial lesions. Coma is produced by mass lesions of the cerebral hemisphere that cause herniation beyond the compartmentalization of the tentorium, thereby compressing the brain stem and the ARAS. Transtentorial herniation is classically described in association with mass lesions occuring in this area. This class of herniation produces two types of clinical syndromes, depending on the location of the supratentorial lesion (Table 15-1). A central downward transtentorial herniation occurs in conjunction with a centrally placed mass, and a medial herniation of the temporal lobe uncus is associated with a laterally situated mass.[6-8]

Infratentorial lesions. Coma may also occur as a consequence of an expanding infratentorial mass. The mass may be of two types: a lesion intrinsic to the brain stem that destroys the ARAS, such as a pontine hemorrhage or paramedian infarction of the midbrain or pons, or a lesion extrinsic to the brain stem that compresses it, such as a cerebellar tumor or a hematoma. Masses of the posterior fossa, such as tumor, hematoma, or metastasis, may cause upward herniation of the superior vermis and blood vessels through the tentorial notch, resulting in midbrain compression. This is referred to as ascending transtentorial herniation[6,7] (Table 15-1).

Compressive lesions of the brain stem are often difficult to distinguish from intrinsic lesions, and cerebellar hemorrhages may mimic a brain stem stroke clinically. The caudal-to-rostral appearance of neurologic signs may resemble the patchy brain stem depression of sedative drug intoxication.

Metabolic abnormalities. Systemic disease may also adversely affect consciousness by interfering with the metabolism of the cerebral cortex and the brain stem or by depriving the brain of essential nutrients. Cerebral metabolism is depressed by endogenous toxins, such as occur in renal and hepatic failure, or by exogenous toxins such as drugs and poisons. Whenever the brain is deprived of the

Table 15-1. Herniation syndromes

Lesions	Underlying pathology	Clinical findings	CT scan findings
Supratentorial			
Central descending transtentorial	Midline mass, downward movement displaces diencephalon caudally, progressive rostral-caudal loss of brain stem function	Reduced consciousness, 1-3 mm reactive pupils, bilateral corticospinal and extrapyramidal signs, decorticate posturing, Cheyne-Stokes respirations	Mass effect, effacement of basal cistern, increased sagittal diameter of brain stem
Uncal transtentorial	Temporal or lateral mass, downward displacement of uncus through tentorial notch compresses midbrain and third cranial nerve	Ipsilateral third cranial nerve palsy, contralateral decerebrate posturing	Lateral mass, distortion of suprasellar cisterns, displacement of brain stem laterally
Infratentorial			
Ascending transtentorial	Posterior fossa mass, herniation of superior vermis through tentorial notch, compresses midbrain	Mild anisicoria to mid-positioned fixed pupils, neurogenic hyperventilation, decorticate/decerebrate posturing	Midbrain compression, quadrigeminal cistern compression
Downward cerebellar tonsillar herniation	Posterior fossa mass, cerebellar tonsils herniate through foramen magnum, compress medulla	Sudden respiratory and circulatory collapse	Unobtainable due to sudden death

essential supply of energy substrates, brain dysfunction and coma may ensue. The metabolic disturbance creates a diffuse cortical or brain stem dysfunction that is frequently reversible. Hypoxia and hypoglycemia induce coma by this mechanism. Rapid restoration of oxygen and glucose supply will offset progressive cerebral injury. Electrolyte disturbances, acid-base abnormalities, hyperosmolality, and hypo-osmolality may alter neuronal excitability.[6]

In metabolic disorders, coma is frequently preceded by irritability and inattentiveness that may progress to delirium, then stupor. Visual hallucinations may occur before the loss of consciousness, and seizures may appear. Metabolic encephalopathy generally produces symmetric neurologic abnormalities; however, focal neurologic deficits can occur confusing the clinical picture. Pupillary reflexes are generally preserved when signs of lower brain stem depression are present, such as apnea, absent oculovestibular reflexes, motor flaccidity, and areflexia. Multifocal myoclonus, tremor, asterixis, and seizures are additional neurologic manifestations. In severe sedative-hypnotic drug overdose, virtually all brain function and cord function are inapparent. Failure to recognize the potential effects of sedative-hypnotic overdose can lead to the mistaken diagnosis of brain death.[9]

Increased intracranial pressure. Mass lesions and metabolic encephalopathy may lead to increased intracra-

nial pressure (ICP) due to space encroachment, cerebral edema, or both. ICP is the common pathway by which various pathologic processes lead to herniation and altered consciousness. The most significant causes are global anoxia, meningoencephalitis, hyponatremia, intracranial trauma, ischemic stroke, brain abscess, extracerebral hematoma, intracerebral hematoma, subdural empyema, subarachnoid hemorrhage, obstructive hydrocephalus, and communicating hydrocephalus.

The pernicious effects of elevated ICP derive from alterations in cerebral perfusion. The brain consists of three fluid compartments that exist in dynamic equilibrium—the cerebrospinal fluid (CSF), circulating blood volume, and parenchymal cellular space. A quantitative increase in any of the fluid compartments or a decrease in available brain space may raise ICP. The volume content of the brain increases when there is an elevation of the blood volume as a consequence of arterial dilatation or venous obstruction. Increased CSF formation or obstruction of flow will raise intracranial volume, while cerebral edema may be the end result of an accumulation of water intracellularly or extracellularly, increasing the overall water content of the brain.[10,11] ICP rises in direct proportion to increases in brain volume that compromise tissue perfusion.

Decreased cerebral perfusion increases cerebral hypoxia and anaerobic metabolism, ultimately resulting in increased vascular permeability and augmented effusion of fluid into the extracellular space. This process initiates a vicious cycle that may culminate in permanent cerebral dysfunction or brain death. If perfusion pressure is maintained, increasing systemic resistance, then adequate perfusion to the brain occurs. If, in addition, the blood is well oxygenated, edema will be diminished.

Cerebral edema may be limited to focal areas of the brain or may be generalized, involving diffuse areas of cortical and subcortical tissues. Both focal and diffuse forms of cerebral edema may produce rising ICP and concomitant signs of cerebral dysfunction. A rise in ICP above 20 mm Hg can produce brain dysfunction and herniation. Several forms of brain herniation are associated with increased ICP and include the previously mentioned downward transtentorial herniation due to centrally and laterally situated masses. In addition, ascending transtentorial herniation and downward cerebellar tonsillar herniation can occur. Brain stem herniation, however, does not necessarily have to be the culmination of cerebral edema. Indeed, focal brain edema may be mild and transient leading to minimal or no increase in ICP. By contrast, diffuse cerebral edema consistently generates elevations in ICP, the degree of elevation depending on the nature and severity of the inciting agent or lesion.[11-13]

Etiology

Approximately 3% of hospital admissions from the emergency department are comatose patients.[14] It is estimated that 10% of patients admitted to the hospital for medical and surgical problems demonstrate a component of altered consciousness.[15] The causes of coma and delirium are numerous but may be simplified by adhering to the conventional categories of supratentorial, infratentorial, and metabolic causes discussed previously (see box on p. 392).

Plum and Posner reported a series of 500 patients whose conditions were categorized as coma of unknown etiology on presentation to a medical facility.[6] Coma as a result of drugs and trauma were excluded. Coma was attributed to supratentorial lesions in 20% of the cases, subtentorial in 13%, diffuse cortical disorder in 65%, and psychiatric in 2%. Thus approximately two thirds of coma cases are due to diffuse cerebral impairment of metabolic and infectious origin while one third are found to result from a structural brain abnormality. Ten percent of comatose patients presenting to the emergency department are victims of trauma.[6]

Initial management

The principal objective in the management of coma is to resuscitate the patient and support respiratory and cardiovascular function, followed by rapid identification and treatment of elevated ICP. Treatable metabolic imbalances should be immediately reversed and potential etiologies defined by a series of diagnostic evaluations. Finally, definitive care is instituted based on information derived from diagnostic evaluation. Foremost in determining a cause is considering whether central nervous system (CNS) dysfunction is due to a structural lesion or metabolic disturbance. Historic features and physical examination may provide clues that are suggestive, but the success of management hinges upon early identification of a structural abnormality if one is present. Therefore performance of the CT scan is the critical point of diagnostic study. The patient's eventual outcome may depend on the rapidity with which definitive therapy is employed in an attempt to remove or neutralize the primary brain insult. Management should proceed quickly through stabilization, diagnosis, and definitive care phases (see box below).

Diagnostic findings

The diagnostic phase includes accumulating historic data when available, performing a thorough physical and neurologic examination, acquiring laboratory data, and completing radiographic studies. These tasks must be carried out rapidly and efficiently so that there is no significant delay in the performance of the cranial CT scan. Diagnosis of the patient presenting to the emergency department frequently challenges clinical acumen. Most often the history is unobtainable because historic sources such as family members are absent. Consequently, reliance on physical examination, laboratory data, and radiographic studies is required to reach a diagnosis.

Coma management

Stabilization

Ensure oxygenation and ventilation
Immobilize cervical spine
Maintain circulation
Administer thiamine (100 mg IV), Narcan (2 mg IV), D50W (50 ml)
Treat elevated ICP: perform endotracheal intubation and hyperventilate (Po_2: 20-25 mm Hg), monitor, and administer mannitol
Treat seizure with anticonvulsants
Control temperature
Treat overdose

Diagnostic evaluation

Take history, perform physical and neurologic examinations
Collect laboratory data
Perform standard radiographs
Order a CT scan
Perform lumbar puncture

Definitive management

Observation (ICU)
ICP monitoring
Surgical decompression
Metabolic and infectious management

Etiology of coma

Supratentorial lesions

Mass lesion with herniation
    Hemorrhage
        Subdural, epidural, subarachnoid
        Intracerebral, basal ganglia, putamen
        Pituitary apoplexy
    Infarction
        Cerebral infarction with edema
    Tumor
        Primary
        Metastatic
    Abscess
        Intracerebral
        Subdural
Destructive lesion
    Bilateral thalamic infarction

Infratentorial lesions

Mass lesion with herniation
    Cerebellum
        Hemorrhage
        Infarction with edema
        Tumor
        Abscess
    Posterior fossa subdural hematoma
    Basilar artery aneurysm

Destructive cerebral lesions

Brain stem
    Hemorrhage
    Infarction
    Tumor
    Abscess
    Demyelination
    Basilar migraine
    Encephalitis

Diffuse cerebral lesions

Closed head injury
Encephalitis
Meningitis
Multiple emboli
Ischemia
Vasculitis
Hypertensive encephalopathy
Subarachnoid hemorrhage

Metabolic causes

Temperature
    Hypothermia
    Hyperthermia
Pulmonary
    Hypoxia
    Hypercapnea
Electrolytes/acid-base osmolality
    Hyponatremia
    Hypernatremia
    Hypercalcemia
    Metabolic acidosis
    Hyperosmolar states
    Osmolar shifts
    Dialysis disequilibrium syndrome
Renal
    Uremia
Hepatic
    Hepatic encephalopathy
    Reye syndrome
Pancreatic
    Pancreatic encephalopathy
Substrate or vitamin deficiency
    Hypoglycemia
    Wernicke syndrome: thiamine deficiency
    Vitamin B_{12} deficiency
Endocrine
    Diabetic ketoacidosis
    Hyperosmolar nonketotic coma
    Myxedema coma
    Hyperthyroidism
    Hypothyroidism
    Addison disease
    Hypopituitarism
Poisons
    Drugs
    Heavy metals
    Solvents

Miscellaneous

Seizure
Post-ictal

Psychiatric

Conversion reaction
Depression
Catatonic stupor

The initial physical survey should focus on discovering evidence of trauma, which includes evaluation of head, body, and extremities for ecchymosis, edema, and deformity. The tympanic membranes, eye grounds, and pharynx are examined as well as the heart, lungs, and abdomen. Even if no evidence of trauma exists but the patient is in a profound coma, it is prudent to assume that trauma may have been the precipitating factor. Thus the cervical spine requires protection by immobilization if overlooked in the initial resuscitation. A neurologic examination is important in determining the depth of unconsciousness, the existence of lateralizing signs, and in specifying the level of the lesion. It is important to assess the level of consciousness according to the Glasgow Coma Scale (see Chapter 3). Respiratory patterns, pupillary responses, oculovestibular reflexes, eye position and movements, motor responses, corneal reflexes, and deep tendon reflexes also require assessment. A rapid search for evidence of lateralizing or focal findings should be completed. Decorticate or decerebrate posture, either occurring spontaneously or in response to noxious stimuli, indicates serious cortical or brain stem dysfunction, respectively. An intracranial mass such as an acute subdural hematoma must be considered. Any suggestion of elevated ICP with possible herniation is sufficient cause to initiate hyperventilation procedures and to administer mannitol.

When focal neurologic deficits exist in the absence of depressed consciousness, vigilance is maintained in anticipation of deterioration of mental status. If no focal findings are present, elevated ICP may nonetheless exist. Metabolic encephalopathy or diffuse cerebral involvement is, of course, a consideration; but more importantly a mass lesion may exist, and a CT scan must be performed to exclude the possibility of structural lesions. Metabolic encephalopathy due to intrinsic systemic failure or extrinsic agents or toxins is a commonly encountered cause of coma. Drugs and toxins always require consideration. An orogastric tube should be inserted and charcoal instilled after the airway has been secured.[16-18]

The alcoholic patient, for example, frequently presents to the urban emergency department with altered consciousness. The patient, although arousable, is often profoundly inebriated with ethanol levels above 300 mg %; has a depressed Glasgow score; may be normotensive, bradycardic or tachycardic; and has malodorous breath. Focal neurologic deficits are typically absent, and signs of trauma may or may not be present. The nature of the alcoholic condition predisposes the patient to potentially significant traumatic experiences. In this setting, serial observation and conservative management is hazardous, placing the patient at risk for delayed recognition of a serious intracranial lesion. These patients generally require airway control, stabilization, metabolic workup, and radiographic assessment including a cervical spine series, chest radiographs, and a CT scan.[19]

Several clinical syndromes emerge when considering the historic features and clinical presentation of a patient. Two distinct presentations of coma may be recognized — a sudden and a subacute onset.[16] In sudden onset, the patient is initially awake and alert, then spontaneously loses consciousness with little or no preceding symptomatology. Although this is most often compatible with cardiac arrest or malignant dysrhythmia, subarachnoid hemorrhage, seizure, pontine herniation, and cerebral trauma may also present suddenly.

Subacute onset of coma transpires over a period of minutes to hours. Several conditions produce this presentation. Acute subdural herniation, metabolic disorders, and drug overdose are examples. Cerebellar hemorrhage may also present similarly. Recognition of cerebellar hemorrhage is extremely important because of its potential for reversibility. Severe headache, nausea, vomiting, and truncal ataxia classically constitute the early presentation. With enlargement of the hemorrhage, coma may follow as the brain stem and ARAS are affected. This lesion is readily detected by a CT scan.

A patient may present with a classic stroke syndrome associated with focal neurologic deficits. A subsequent depressed level of consciousness develops and coma may follow. This presentation is usually the result of an isolated mass lesion such as an intracerebral hemorrhage that has progressed to a herniation syndrome or a massive infarction with co-existent massive brain swelling. The process may continue to profound coma, accompanied by decerebrate posturing and loss of brain stem function. Hemodynamic and respiratory instability are preterminal events.

The evaluation and treatment of delirium are not dissimilar to that for coma; however, several features require emphasis to avoid pitfalls. Although metabolic encephalopathy is the most frequent cause of delirium, an intracranial lesion remains the greatest threat to brain stability and function. Therefore resuscitation and stabilization should proceed rapidly followed by an urgent CT scan to rule out an intracranial hemorrhage. A false sense of security should not be derived from the fact that delirium is likely due to PCP intoxication, narcotics, or other drugs or poisons. The very nature of drug and poison intoxication predisposes the patient to trauma and, in some instances, hypertensive emergencies, all of which may produce intracranial neuropathology. An inebriated patient who has suffered what appears to be minor trauma and appears to awaken after Narcan administration may harbor an epidural hematoma. The improvement in mental status merely represents the lucid interval. Extreme caution must be exercised, and this patient should not be dismissed as just another drug addict.

To effectively carry out an adequate clinical evaluation, the incoherent, agitated, combative patient must frequently be immobilized by physical or pharmacologic means. Although generally it is undesirable to dispense sedation when the cause of mental disturbance is unknown because potential alterations in the patient's neurologic findings may be induced, from a practical standpoint such sedation may represent the only means to successfully manage the patient. Performance of a lumbar puncture and a CT scan require the patient to lie motionless. Haldol (5 to 10 mg intravenously or intramuscularly) and droperidol (2.5 mg intravenously) are butyrophenones that have been recommended as effective sedation in selected head trauma victims as well as in agitated patients with delirium.[20,21]

Further evaluation of altered consciousness should include laboratory analyses that provide information regarding metabolic derangements. Blood samples are drawn for complete blood count, electrolytes, blood urea nitrogen (BUN), creatinine, calcium, magnesium, phosphorus, carbon monoxide, liver function test, urinalysis, toxicology screen, and arterial blood gas. Lumbar puncture and blood cultures are performed whenever systemic infection is a consideration. However, if there is a high possibility that meningitis exists on the basis of fever and altered mental status, antibiotics may be initiated early; lumbar puncture can be performed after the CT scan, thereby treating the CNS infection and potentially avoiding the sequelae of brain herniation. Immunocompromised patients such as the patient with AIDS or other immunosuppressed patients, such as the diabetic or the alcoholic patient, possess a higher than normal risk of developing CNS infection. Therefore one must aggressively search for these infections.

Prothrombin time, partial thromboplastin time, and coagulation profile should be ordered to eliminate an underlying bleeding disorder. The alcoholic patient with platelet dysfunction, the anticoagulated patient, and the hemophiliac patient are all at risk of developing spontaneous bleeding or bleeding secondary to incidental trauma. Persistent bleeding after insertion of an intravenous needle, evidence of ecchymosis, petechiae, or purpura should raise suspicion of bleeding abnormalities. A bleeding diathesis may require correction with vitamin K, fresh frozen plasma (FFP), cryoprecipitates, or specific factor therapy.

Radiographic evaluation

Radiographic studies begin with an evaluation of the lateral cervical spine. A portable chest radiograph is indicated in the initial evaluation of the comatose patient. Although it is uncommon that the chest radiograph will provide information suggesting the underlying causes of coma, it serves as a baseline evaluation and assesses cardiac and pulmonary status.[22] Endotracheal tube, nasogastric tube, and central line positions may be confirmed. Occasionally specific cardiopulmonary conditions cause systemic hypoxia or low flow states. Congestive heart failure, pulmonary edema, pneumonia, and pneumothorax may lead to altered consciousness and are readily demonstrated radiographically. Aspiration is an additional finding that may be revealed on the chest radiograph.

The patient with hepatic disease and a portocaval shunt or splenorenal shunt may develop coma as a result of a high protein meal or hepatic encephalopathy. Clinical evidence of jaundice may be absent. Metallic clips radiographically visible below the diaphragm may be the only clue to a prior surgical procedure. Multiple rib fractures in various stages of healing are an associated finding in alcoholic patients vulnerable to falls and violent encounters. The chest radiographic finding suggestive of a lung mass or neoplasm raises the possibility of paraneoplastic syndromes that may contribute to onset of altered consciousness. Among other possible disorders producing coma are metastatic brain tumor, marantic endocarditis with embolism, disseminated intravascular coagulation (DIC) with thrombosis, hypercalcemia, hypoglycemia, hyponatremia, and progressive multifocal leukoencephalopathy (PML).[22]

Infants with intracranial or systemic arteriovenous malformation may demonstrate an enlarged cardiac silhouette. It should also be noted that an infant may lose over one half of the normal blood volume in a cephalohematoma, subgaleal herniation, or subdural hematoma. In this instance, the heart will appear small due to volume loss.

Pleural and pericardial effusions can be found in combination with conditions such as myxedema, malignancy, uremia, hepatic failure, and parasitic cysts. Twenty percent of cerebral abscesses originate from pulmonary infection. Pneumonia or lung abscess may be the source of a co-existing meningitis or cerebral abscess.[23]

The chest radiograph and abdominal radiograph may be helpful by identifying radio-opaque substances in the stomach or gastrointestinal tract from poisoning and overdose. Examples of radio-opaque drugs include chloral hydrate, hydrocarbons, iron, phenothiazines, enteric-coated drugs, and salicylates.[24]

Computed tomography. Standard CT scans should be performed on patients to evaluate states of altered consciousness. The CT scans are performed at a plane that runs at an angle of 15 degrees above the orbitomeatal line. This position allows the smallest number of slices, providing the most information and reducing scanning times and radiation exposure. The initial slice begins with the foramen magnum (base of the skull) and progresses cephalad to the vertex of skull. The posterior fossa is not examined in detail by this technique; a posterior fossa examination must be ordered when information relevant to this area is required.[5]

The head CT scan includes approximately 10 slices with a range of 8 to 10 mm in thickness. The number of slices depends on the head size and shape. Posterior fossa imaging is performed using a 4 to 5 mm slice thickness. A normal CT scan at 80 mA requires an exposure time of 4.6 seconds, and a complete study requires approximately 20 minutes. Contrast enhancement prolongs the study. The time factor must be considered when electing to administer contrast material. The patient is at risk of deteriorating neurologically or cardiovascularly while in the radiology suite and therefore must be monitored and accompanied by a physician who is prepared to resuscitate or stabilize the patient while the examination is being completed.[25]

Indications for administering contrast material. The addition of intravenous contrast material is often helpful in enhancing and clarifying specific intracranial lesions. It may provide useful information with regard to mass effect, edema, and low-density or high-density areas that may otherwise be imperceptible on nonenhanced scans. Specific brain lesions may be diagnosed according to characteristic enhancement patterns. The dilemma lies in recognizing the specific instances when an enhanced CT scan will provide superior information to a nonenhanced scan. Argument abounds as to the proper indications for administering contrast material. It has been suggested that both nonenhanced and enhanced scans should always be performed in the diagnostic evaluation of nontraumatic coma. Conventional practice promotes performing a nonenhanced CT scan to detect midline shift, cerebral edema, mass lesions, and enlarged ventricles. The enhanced scan is delayed unless a specific lesion is suspected or a suspicious finding on the nonenhanced CT scan necessitates enhancement for further elucidation.

Although in many medical centers enhanced CT scans are not ordered, there are specific indications relevant to coma evaluation that justify the ordering of an enhanced scan[5]:

- If the nonenhanced CT scan displays either ventricular dilatation or mass effect and the patient is exhibiting evidence of intracranial hypertension without other neurologic abnormalities.
- In selected patients with suspected stroke syndromes. Approximately 10% to 25% of patients with cerebral ischemia or infarction demonstrate an isodense lesion that enhances. All acute intracerebral hematomas that are clinically symptomatic can be recognized on a nonenhanced CT scan. However, delayed presentations may require contrast to enhance and delineate the lesion.
- If either the clinical presentation or the nonenhanced CT scan are suggestive of aneurysm or arteriovenous malformation. Characteristic findings of the intravascular component of the lesion may be revealed with enhancement.
- Patients with acute head trauma who do not require an enhanced CT scan in the acute setting. A nonenhanced CT scan yields appropriate diagnostic information, while an enhanced CT scan may cause neurotoxicity by exposing the patient to contrast when the blood-brain barrier is disrupted. A patient who is studied a week after the trauma may require contrast enhancement to detect an isodense subdural hematoma. An enhanced CT scan enables identification of isodense subdural hematomas or ring enhancement of hemorrhagic contusions.
- In suspected inflammatory lesions, which are best evaluated by an enhanced CT scan. Included in this category are cerebritis, abscess, and infarction due to vasculitis.

The administration of IV contrast material is accompanied by an inherent risk of adverse reactions that range from mild to potentially fatal. Diatrizoate (Renografin, Hypaque), metrizoate (Isopaque), and iothalamate (Conray) are the iodide contrast agents most commonly employed. The occurrence of complications depends on the route of administration, type of study performed, and the patient's condition. The dose of contrast material depends on the structures requiring enhancement. Generally, 30 to 40 g of iodine are required to enhance vascular structures. One half of a solution containing 42 g of iodine (300 ml of 30% or 150 ml of 60% contrast material) is rapidly delivered intravenously before scanning. The remainder is infused slowly during the scan. The following complication rates have been reported—intravenous urography (5.6%), intravenous cholangiography (10%), and cerebral angiography (2.3%). An enhanced CT scan of the brain and orbits has been associated with an adverse reaction rate of 2.2% to 3.4%.[26,27]

Although most adverse reactions occur within minutes of administration, occasionally delayed reactions occur within 30 to 60 minutes. Most commonly, nausea and vomiting are experienced and result from histamine release. Treatment is initiated by removing the patient from the CT scanner to prevent aspiration and discontinuing administration of contrast material. Benadryl and Tagamet given IV may be helpful. Idiosyncratic and anaphylactic reactions may also be experienced. Hives and flushing may herald the onset of a major allergic response. Laryngeal edema may rapidly follow. In this case urgent treatment is indicated with epinephrine and steroids. Instillation of IV contrast material can evoke cardiovascular responses. An acute vagal reaction is characterized by a decrease in blood pressure with bradycardia. The reaction is treated with atropine.

Neurologic complications can be anticipated and may complicate the course of the comatose patient. Impairment of the blood-brain barrier as a result of increased capillary permeability leads to extravasation of contrast material into the brain parenchyma. Neurotoxicity is manifested by the sudden onset of convulsions, paralysis, and a worsening in the level of consciousness. Neurologic disturbances typically occur immediately but may be delayed and occur up to 24 hours later.[28]

Renal toxicity is a well-recognized complication of contrast material administration. Specific risk factors predisposing to the development of renal impairment are diabetes mellitus, multiple myeloma, underlying renal failure (creatinine level greater than 4.5 mg), and dehydration.[27]

CT findings. It has become increasingly evident that the value of the CT scan is limited by the expertise of the interpretation. At most major medical centers the CT scan is read by an experienced radiologist who provides timely and accurate feedback. Unfortunately, this service is not consistently provided around the clock at all medical centers. The initial clinical interpreter must possess a basic familiarity with interpreting CT scans in order to detect

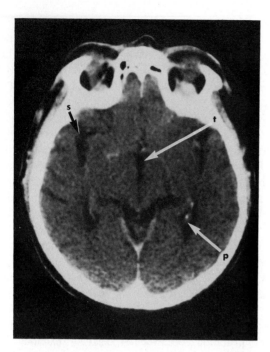

Fig. 15-1. CT scan of normal neuroanatomy: *s*, sylvian fissure; *t*, third ventricle; *p*, posterior horn of lateral ventricles.

CT scans findings in intracranial lesions

High-density lesions

Hemorrhage
Calcification

Isodense lesions

Subacute hematoma

Low-density lesions

Infarction
Abscess
Tumor
Edema
Cyst
Hygroma

Contrast enhancement

Vasogenic edema
Isodense hematoma
Tumor
Abscess
Vascular anomalies

---

gross abnormalities. Evidence of increased ICP and herniation must be appreciated, as well as identification of the etiology whether it be a mass lesion or diffuse or focal cerebral edema. If an intracranial mass exists, such as an intracerebral hemorrhage, the character, location, and extent require documentation so that the appropriate steps in management may be pursued.

Interpreting a CT scan requires recognition of basic neuroanatomy. The ventricular system serves as a structural landmark by which CT scan levels are defined. Specific CT scan levels are represented by four regions with respect to the ventricular system—infraventricular, low ventricular, high ventricular, and supraventricular levels. The cranial slices will reflect high and low areas within each of these levels. To identify increased ICP and herniation and to further identify pathology, a knowledge of basic neuroanatomy is mandatory. Recognition of the following structures is of paramount importance—cortical, subcortical and brain stem structures; ventricular system; subarachnoid spaces; vascular structures (veins and sinuses); and midline and positional landmarks (interhemispheric fissures, sylvian fissure, and major sulci)[29,30] (Fig. 15-1).

The recognition of pathologic findings includes identifying midline shifts of the interhemispheric fissures, distortion of the central and sylvian fissures, and location of the pineal gland. The ventricles are evaluated for evidence of dilatation, diminution, and distortion. The cisterns are evaluated for compression or effacement signifying increased ICP. Compression and distortion of cortical brain stem structures are visualized. Extra-axial masses in the form of hemorrhages, tumors, empyema, abscesses, or

cysts are searched for, and similar lesions are sought in intracerebal locations. Based on the recognition of hemorrhage, infarction, tumor, or abscess, locations can be assigned to either brain stem, thalamic, basal ganglia, subcortical, or cortical tissue. Sulci and glia are evaluated for prominence and alteration in contour. Distortion may represent mass lesions, cerebral edema, or increased ICP. Extracerebral mass lesions and diffuse and focal intraparenchymal lesions are described according to whether they are qualitatively of high density, isodensity, or low density in comparison with surrounding brain tissue on the CT scan (see the box above). High-density lesions usually represent hemorrhage or calcification whereas low-density lesions are consistent with edema, infarction, tumor, abscess, cyst, empyema, or granuloma. Specific primary neoplasms and metastatic lesions may appear isodense and occasionally of high density. Isodense lesions may escape detection without contrast enhancement. For example, the rare presentation of a subacute subdural hematoma may appear isodense with surrounding brain parenchyma. Without enhancement, the possibility of missing an isodense lesion is conceivable. This supports the contention that nonenhanced and enhanced scans should be routinely performed in nontraumatic coma.

A CT scan in the comatose patient is performed to reveal evidence of increased ICP and herniation caused by a primary lesion that compresses the brain stem. A primary lesion that affects the integrity of the ARAS along its ascending tract may alternatively be demonstrated. At minimum, a surgically correctable lesion must be excluded. The absence of such a lesion on a CT scan is acceptable evidence that a

CT scan findings in altered consciousness

Extra-axial mass
   Subarachnoid hemorrhage
   Epidural hematoma
   Subdural hematoma
   Subdural empyema
Intra-axial mass
   Intracerebral hemorrhage
   Infarction
   Tumor
   Abscess
   Cyst
Herniation
Cerebral edema
Hydrocephalus
Cerebral atrophy
Normal

In herniation

Shift of midline structures
Ventricular dilatation or compression
Cistern effacement
Masses
   Extra-axial
   Intra-axial
Cerebral edema

In cerebral edema

Diffuse swelling
   Loss of sulci, cisterns, and fissures
   Small or absent ventricles
Focal swelling
   Unilateral loss of sulci and fissures
   Unilateral hemispheric enlargement
   Loss of cisterns
   Unilateral mass effect with midline shift
Obstructive hydrocephalus
   Periventricular white matter edema

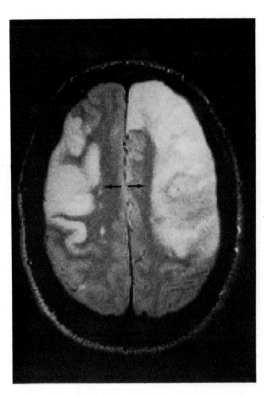

Fig. 15-2. Proton-density MRI image of bilateral infarction of parietal lobes demonstrates bilateral areas of increased signal intensity *(arrows).*

neuropathologic lesion is not responsible for the patient's comatose condition. In the unusual circumstance of an isodense lesion or delayed CT scan appearance of the lesion, the initial CT scan may not reveal the causal lesion.[29]

The CT scan will either be normal or will generate 18 recognizable abnormal patterns as described by Moody et al.[31] These patterns may be consolidated into six pathologic categories (see the box above). The CT scan may demonstrate extra-axial mass, intra-axial mass, herniation, cerebral edema, hydrocephalus, cerebral atrophy, or some combination of these findings.

Magnetic resonance imaging. MRI is an exciting and rapidly developing imaging modality that has potential application in the evaluation of CNS-injured patients. This imaging technique is discussed in greater detail in the Appendix.

MRI results from the absorption or emission of electromagnetic radiation by a nucleus of atoms under the influence of a static magnetic field. The spectrum of absorbed or emitted electromagnetic radiation is determined by the nature of the nucleus and the surrounding chemical environment. The nuclei of tissues are exposed to a series of electromagnetic fields. The first electromagnetic field is applied, causing the nucleus to align along the direction of the electromagnetic field. A second short radiofrequency pulse creates a second electromagnetic field at right angles to the first. When the second field is removed, the nuclei reorient toward the first field, emitting energy in the process. The energy cycle is defined by two time constants, T1 and T2, during the nuclei alignment and realignment. Nuclear alterations generate small electrical voltages. The voltage is received by a surface coil receiver and transmitted to a computer. The computer analyzes signals received from the response of nuclei to the magnetic fields. Images are reconstructed depending on how an element is distributed within the tissue examined and its response to magnetic alteration.[31a,31b]

MRI permits the greatest differentiation between intracranial gray and white matter. It has been established as a superior diagnostic tool in the detection of brain tumor, infarctions, and multiple sclerosis (Fig. 15-2). Useful information is obtained from MRI when posterior fossa lesions are suspected. Brain tumors are accurately identified, and

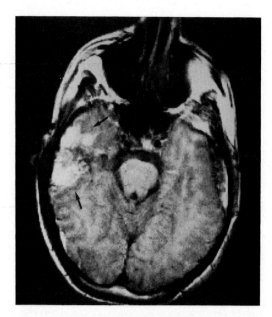

Fig. 15-3. T$_1$-weighted MRI image of hemorrhagic contusion of the right temporal lobe *(arrows)* demonstrates an irregular area of high signal intensity.

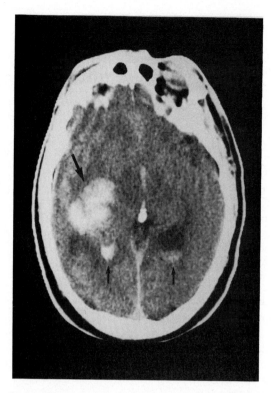

Fig. 15-4. CT scan of acute subarachnoid hemorrhage demonstrates an irregular high-density area within the right temporoparietal lobes *(large arrow)* and posterior horns of the lateral ventricles *(small arrows).*

MRI also distinguishes extra-axial from intra-axial posterior fossa space-occupying lesions.

MRI may have application in the diagnosis of intracranial trauma; however, the CT scan remains the modality of choice since it permits rapid examination of critically ill patients. MRI has the capacity to reveal intracranial hemorrhage, cerebral contusions, and isodense lesions (Fig. 15-3). This modality possesses the additional capability of providing views in the sagittal, coronal, and transaxial planes and with better contrast resolution.[32]

MRI presently is not incorporated in the initial evaluation of altered consciousness. Currently, technical and clinical limitations prevent this application. However, it is anticipated that MRI technology will become increasingly available and less cumbersome with continued development.

Brain hemorrhage

Brain hemorrhage may be induced by trauma, vascular malformation, or aneurysm, or it may be associated with hypertension and disturbances of the clotting mechanism. Intraparenchymal hemorrhage may cause coma depending on the location and size of the bleeding. For example, brain stem hemorrhages commonly result in coma whereas cortical hemorrhages tend to cause coma only when extensive.

Subarachnoid hemorrhage. Subarachnoid hemorrhage (see Chapter 17) most commonly occurs after significant head trauma and in many instances escapes medical detection due to low-grade symptomatology, especially in minimal-to-moderate bleeding. Spontaneous subarachnoid

hemorrhage most commonly results from a ruptured vascular aneurysm. In the early stages, the only prodromal symptoms may be a severe headache that is often mistakenly presumed to be a migraine. Bleeding in the subarachnoid space leads to meningeal irritation, headache, back pain, stiff neck, and vomiting. Fifty percent will experience altered consciousness in association with headache. A dramatic presentation is that of sudden onset of headache, vomiting, and loss of consciousness (LOC), with or without pupillary changes. An additional presentation is that of seizure with recovery of consciousness. In the patient who is alert and is suspected of having a subarachnoid hemorrhage without neurologic deficits, the most sensitive diagnostic procedure is the lumbar puncture. These cases are more likely to involve small hemorrhages in which the CT scan may be interpreted as normal. Omission of a lumbar puncture in this setting would be considered an insufficient diagnostic investigation. The CT scan is performed in this setting to assess baseline ventricular size, determine the presence and location of the intracerebral hemorrhage, and the presence of complications. The typical CT scan demonstrates high-density material in the interhemispheric or sylvian fissures, cerebral sulci, basilar cisterns, or ventricles (Figs. 15-4 and 15-5). Occasionally it is difficult to distinguish interhemispheric blood from a dense falx.[33]

Diffuse or localized subarachnoid hemorrhage is confir-

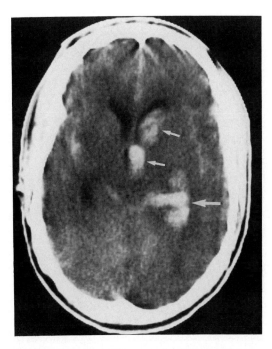

Fig. 15-5. Nonenhanced CT scan of subarachnoid hemorrhage shows high-density blood within the lateral and third ventricles *(small arrows)* due to hemorrhage from an arteriovenous malformation fed by the choroidal artery on the left *(large arrow)*.

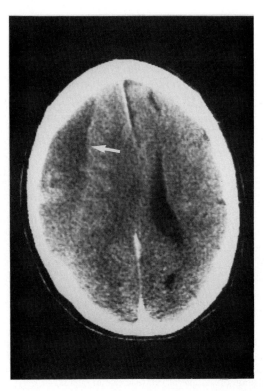

Fig. 15-6. Enhanced CT scan of subdural hematoma demonstrates a moderately well defined area of decreased density adjacent to the right parietal bone *(arrow)*. There is mass effect with shift of the midline structures and obliteration of the right lateral ventricle.

matory evidence of aneurysmal subarachnoid hemorrhage. Extensive opacification on a CT scan is more representative of an aneurysmal hemorrhage, whereas local opacification is more consistent with trauma. Further confirmation is established by angiography. Angiography allows determination of the nature of the vascular lesion as well as the surrounding vessels. Ordinarily a delayed angiogram is performed but early angiography is indicated when immediate surgery is contemplated to correct associated complications. Most patients with intracerebral or intraventricular hematoma visualized on a CT scan will exhibit depressed consciousness and focal neurologic deficits. The reliability of a CT scan for detecting subarachnoid hemorrhage due to ruptured aneurysm has ranged from 55% to 95%.[34] A CT scan performed on a high-resolution scanner on the day of subarachnoid hemorrhage will detect 95% of cases. This number decreases to 67% by the third day following subarachnoid hemorrhage.[35,36]

Subarachnoid hemorrhages are graded from I to V. Grades IV and V are massive hemorrhages and will be accompanied by positive neurologic findings. A CT scan will not only assist in procuring a diagnosis but will also reveal associated complications that may require immediate surgery or ICP monitoring. Intracranial hematomas, basal cistern clots, intracerebral hemorrhages, and hydrocephalus may occur in conjunction with subacrachnoid hemorrhage. Mortality in the first 24 hours is related to the development of these complications. Early recognition prompts expedi-

tious surgical intervention and obviates fulminant clinical deterioration. Subdural hematoma displayed in the context of an existing subarachnoid hemorrhage is usually due to rupture of an aneurysm.[35]

Subarachnoid hemorrhages occurring in intravenous drug abuse should arouse the suspicion of a mycotic aneurysm. Fever, sepsis, bacterial endocarditis, and meningitis are found in association with or antedating the development of a mycotic aneurysm. Blood vessels damaged by inflammatory arthritis can also lead to aneurysmal rupture.[37]

Subdural hematoma. A subdural hematoma may be an isolated finding following the rupture of an aneurysm or an arteriovenous malformation. Acute subdural hematoma is most often discovered in relation to acute head trauma. Subdural veins tear in response to shearing forces in the cranial vault. Ruptured vessels at the site of contusion and tears in small cortical arterial branches also produce subdural hematomas. Acute subdural hematoma appears on a CT scan as crescentic high-density tissue mass with smooth, well demarcated borders adjacent to the inner table of the skull (Fig. 15-6). Subdural hematoma usually occurs over a unilateral parietal or frontal convexity; in 25% of patients, they occur over bilateral convexities. A subdural hematoma compresses the lateral ventricles, ef-

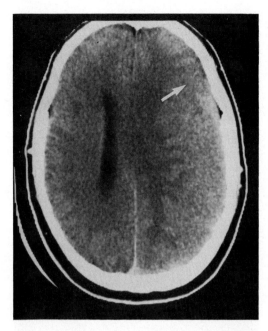

Fig. 15-7. Nonenhanced CT scan of isodense hematoma demonstrates a slightly increased density of the lateral aspect of the brain *(arrow)* adjacent to the left parietal bone, with obliteration of the lateral ventricle due to edema.

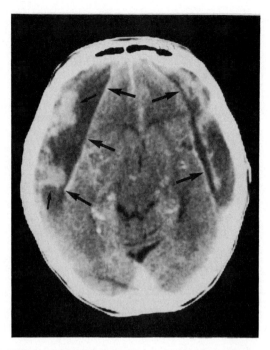

Fig. 15-8. Nonenhanced CT scan shows bilateral subdural hemorrhage *(large arrows)*. Areas of high density *(small arrows)* indicate acute bleeding superimposed on chronic low-density hematomas adjacent to the parietal bones.

faces cortical sulci, and displaces midline structures except when the brain is atrophic or the hematoma is small.[38-40]

Subdural hematoma may occur in the interhemispheric fissure. In a child with nonaccidental trauma (NAT) caused by severe shaking, an interhemispheric subdural hematoma results when bridging veins tear at their points of attachment to the superior sagittal sinus.[41,42] Up to 50% of patients with subdural hematomas have intracranial abnormalities identified on a CT scan, including contusion, edema, and associated hematomas. The high-density appearance of intracranial hemorrhage is due to the heme component of the blood clott. As hemoglobin is degraded, attenuation of the clot decreases causing the hematoma to become isodense in appearance. This process usually takes place in 1 to 3 weeks. An acute subdural hematoma in anemic patients and in patients with clotting abnormalities may initially appear isodense. An isodense hematoma may cause ventricular compression or midline shift. Newer CT scanners can distinguish isodense hematoma by displaying a pattern in the hematoma that is distinctive from surrounding cortical tissues (Fig. 15-7). Bilateral isodense subdural hematomas produce little or no shift. Ventricular distortion may be the single most suggestive finding. A suspected isodense hematoma may be demonstrated by contrast enhancement. Contrast material enhances the richly vascular membrane that develops around the subdural hematoma 1 to 4 weeks after injury.[43,44]

Chronic subdural hematomas develop over a 4 to 6 week period as cellular elements break down and fluid per-

fuses into the area by osmosis. The hematoma appears as a low-density area compared with surrounding brain tissue. Sulcal effacement, midbrain shift, and ventricular distortion may also be seen as well (Fig. 15-8).

Epidural hematoma. Epidural hematoma (see Chapter 17) is most commonly due to skull fractures over the temporal region that lacerate the underlying middle meningeal artery. Blood dissects the dural from the inner table of the skull. Rarely venous bleeding from the calvarial diploe through a fracture or a dural sinus tear may cause an epidural hematoma. Skull fracture is demonstrated in 85% of patients. Because blood accumulates rapidly under high pressure, coma rapidly ensues. The CT scan shows a focal, biconvex smoothly marginated high-density tissue mass adjacent to the inner table of the skull. Sulcal effacement, ventricular compression, and midline shift are frequent findings. A skull fracture may also be seen on a CT scan.[45]

Intracerebral hemorrhage. Intracerebral hemorrhage may occur as a result of trauma, surgery, hypertension, vascular malformation, mycotic aneurysm, or berry aneurysm. The location of the hemorrhage on a CT scan is helpful in determining the etiology. The CT scan is reliable in detecting the majority of these cases. The sudden development of a neurologic deficit accompanies most intracerebral hemorrhages. A maximal deficit occurs at onset in 34% of these patients, or gradual progression of the deficit occurs over several hours. Blood leaks from small penetrating arterioles into brain parenchyma over several minutes to hours. On a CT scan, acute hemorrhages are seen

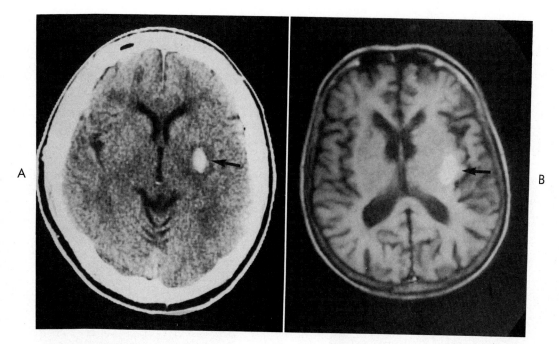

Fig. 15-9. A, Nonenhanced CT scan of hypertensive hemorrhage in the region of the putamen *(arrow)* demonstrates high-density blood. **B,** T$_1$-weighted MRI image of putamen hemorrhage shows a well defined area of increased signal intensity *(arrow).*

as round or irregularly shaped homogenous, high-density lesions. The margination is usually smooth but may be irregular. The central portion of the hematoma may be denser and more homogenous. Hematomas are surrounded by a periphery of vasogenic edema. Mass effect caused by large hemorrhages creates midline shift and displacement of the ventricles. Bleeding may also extend into the ventricles. Subacute hematomas may become isodense or be of low density.[46,47]

The putamen is the most frequent site of hypertensive hemorrhage. Depending on whether the bleeding presents medially or laterally, a clinical syndrome with headache, varying degrees of impaired consciousness, hemiparesis, hemianesthesia, and conjugate lateral gaze palsy develops. Medial hemorrhages have a greater tendency to rupture into ventricles and cause transtentorial herniation. As a consequence, medial bleeding has a poorer prognosis when compared to lateral bleeding. When medial hemorrhage is discovered in the normotensive patient less than 40 years of age, it is most likely due to substance abuse. The CT scan shows a high-density mass in the region of the putamen (Fig. 15-9). The mass may show extension into the internal capsule, thalamus, ventricles, or cortical area.[48]

The second most common site of hypertensive bleeding is the thalamus, representing 10% to 15% of hypertensive hemorrhages. About 25% of hemorrhages detected by a CT scan are thalamic. Approximately 84% of patients are hypertensive and clinically manifest headache, altered consciousness, papilledema, lateralizing signs, hemiparesis,

and hemianesthesia. Massive thalamic hematoma causes third ventricle displacement and intraventricular hemorrhage and dilatation. Headache and vomiting ensue followed by progressively diminished consciousness and hemiparesis. Downward ocular deviation, restricted gaze, ipsilateral miotic pupils that are poorly reactive may be seen. Smaller hemorrhages in the thalamic area may not be manifested by headache or altered consciousness. The presentation may be marked by an isolated neurologic deficit. A massive hemorrhage has an associated high mortality. The CT scan displays a high-density lesion, which can be irregularly marginated and round, oval, or linear. The lesion ranges in size from 1.0 to 7.0 cm. Large hematomas possess a low-density region peripherally that represents edema. Massive hemorrhages may produce mass effect with distortion, displacement, and elevation of the third ventricle.[49,50]

Primary pontine hemorrhages occur most commonly at the junction of the basis pontis and tegmentum. The pons is disrupted by several mechanisms. Injury occurs due to selective bleeding in the brain stem or a contiguous intraparenchymal hemorrhage. Secondary petechial hemorrhages due to mass effect, herniation, and brain stem contusion caused by trauma are known mechanisms. The clinical features are recognizable and include rapid onset of coma, quadriplegia, bilateral positive Babinski signs, miotic pupils, absent horizontal eye movement, absent caloric response, and irregular respiratory pattern. Ninety percent of patients will have blood in the CSF. In decreasing frequency the causes are hypertension, vascular mal-

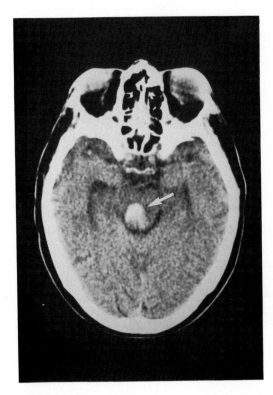

Fig. 15-10. Nonenhanced CT scan of hypertensive brain stem hemorrhage demonstrates high density blood within the brain stem *(arrow)*.

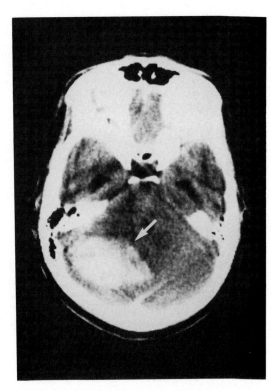

Fig. 15-11. Nonenhanced CT scan of hemorrhage in the cerebellum *(arrow)* demonstrates high-density blood.

formation, and basilar artery aneurysm. The CT scan displays a round or comma shaped irregularly marginated high-density lesion. Hemorrhage may extend cephalad, caudad, or into the fourth ventricle. Basilar cisterns are effaced[51,52] (Fig. 15-10).

Cerebellar hemorrhage. Cerebellar hemorrhage is an important pathologic entity that requires rapid recognition to achieve successful surgical correction. It comprises 10% to 15% of spontaneous intracranial hemorrhages. Generally, if surgery is performed before the onset of brain compression, the outcome will more likely be successful. The associated clinical syndrome appears in an acute and subacute form. The acute presentation consists of headache, vomiting, dizziness, and gait disturbance. In addition, the level of consciousness deteriorates precipitously. The physical evaluation reveals signs of brain stem compression that include miotic pupils, lateral gaze palsy, sixth and seventh nerve paresis, and bilateral positive Babinski signs. The subacute presentation is marked by prominence of gait instability with a distinct absence of signs of brain stem compression. CSF examination reveals serosanguineous fluid under increased pressure. Bleeding may extend into cerebellar hemispheres, the brain stem, and the fourth ventricle. A CT scan in the acute syndrome shows a large cerebellar hematoma and obstructive hydrocephalus with effacement of the fourth ventricle and basilar cisterns. The subacute presentation will result in CT scan findings consis-

tent with a smaller hematoma and no mass effect. The presence of coma is associated with a mortality of 75%[53,54] (Fig. 15-11).

Intracerebral hemorrhage and hypertension. From 15% to 25% of nontraumatic intracerebral hemorrhages (see Chapter 17) are located in the cerebral hemispheric white matter. Hypertension is less often a contributing factor. Discovery of a hemorrhage in this area should raise suspicion of angioma, aneurysm, neoplasm, blood dyscrasia, cerebrovascular accident (CVA), or cortical vein or dural sinus thrombosis. In the Weisberg series,[53] only 10% of patients had a specific cause identified. Sixty-four percent of hemorrhages occurred in normotensive patients. Locations included frontal (22%), frontotemporal (8%), temporal (10%), temporopontine (10%), parietal (30%), and occipital areas (14%).[5] Headache, vomiting, and seizures are typical early symptoms followed by neurologic deterioration. The severity appears greater in the hypertensive group as compared to the normotensive group. Hematomas are accessible to surgical evacuation, and decompression may prevent development of neurologic sequelae. The CT scan findings reveal a high-density lesion in the cerebral hemisphere subcortical white matter. A large hematoma may have a surrounding halo of low-density edema, and the hematoma may extend into the ventricles. Lobar hematomas are caused by anticoagulants. Hemorrhagic infarctions are often caused by embolic phenomena.

Multiple spontaneous hemorrhages can occur but usually are not due to hypertensive disease. The likely causes include neoplasms, blood dyscrasia, vasculitis, venous sinus thrombosis, and herpes simplex encephalitis. Three percent of patients with intracranial hemorrhage will demonstrate multiple hematomas.[55]

Intraventricular hemorrhage. Intraventricular hemorrhage occurs by two mechanisms. Either blood extends into the ventricle from a contiguous hemorrhage, or there is rupture of anomalous vessels located within the ventricular wall or choroid plexus. Clinical findings in primary ventricular bleeding are seizures, altered consciousness, nuchal rigidity, high fever, extensor spasms, and bilateral Babinski signs.

Anticoagulated patients are at risk of developing intracranial bleeding. Bleeding can occur either spontaneously or in response to minor trauma. Hemorrhage can be intracerebral, subdural, intraventricular, or subarachnoid. On a CT scan, a characteristic hematoma appears as a fluid-blood interface. The interface reflects layering of blood and separation from the plasma component. An isodense or normal-appearing CT scan may also be encountered. A normal CT scan may not be conclusive evidence of the absence of an intracranial hemorrhage.[56]

The conversion of a dry infarction into a hemorrhagic infarction is most frequently seen in patients with embolic infarctions emanating from the heart. Anticoagulation and bleeding diathesis increase the likelihood of this transformation; however, hemorrhagic infarction may result without an identifiable bleeding tendency. Transition to hemorrhagic infarction requires an average of 4 days.

The alcoholic patient exhibits a higher incidence of intracranial hemorrhage than other patients. Coagulation defects and impaired platelet function cause bleeding diathesis. Alcoholic cerebral atrophy exposes cerebral blood vessels to a greater vulnerability to trauma. Frequent falls and violent encounters due to the effect of alcohol on the patient's mental status and behavior increase the potential for intracranial trauma. Intracerebral hematomas typically occur in subcortical white matter. Bleeding may be massive; however, the mass effect may be less pronounced because of the underlying cerebral atrophy. Trauma-induced contusions are distinctively different lesions in that they are small, superficial, and multiple.

Intracerebral hematomas may accumulate after significant head trauma. Blood vessels are subjected to shearing forces causing tears and extravasation of blood. Frontal and temporal regions are most commonly involved, and the bleeding tends to remain superficial. Delayed intracerebral hematomas may develop up to 2 weeks after the initial head trauma.

Intracranial hemorrhages are reported in 4% to 10% of patients with hemophilia. Most of the episodes are recognized in patients below the age of 12. One third of patients are younger than 3 years. Head trauma is a frequent causative factor. A period of up to 7 days may transpire before the onset of neurologic symptoms. Similar to the patient on anticoagulants, bleeding may occur in any intracranial location. Intracerebral hemorrhages, however, have the worse prognosis, with a mortality of 30% to 40%.[57]

Cerebral infarction

The usefulness of the CT scan is related to its ability to differentiate the hemorrhagic lesion from the cerebral infarction. The management options are distinctly different. The therapeutic considerations for intracerebral hemorrhage are surgical evacuation, ICP monitoring, and observation. The management of cerebral infarction includes consideration of anticoagulation therapy. Surgical intervention and ICP monitoring are less likely with cerebral infarction. Hemorrhagic stroke is more likely to be associated with coma when compared to cerebral infarction. Whenever coma is a feature of cerebral infarction, the implication is that an extensive area of the brain is involved with shift of midline structures. Infarction localized to the diencephalon may also produce coma. McDowell[58] reported that fewer than 20% of patients with cerebral infarction lose consciousness at the onset and many recover within an hour. Brain stem infarction may cause coma, but the majority of the various vascular brain stem syndromes do not include loss of conciousness or coma. Vertebrobasilar insufficiency occurs distinctively in the absence of coma. Bilateral pontine infarctions are particularly likely to induce coma. Unilateral pontine infarction, by contrast, will cause altered consciousness ranging from normal to coma. In the majority of cases no change in mental status is experienced. Central tegmental infarction, on the other hand, consistently produces coma, as does hemorrhage in this region.[58,59]

The "locked-in" syndrome is an uncommon syndrome that presents with clinically unique features. The brain stem infarction involves the basis pontis. These patients present in a comatose-like state but demonstrate preservations of eyelid and limited extraocular movement (EOM). The patient is otherwise without speech or movement.

Cerebral infarction is a vaso-occlusive phenomenon that generates ischemic edema. The initial stage of the edema is characterized by localized cellular swelling. The CT scan demonstrates a homogenous, low-density area with indistinct adjoining margins. The gyri are compressed and the sulci effaced.

Brain tumor

Brain neoplasms (see Chapter 17) may be classified according to location: supratentorial, infratentorial, or midline. The neoplasm may be located extra-axially or intra-axially. In the extra-axial location, meningiomas are the most frequently encountered neoplasms whereas gliomas and metastases are the most frequent intra-axial neoplasms. In the infratentorial region, intra-axial masses involve the brain stem and the cerebellar, frontal, and ventricular areas. Extra-axial lesions are located at the cere-

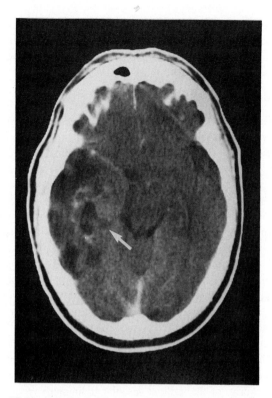

Fig. 15-12. Enhanced CT scan of an irregular low-density area in the right temporal lobe, with mass effect causing midline shift *(arrow)*. Glioblastoma multiforme was found.

bellopontine angle. The lesions commonly found in this region are acoustic neuromas, meningiomas, dermoids, and subarachnoid cysts.[60]

The clinical presentation in brain tumor is most commonly a gradual onset of neurologic symptoms that may progressively worsen. The presentation may mimic a stroke syndrome. Sudden onset of clinical symptoms is less common. Acute onset of neurologic deterioration accompanying intracranial neoplasms occurs due to several mechanisms: (1) peritumoral hemorrhage, (2) seizure activity, (3) mechanical compression of the arterial or venous blood vessels by tumor causing necrosis or hemorrhage, and (4) sudden shifts in ICP due to mass effect. Neoplasms may cause CSF obstruction, herniation, and tissue infiltration. The type and locations of the tumor determine the onset of presentation and the character of the neurologic symptoms. Meningiomas and gliomas usually cause both mass effect and CSF obstruction. Similar lesions will produce early intracranial hypertension and obstructive hydrocephalus.[60]

Meningiomas most commonly occur in intracranial areas with significant arachnoid tissue. The parasagittal zones, the falx, cerebral convexity, sphenoid ridge, and olfactory groove are common locations. The benign lesions are extra-axial in location and are encapsulated. On a nonenhanced CT scan, they appear as homogenous, speckled, high-density lesions that are regular in shape and sharply marginated. One third of these lesions are isodense but nonetheless discernible from surrounding brain tissue. Meningiomas usually show intense contrast enhancement,

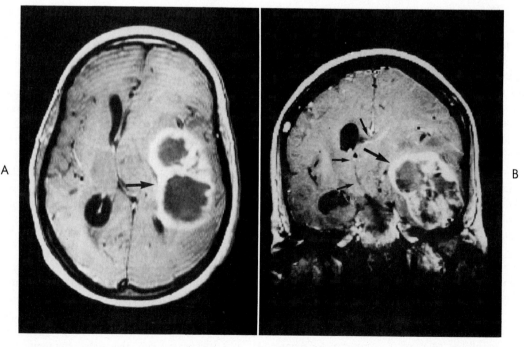

Fig. 15-13. A, Axial T_1-weighted MRI image of glioblastoma multiforme shows an irregular low-signal mass in the left temporal lobe *(arrow)*, with a high-signal rim. There is significant mass effect and midline shift. **B,** Coronal T_1-weighted MRI image of the same mass *(large arrow)* demonstrates brain herniation across the midline *(small arrows)*.

appearing as homogenous lesions that are sharply marginated. Vascular anatomy is usually defined by angiography preoperatively.

Gliomas represent malignant intracerebral neoplasms. These tumors may originate in the cerebral cortex and extend into the corpus callosum, basal ganglia, or thalamus. Classification of gliomas includes low-grade astrocytoma, anaplastic astrocytoma, and gliobastoma multiforme. Glioblastoma multiforme is characteristically seen as a heterogeneous mixed-density or low-density lesion with significant mass effect. An enhanced CT scan or MRI demonstrates irregularly shaped ring enhancement (Figs. 15-12 and 15-13).

From 20% to 30% of patients with systemic carcinoma are reported to develop intracranial metastases. Intracerebral metastases are commonly located at the junction of gray and white matter or in the superficial cortex. Tumor nodules may be small and discrete yet can be accompanied by extensive peritumor edema. Metastatic tumors are most frequently found in the territory of the middle cerebral artery because metastatic deposits are hematogenous and follow the cerebral flow distribution. About 80% are located supratentorially, 20% infratentorially, and 35% are multiple. Neurologic symptoms may be insidious or rapid in onset, usually characterized by a stroke-like syndrome. Neurologic deterioration occurs due to peritumoral edema or hemorrhage into the metastatic tumor.[60]

Intracranial metastases detected by a CT scan even when less than 10 mm in size may have variable presentations. The CT scan may demonstrate a low-density lesion

with projections representing peritumor edema (Fig. 15-14). There may be a peripheral, small, high-density nodule that densely enhances with contrast. Ring enhancement may be displayed. When metastatic lesions are a consideration, it is important to perform an enhanced CT scan because many lesions are isodense. In clinically symptomatic patients the initial enhanced CT scan is occasionally negative. A follow-up scan in approximately 2 weeks may demonstrate the lesions.

Infection

Infectious sources (see Chapter 17) can be significant causes of CNS pathology, resulting in altered sensorium from systemic toxicity or mass effect. Mass effect arises secondary to abscess formation or brain edema and may further progress to produce a herniation syndrome. Viral, bacterial, fungal, and protozoan infections may occur causing focal suppurative cerebritis, brain abscess, and empyema located in subdural or epidural spaces. Focal cerebritis and brain abscess are infectious conditions that develop in the brain parenchyma as a consequence of contiguous extension from sinusitis or mastoiditis, hematogenous dissemination of systemic illness, or generalized sepsis. Pathologic tissue changes are characterized by tissue necrosis, polymorphonuclear (PMN) response, petechial hemorrhage, and local edema. The suppurative area may become an encapsulated abscess. Lesions are typically larger than 7 mm and may be single or multiple depending on the source of infection. The center of the abscess contains necrotic tissue and bacteria. This area is surrounded by a low-density periphery that represents brain edema with mass effect.[61]

Meningeal symptoms of cerebritis and abscess are accompanied by neurologic deficit or seizure. Mass effect

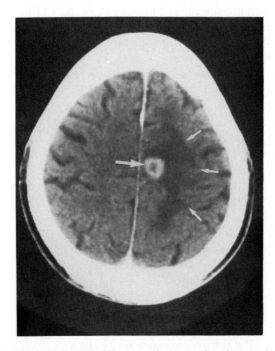

Fig. 15-14. Enhanced CT scan of metastatic adenocarcinoma with an area of low-density edema *(small arrows)* surrounding a more central high-density lesion *(large arrow)* in the left parietal lobe.

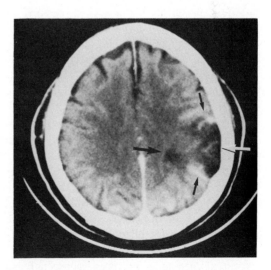

Fig. 15-15. Enhanced CT scan of brain abscess in a patient with IV drug abuse demonstrates an area of low density *(large arrows)* within the left parietal lobe, with high-density enhancement peripherally *(small arrows)*.

and seizure may produce mental status changes. CSF study reveals pleocytosis, elevated protein count, normal glucose concentration, and negative bacteria cultures. Although infrequently performed, a radionuclide brain scan may be helpful in the diagnosis, and the electroencephalogram (EEG) will show a focal slow wave pattern. Nonenhanced and enhanced CT scans are done when brain abscess is the suspected diagnosis. The nonenhanced scan shows a low-density lesion surrounded by a low-density rim. A central low-density core is recognized. Most brain abscesses enhance following contrast material infusion, demonstrating a ring of enhancement as the hallmark finding (Fig. 15-15). Multiple lesions, mass effect, and hydrocephalus may also be demonstrated. The ring enhancement of abscesses must be differentiated from that of neoplasms in which the enhancement tends to be more complex and irregularly marginated. Infarctions and hematomas may also form a ring of enhancement but are readily differentiated by their characteristic CT scan patterns. Abscess formation is always preceded by a stage of focal cerebritis. The CT scan is sensitive enough to detect cerebritis before significant suppurative formation. Consequently, antibiotics may be administered early in the course, potentially preventing the development of abscess. If abscess formation develops (especially when large), surgical drainage and decompression are indicated. Steroids and antibiotics may assist in management, but surgery is frequently required.[62-64]

Subdural empyema results from penetration of the dura by frontal sinusitis, by septic thrombophlebitis of emissary veins, or by infection of a subdural effusion. The clinical syndrome is similar to and the clinical findings simulate brain abscess. A sinus radiograph, EEG, and lumbar puncture may be helpful in the preliminary diagnosis. An associated high mortality results from diagnostic delay. The most common initial diagnosis is meningitis or brain abscess. CT scan findings reflect the pathologic effects of subdural empyema on the brain, such as cerebral edema ischemia, subdural fluid collection, and, within several weeks, a highly vascular enveloping membrane (Fig. 15-16). Empyema is usually of low density, although isodense and high-density lesions do occur. Mass effect, unilateral gyral enhancement, and low-density gray matter are additional findings on the CT scan.[65,66]

Several infectious agents deserve mention because of their increased prevalence and propensity to cause mental status changes. Cryptococcus, toxoplasmosis, and herpes simplex produce meningoencephalitic syndromes, particularly in patients with varying degrees of immunocompromise. Alterations in brain physiology, resulting from the direct effect of lesions, seizures, or cerebral edema producing a mass effect, may be detected (see Chapter 26).

Cryptococcal meningitis has been increasingly recognized in patients suffering from acquired imunodeficiency syndrome (AIDS) and other immunocompromised states. A subacute or chronic meningitis syndrome, focal neuro-

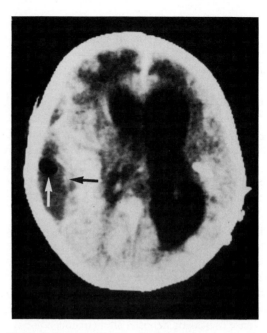

Fig. 15-16. Enhanced CT scan of subdural empyema adjacent to the right parietal bone *(black arrow),* with marked mass effect causing shift of the midline and impingement on the lateral ventricle. Air is seen within the subdural empyema *(white arrow).*

logic deficits, and seizures are common manifestations. Intracranial hypertension typically occurs late in the disease course. A basilar granulomatous meningitis is characteristic of cryptococci. Small, multiple nodules may form, representing small subcortical cysts with minimal gliosis or capsule formation. One half of cases are seen in immunocompromised patients, whereas the remaining cases occur in patients who are normal. The CSF evaluation reveals lymphocytic pleocytosis, diminished glucose concentration, positive India ink (25%), elevated protein level, and positive fungal cultures.[67]

The CT scan findings may be normal in uncomplicated cryptococcal infections. The formation of intracranial granulomas as coalescing existing lesions can be demonstrated by a CT scan that shows the granulomas as isodense lesions with nodular or ring enhancement (Fig. 15-17). This is a nonspecific pattern requiring brain biopsy to confirm the diagnosis. Multiple coalescing, subcortical, low-density, nonenhancing lesions represent multiple cysts. Abscess and granuloma may develop a distinct mass of necrotic tissue, and granuloma formation constitutes a cryptococcoma, readily demonstrated on a CT scan as an isodense lesion with nodular or ring enhancement [67] (see Chapter 26).

Immunologically suppressed patients are also predisposed to developing CNS infection as a result of toxoplasmosis. The typical presentation is a subacute meningoencephalitis. Multiple necrotic granulomas may be scattered throughout the cerebral hemispheres. A CT scan may show nodular or ring-enhancing lesions similar to pyo-

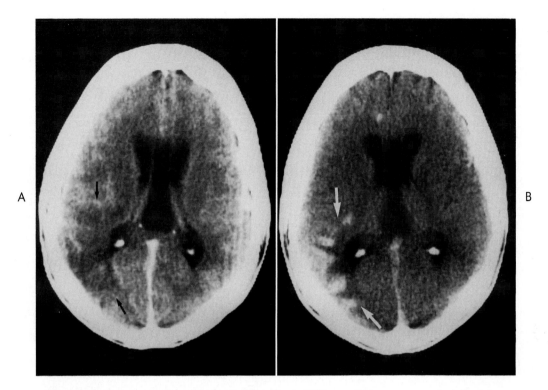

Fig. 15-17. Cryptococcal meningitis. **A,** Nonenhanced CT scan demonstrates poorly defined area of low density in the right posterior parietal region *(arrows).* **B,** Enhanced CT scan shows areas of enhancement in the right posterior parietal region *(arrows).*

genic abscess, tuberculomas, or sarcoidosis (Fig. 15-18). Brain biopsy is required to establish the diagnosis. Intracranial calcifications throughout the brain may be seen on a nonenhanced CT scan, particularly in congenital forms of toxoplasmosis.[68]

Herpes simplex encephalitis is an infection of the CNS that may create considerable damage to the cerebral tissue. A necrotizing hemorrhagic lesion is produced that has the potential for immediate complications as well as long-term effects. Mortality has been reported as high as 70%. The infection demonstrates an affinity for the temporal or frontal areas. Widespread involvement may be encountered in the pediatric population. The initial symptoms are consistent with a typical viral syndrome that includes fever, headache, and myalgias. As temporal lobe necrosis develops, psychomotor seizures, olfactory hallucinations, amnesia, confusion, aphasia, visual field deficits, and psychiatric symptoms may develop. Hemorrhage, edema, and necrosis then leads to elevated ICP and transtentorial herniation.

The diagnosis is established by brain biopsy, which demonstrates characteristic histopathologic changes, positive immunofluorescent herpes simplex virus stains, and positive viral cultures. The CSF study usually shows lymphocytic pleocytosis with red blood cells, elevated protein concentration, and diminished glucose concentration. The EEG may show unilateral or bilateral temporal slowing.

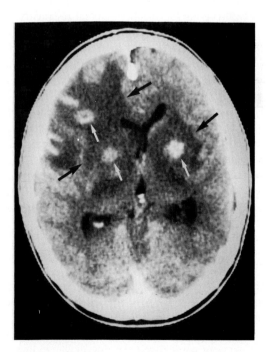

Fig. 15-18. Enhanced CT scan of toxoplasmosis secondary to AIDS. There are multiple intracerebral abscesses that enhance with IV contrast material *(small arrows).* Surrounding low-density edema is seen *(large arrows).*

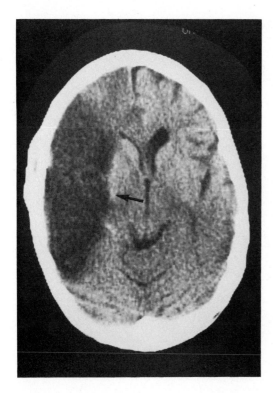

Fig. 15-19. Nonenhanced CT scan of herpes encephalitis demonstrates a large low-density area in the right temporal region *(arrow)* with a mass effect demonstrated by shift of the midline structures to the left and compression of the anterior horn of the right lateral ventricle.

Although infrequently performed, radionuclide brain scan shows frontotemporal uptake. On a CT scan, a high-density area involving the medial temporal regions is demonstrated. High-density areas representing hemorrhage are interspersed with low-density areas (Fig. 15-19). Edema and mass effect are reported in 80% of cases. Contrast material infusion results in enhancement in 50% of the cases.[69]

The CT scan is the primary diagnostic procedure that should be performed when there is suspicion of herpetic encephalitis. In many instances the findings are nonspecific but may localize to the specific area in which surgical biopsy is warranted. If the patient's neurologic status rapidly deteriorates, then surgical decompression is indicated. Antiviral therapy with acyclovir has been beneficial. Therapy should be initiated as early as possible on the basis of clinical presentation or a suggestive findings on the CT scan.[70,71]

Coma in the pregnant patient

The pregnant comatose patient requires a separate series of considerations. A CVA is a possible complication during pregnancy. In addition to the indicated differential diagnosis, possible causes are toxemia of pregnancy and venous sinus or cortical vein thrombosis due to hypercoagulable states. Other causes include cardiac-generated embolus from endocarditis, amniotic fluid embolism, choriocarcinoma causing tumor embolus, intracerebral hemor-

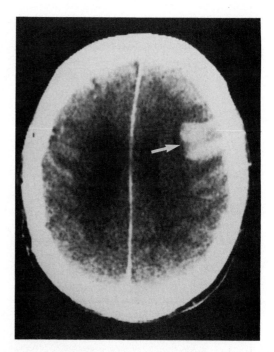

Fig. 15-20. Nonenhanced CT scan shows an area of high density within the left parietal lobe *(arrow)*, representing an hemorrhagic infarction. Subsequent angiography revealed thrombosis of the superior sagittal sinus.

rhage, or artero-occlusive disease. Oral contraceptives predispose to venous or occlusive disease.[72,73] Dural venous sinus thrombosis and cerebral vein thrombosis may occur due to a localized or systemic infection or miscellaneous conditions including: pregnancy, use of oral contraceptives, dehydration, hematologic disorders, polycythemia, leukemia, sickle cell disease, disseminated intravascular coagulation, head trauma, or neoplasm. The accompanying neurologic syndrome depends on the location, extent of thrombosis, presence of venous infarction, brain inflammatory process, or brain hemorrhage. The brain appears edematous due to diminished venous outflow. The symptomatology of venous-induced hemorrhagic infarctions depends on the specific venous system involved. The dural sinus or superior sagittal sinus is the most common site of venous thrombosis. Associated symptoms are headache, diplopia, and vomiting. Papilledema and abducens nerve palsy may be recognized as well as depressed consciousness and paraparesis. Nonenhanced CT scan findings include hemorrhagic infarctions, intracerebral hematoma, and compressed ventricles that are highlighted by the demonstration of a high-density lesion within the straight sinus. An enhanced CT scan may show filling defects within the contrast-filled sinus caused by venous clot. Diagnosis is established when carotid angiography reveals nonfilling of the venous sinus and cortical veins (Fig. 15-20).

Lateral sinus thrombosis most commonly results from mastoiditis and otitis media. The lateral sinus is located posterior to the mastoid. The enhanced CT scan shows a

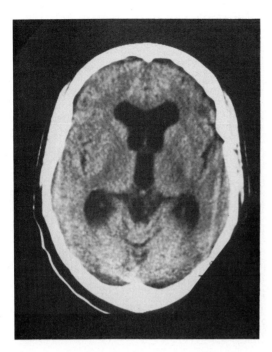

Fig. 15-21. Nonenhanced CT scan demonstrating hydrocephalus with dilatation of the lateral ventricles and third ventricle.

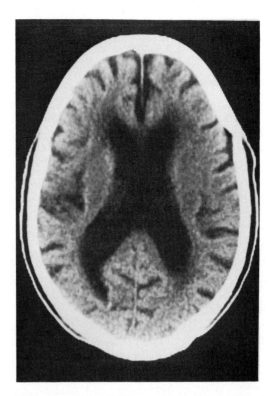

Fig. 15-22. Nonenhanced CT scan of cerebral atrophy demonstrates enlargement of the lateral ventricles and prominence of the cortical sulci.

filling defect in the lateral sinus. Infection localized to the orbit or paranasal and meningeal region may lead to cavernous sinus thrombosis.[74,75]

Hydrocephalus

The CT scan definitively identifies ventricular enlargement. Ventricular enlargement may result from either hydrocephalus or cortical atrophy. Hydrocephalus denotes increased intraventricular pressure that causes compression of adjacent brain tissue, whereas cerebral atrophy causes ventricular enlargement by ventricular expansion into the degenerative brain. Obstructive hydrocephalus is the most common cause of ventricular enlargement and may be subdivided into communicating and noncommunicating. Communicating hydrocephalus occurs as a result of obstruction of CSF absorption, whereas noncommunicating hydrocephalus implies obstruction to flow within the ventricular system.

Communicating hydrocephalus results when flow through the subarachnoid spaces or reabsorption of CSF by arachnoid villi is diminished. The subarachnoid space is obliterated or the subarachnoid villi are altered and dysfunctional. A few conditions associated with the development of communicating hydrocephalus are meningeal carcinomatosis, dural venous thrombosis, subdural hematoma, subarachnoid hemorrhage, and meningitis. The CT scan shows symmetric enlargement of the lateral third and, frequently, fourth ventricles with effacement of cerebral sulci (Fig. 15-21). CSF under elevated pressures may leak into adjacent brain tissue. This is demonstrated on a CT scan as periventricular white matter lucency indicative of interstitial edema.

Noncommunicating hydrocephalus similarly demonstrates enlarged lateral ventricles and effaced cerebral sulci. Obstruction may result from colloid cyst, congenital malformation, inflammation, tumor, or intraventricular hemorrhage. CSF blockage arises at several points in the ventricular system The CT scan findings differ from communicating hydrocephalus in that ventricular dilatation is found distal to the obstuction while ventricular contraction occurs proximally. Obstruction between the lateral and third ventricles results in dilatation of the lateral ventricles and diminution of the third ventricle.[76,77]

Diffuse brain atrophy is a finding that may be encountered on a CT scan in the patient with altered consciousness. Cerebral atrophy is an irreversible loss of brain substance that results in enlarged ventricles and sulci. Atrophy may result from trauma, inflammation, demyelinating disease, radiation, chemotherapy, alcoholism, hypoxia, and Alzheimer's disease. The importance of this CT scan finding is the differentiation of ventricular enlargement resulting from cerebral atrophy compared to that resulting from hydrocephalus (Fig. 15-22). The distinction is that enlarged sulci are associated with cerebral atrophy, whereas small effaced sulci characterize hydrocephalus. When cerebral atrophy is the CT scan diagnosis, evaluation is pursued to isolate a metabolic or toxic cause. For hydrocephalus, a shunting procedure may be required. Normal CT scan findings would likewise essentially eliminate a structural lesion as the cause of altered consciousness. Thorough medical evaluation is indicated to detect diffuse cerebral impairment based on systemic infection or metabolic abnormalities.[78]

Pediatric considerations

Altered consciousness in the child does not substantially differ from that experienced in the adult population. A deteriorating neurologic condition must be interpreted as potentially life threatening. The Glasgow Coma Scale must be modified in order to recognize differences in infant neurologic responses. Of course, dosages of therapeutic medications must also be altered. Disorders unique to the pediatric population should always be considered.

Coma in children can be divided into three etiologic categories: supratentorial lesions, infratentorial lesions, and metabolic encephalopathy. Trauma is the most common cause of coma in children. Aside from accidental and nonaccidental head trauma, metabolic abnormalities and infection constitute the other major causes of altered neurologic function. The important causes of supratentorial mass lesions in children that produce progressive deterioration include cerebral hyperemia resulting from head trauma, epidural and subdural hematomas, intracerebral hemorrhage, acute hydrocephalus, and subdural empyemas. The most common clinical situations associated with acute supratentorial lesions are accidental and nonaccidental head trauma, severe systemic hypertension, obstruction of an existing ventricular peritoneal shunt, or a bleeding arteriovenous malformation. Infratentorial lesions may also cause coma by destroying the ARAS or by compressing the brain stem. Coma resulting from infratentorial lesions can be differentiated from that resulting from supratentorial lesions if localizing brain stem signs precede the onset of coma. Infratentorial lesions commonly recognized in the pediatric population are brain stem contusions associated with head trauma, basilar artery thrombosis (rare), cerebellar hemorrhage, tumor with secondary hydrocephalus, and brain stem encephalitis. Midbrain or pontine lesions rarely lead to abrupt coma in the pediatric population. However, lesions in the infratentorial region may produce central neurogenic hyperventilation, absent oculovestibular reflexes, pinpoint pupils, and decerebate rigidity. Metabolic disorders, such as hyponatremia and hypoglycemia, are common causes of pediatric coma, whereas hepatic and renal failure are rarely responsible for altered conciousness.[79,80]

Illicit drug abuse is increasingly recognized in the pediatric population as a cause of coma; however, two distinct etiologies that are pre-eminent considerations in altered consciousness are Reye's syndrome and nonaccidental trauma (NAT). Reye's syndrome occurs in association with hepatic dysfunction and causes diffuse brain swelling that results in increased ICP and coma. Fever and altered mental status prompt suspicion of an infectious central nervous system process such as bacterial meningitis or herpes encephalitis. If ICP elevation is not evident, lumbar punc-

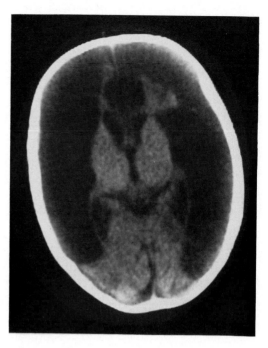

Fig. 15-23. Nonenhanced CT scan demonstrates cerebral anoxia in a battered child with large areas of low density within temporal, frontal, and parietal lobes. These areas represent infarction in the distribution of the internal coratid arteries bilaterally.

ture is performed to exclude CNS infection. Metabolic screening tests, including liver function and a serum ammonia, are indicated.[79,80]

Nonaccidental trauma is frequently a diagnostic dilemma. Unsuspected cerebral injury can rapidly lead to disability and death. A vague clinical presentation, absence of bruising, and the presence of significant intracranial bleeding without external evidence of trauma frequently make the diagnosis elusive. Severe head injuries in the first year of life are usually due to NAT. The shaking injury is the most frequently encountered source of damage. Shaking injuries create tremendous neurologic damage and therefore significant risk of death, as well as a high incidence of mental retardation and neurologic deficits. Signs and symptoms are sparse. The presentation may mimic infection, intoxication, or metabolic abnormalities. Diagnosis depends on recognizing high-risk environments. Physical findings include a bulging fontanel, head circumference greater than the 90th percentile, and retinal hemorrhages. The finding of bloody fluid from a lumbar puncture is suggestive. Diagnosis is confirmed by a CT scan demonstrating an intracranial hemorrhage, usually a subdural hematoma[81] (Fig. 15-23).

Generalized seizures may cause alterations in consciousness. Recovery may be delayed when prolonged post-ictal periods occur. Prolonged unresponsiveness after seizure may also represent continued, clinically inapparent seizure activity.

SUMMARY

The CT scan has revolutionized the diagnostic evaluation of the comatose patient. It is anticipated that advances in the CT scan and MRI will tremendously advance the sophistication with which neuropathology is diagnosed. This progress in the technical realm of neurodiagnosis, however, has not been accompanied by substantial change in the overall management of disorders of consciousness. The thrust of management is still to rapidly identify and remove the injurious cause and to reverse progressive injury to the brain. Ultimately, preservation of brain function is the goal. This is best accomplished by rapidly instituting cardiovascular and brain resuscitation measures to assure adequate brain perfusion. An inciting agent must be anticipated. This can only be discovered by ascertaining the nature of the lesion. Consequently, A CT scan is the crucial diagnostic step. The preservation of normal brain tissue and the potential of restoring normal brain function depends on appropriate resuscitation, accurate diagnosis, and rapid implementation of definitive management.

SYNCOPE
Definitions

Syncope is a sudden loss of consciousness in response to an impairment in cerebral metabolism or sudden deprivation of essential nutrients, including oxygen and glucose. It is symptomatic of potentially serious disorders. Ironically, syncope may also represent a benign self-limited disturbance completely devoid of serious implications. In effect, syncope is representative of a constellation of disorders that range from the trivial to life threatening. The diagnostic challenge lies therein. Life-threatening causes of syncope such as cardiac dysrhythmias require differentiation from those clinical entities that pose a minimal threat to overall health. As an isolated symptom, syncope provides little clue as to the severity of the underlying problem.[82] The endpoint of diagnostic evaluation is to establish whether the seriousness of presentation warrants hospitalization or whether discharge from the emergency department may be accomplished confidently and safely. The final decision is based on a logical analysis of clinical information so that selected diagnoses may be excluded or eliminated. The likelihood that the patient will suffer significant morbidity or mortality if discharged is the ultimate consideration that should sway decision-making toward admission.

The magnitude of identifying life-threatening causes of syncope is reflected in the Kapoor et al. study[83] in which patients with cardiovascular origins of syncope were found to have mortality rates of 30% ($\pm$ 6.7%) compared with the lower mortality rates for patients with syncope of noncardiovascular origin (12.2% $\pm$ 4.4%) and of unknown origin (6.4% $\pm$ 2.8%).[83] The effectiveness of pinpointing various disorders within the cardiovascular category depends on a thorough clinical evaluation, the basis of which is the patient's history and physical examination. History and physical examination have been reported to be contributory to the final diagnosis in 85% of patients with diagnosed syncope.[84] Radiographic intervention fails to significantly contribute to the diagnosis in the majority of cases. However, in isolated circumstances, radiographic studies may assist in clarifying specific clinical problems.

Pathophysiology

In patients with syncope the brain is briefly deprived of essential nutrients, specifically oxygen and glucose by one of four mechanisms[85]:

- Diminution or loss of intrinsic cerebral circulation.
- Transient decrease in cardiac output.
- Decrease in systemic arterial pressures that compromises cerebral perfusion.
- Insufficient concentration of energy substrates within blood transported to the brain (i.e., hypoglycemia or hypoxemia).

Obstruction of cerebral blood flow occurs as a consequence of a fixed lesion in the cerebral vessels leading to transient ischemic attacks (TIAs) or stroke. Cardiogenic causes of syncope are due to disturbances in rate or rhythm, dysfunction of valves, wall motion abnormalities, and obstruction to inflow, outflow, or ventricular activity. Tachycardia, bradycardia in the form of sinus node dysfunctions, and the Stokes-Adams syndrome are other identifiable causes. Addtional causes are aortic stenosis, idiopathic hypertrophic subaortic stenosis (IHSS), and atrial myxoma.

Decreases in blood pressure result from decreased cardiac output and diminished total peripheral resistance. Stroke volume and heart rate are important components of cardiac output. Extreme increases or decreases in heart rate may be accompanied by hypotension and syncope. Alteration of systemic vascular resistance by autonomic dysfunction or drugs may likewise diminish pressure. Hypovolemia implies a reduced circulating volume associated with lowered cardiac output and blood pressure. Occult bleeding is an important consideration, and syncope may be the premonitory sign indicating impending rupture or exsanguination. Fluid loss on the basis of vomiting, diarrhea, urinary losses, and third spacing frequently cause hypovolemia; lack of venous tone may decrease blood pressure by decreasing venous return.

A decrease in systemic vascular resistance reflects direct vascular actions. Alterations in vasomotor tone occur as a result of extrinsic agents such as drugs or intrinsic alterations of autonomic regulation.

Adequate cerebral perfusion does not ensure a sufficient supply of energy substrate to the brain. Oxygen distribution may be diminished by intrinsic respiratory or cardiac disease. Oxygen-carrying capacity may be reduced by anemia. Glucose may become unavailable due to fasting, hypoglycemic medications, or alcohol use.

Etiology

The most common cause of syncope is the vasovagal or vasodepressor syndrome. This syndrome is thought to be due to autonomic overactivity that produces symptoms including pallor, sweating, and gastrointestinal disturbances. These symptoms are noted before the onset of the syncopal episode and contrast with that of cardiac etiologies.[85-87] Cardiac-related syncope may occur suddenly in the absence of prodromal autonomic symptomatology.

Although the mechanisms contributing to transient loss of consciousness overlap significantly, the causes of syncope have traditionally been classified according to broad categories: cardiac, neurologic, vascular, psychogenic,

and idiopathic (see the box below). The pre-eminent consideration is recognizing immediately life-threatening causes, such as occult bleeding, or primary cardiac disturbances, such as malignant dysrhythmia or myocardial infarction. In 20% to 50% of patients a diagnosis will not be established.[83,84,88,89] Martins et al.[84] in evaluating 174 patients in the emergency department found 37% of the cases to be vascular, 8% cardiac, and 9% neurologic, with the remainder being idiopathic.[84]

Syncope presents a significant diagnostic dilemma in the elderly. There is a greater likelihood that cardiac abnormalities underlie the onset of syncope. The elderly are also more likely to have underlying cerebrovascular disease, multisystem disease, and to be taking medications affecting cerebral and cardiac perfusion. This combination of factors broadens the range of differential considerations and increases the diagnostic dilemma. In deciding on a probable cause, a cardiac etiology is far more likely in the older than in the younger population.[90,91]

Initial management

The initial evaluation and management of syncope should ensure hemodynamic and cardiac stability and exclude life-threatening events. Instability in the form of hypotension or cardiac dysrhythmia requires immediate resuscitative measures. Upon presentation after syncope, the patient is rapidly assessed for evidence of ongoing vasomotor instability and evidence of trauma resulting from the fall. If instability exists, oxygen is provided, the cervical spine is immobilized, and, if indicated, a large-bore intravenous line is inserted while routine blood samples are drawn. Fluids are administered as a bolus and the patient's response is monitored. Cardiac monitoring is initiated to evaluate for cardiac rhythm abnormalities.

High-grade cardiac dysrhythmias may be treated according to the indicated medical protocol. Orthostatic hypotension, persistent hypotension, or tachycardia potentially indicate a volume deficit attributable to blood loss or fluid depletion, often requiring crystalloid or blood infusion. Hypotension may also reflect cardiac tamponade, right ventricular failure, cardiogenic shock, or pulmonary embolus.

When blood loss is a consideration, the origin may be intra-abdominal, retroperitoneal, or pelvic in location. Although hypotension may be exhibited on the basis of fluid loss, autonomic dysfunction, caused by medications, sepsis, or an endocrine disorder, often occurs.

A gastrointestinal hemorrhage may be the suggested diagnosis after a patient history of peptic ulcer disease, aspirin use, or steroid use is revealed. In the woman of reproductive age there may be risk of an ectopic pregnancy or ruptured ovarian cyst. A presentation of abdominal pain followed by syncope in these patients is suggestive of these disorders.

Diagnostic findings

In most instances the patient is hemodynamically stable and a thorough history and physical examination can be

---

Differential considerations of syncope

Cardiac
  Dysrhythmia
  Valvular heart disease
  Aortic stenosis
  Idiopathic hypertrophic subaortic stenosis (IHSS)
  Myocardial infarction
  Myocardial contusion
  Pulmonary hypertension
  Pulmonary embolism
  Atrial myxoma
  Pericardial tamponade
  Dissecting aneurysm
Neurogenic
  Central
    Cerebral ischemia
    Transient ischemic attack (TIA)
    Seizure
  Vasodepressor
    Vasovagal syndrome
  Carotid sinus disorder
Vascular
  Hemorrhage
  Fluid depletion
    Vomiting
    Diarrhea
    Diuresis
    Third spacing
Venous insufficiency
Autonomic insufficiency
  Diabetic neuropathy
  Polyneuropathy
Drugs and toxins
  Antihypertensives
  Nitrates
  Antidysrhythmics
  Antidepressants
Metabolic
  Hypoglycemia
  Hypoxemia
Psychogenic
Idiopathic

obtained and constitute the foundation of the evaluative process. The history and physical examination may assist in diagnosing the cause of syncope in 25% to 70% of patients. Crucial aspects of preliminary evaluation are careful history, orthostatic vital signs, and complete cardiac and neurologic examinations.[92] A complete history should include questions regarding prodromal symptomatology and a description of onset, duration, and recovery. Persistent symptoms need to be documented. Prior episodes of syncope and a thorough past medical history, including medications, may provide additional information. In obtaining a history, drop attacks and seizures are to be distinguished from syncope. Any neurologic symptoms such as aphasia, weakness, or visual changes should also be noted. Ascertaining neurologic elements in the history assists in determining the value of a CT scan in the patient's assessment.[89] Finally, evidence of injury from trauma or a fall should be sought. Elderly patients are especially prone to develope hip fracture, rib fractures, and skull injuries.[93]

The physical examination is highlighted by the performance of orthostatic vital signs and meticulous heart, lung, abdominal, and rectal examinations, including testing for occult blood. A complete neurologic examination is essential. A musculoskeletal survey is performed to search for evidence of bony injuries requiring radiographic assessment.[84]

Radiographic evaluation

Following the history and physical examination, if it is established that the patient is at risk but is stable, a preliminary laboratory screen of blood (hematocrit, glucose), an ECG, and radiographs are obtained. Hemodynamically unstable patients require empiric intervention. A chest radiograph assists in evaluation of cardiac size. Cardiac enlargement may result from valvular heart disease, congestive heart failure, or pericardial effusion, whereas widening of the mediastinum indicates a possible dissecting thoracic aortic aneurysm (see Chapters 10 and 12). Lung fields are examined for gross infiltrates, atelectasis, and collapse. Radiographs of the hip or extremities may be indicated when a fall results in injury or if blood loss is suspected on the basis of trauma. A CT scan is not done unless the history suggests a TIA, CVA, drop attack, seizure, or a neurologic deficit is found on examination. Kapoor et al.[83,94] and Day[95] have suggested that the yield in performing CT head scans in the absence of focal neurologic findings is low.[83,94,95]

Several medical disorders are manifested by syncope; radiographic or ultrasonographic procedures may assist in early diagnosis. Syncope is a presenting symptom in 13% of patients with acute pulmonary embolism.[96,97] In pulmonary embolism, syncope occurs in response to pulmonary vascular obstruction, pulmonary hypertension, autonomic discharge, right heart failure, diminished cardiac output, and subsequent compromised cerebral perfusion. Syncope in association with pulmonary embolism is typified by a myriad of symptoms and signs, including chest pain, dyspnea, hemoptysis, and tachypnea. It is unusual to experience syncope in this setting as an isolated symptom although there is one reported case.[97]

A ventilation/perfusion (V/Q) scan may be obtained to diagnose pulmonary embolism (Fig. 15-24). There is a greater than 90% probability of pulmonary embolism if the lung scan shows multiple segmental and lobar perfusion defects with normal ventilation.[98] A normal perfusion scan virtually excludes pulmonary embolism. Cheerley et al. recommended that patients who do not fall into the high-probability or low-probability group should undergo pul-

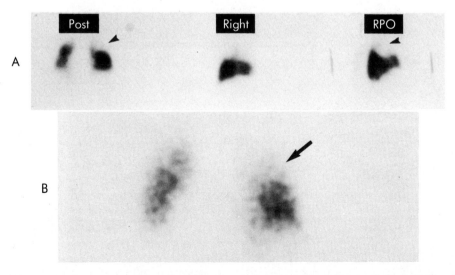

Fig. 15-24. **A,** Perfusion (Q) scan demonstrates a large perfusion defect involving the entire right upper lobe *(arrowheads)*. **B,** Accompanying ventilation (V) scan shows the same defect *(arrow)*.

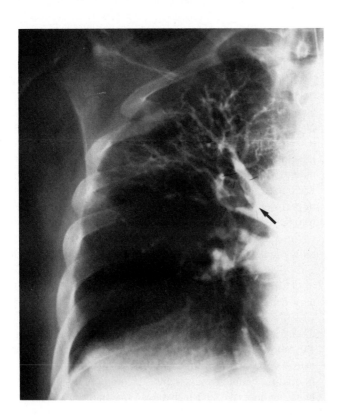

Fig. 15-25. Pulmonary angiography demonstrates a large embolus within the right upper lobe pulmonary artery *(arrow)*.

Fig. 15-26. Echocardiography of large pericardial effusion. **A,** Apical four-chamber view demonstrates compression of the right atrial wall *(large arrow)*. *PE*, pericardial effusion; *TV*, tricuspid valve *(small arrow)*; *RV*, right ventricle; *RA*, right atrium; *LV*, left ventricle; *LA*, left atrium. **B,** Parasternal long axis view shows pericardial effusion with fibrinoid (white) strands *(small arrows)* within. Note compression of the right ventricle *(large arrow)*. *PE*, pericardial effusion; *LV*, left ventricle; *RV*, right ventricle; *AV*, aortic valve *(small arrow)*; *LA*, left atrium. **C,** Parasternal short axis view of left ventricle demonstrates surrounding pericardial effusion. *PE*, pericardial effusion; *LV*, left ventricle; *RV*, right ventricle; *PM*, papillary muscles *(small arrows)*.

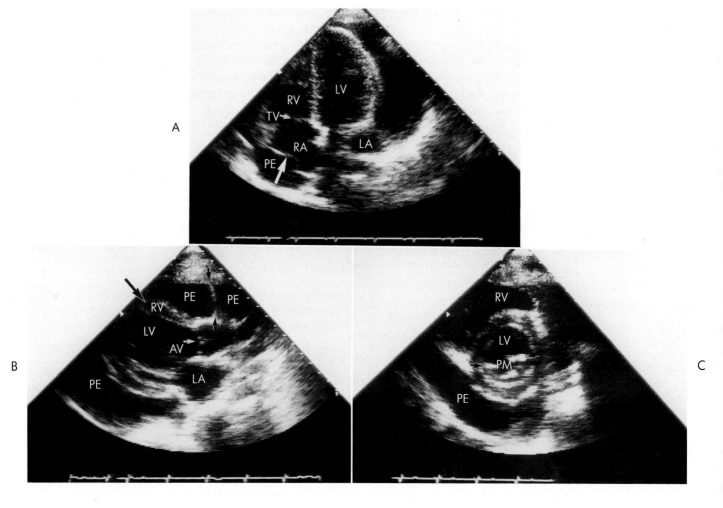

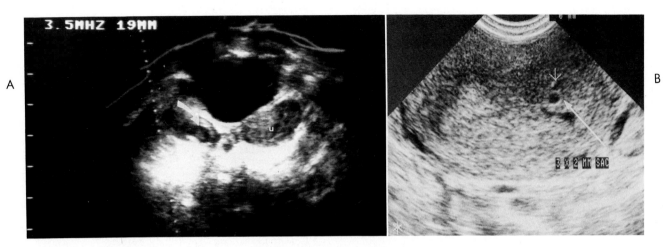

Fig. 15-27. A, Static transverse oblique ultrasonogram of a right tubal gestational sac containing a living fetus *(arrow)* with a dilated proximal tube and an empty uterus, *u.* **B,** Real-time sector ultrasonogram of a 4-week, 4-day pregnancy *(long arrow)* after administration of clomiphene citrate. The 6 mm chorionic sac is clearly defined, and there is a thick decidual reaction. The lacunar spaces *(short arrow)* evident in the decidua are often apparent at this stage. The beta human chorionic gonadotropin (β-hCG) was already 1800. (Reproduced from Hagen-Ansert S: Textbook of diagnostic ultrasonography, ed 3, St. Louis, 1989, CV Mosby.

monary angiography.[99] The risks of pulmonary angiography are less that those of long-term anticoagulation therapy. When a massive pulmonary embolism develops, a V/Q scan may be nondiagnostic due to an overall decrease in pulmonary arterial flow. Pulmonary angiography may then be required to confirm the diagnosis (Fig. 15-25).

Echocardiography is often accessible and may be used for the evaluation of suspected pericardial and cardiac pathology. Hypotension, neck vein distention, distant heart sounds, and syncope may indicate cardiac tamponade. Right ventricular infarction, pulmonary embolism, valvular dysfunction, and tension pneumothorax may provide a similar picture. M-mode or two-dimensional echocardiography on an emergent basis may provide valuable information regarding the pericardial space, ventricular wall motion, and valve function[100] (Fig. 15-26). If the patient's stability permits, a complete study may reveal decreased right ventricular end diastolic dimensions during inspiration associated with pericardial tamponade and a shift of the intraventricular septum towards the left ventricular cavity.[100] One of the most sensitive findings is early diastolic collapse of the right ventricle.[101] Valvular and aortic disease should also be investigated (see Chapters 10 and 12).

Ultrasonography is employed in the evaluation of the stable female patient with a positive serum pregnancy test who is suspected of having an ectopic pregnancy (Fig. 15-27, A). Fifteen percent of ectopic pregnancies are associated with syncope, but most patients experience some combination of abdominal pain, amenorrhea, and vaginal bleeding. Ultrasonography can reliably detect a gestational sac at 5 weeks (Fig. 15-27, B) and a fetal heart rate at 6 weeks, thereby confirming an intrauterine pregnancy or differentiating an ectopic pregnancy from an adnexal mass.[102-104] Dates are established by the last normal period. When dates are unavailable, a quantitative human chorionic gonadotropin level greater than 6500 is usually associated with an identifiable pregnancy by ultrasonography (see Chapter 21).

SUMMARY

Syncope may result from a variety of medical and traumatic conditions. Plain radiography may be useful in the initial evaluation of cardiac and pulmonary disease or musculoskeletal injury. Further diagnostic studies must focus on excluding specific diagnoses.

REFERENCES

1. Fineberg HV, Bauman R, and Sosmun M: Computerized and cranial tomography: effect on diagnosis and therapeutic plans, *JAMA* 238:224, 1977.
2. Roberson PC, Kishore PRS, Miller JO et al: The value of serial computerized tomography in the management of severe head trauma, *Surg Neurol* 12:161, 1979.
3. Saul TG, Ducker TB: The role of computerized tomography in acute head injury, *CT* 4:296, 1980.
4. Baker HL: CT and neuroradiology: a fortunate primary union, *Am J Roentgenol* 137:101, 1976.
5. Weisberg L, Nice C: *Cerebral computed tomography: a text atlas,* ed 3, Philadelphia, 1989, WB Saunders.
6. Plum F, Posner JB: *The diagnosis of coma,* ed 3, Philadelphia, 1983, FA Davis.

7. Daube JR et al: The consciousness system. In Daube JR et al, eds: *Medical neurosciences: an approach to anatomy, pathology, and physiology by systems and levels,* Boston, 1978, Little, Brown.
8. Osborn AG: Diagnosis of descending transtorial herniation by CCT, *Radiology* 123:93, 1977.
9. Beecher HK: A definition of irreversible coma: report of the Ad Hoc Committee of the Harvard Medical School to examine the definition of brain death, *JAMA* 205:85, 1968.
10. Klatzo I: Neuropathological aspects of brain edema, *J Neuropathol Exp Neurol* 26:1, 1977.
11. Greenberg JO: Neuroimaging in brain swelling, *Neurol Clinic* 2(4):677, 1984.
12. Bucy PC, Winston SP: Cerebral edema, *Mod Treat* 9:90, 1977.
13. Overgaard J, Tweed WA: Cerebral circulation after head injury. Part I: Cerebral blood flow and its regulation after closed head injury with emphasis on clinical correlations, *J Neurosurg* 41:531, 1974.
14. Ropper AH, Martin JB: Coma and other disorders of consciousness, In Petersdorf RG, Adams RD, Braunwald E et al, eds: *Principles of internal medicine,* ed 10, vol 1, New York, 1983, McGraw-Hill.
15. Pruitt A: Approach to the patient with altered consciousness. In Wilkins EW, ed: *Emergency medicine,* ed 3, Baltimore, 1989, Wilkins & Wilkins.
16. Edelsohn L: Coma, *Primary Care* 13(1):63, 1986.
17. Miller BL, McEntyre HB: Evaluation of the comatose patient, *Primary Care* 11(4):693, 1984.
18. Caronna JJ, Hagar EL, and Graham D: Clinical diagnosis of the comatose patient: a forgotten art, *Emerg Med Rep* 6(15):113, 1985.
19. Landers DF: Alcoholic coma and some associated conditions, *AFP* 28(4):219, 1983.
20. Clinton JE, Sterner S, Stelmucher Z et al: Haloperidol for sedation of disruptive emergency patients, *Ann Emerg Med* 16:319, 1987.
21. Van Leeuwen AMH, Molders J, Sterkmans P et al: Droperidol in acutely agitated patients—a double blind placebo-control study, *J Nerv Ment Dis* 164:280, 1977.
22. Moody DM, Laster DW, and Marshal BR: Emergency plain film radiology of the nontraumatized patient with altered consciousness, *Radiol Clin North Am* 14(1):49, 1978.
23. Harriman DGF: Bacterial infections of the CNS. In Blackwood W, Corsellis JAW, eds: *Greenfield's neuropathology,* Chicago, 1976, Mosby–Year Book.
24. Haddad LM: A general approach to the emergency management of poisoning. In *Clinical management of poisoning and drug overdose,* Philadelphia, 1983, WB Saunders.
25. Bradshaw JR: *Brain CT: an introduction,* Bristol, England, 1985, John Wright and Sons.
26. Burman S, Rosenbaum AE: Rationale and techniques for intravenous enhancement in CT, *Radiol Clin North Am* 20:15, 1982.
27. Shehadi WH: Adverse reactions to intravascularly administered contrast media: a comprehensive study based on a prospective survey, *Am J Roentgenol* 124:145, 1975.
28. Melartin E, Taohimac PJJ, and Dabb R: Neurotoxicity of iodothalamates and diatrizoates. I. Significance of concentration and reaction, *Invest Radiol* 5:22, 1970.
29. Daniels DL: Normal cerebral anatomy. In *Cranial computed tomography: a comprehensive text,* St Louis, 1985, CV Mosby.
30. Gado M, Hanaway J, and Frank R: Functional anatomy of the cerebral cortex by computed tomography, *Comput Assist Tomogr* 3:1, 1979.
31. Moody DM, Buananno FS, and McWhorter JM: The radiology of nontraumatic coma, *Neurol Clin* 2(4):637, 1984.
31a. Rosenbloom SA: NMR: a realistic appraisal of a revolutionary imaging technique, *Emerg Med Rep* 6(25):193, 1985.
31b. Paushter DM, Modic MT, Burkowski DM et al: Magnetic resonance: principles and applications, *Med Clin North Am* 68(6):1393, 1984.
32. Han JS, Kaufman B, Alfidi RJ et al: Head trauma evaluated by magnetic resonance and computed tomography: a comparison, *Radiology* 150:71, 1984.
33. Adams HP, Kassell NF, Tomer JC et al: CT and clinical correlations in recent aneurysmal SAH, *Neurology* 33:981, 1983.
34. Weisberg LA: Computed tomography in aneurysmal subarachnoid hemorrhage, *Neurology* 29:802, 1979.
35. David KR, Kastler JP, and Herod RC: *Radiol Clin North Am* 20:87, 1982.
36. Gurusinghe NT, Richardson AE: The value of CT in aneurysm and SAH, *J Neurol* 60:763, 1984.
37. Morowetz RB, Karp RB: Evolution and revolution of intracranial bacterial mycotic aneurysm, *Neurosurgery* 15:43, 1984.
38. Perini S, Beltramello A, Pasut ML et al: CNS trauma: head injuries, *Neurol Clin* 2:4, 719, 1984.
39. Zimmerman RD, Danriger A: Extracerebral trauma, *Radiol Clin North Am* 20:105, 1982.
40. Stone JL, Rifai MHS, Sugar D et al: Subdural hematomas, *Surg Neurol* 19:216, 1983.
41. Glista GG, Reichman OH, Brumlik J et al: Interhemispheric subdural hematoma, *Surg Neurol* 10:119, 1978.
42. Bergstrom M, Ericson K, Levander B et al: Computed tomography of cranial subdural and epidural hematomas: variation of attenuation related to time and clinical events such as rebleeding, *J Comput Assist Tomogr* 1:449, 1977.
43. Weisberg LA: Bilateral isodense subdural hematomas, *Comput Radiol* 10:245, 1986.
44. Markwalder TM: Chronic subdural hematomas: a review, *J Neurosurg* 54:637, 1981.
45. Cordobes F, Lobato R, and Rivas JJ: Observations on 82 patients with extradural hematoma, *Neurosurgery* 54:179, 1981.
46. Weisberg LA: Computed tomography in intracranial hemorrhage, *Arch Neurol* 36:422, 1979.
47. Kelley RE, Berger JR, and Scheinberg D: Active bleeding in hypertensive intracerebral tumor: computed tomography, *Neurology* 32:852, 1982.
48. Hier DB, Davis KR, and Richardson ED: Hypertensive putaminal hemorrhage, *Ann Neurol* 1:152, 1977.
49. Weisberg LA: Thalamic hemorrhage: clinical CT correlations, *Neurology* 36:1382, 1986.
50. Walshe TM, David KR, and Fisher CM: Thalamic hemorrhage: computed tomographic clinical correlations, *Neurology* 27:217, 1977.
51. Goto N, Kaneko M, and Hosaka Y: Primary pontine hemorrhage: clinicopathological correlations, *Stroke* 11:84, 1980.
52. Weisberg LA: Primary pontine hemorrhage: clinical computerized tomographic correlations, *J Neurol Neurosurg Psychiatry* 49:346, 1986.
53. Weisberg LA: Cerebellar hemorrhage in adults, *Comput Radiol* 6:75, 1982.
54. Ott RH: Cerebellar hemorrhage diagnosis and treatment, *Arch Neurol* 31:160, 1974.
55. Weisberg LA: Subcortical lobar intracerebral hemorrhage: clinical-computed tomographic correlations, *J Neurol Neurosurg Psychiatry* 48:1078, 1985.
56. Weisberg LA: The fluid blood level in intracranial hematoma due to anticoagulant medication, *Comput Radiol* 11:175, 1987.
57. Eyster ME, Gill FM, and Blat PM: Central nervous system bleeding in hemophiliacs, *Blood* 81:1179, 1978.
58. McDowell FH: *Cerebrovascular diseases,* New York, 1961, Grune.
59. Davis KR, Taveras JM, New PFJ et al: Cerebral infarction diagnosis by computerized tomography: analysis and evaluation of findings, *Comput Tomogr* 124:643, 1975.
60. Weisberg LA: Intracranial neoplasm, *Neurol Clin* 2(4):695, 1984.
61. Heineman HS, Braude AI, and Osterholm JL: Intracranial suppurative disease: early presumptive diagnosis and successful treatment without surgery, *JAMA* 218:1542, 1971.

62. Enzmann D: *Imaging of infections and inflammation of the CNS: CT, ultrasound, and nuclear magnetic resonance,* New York, 1984, Raven Press.

63. Weisberg LA: Cerebral computerized tomography in intracranial inflammatory disorders, *Arch Neurol* 37:137, 1980.

64. Samson DS, Clark: A current review of brain abscess, *Am J Med* 54:201, 1973.

65. Luken MG, Whelan MA: Recent diagnostic experience with subdural empyema, *J Neurosurg* 52:764, 1980.

66. Moseley IF, Kendell BF: Radiology of intracranial empyemas with special reference to computed tomography, *Neuroradiology* 26:333, 1984.

67. Weisberg LA, Garcia C, and Lacorte W: CT findings in intracranial cryptococcal disease, *Neurology* 35:731, 1985.

68. Weisberg LA, Dunn DW: CT finding in intracranial toxoplasmosis, *Comput Radiol* 8:133, 1984.

69. Davis JM, Davis KR, Kleinman GM et al: Computed CT tomography of herpes simplex encephalitis with clinicopathology correlation, *Radiology* 129:409, 1978.

70. Dutt MK, Johnston IDA: Computerized tomography and EEG in herpes simplex encephalitis, *Arch Neurol* 39:99, 1982.

71. Zimmerman RD, Russell EJ, and Leeds NE: CT in early diagnosis of herpes encephalitis, *Am J Radiol* 134:61, 1980.

72. Wieberg DO: Ischemic cerebrovascular complications of pregnancy, *Arch Neurol* 42:1106, 1985.

73. Colosimo C, Fileni A, Moschini M et al: CT finding in eclampsia, *Neuroradiology* 27:313, 1985.

74. Ahmadi J, Keane JR, Segall HD et al: CT observation pertinent to septic cavernous sinus thrombosis, *Am J Neuroradiol* 6:755, 1985.

75. Rao KCVG, Knipp HC, and Wagner EJ: Computed tomographic findings in cerebral sinus and venous thrombosis, *Radiology* 140:391, 1981.

76. Fitz CR, Harwood-Nash DC: Computed tomography in hydrocephalus, *CT* 2:91, 1978.

77. Naidich TP, Schott LG, and Baron RL: Computed tomography in the evaluation of hydrocephalus, *Radiol Clin North Am* 20:143, 1982.

78. Hughes CP, Cado M: Computed tomography and aging of the brain, *Radiology* 139:391, 1981.

79. Humphreys P: Coma in infancy and childhood. In Ivan LP, Bruce DA, eds: *Coma physiopathology: diagnosis and management,* Springfield, Ill, 1982, Charles C Thomas.

80. Chuang S: Neuroradiological findings in the comatose child. In Ivan LP, Bruce DA, eds: *Coma physiopathology: diagnosis and management,* Springfield, Ill, 1982, Charles C Thomas.

81. Humphreys P, Coffey J: Coma in infancy and childhood: the whiplash shaken infant syndrome, *Pediatrics* 54:396, 1974.

82. Savage DD, Corwin L, McGee DL et al: Epidemiologic features of isolated syncope: the Framingham Study, *Stroke* 16(4):626, 1985.

83. Kapoor WN, Karf M, Wieand S et al: A prospective evaluation and follow-up of patients with syncope, *N Engl J Med* 309:4, 197, 1983.

84. Martin GJ, Adams SL, Martin HG et al: Prospective evaluation of syncope, *Ann Emerg Med* 499, 1984.

85. Noble RJ: The patient with syncope, *JAMA* 247:13, 1372, 1986.

86. Wright KE Jr, McIntosh HD: Syncope: a review of pathophysiological mechanisms, *Prog Cardiovasc Dis* 13:580, 1971.

87. Wayner HH: Syncope, *Am J Med* 30:418, 1961.

88. Silverstein MD, Singer DE, Mulle AG et al: Patients with syncope admitted to medical intensive care units, *JAMA* 248:1185, 1982.

89. Gendelman HE, Liner M, Gabelman M et al: Syncope in a general hospital population, *NY State J Med* 83:1161, 1983.

90. Lipsitz LA: Syncope in the elderly, *Ann Intern Med* 99:92, 1983.

91. Kapoor WN, Snustad D, and Peterson J: Syncope in the elderly, *Am J Med* 80(3):419, 1986.

92. Liner M: Syncope, *South Med J* 80(5):545, 1987.

93. Whiteside-Yim C: Syncope in the elderly: a clinical approach, *Geriatrics* 42(4):37, 1987.

94. Kapoor WN, Karpf M, Maher Y et al: Syncope of unknown origin, *JAMA* 247:2687, 1982.

95. Day SC, Cook EF, Funkenstein H et al: Evaluation and outcome of emergency room patients with transient loss of consciousness, *Am J Med* 73:15, 1982.

96. Soloff, Rodman T: Acute pulmonary embolism. II, *Clin Am Heart J* 74:710, 1967.

97. Oster MW, Leslie B: Syncope and pulmonary embolus, *JAMA* 224(5):630, 1973.

98. Thames MD, Alpert JS, and Dalen JE: Syncope in patients with pulmonary embolism, *JAMA* 238:2509, 1977.

99. Cheerley R, McCarthey WH, Perry JR et al: The role of noninvasive tests versus pulmonary angiography in the diagnosis of pulmonary thromboembolism, *Am J Med* 70:17, 1981.

100. Horowitz MS, Schultz CS, Stinson EB et al: Sensitivity and specificity of echocardiographic pericardial effusions, *Circulation* 50:239, 1974.

101. Armstrong WF, Schilt BF, Helper DJ et al: Diastolic collapse of the right ventricle with cardiac tamponade: an echocardiographic study, *Circulation* 65:1491, 1982.

102. Gleicher N, Giglia RV, Deppe G et al: Direct diagnosis of unruptured ectopic pregnancy by real-time ultrasonography, *Obstet Gynecol* 61:425, 1983.

103. Weckstein LN, Boucher AR, Tucker H et al: Accurate diagnosis of early ectopic pregnancy, *Obstet Gynecol* 65:393, 1985.

104. Romero R, Kadar N, Jeanty D et al: Diagnosis of ectopic pregnancy: value of the discriminating human chorionic gonadotropin zone, *Obstet Gynecol* 66:357, 1985.

Seizures

John B. McCabe
Leo Hochhauser

Seizure disorders are a common medical problem. A seizure is such a dramatic and frightening experience to most patients and observers that they seek immediate medical attention.

The risk of having a seizure at some point in life is estimated to be 8.8%.[1] Epilepsy, defined as recurrent seizures not resulting from fever or acute cerebral injury, is less prevalent. It is estimated to be present in 0.65% to 1.0% of the population.[1,2] Up to 5% of all children will experience a febrile seizure.[3]

In one recent study in an urban community hospital,[4] 0.7% of emergency department visits over a 6-month period were for seizures. Of these, 34.5% were for new onset seizures, 15% for febrile seizures, and 46% for seizures that occurred in patients with epilepsy taking prescribed antiepilepsy drugs. In particular, patients with first time major motor seizures present a particular diagnostic challenge to the emergency physician. This group represents a diverse set of causes that ranges from relatively benign and self-limited disorders to malignant and rapidly fatal conditions[5-8] (Table 16-1). Diagnostic radiology plays a key role in the evaluation of such patients and in the ability of the emergency physician to differentiate benign self-limited disorders from life-threatening conditions.

ANATOMIC AND PHYSIOLOGIC CONSIDERATIONS

There are many descriptions of seizure type and confusion may result from inappropriate use of seizure terminology.[9] An abbreviated form of the international classification of epileptic seizures is presented in the box on the left on p. 420, dividing seizures into two major types: partial and generalized.[10] Distinction between seizure types is important because the underlying causes are different and the yield of diagnostic evaluation, both laboratory[11] and radiographic,[12] varies depending on seizure type. History and neurologic examination remain the mainstay in making an appropriate diagnosis in the seizure patient.

Technically, a seizure is an abnormal discharge of electrical activity from the gray matter of the brain, resulting in alteration of normal brain function. Although this definition includes both an electrophysiologic and clinical component, the emergency department diagnosis of a seizure is always based on the clinical component alone. As such, it is sometimes difficult to determine if a seizure has, in fact, occurred. The spectrum of clinical presentation of seizure disorders is much wider than the dramatic tonic-clonic major motor seizure. Some of the subtleties of clinical history and examination that may be useful to the emergency physician are discussed in the box on the right on p. 420. Additionally, an understanding of the most common causes of seizure in each age group may help to delineate possible causes and adjust the appropriate diagnostic and radiographic evaluation (Table 16-2). For instance, the adult patient with a first time seizure is more likely to have a positive yield from emergent radiographic investigation than is the adolescent with a first time seizure.

The emergency department physician must approach a seizure patient with the following questions in mind: (1) has a seizure occurred? (2) what type of seizure has occurred? (3) does the patient have a life threat and require immediate therapy? (4) does the history or examination suggest an underlying cause? (5) are there complications of the seizure that require investigation (i.e., head

Table 16-1. Causes of seizure disorders

Causes of seizures	Description
Acquired	
Congenital and hereditary	Microgyria, porencephaly, congenital infections (toxoplasmosis, cytomegalovirus, syphilis), phenylketonuria, Niemann-Pick syndrome, Tay-Sachs syndrome, tuberous sclerosis, Sturge-Weber syndrome
Antenatal and perinatal	German measles, toxoplasmosis, cytomegalovirus, meningitis, severe toxemia, anoxia, drugs, placental abnormalities
Metabolic	Hypoglycemia, hypocalcemia, hyponatremia, pyridoxine deficiency, porphyria
Febrile	Threshold elevated with age
Traumatic	If dura is penetrated, greater than 30% incidence
	If dura is intact, greater than 10% incidence (World War II veterans)
Subarachnoid hemorrhage	In 19%-26% of cases, does not correlate with prognosis or site; occurs later with rebleeding
Heredofamilial and degenerative diseases	
Youth	Tuberous sclerosis, Sturge-Weber syndrome, neurofibromatosis
Old age	Alzheimer disease, Pick disease
Intoxication	
Drugs	Tricyclics, phenothiazines, lidocaine, aminophylline, IV penicillin, propranolol, metoclopromide, propoxyphene hydrochloride, lithium, isoniazid, cocaine, LSD, phencylidine, amphetamines, scopolamine and salicylamide (Sominex), pentylentetrazol
Toxins	Picrotoxin, camphor, strychnine, lead, carbon monoxide, mercury, iron, methyl bromide, phenol, parathion, ammonia, chlorinated hydrocarbons, organophosphate insecticides
Withdrawal	Barbiturates, alcohol (usually within 48 hours; one third go on to experience delirium tremens), all anticonvulsants, most sedatives
Brain tumors	
Seizures developing later in life	Approximately 16% of patients will have tumor; the most likely site is the rolandic area; least likely site is the occipital
	Highest incidence of tumors: meningiomas, astrocytomas, oligodendrogliomas, metastases (lung, breast, melanoma)
Cerebral infections	
Meningitis	Bacterial or viral
Encephalitis	St. Louis, California, herpes
Parasites	*Schistosoma japonicum*, cysticercosis
Brain abscess	Rare, usually associated with early phase
Immunization	Smallpox, pertussis, typhoid
Vascular	
Cardiac arrest	Venous thrombosis, common with vascular malformations; seizure not common in "usual" cerebral thrombosis
Vasodepressor syndrome	
Thrombosis or hemorrhage	Most common cause of seizure over age 50 years
Sequelae of cardiac arrest	30% of cardiac arrest survivors will have a seizure, usually within 24 hours, but some seizures may occur or recur up to 2 weeks
	Epilepsy is very rare (only 2% after discharge)

Modified from Henry GL, Little N: *Neurologic emergencies*, New York, 1985, McGraw-Hill.

International classification of seizures

I. Partial (focal, local)
  A. Simple partial (consciousness not impaired)
    1. With motor signs
      a. Focal motor without march
      b. Focal motor with march (rolandic)
      c. Versive
      d. Postural
      e. Phonatory (vocalization or arrest of speech)
    2. With somatosensory or special sensory symptoms (simple hallucinations: tingling, light flashes, buzzing)
      a. Somatosensory
      b. Visual
      c. Auditory
      d. Olfactory
      e. Gustatory
      f. Vertiginous
    3. With autonomic symptoms or signs (including epigastric sensation, pallor, sweating, flushing, piloerection, pupillary dilatation)
    4. With psychic symptoms or disturbance of higher cerebral function (symptoms rarely occur without impairment of consciousness and are much more commonly experienced as complex partial seizures)
      a. Dysphasic
      b. Dysmnesic (déjà vu)
      c. Cognitive (dreamy states, distortions of time sense)
      d. Affective (fear, anger)
      e. Illusions (macropsia)
      f. Structured hallucinations (music, scenes)
  B. Complex partial (includes symptoms of simple partial seizure and impairment of consciousness)
    1. Simple partial onset followed by impairment of consciousness
    2. With impairment of consciousness at onset
  C. Partial evolving to secondarily generalized seizures

Modified from The Commission on Classification and Terminology of the International League Against Epilepsy: *Epilepsia* 22:489, 1981.

Clinical seizure symptomatology

Partial seizures

With elementary symptomatology (motor; jacksonian)	Usually begins distally with proximal spread, starting in thumb and index finger or angle of mouth, and spreads proximally
Somatosensory	Numbness, alterations of sensation
Uncinate	Hallucinations of smell
Auditory	Primary and secondary auditory areas; hissing or ringing, association areas; can be orchestra playing
Visual	Flashes of light (commonly red) from 1-degree and 2-degree association areas; formed complex hallucinations
Autonomic	Pupillary change, sweating (rarely as isolated)
Compound	Combinations of above
With complex symptomatology	Consciousness usually impaired Semiautomatic behavior (automatism or lip smacking inappropriate to time and place); all capacity to react to environment is not completely lost; may have déjà vu, jamais vu

Generalized seizures

Absences (petit mal): children; uncommon after age 20; rarely after 30 years of age; 10 to 200 attacks daily lasting 10 to 30 sec; fixed vacuous stare, possibly fluttering eyelids, speech arrest, can be with a few myoclonic jerks

Tonic-clonic (grand mal): prodrome (hours to days), aura, cry, loss of consciousness (LOC), tonic (2 to 3 min), clonic, postictal

Reflex epilepsy

Visually induced: photic, pattern, eye closure, color, object
Auditory evoked: startle, musicogenic, voice
Language evoked: reading, decision evoked
Eating evoked

Modified from Henry GL, Little N: *Neurologic emergencies,* New York, 1985, McGraw-Hill.

---

trauma)? and (6) what diagnostic studies may be helpful?

Radiographic studies are most helpful in the adult patient with new onset seizure, in patients with focal epilepsy,[13] and in those with persistent abnormal postictal neurologic findings[14,15] (see box on p. 421).

INDICATIONS FOR RADIOGRAPHIC EVALUATION

Fig. 16-1 indicates a diagnostic and therapeutic approach to seizure management in the emergency department. The role of radiographic evaluation is to (1) clarify a diagnosis in the patient with recurrent seizure, (2) find a cause in the patient with a new onset seizure, or (3) differentiate seizure from other disorders.

Many diagnostic procedures are available to the emergency physician. Before discussing the advantages and dis-advantages of each technique, certain caveats are worthy of mention. First, the patient experiencing seizures may require multidisciplinary care. Often, the emergency physician, neurologist, neurosurgeon, and radiologist together may be in the best position to determine the appropriate approach to patient diagnosis and management. Second, the extent and type of radiographic workup will depend on the hospital setting, availability of imaging modalities, and the level of interest and expertise of the radiology consultant. Finally, the technology of radiographic imaging continues to change at a very rapid pace. Therefore the approach to the evaluation of the patient with seizures will be a dynamic process that changes with time.

Table 16-2. Causes of seizures in different age groups

Age of onset	Probable cause
Neonatal period	Congenital maldevelopment, birth injury, anoxia, metabolic disorders (hypocalcemia, hypoglycemia, vitamin B_6 deficiency, phenylketonuria)
Infancy (1-6 mo)	Infantile spasms (see also Neonatal period)
Early childhood (6 mo-3 yr)	Infantile spasms, febrile convulsions, birth injury and anoxia, infections, trauma
Childhood (3-10 yr)	Perinatal anoxia, injury at birth or later, infections, thrombosis of cerebral arteries or veins, or indeterminate cause ("idiopathic" epilepsy)
Adolescence (10-18 yr)	Idiopathic epilepsy, including genetically transmitted types, trauma
Early adulthood (18-25 yr)	Idiopathic epilepsy, trauma, neoplasm, alcohol or other sedative-hypnotic drug withdrawal
Middle age (35-60 yr)	Trauma, neoplasm, vascular disease, alcohol or other drug withdrawal
Later life (over 60 yr)	Vascular disease, tumor, degenerative disease, trauma

From Adams RD, Victor M: *Principles of neurology*, ed 3, New York, 1985, McGraw-Hill.

Note: Meningitis and its complications may be a cause of seizures at any age. In tropical and subtropical countries, parasitic infection of the central nervous system is a common cause.

Available radiographic modalities useful in the evaluation of the seizure patient are illustrated in Table 16-3 and discussed in the paragraphs following.

Plain skull radiographs are easy to perform and relatively inexpensive. Radiation doses for a radiographic skull series is low (approximately 1 rad). However, plain skull radiographs are rarely helpful in the differentiation of the causes of seizure because they do not give definitive information about the anatomy of the brain or cerebrospinal fluid (CSF) spaces. They may be useful in the detection of other injuries associated with seizure such as skull fracture. Rarely, the presence of a shifted calcified pineal gland may suggest an intracranial mass lesion. Other abnormal calcifications may suggest malignancy or congenital vascular malformations.[16,17] Finally, abnormalities of the cranium associated with primary malignancy such as multiple myeloma or secondary metastatic disease may be seen on skull radiographs. Skull radiographs are indicated in the patient with serious head trauma as a result of seizure, employing the usual head trauma indications,[18] or when the history or physical examination suggests a fracture. Routine use of skull radiographs in the evaluation of the patient with seizures in the emergency department cannot be justified (see Chapter 3).

Clues suggesting structural causes of seizure disorders

History

First seizure, whether of the partial or secondarily generalized type, occuring in adult life

Uncinate seizures (complex partial with olfactory or gustatory aura) may be associated with a high incidence of glioma in the temporal lobe

Post-ictal focal symptoms (e.g., hemiparesis, dysphasia, unilateral hypethesia) are present

Associated neurologic symptoms of recent onset including headaches, nausea or vomiting, dysphasia, and weakness or numbness

Examination

Signs of increased intracranial pressure (e.g., papilledema, lethargy, irritability) are present

Signs of meningeal irritation (e.g., stiff neck, Kernig or Brudzinski signs) are present

Focal neurologic deficits (e.g., hemiparesis, hemianesthesia, dysphasia, or dyspraxia, visual field defect, hyper-reflexia, Babinski reflex) are experienced

Unilateral post-ictal (Todd) paralysis is present

CT scan is the single most readily available and useful radiographic study in the emergency department for the patient with a seizure disorder. A CT scan is relatively easy to perform, requires a moderate radiation dose, and yields minimal complications. The technique is extremely sensitive for structural abnormalities, with a sensitivity approaching 100% for the detection of brain abscess, neoplasm, acute hemorrhage, and hydrocephalus.[19] Numerous studies have demonstrated the use of the CT scan in the evaluation of the patient with a seizure disorder (Table 16-4). Eisner et al[11] showed that the CT scan changed the diagnosis in 44% of patients in a series of 163 seizure patients presenting to a city emergency department. A CT scan is indicated for all patients with new onset seizures. Additionally, any patient in whom an intracranial structural lesion is suspected on the basis of history and physical examination should have a CT scan performed. This includes patients with altered neurologic findings, focal seizure, or a history of a chronic seizure disorder with recent change in seizure activity. When possible, both enhanced and nonenhanced CT scans should be performed. A normal CT scan result, however, does not rule out the possibility of significant pathologic states, such as infection, infarction, and some neoplastic diseases that may be missed when the CT scan is the only imaging modality used.[34]

Magnetic resonance imaging (MRI) of the brain is a newer technique that, similar to the CT scan, produces images of striking detail and clarity. It has a better safety profile than invasive imaging techniques and does not expose the patient to ionizing radiation. It is sensitive to physical and chemical characteristics of cells and tissues as well as

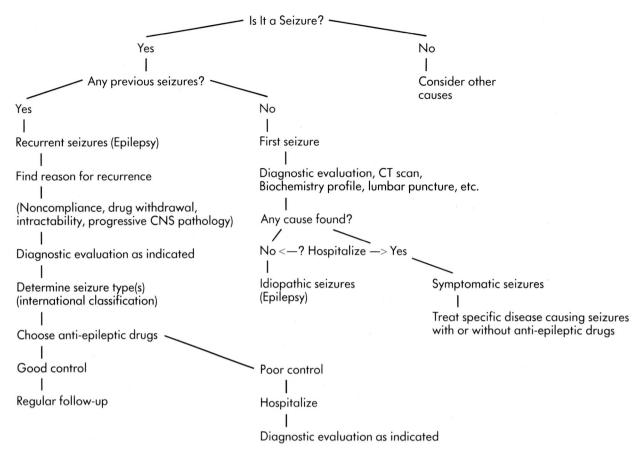

Fig. 16-1. Algorithm for the evaluation of patients with seizures in the emergency department.

Table 16-3. Available radiographic studies for seizure evaluation

Imaging Characteristics	Plain skull radiographs	Computed tomography	Radionuclide brain scan	Cerebral angiography	Magnetic resonance imaging
Advantages	Directs CT scan Defines air-fluid levels, depressed fractures Nature of intracranial calcifications	Sensitive and often specific noninvasive screening test for variety of neurologic problems	Adjunct to normal CT scan Defines patency of dural sinuses Occasionally more sensitive than CT scan in diagnosing herpes encephalitis, superficial vascular processes	Adds specificity to CT scan Evaluates arteriovenous malformations, aneurysms, and other vascular lesions Normal CT scan but patient deteriorating (e.g., isodense SDH suspected)	Adds specificity to CT scan evaluation of structural lesions
Limitations	Does not give information about anatomy of brain or CSF spaces	Artifacts common, particularly in posterior fossa Small lesions, leptomeningeal processes missed Limited detail of vascular lesions and structures	Nonspecific; edema, mass shift, hydrocephalus, midline abnormalities not detected	Invasive Needs highly trained personnel	Availability limited
Radiation dose	1 rad Depends on number of radiographs and technical factors	3.5 rad Varies with different scanners	0.2 rad to body 1 rad to bladder	1.5 rad/vessel injected plus 1.5-6 rad/min for fluoroscopy	None
Complications	None	Contrast material reaction (if used)	None	Stroke Contrast material reaction Femoral artery embolus or thrombosis	Contrast material reaction (if used)

Table 16-4. Incidence of abnormalities detected on CT scan by seizure type*

Series	Patient's age	Generalized tonic-clonic seizures	Partial elementary	Partial complex	Secondary generalization	Total	Absence of seizures
Bogdanoff et al. (1975)[13]	All ages	—	13 (?)	18 (?)	19 (?)	50 (35%)	—
Gastaut and Gastaut (1976)[20]	All ages	24 (4%)	69 (66%)	84 (60%)	45 (64%)	198 (63%)	20 (10%)
Caille et al. (1976)[21]	All ages	—	—	—	—	66 (46%)	—
Bachman et al. (1976)[22]	3 mo-20 yr	23 (32%)	14 (43%)	42 (27%)	—	56 (31%)	1 (0%)
Janz (1977)[23]	20 yr and above	97 (40%)	39 (82%)	66 (39%)	44 (52%)	149 (55%)	—
Gastaut and Gastaut (1977)[24]	All ages	28 (3.5%)	—	—	—	490 (63%)	21 (9%)
Scollo-Lavizzari et al. (1977)[25]	11-79 yr	59 (34%)	16 (62%)	16 (19%)	—	32 (40%)	—
Zimmerman et al. (1977)[26]	0-40 yr	—	—	—	—	—	—
Carrera et al. (1977)[27]	21-75 yr	—	—	22 (0%)	—	—	—
Ghazy et al. (1978)[28]	10-79 yr	40 (35%)	12 (58%)	5 (40%)	—	17 (52%)	3 (33%)
Reisner et al. (1978)[29]	3-15 yr	63 (83%)	65 (71%)	26 (31%)	—	91 (60%)	41 (49%)
Ratzka et al. (1978)[30]	All ages	211 (48%)	98 (71%)	91 (61%)	52 (82%)	241 (70%)	—
McGahan et al. (1979)[31]	All ages	77 (38%)	12 (58%)	28 (32%)	17 (71%)	57 (49%)	—
Lagenstein et al. (1979)[32]	Children	—	—	—	—	—	49 (41%)
Ladurner et al. (1979)[33]	All ages	173 (29%)	—	—	—	35 (62%)	—

*Values are the number of patients studied in each category; in parentheses are the percentages of patients with the abnormality.

to structural lesions. Thus it may have certain advantages in the detection of some lesions and disease states[35] not detected by the CT scan. The use of MRI in patients with seizures has been directed more toward patients with partial seizures, with partial seizures refractory to therapy, or with nondiagnostic CT scans (Table 16-5). In such patients with focal seizure, MRI abnormalities may be detected in 20% to 90% of patients. In patients with a normal CT scan, MRI identifies lesions in 15% to 30% of patients.[37] Although MRI detects more abnormalities than does the CT scan[42] and better localizes seizure foci, especially in the absence of a mass lesion, its effect in acutely changing patient management and outcome is not well documented. Additionally, the high cost and limited availability of MRI scanners relegate MRI to a secondary diagnostic technique in treating the patient with seizures in the emergency department. MRI is indicated to assist in localization of the seizure focus in the patient with a negative CT scan finding in whom a structural lesion is suspected as the cause of a refractory partial seizure disorder.

Before the introduction of the CT scan, the radionuclide brain scan was the radiographic screening examination of choice. It has the advantage of little or no risk since no contrast material is used. It is sensitive for the detection of structural lesions but is less specific than the CT scan. The dynamic demonstration of the vascularity of the brain makes it useful in the diagnosis of stroke, arterio venous malformation, encephalitis, and other inflammatory disorders. It may be useful in patients in whom a vascular-related cause is suspected and in those with known allergies to contrast material necessary for an enhanced CT scan.

Cerebral angiography is a procedure of significant expense, radiation exposure, and potential complications.[37a] In the emergency department setting, it is a useful adjunct to other radiographic diagnostic studies for the clarification and delineation of the CT scan or MRI findings. It provides information to assist in anatomic localization for surgical procedures and can assist in definition of the extent of vascular lesions such as arteriovenous malformations. This technique, however, is not part of the primary diagnostic evaluation of the emergency department patient with seizure.

NORMAL RADIOGRAPHIC ANATOMY

In the evaluation of the emergency seizure patient, the CT scan will most likely yield positive findings. Therefore the normal anatomy of the intracranial contents in relation to the CT scan appearance will be identified. Normal CT scan and skull radiographic findings can also be reviewed in Chapter 3.

The CT scan consists of a series of slices obtained in sequence, usually from the base of the skull to the vertex of the cranial vault. What follows is a brief description of representative CT scan slices and their appearance at different axial levels. The discussion is designed to emphasize the features of each slice that enable its correct position to be identified in the sequence of slices making up the entire study.

For diagnostic purposes, the CT scans can be divided into infraventricular, ventricular, and supraventricular sections, depending on the presence of the lateral ventricles on the image (Fig. 16-2).

Infraventricular images are shown in Fig. 16-2, *A*. Often on the lowest slices, the petrous and occipital bones outline the posterior fossa and temporal fossa. Cerebellar hemispheres are separated from the brain stem anteriorly by the inferior aspect of the fourth ventricle level, which often appears slitlike on the CT scan.

On the next higher slice shown in Fig. 16-2, *B*, the bony portion of the sella is evident. The pons is visualized and the fourth ventricle appears more oblong. The frontal lobes are included, and the suprasellar and sylvian cisterns are identified.

Fig. 16-2, *C* and *D*, demonstrates low ventricular slices. These are above the level of the petrous bones. They demonstrate parts of the frontal horns and posterior

Table 16-5. Magnetic resonance imaging in seizure disorder

Series	Seizure type	Total number of patients	Number of patients with negative CT scan and positive MRI	Number of patients with structural lesions
Ormson et al. (1986)[36]	Partial seizure	25	4	12
Latack et al. (1986)[37]	Partial seizure	50	10	0
Jabbari et al. (1986)[38]	Partial seizure	30	13	0
Sperling et al. (1986)[39]	Refractory partial seizure with negative CT scan findings	35	—	7 (tuberous sclerosis, astrocytoma, hamartoma)
Lesser et al. (1986)[40]	Refractory partial seizure with negative CT scan findings	12	3	0
Theodore et al. (1986)[41]	Partial seizure	36	20	0
Baker et al. (1985)[42]	Mixed seizure types	60	14	4 (glioma)
McLachlan et al. (1985)[43]	Partial seizure	16	14	0

horns of the lateral ventricles. They may include basal ganglia. The superior cerebellar cistern and third ventricle are also identified, and the sylvian fissure is well demonstrated.

More cephalad levels include additional visualization of the frontal horn of the lateral ventricles and identification of the caudate and lentiform nuclei. Fig. 16-2, *E* and *F*, represents typical ventricular slices. These illustrate the

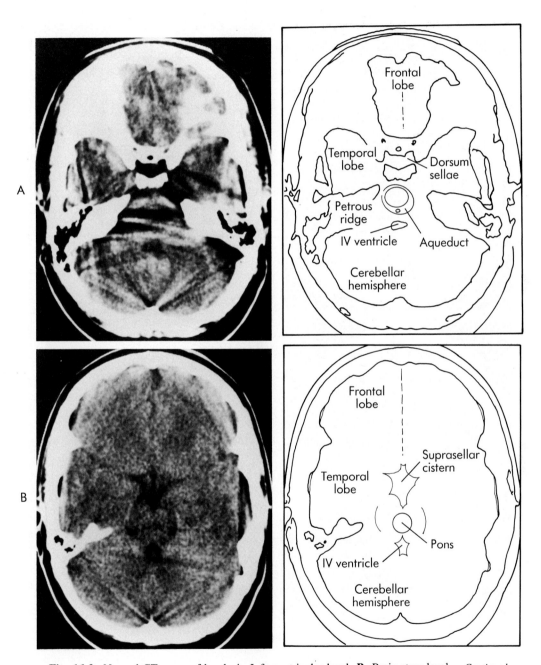

Fig. 16-2. Normal CT scans of head. **A,** Infraventricular level. **B,** Brain stem level.   *Continued.*

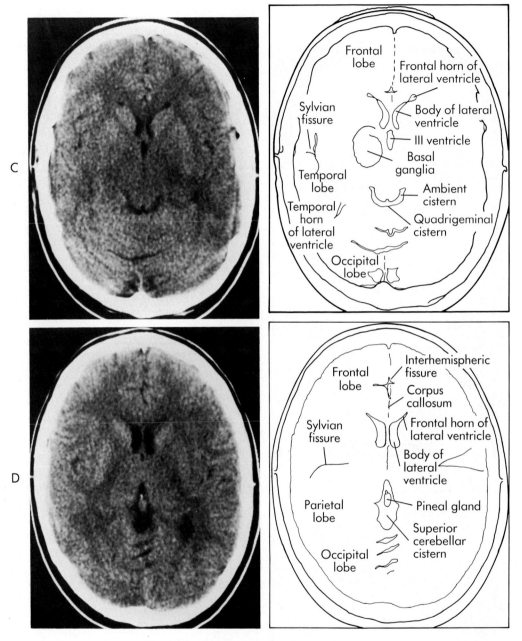

Fig. 16-2, cont'd.   C and **D,** Low ventricular level.

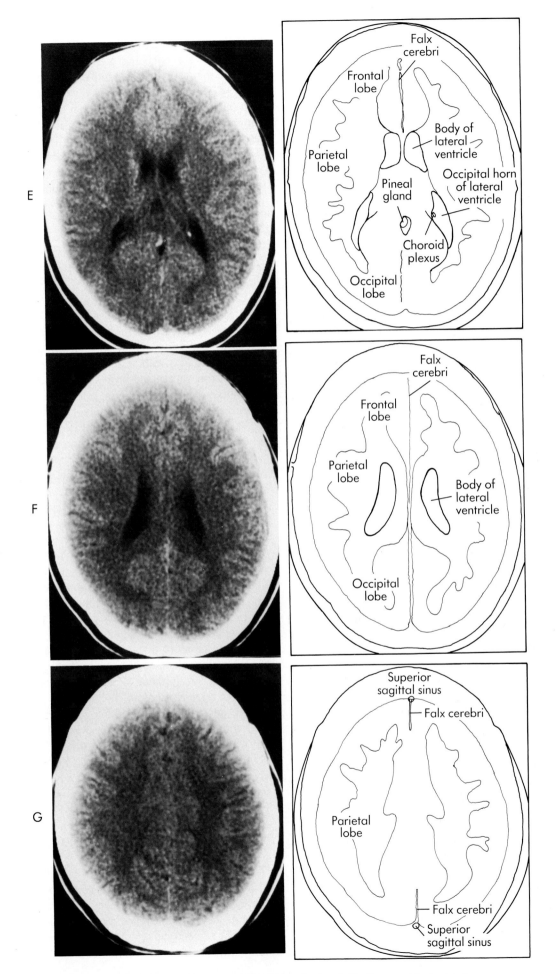

Fig. 16-2, cont'd. E and F, Ventricular level. G, Supraventricular level.

Causes of brain atrophy

Focal

Post-trauma
Post-infarction
Post-inflammation
Vascular anomalies
Cerebellar factors

Diffuse

Alzheimer disease
Pick disease
Multifocal infarction
Huntington disease
Parkinson disease
Wilson disease
Cerebral anoxia
Binswanger disease
Jakob-Creutzfeldt disease
Neoplasia and metabolic disorder
Drug-related atrophy
Demyelinating disease
Chronic schizophrenia

---

lateral ventricles well and show separation of the lateral ventricles by the corpus callosum.

Finally, a supraventricular slice is illustrated in Fig. 16-2, *G*. Such slices show the sulci well; no central CSF space is evident.

RADIOGRAPHIC FINDINGS

Many lesions readily identifiable on radiographic examination may be the cause of a seizure disorder in the patient in the emergency department.

Primary idiopathic seizure

Patients with documented seizure disorder who undergo diagnostic evaluation without demonstrable causes for seizures are said to have idiopathic epilepsy. By definition, abnormal structural lesions are not detected on a CT scan or other diagnostic evaluations. However, such patients, especially those with prolonged seizure history, frequently have abnormal CT scans.[44] The most common nonetiologic finding associated with longstanding epilepsy is brain atrophy, either generalized or focal.[31,44,45]

Brain atrophy is defined as a loss of brain substance that may involve white matter, gray matter, or both in a generalized or focal manner. Focal atrophy presents as a region of low density within brain parenchyma or as a focal dilatation of a part of the ventricular or subarachnoid space. Both components may be present.

Diffuse atrophy may have many specific causes or may be nonspecific (see the box above). It may also involve gray or white matter but is usually mixed. Atrophy may be either central, in which ventricular enlargement is more

marked than the widening of sulci, or cortical, in which the sulci are wide in relation to the ventricular enlargement (Fig. 16-3). Generalized atrophy is common in patients with idiopathic seizures. McGahan[31] found generalized atrophy in 20 of 150 patients evaluated by a CT scan. Such atrophy may be associated with a longstanding history of seizure disorder and its treatment, rather than a specific cause. The association between cerebellar atrophy and prolonged use of phenytoin (Dilantin) has been documented.[46]

Degenerative disease

Degenerative disease is more frequently associated with progressive dementia or neurologic deficit than with seizure. A large group of degenerative disorders may be found on the CT scans of patients with seizure, particularly elderly patients (those greater than 60 years of age), but the role of these disorders as the cause of seizures is not clear.

Cerebral atrophy, as previously described, is a frequent finding in patients with seizure. It is generally idiopathic. The CT scan appearance includes ventricular enlargement with increased prominence of sulci and large basal cisterns. The role of atrophy as an etiologic factor in producing seizures in these patients is not clear.

Alzheimer disease is a diffuse form of cerebral atrophy with predominant gray matter involvement. The CT scan reveals symmetrically enlarged ventricles with prominent central sulci. This finding is nonspecific for Alzheimer disease since Pick disease displays similar atrophy. However, Pick disease more frequently involves the temporal and frontal lobes. Both diseases can be a cause of seizure.

Parkinson disease predominantly involves subcortical regions resulting in degeneration of the corpus striatum, globus pallidus, and substantia nigra. The CT scan findings include enlarged ventricles and often calcification of the basal ganglia. Severity of symptoms cannot be correlated with the CT scan findings.

A large group of diseases can be classified as leukoencephalopathies. These diseases predominantly affect the white matter of the brain. They are not commonly associated with seizure disorders. These include such diseases as the leukodystrophies and multiple sclerosis. All are associated with white matter loss and increased fluid content of the white matter, resulting in low-density areas on the CT scan. These conditions are bilateral, patchy, and progressive. They are not associated with surrounding edema. All are recognizable by both a CT scan and MRI (Fig. 16-4). Particularly with multiple sclerosis, MRI is the imaging technique of choice because it is superior in the detection of multiple sclerosis plaques.[47]

Abscess and infection

Intracranial infection is an uncommon but important cause of seizure in the emergency department patient. The value of the CT scan varies, depending on the type of lesion. Other neuroradiographic modalities have minimal

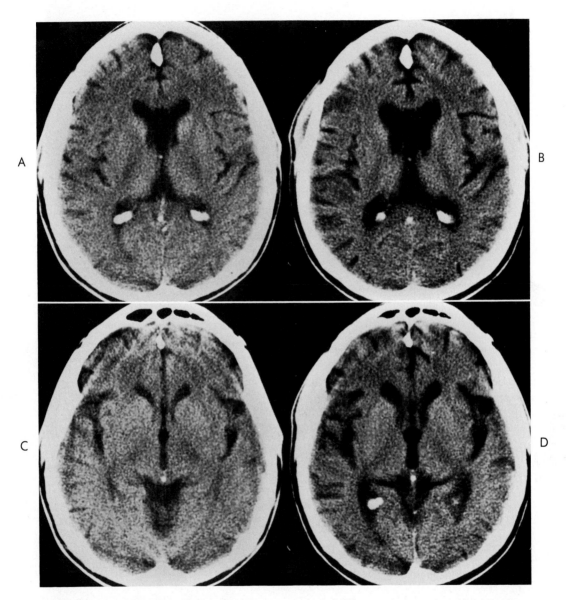

Fig. 16-3. A to **D,** CT scans demonstrating progression of diffuse cortical atrophy with widening of sulci and ventricular dilatation in a patient with HIV infection. There is greater hydrocephalus in **B** and **D** than in **A** and **C.**

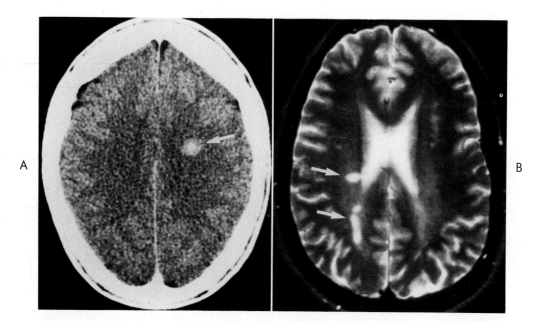

Fig. 16-4. A, CT scan with double-dose contrast enhancement and thin sections. Well-defined contrast enhancement in left periventricular region represents an area of acute demyelination with disruption of blood-brain barrier in a patient with multiple sclerosis *(arrow).* **B,** MRI showing multiple plaque lesions in the periventricular region and throughout the white matter *(arrows)* in a patient with multiple sclerosis.

emergent application. Intracranial infections include abscess, encephalitis, and meningitis.

Brain abscess is commonly associated with seizures. On the CT scan, it may be mistaken for neoplasm. Abscess may occur anywhere in the brain parenchyma or subdural space. The frontal and temporal lobes are frequent sites. The CT scan shows a low-density lesion with an enhancing, thin rim that has smooth margins (Fig. 16-5). Abscesses may be single or multiple. Extraparenchymal abscesses in the epidural or subdural space are usually caused by direct extension of a paranasal sinus infection. These may be associated with bony or soft tissue infection as well.

Patients with viral encephalitis may present with seizure. Herpes simplex virus type 1 is the most common cause of sporadic viral encephalitis in the United States. Herpetic encephalitis is characterized by petechial hemorrhages, predominantly in the subfrontal and medial temporal lobes. The CT scan findings include poorly marginated low-density areas, mass effect, and nonhomogeneous contrast enhancement[48] (Fig. 16-6). The CT scan changes are usually not seen in the first 5 to 7 days, and contrast enhancement may persist for prolonged times after the onset of the disease.

Patients with pyogenic meningitis may present with seizure. Early in this disease the underlying brain may be normal and the CT scans nondiagnostic. With progressive disease, inflammatory changes in the subpial cortex and ependymal linings of the ventricles can occur and there can be focal areas of edema. The CT scan may be useful in the detection of complications of meningitis, such as subdural effusions; however, this is probably of little rele-

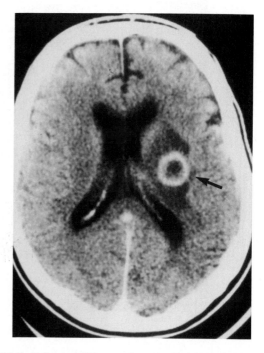

Fig. 16-5. Enhanced CT scan demonstrating a capsular or ring-enhancing lesion in the left parietal lobe *(arrow)* with surrounding edema in a patient with subacute bacterial endocarditis.

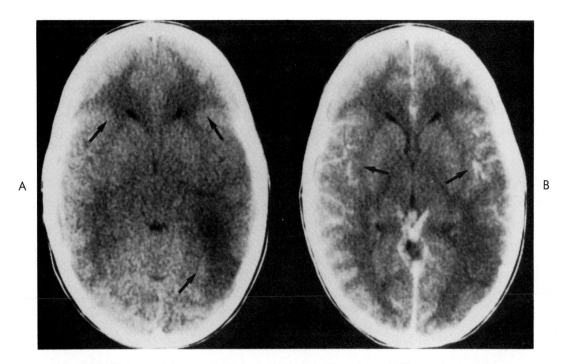

Fig. 16-6. Patient with herpes simplex encephalitis. **A,** Nonenhanced CT scan shows poorly defined low-density areas in the left parietal and both frontal areas *(arrows)*. **B,** Enhanced CT scan shows patchy areas from necrotizing vasculitis *(arrows)*.

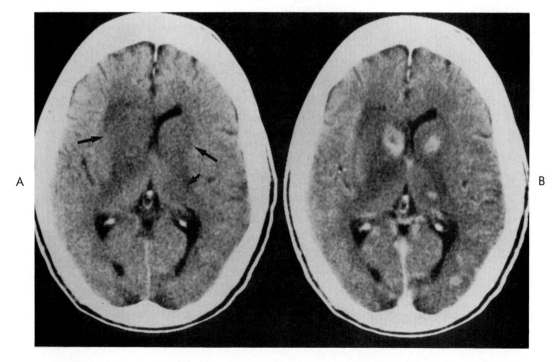

Fig. 16-7. Nonenhanced **(A)** and enhanced **(B)** CT scans of AIDS patient with toxoplasmosis demonstrate basal ganglia abscesses *(arrows)* with edema and mass effect. Also note infectious focus in left thalamus *(small arrow)*.

vance to the acute management of the patient with seizures in the emergency department.

In the patient with acquired immunodeficiency syndrome (AIDS), the cause of new-onset seizure is likely to be infectious, although hemorrhage and neoplasm are also common. The infectious cause is most frequently an opportunistic organism. Toxoplasmosis is the most common infectious agent in these patients.[49] The CT scan findings consist of multiple intraparenchymal lesions with ring or nodular contrast material enhancement and low-density areas, usually in the gray matter, cortical medullary junction, and basal ganglia[50] (Fig. 16-7).

Toxic and metabolic disease

Toxic and metabolic abnormalities make up a small percentage of the causes of seizures in emergency patients. Rosenthal noted a 4% incidence of metabolic causes and a 3% incidence of drug-related seizures in a series of 91 patients.[51]*

Endogenous and exogenous toxic causes are generally not evidenced on the CT scan. Exceptions include hypoxia and carbon monoxide poisoning. Anoxia may be caused by respiratory failure from associated disease or from toxins such as narcotics or barbiturates. The most commonly

---

*Those departments with larger populations of drug abusers will see a higher incidence of toxic seizures.

involved areas include the periventricular white matter in the basal ganglia.[52] Although the early CT scan findings may show only edema, within 24 to 48 hours the CT scan demonstrates low-density areas. Hyperemia in the early post-anoxic phase may lead to areas of contrast enhancement (Fig. 16-8).

Patients with acute carbon monoxide poisoning present with bilateral low density areas in the basal ganglia, most notably in the region of the globus pallidus. Diffuse low density areas in cerebral white matter is also common.[53] The findings are similar to those for anoxic central nervous system injury (Fig. 16-9).

Endogenous metabolic causes of seizures such as hypoglycemia, hyponatremia, and uremia are usually clinically obvious. If not, laboratory investigation is considerably more useful than radiographic evaluation in these patients.

Neoplastic disease

Neoplastic disease is an important cause of seizures in the emergency department patient. Many studies have evaluated the use of the CT scan in patients with seizures (see Table 16-4) and newly diagnosed neoplastic disease appears to be found in approximately 8% to 10% of patients, regardless of patient age or type of seizure. In patients with chronic seizure disorder, the yield is somewhat less. In Jabbari's series of 162 patients with chronic seizure disorder, four newly diagnosed malignancies were

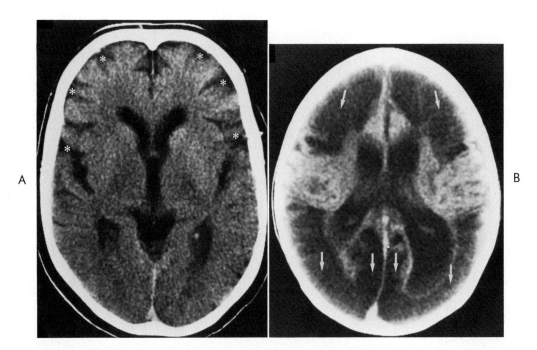

Fig. 16-8. A, CT scan of anoxic central nervous system injury marked by low-density lesions in area of basal ganglia and frontal lobes *(asterisks)* in 60-year-old patient with aspiration. **B,** CT scan of anoxic central nervous system injury in an 8-month-old child caused by nonaccidental trauma (NAT) or "shaken baby syndrome." CT scan shows bilateral cortical infarctions and atrophy *(arrows)* resulting in ventricular dilatation.

discovered by the CT scan.[54] The duration of seizure disorders in this series was 8 to 21 years.

Factors reported to increase the likelihood of tumor as a cause of seizure include the following: (1) age greater than 20 years,[13,20,31] (2) presence of abnormal neurologic signs,[13,31] and (3) partial seizure or a generalized seizure with a focal component.[31] False-negative CT scan findings have been reported with posterior fossa and parasellar lesions.[34] However, the incidence of seizure with lesions in these areas is considerably less than that for supratentorial neoplastic lesions.[55]

The appearance of neoplastic disease varies depending on the tumor type and location. The classic description of a neoplastic lesion on a CT scan is that of an area of diminished density that enhances with contrast material administration. Such tumors frequently are associated with a mass effect that distorts or obliterates the adjacent CSF-containing structures such as the sulci, subarachnoid cisterns, or ventricles. Focal areas of hemorrhage, calcification, or edema may be prominent.

Table 16-6 illustrates typical findings on the CT scan for various types of neoplastic disease.

Gliomas of the temporal lobe are a frequent cause of seizure (Fig. 16-10). Intracerebral metastatic disease is frequently identified by multiple lesions, which are often associated with significant edema (Fig. 16-11). Tumor hemorrhage is also frequent (Fig. 16-12). Meningeal carcinomatosis may occur with or without parenchymal metastasis. Contrast material enhancement is required to identify this condition. Patients with such lesions present with intense enhancement of the sulci and adjacent cisterns (Fig.

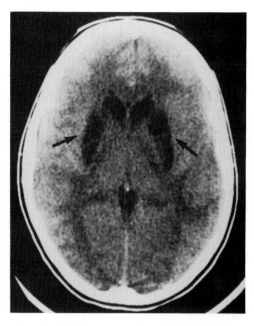

Fig. 16-9. Acute anoxia following cardiac arrest. CT scan of a 14-year-old male shows bilateral low-density areas in the basal ganglia *(arrows)*. Findings are also consistent with acute carbon monoxide intoxication.

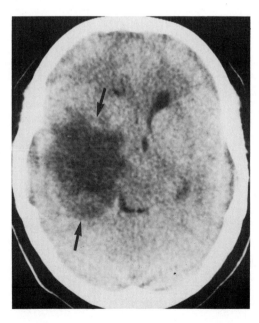

Fig. 16-10. CT scan of low-grade astrocytoma without evidence of enhancement in the right temporal lobe *(arrows)*. There is a mild-to-moderate mass effect.

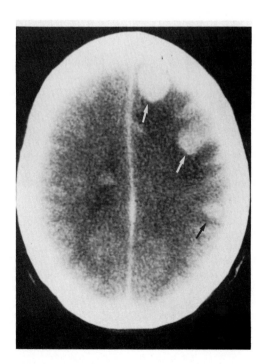

Fig. 16-11. Enhanced CT scan demonstrates multiple intracranial metastatic lesions *(arrows)* in the corticomedullary junction from an oat cell carcinoma.

Table 16-6. CT scan findings of neoplastic disease

Tumor	Initial density	Frequency calcification	Edema	Enhancement pattern	Age/sex group	Location	Other findings
Extra-axial							
Meningioma	↑	20%	+1	+3 H	A/F	Dural attachment	Occasional hemorrhage
Pinealoblastoma	↑	Rare	0	+3 M	P/M	Pineal region	Irregular margin and low-density center
Choroid plexus papilloma	↑	Rare	0	+3 H	P	Ventricular system	Occasional hemorrhage
Choroid plexus carcinoma	↑	Rare	0	+3 H	P	Ventricular system	Irregular margin
Colloid cyst	↑	0	0	0/+1 H	A	Anterior third ventricle	
Germinoma	↑/↔	Rare	0	+3 H	A/M	Pineal region	Meningeal and ependymal seeding
Pituitary adenoma	↔/↑	<5%	0	+3 H	A	Sella	Rare hemorrhage or infarction
Neuroma	↔/↑	0	+1	+3 H	A	Cerebellopontine angle	Occasionally cystic
Pinealocytoma	↔/↑	Rare	0	+2 H	P	Pineal region	
Craniopharyngioma	↔/↓	30%-80%	0	+2 M/R	A/P	Suprasellar	Some cystic
Teratoma	↓	Frequent	+1/0	0	P/A/M	Midline supratentorial	Some cystic, rupture, seeding
Dermoid	↓	Frequent	+1/0	0	P/A/F	Posterior fossa base of skull	Some cystic
Epidermoid	↓	Frequent	+1/0	0	P/A	Posterior fossa base of skull	Some cystic
Lipoma	↓	Rare	+1/0	0	P/A	Midline supratentorial	
Intra-axial							
Primary lymphoma	↑/↔	0	+2	+2/+3 H	A	Peripheral and deep structures	Irregular margin, multiplicity
Medulloblastoma	↑	10%	+2	+2 H	P	Vermis	Irregular margin
Oligodendroglioma	↑	>90%	+1	+2 M	A	Supratentorial	Irregular margin
Ependymoma	↔/↑	30%-40%	+2	+2 H	P	Fourth ventricle	Irregular margin
Embryonal cell carcinoma	↑/↓	Rare	+1	+3 H	P	Pineal region	
Hemangioblastoma	↔	0	+1	+3 H	A	Posterior fossa	Cystic, mural nodule
Ganglioglioma	↓/↔	>30%	0	+1 M	P/A	Temporal lobe	Irregular margin, cystic
Neuroblastoma	↔/↓	Common	+2	+2 M	P	Supratentorial	Hemorrhage
Low-grade astrocytoma	↔/↓	<30%	+1	0/+1 M	A	Supratentorial	Indistinct margin
High-grade astrocytoma (glioblastoma)	↔/↓	Rare	+2	+2-3 M/R	A	Supratentorial	Can be cystic, irregular margin
Brain stem glioma	↓/↔	0	0	+1 M	P	Brain stem	Indistinct margin
Cystic astrocytoma	↓	Rare	+1	+1 H	P	Posterior fossa	Mural tumor nodule

From Lee SH, Rao KL, eds: *Cranial computed tomography and MRI*, ed 2, New York, 1987, McGraw-Hill.

↑ = High density	H = Homogeneous
↔ = Isodensity	M = Mixed
↓ = Low density	R = Ring pattern
+1 = Minimal enhancement	A = Adult; P = Pediatric
+2 = Moderate enhancement	M = Male predominance
+3 = Intense enhancement	F = Female predominance

16-13).[56] There is little role in the emergency department for other diagnostic modalities in the patient with seizures in whom neoplastic disease is suspected. MRI and angiography have value in further helping to define the anatomic location and extent of the tumor, but they provide little advantage over a CT scan in the initial diagnosis of the seizure patient. Radionuclide brain scan may be useful in the

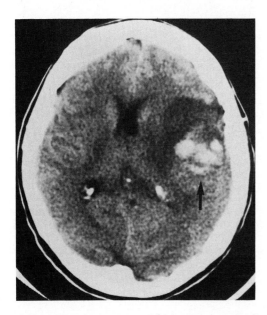

Fig. 16-12. CT scan of a hemorrhage within an oligodendroglioma (intracranial metastatic lesion) *(arrow)* with focal edema in the left frontotemporal region.

patient with a documented contrast material allergy in the absence of MRI availability because it is a sensitive modality in the detection of intracranial tumor lesions.[56a]

Trauma

A seizure is frequently a secondary insult in the patient with severe head trauma. In fact, most current teaching regarding severe head injury suggests that anticonvulsant therapy be instituted to prevent such seizures.[57] Patients with focal neurologic findings, including seizures, have a higher incidence of associated intracranial pathologic conditions. Such pathologic lesions are best diagnosed using a CT scan. The CT scan has virtually replaced all other diagnostic modalities in this regard.

Before the advent of the CT scan, skull radiography was the primary diagnostic mode in the head-injured patient. However, even then it was clear that skull radiography did not affect patient outcome.[58] Although basal skull fractures not detected by a CT scan may occasionally be seen on plain radiographs, skull radiography does not reveal the presence of intracranial pathology. Only indirect signs of intracranial pathologic states can be identified on radiographs (e.g., fluid-filled sphenoid sinus, depressed fracture, soft tissue injury, foreign body).

MRI in head-injured patients, on the other hand, demonstrates abnormalities that are not identifiable on a normal CT scan.[59] However, the clinical use of this information in day-to-day emergency department management is unclear. The acutely head-injured patient with seizure as a result of intracranial pathology often requires resuscitation

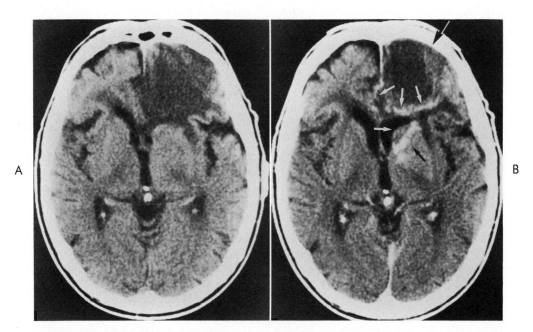

Fig. 16-13. Nonenhanced **(A)** and enhanced **(B)** CT scans of leptomeningeal carcinomatosis. **B** demonstrates ependymal and periependymal enhancement *(white arrows)* in a patient with proved leptomeningeal lymphoma. Note the anterior limb of the left internal capsule enhances with contrast material *(black arrow)*.

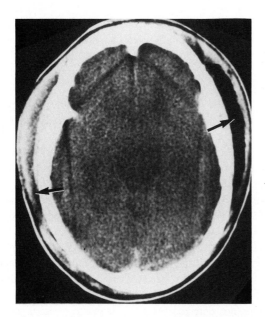

Fig. 16-14. CT scan of traumatic cerebral edema in 25-year-old patient with head trauma. Subcutaneous emphysema is present *(arrows),* and there is effacement of the cisterns with ventricular compression. Differentiation of white and gray matter is impossible.

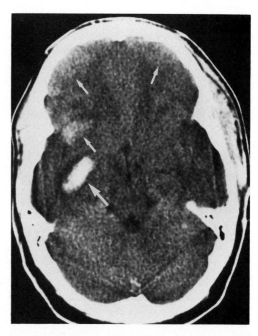

Fig. 16-15. CT scan of post-traumatic intracranial contusion in a patient with closed head trauma. Findings include bilateral frontal contusions with patchy increased density *(small arrows)* and a traumatic hematoma in the right temporal lobe *(large arrow).*

and life support, which precludes the emergent use of MRI. Therefore the CT scan is the accurate method for diagnosis of such major intracranial lesions and remains the diagnostic examination of choice in the head-injured patient with neurologic deficit or seizure.

Most seizures in the head-injured patient are associated with significant intracranial traumatic pathology.[60] Such lesions include cerebral edema, contusion, intracerebral hematoma, and epidural or subdural hematoma.

Edema appears as low-density zones on a CT scan. This may be focal, multifocal, or diffuse. When diffuse, edema may be manifest only by generalized compression of the brain with a decrease in ventricular size (Fig. 16-14). Such low-density areas must be distinguished from ischemic infarction.

Contusion of the brain substance can be multiple or single. It most frequently occurs in the frontal and temporal lobes. Contusions appear as nonhomogeneous areas of increased density, representing small areas of hemorrhage interspersed with areas of edema and tissue necrosis. The margins of these lesions are poorly defined (Fig. 16-15).

Intracerebral hematoma is seen as a well-circumscribed high-density lesion that is usually surrounded by low-density areas caused by edema. Such hematomas may occur in any location, but they are most frequent in the temporal and frontal areas (Fig. 16-16).

Acute subdural hematoma appears as a peripheral zone of increased density with concave inner margins and a convex outer margin adjacent to the inner table of the skull (Fig. 16-17). Subdural hematoma is frequently associated with a mass effect, and the absence of a midline shift with

these lesions should raise suspicion of the presence of a contralateral lesion.[61]

Epidural hematoma is usually seen as a biconvex, peripheral, high-density lesion (Fig. 16-18). The most frequent site is the temporal or frontal region. Epidural hematoma is most often of arterial origin. If so, it can be associated with significant edema and mass effect. The classic descriptions of subdural and epidural hematomas were given previously. Often, it may be difficult to differentiate subdural and epidural hematomas; in up to 20% of head-injured patients, both may co-exist.[62]

Direct bony injury to brain parenchyma caused by a depressed fracture may also cause seizure in the head-injured patient even in the absence of identifiable localized hemorrhage. Such a depressed skull fracture may be easily identified on the CT scan (Fig. 16-19) or on skull radiographs.

Most emergency department series of seizure patients include those with CT scan findings of subacute or chronic subdural hematomas caused by a history of remote head trauma.[63] With time, the attenuation coefficient of an acute subdural hematoma decreases. The progression to a low-density or isodense area on the CT scan varies both with the size of the initial lesion and with the presence of CSF in the initial clot (Fig. 16-20). An isodense lesion may not be visible on nonenhanced CT scans if significant mass effect is not present. Enhanced CT scans are useful in the clinical setting of seizure in the patient with a history of head trauma in the past. MRI may offer some advantage in

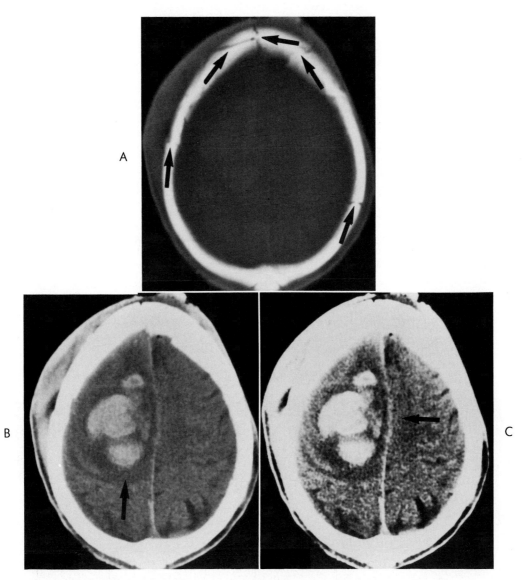

Fig. 16-16. Traumatic intracerebral hematoma in patient with closed head injury. Multiple CT scan windows show **(A)** fractures of frontal bones, right and left parietal bones *(surrounding arrows)*, **(B)** hemorrhage with surrounding edema in the right cortex *(vertical arrow)* and **(C)** mild indentation of the falx *(horizontal arrow)*.

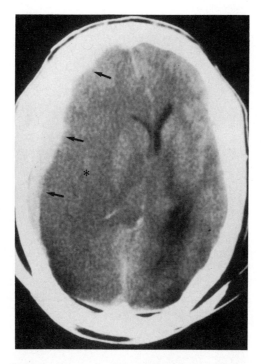

Fig. 16-17. CT scan of an acute traumatic right subdural hematoma *(arrows)* showing a classic semilunar shape from rupture of the bridging veins. Also present is a right hemispheric infarction *(asterisk)* resulting from middle cerebral artery compression caused by the mass effect.

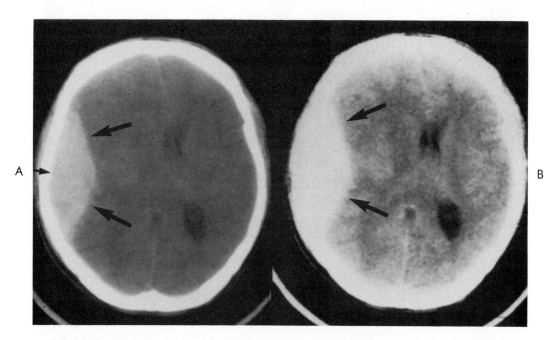

Fig. 16-18. Right convex hemorrhage of acute traumatic epidural hematoma *(large arrows)* with compression of the right lateral ventricle and a midline shift to the left. **A,** CT scan at wide window setting better distinguishes the interface between the dense clot and the equally dense bone *(small arrow).* **B,** CT scan at soft tissue window setting is used for evaluation of brain tissue.

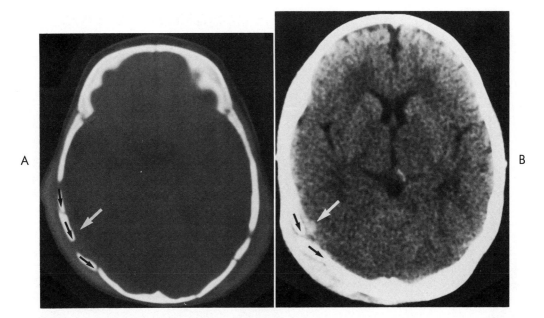

Fig. 16-19. CT scans at bone window setting **(A)** and brain tissue setting **(B)** demonstrate comminuted depressed skull fractures of right temporal and occipital bones *(small arrows)* with a small subdural hematoma *(large arrows).*

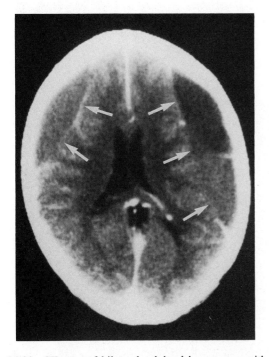

Fig. 16-20. CT scan of bilateral subdural hematomas with subacute on the right, subacute or chronic on the left *(arrows).* Improved image resolution with fourth generation CT scanners and added benefit of contrast material enhancement almost always permits detection of the interface of the cortex vs. the isodense subdural hematoma. There is medial displacement of the cortical hemispheres on both sides.

the diagnosis of isodense subdural hematoma because of the lack of bone artifact and the excellent visualization of soft tissues[64] (see Chapter 15).

Vascular abnormalities

Another group of patients who may present with seizures includes those with vascular abnormalities in the CNS. These include arteriovenous malformation, infarction, and hemorrhage.

Previously undetected intracranial vascular malformation is a common cause of seizure.[65] There are four distinct groups of such malformations: capillary telangiectasia, cavernous angioma, arteriovenous malformation, and venous malformation.

Capillary telangiectasia is a relatively common incidental finding on autopsy and is rarely symptomatic.

Cavernous angiomas are rare, but frequently they can be associated with seizure. They are composed of large sinusoidal vascular spaces clustered together, often with abnormal calcification. The CT scan shows a high-density lesion, often calcified with minimal or no contrast enhancement (Fig. 16-21). This lesion is rarely associated with edema or a mass effect.[66]

Arteriovenous malformation (AVM) is the most common form of vascular malformation and is often symptomatic. Approximately one third of patients with AVM will initially present with seizure.[67] These lesions may occur anywhere in the central nervous system but are most frequently found in the distribution of the middle cerebral artery. An AVM without hemorrhage reveals an area of mixed density on the nonenhanced CT scan. Margins of

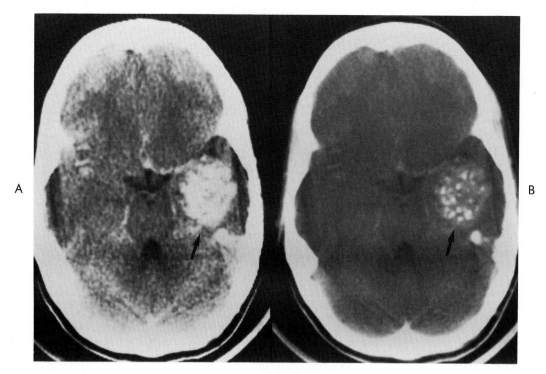

Fig. 16-21. Nonenhanced **(A)** and enhanced **(B)** CT scans of a high-density calcified cavernous hemangioma of the left temporal lobe *(arrows)*.

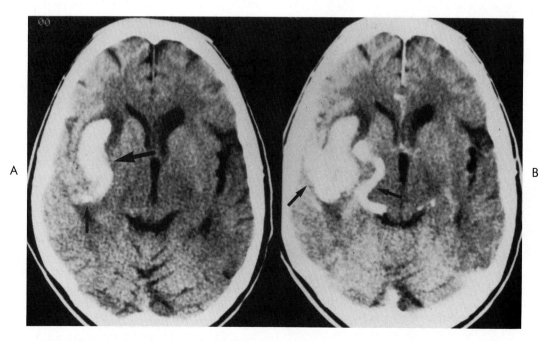

Fig. 16-22. A, Nonenhanced CT scan shows calcified lesions *(small arrow)* of an arteriovenous malformation with a hematoma *(large arrow)* in the right temporal lobe. **B,** Enhanced CT scan shows tangle of vessels and large draining veins *(small arrows)* just medial to the area of hemorrhage.

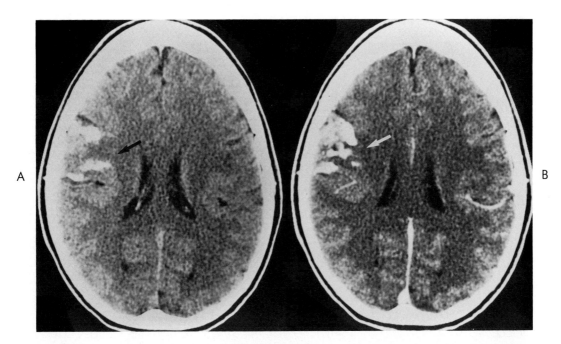

Fig. 16-23. Nonenhanced **(A)** and enhanced **(B)** CT scans of venous angioma *(arrows)* of the right temporal lobe. Angioma is seen as an area of increased density. There is no edema or mass effect.

the lesion are generally poorly defined and irregular. With contrast enhancement, the lesion shows nonhomogeneous enhancement (Fig. 16-22). A significant percentage of AVMs are apparent on enhanced CT scans, and thus contrast material enhancement must be routine in the evaluation of seizures when AVM is suspected.[68]

Up to one half of patients with AVM present with hemorrhagic lesions.[67] Hemorrhage often occurs in the subarachnoid space or ventricular system and less often in the parenchyma.

Venous angiomas are the rarest form of AVM, and patients with this disorder may present with seizure.[69] Venous angiomas frequently are associated with hemorrhage. The nonenhanced CT scan is usually normal. Enhancement shows a rounded or linear area of enhancement without mass effect or edema (Fig. 16-23).

The CT scan should be the initial imaging study performed in patients with seizure when AVM is suspected. Both nonenhanced and enhanced CT scans are required. Angiography may be required to document the extent, nature, and exact anatomy of such lesions.

Most patients with ischemic stroke eventually develop positive findings on the CT scan. The CT scan may yield such findings as early as 3 hours following the onset of symptoms. However, the classic low-density lesion usually develops between 24 and 72 hours.[70] The size and location of the infarction, as well as the spatial and contrast resolution capability of the CT scanner in use will determine the ability to detect ischemic lesions early.

Fig. 16-24 shows the progress of the CT scan findings

in ischemic infarction. In the first 24 hours, a nonenhanced CT scan may reveal an area of low density that becomes more distinct during the next 48 to 72 hours. A mass effect may be present in up to 70% of ischemic infarctions and is most marked between days 3 and 5. Enhancement of an ischemic infarction lesion may be seen early, but it is often not seen until a few days following the onset of symptoms. Patterns of enhancement vary widely. Markedly enhancing lesions often are more prone to significant necrosis. Occasionally, enhancement is the only method of identifying an ischemic lesion early (Figs. 16-25 and 16-26).

Hemorrhagic infarction is most frequently associated with embolic stroke. The CT scan image is characteristically different from intracerebral hematoma in that it primarily involves the cortex and has unsharp margins, with a low-density area surrounding light matter in a distribution that matches the anatomic vascular distribution (Fig. 16-27).

Patients with spontaneous intracerebral hematoma may present with sudden neurologic symptoms and seizures. It is most common in elderly hypertensive patients. The CT scan is the preferred diagnostic modality. Most of these hemorrhages occur in the basal ganglia or centrosylvian areas. The CT scan shows an area of increased density. Mass effect and associated edema vary, depending on the location and extent of the hemorrhage (Fig. 16-28).

Miscellaneous

Two neurocutaneous syndromes are frequently associated with seizures—tuberous sclerosis and Sturge-Weber syndrome. *Text continued on p. 447.*

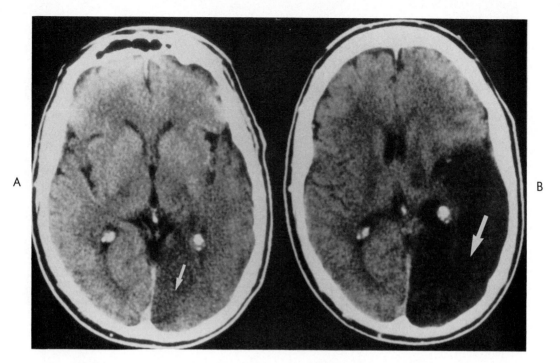

Fig. 16-24. A, CT scan of ischemic infarction at 12 hours demonstrates low-density region *(arrow)* in the left posterior parietal area caused by a left middle cerebral artery stroke. **B,** CT scan 4 days later demonstrates the margins of the infarction as clearer *(arrow),* and the affected area shows increased low density.

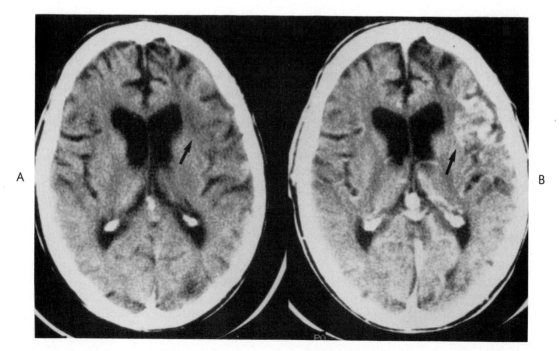

Fig. 16-25. Acute ischemic infarction with enhancement. **A,** Nonenhanced CT scan demonstrates a questionable area of low density in the left frontal parietal region *(arrow).* **B,** Enhanced CT scan demonstrates an obvious area of high density *(arrow)* in the same region.

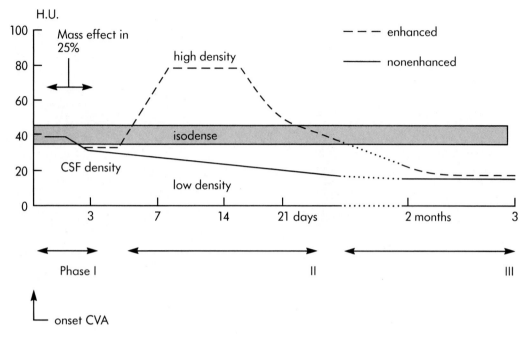

Fig. 16-26. Temporal development of the CT scan image of infarctions. (Modified from Valk J: *Computed tomography and cerebral infarctions,* New York, 1980, Raven Press.)

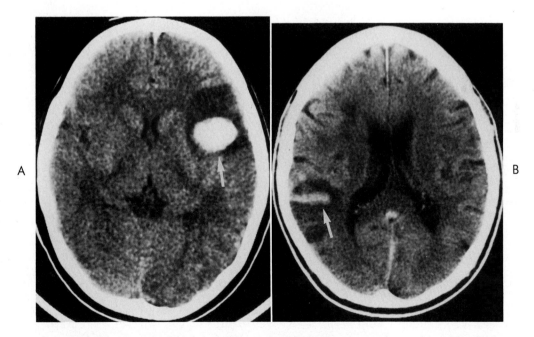

Fig. 16-27. A, CT scan of a left frontal hemorrhagic infarction *(arrow)* in a patient with aplastic anemia. **B,** CT scan of a hemorrhagic infarction *(arrow)* in right temporal parietal area with a surrounding area of edema.

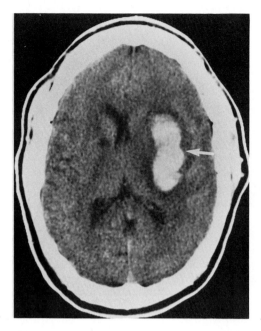

Fig. 16-28. CT scan of left basal ganglia hemorrhage *(arrow)* in a hypertensive patient.

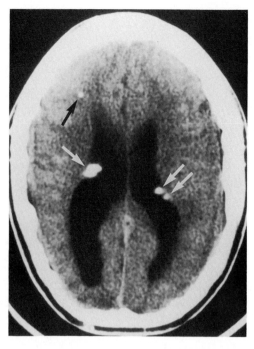

Fig. 16-29. Tuberous sclerosis. CT scan of a calcified hamartomas within the parenchyma and along the ependymal surface of the ventricles *(arrows)*.

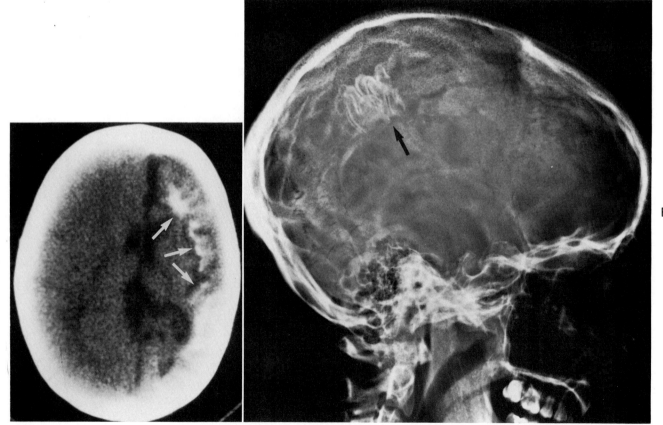

Fig. 16-30. Sturge-Weber syndrome. **A,** Nonenhanced CT scan demonstrates a typical calcification *(arrows)* in the left parietal convexity. **B,** Skull radiograph shows the calcified cortex *(arrow)*.

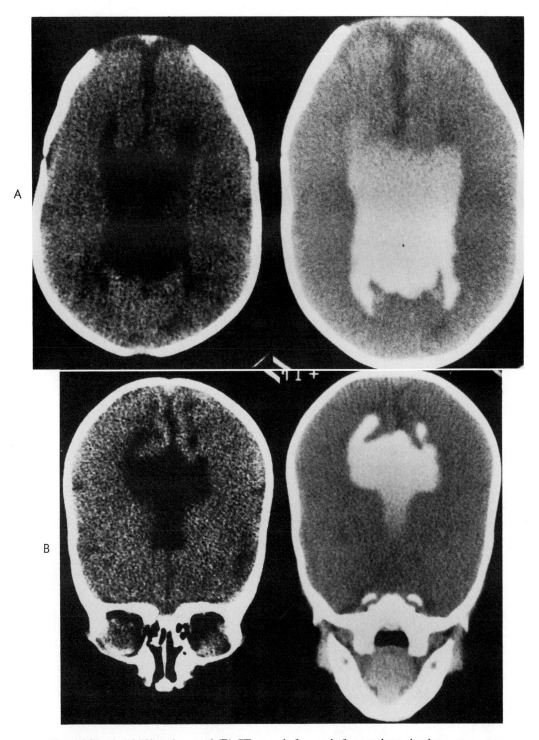

Fig. 16-31. Axial (**A**) and coronal (**B**) CT scans before and after myelography demonstrate agenesis of the corpus callosum. The bodies of the lateral ventricles are widely separated, resulting in a concave configuration of the lateral ventricles. *Continued*.

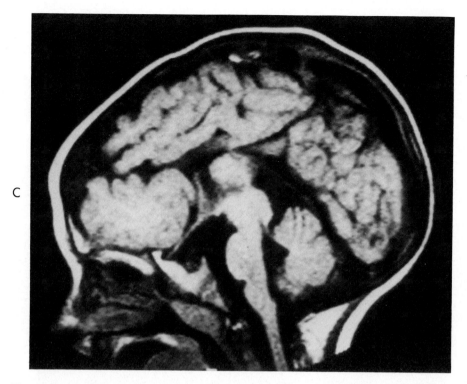

Fig. 16-31, cont'd. (C) Sagittal T$_1$-weighted MRI image also shows absence of the corpus callosum.

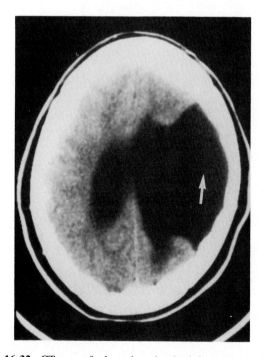

Fig. 16-32. CT scan of a large low-density left parietal area representing a porencephalic cyst *(arrow)* as a result of old trauma.

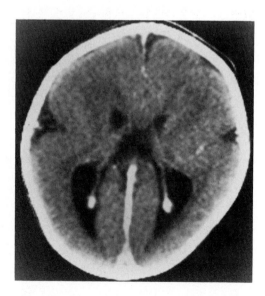

Fig. 16-33. CT scan demonstrating lissencephaly. Note absence of identifiable cerebral sulci, sometimes referred to as "smooth brain."

Tuberous sclerosis is characterized by hamartomas in multiple organs, including the brain. The most common site of intracranial hamartoma is the cerebrum, although the cerebellum and even the spinal cord may be involved.[71] The CT scan shows calcified, dense, rounded glial masses on the inner border of the ventricular system (Fig. 16-29). Lesions may sometimes be dense enough to be seen on plain skull radiographs.

Sturge-Weber syndrome includes port wine nevi of the face, seizures, leptomeningeal angiomatosis, hemiatrophy, and hemiparesis. The CT scan usually shows calcification involving the periphery of the cerebral hemispheres in a gyral pattern (Fig. 16-30, *A*). Plain skull radiographs often demonstrate the calcifications (Fig. 16-30, *B*).

Congenital lesions, such as agenesis of the corpus callosum, can cause seizures. This appears as a wide separation of the frontal horns of the lateral ventricles and a high position of the third ventricle (Fig. 16-31, *A* and *B*). It is well demonstrated on the MRI (Fig. 16-31, *C*). Congenital or posttraumatic cystic lesions may also be a cause of persistent or new seizure. These appear as large, low-density lucent areas (Fig. 16-32).

Lissencephaly is a rare malformation in which the telencephalon remains in a primitive form without gyri. This is due to a disturbance of cell migration.[72] The CT scan shows a relatively thickened cortex with sparse white matter. Cerebral fissures are malformed and cerebral sulci cannot be identified (Fig. 16-33). Patients have mental retardation and often have seizures.[73]

SUMMARY

Patients with seizures commonly present to the emergency department requiring stabilization and expeditious evaluation. Radiographic evaluation is essential in excluding anatomic causes of seizures, either on an acute, chronic, or recurrent basis. Several imaging modalities may be considered in the initial patient evaluation; specific indications should determine the approach to assessment.

REFERENCES

1. Hauser WA, Annegers JF, and Anderson VE: Epidemiology and the genetics of epilepsy. In Ward AA, Penry JK, and Purpura D, eds: *Epilepsy,* New York, 1983, Raven Press.
2. Forster FM, Booker HE: The epilepsies and convulsive disorders. In Baker AB, Baker LH, eds: *Clinical neurology,* New York, 1983, Harper & Row.
3. Gorman RJ et al: Febrile seizures, *Am Fam Physician* 19:101, 1979.
4. Krumholz A, Grufferman S, Orr ST et al: Seizures and seizure care in an emergency department, *Epilepsia* 30(2):175, 1989.
5. Berlin L: Significance of grand mal seizures developing in patients over 35 years of age, *JAMA* 152:794, 1953.
6. Douglas D: Interval between first seizure and diagnosis of brain tumor, *Dis Nerv System* 32:255, 1971.
7. Korczyn F, Bechar M: Convulsive fits in thyrotoxicosis, *Epilepsia* 17:33, 1976.
8. Livingston S: Etiologic factors in adult convulsions, *N Engl J Med* 254:1211, 1956.
9. Glaser G: Convulsive disorders. In Merritt HH, ed: *A textbook of neurology,* Philadelphia, 1975, Lea & Febiger.
10. Commission on Classification and Terminology of the International League Against Epilepsy: Proposal for revised clinical and electroencephalographic classification of epileptic seizures, *Epilepsia* 22:489, 1981.
11. Eisner RE, Turnbull TL, Howes DS et al: Efficacy of a standard seizure workup in the emergency department, *Ann Emerg Med* 15:33, 1986.
12. So LE, Penry JK: Epilepsy in adults, *Ann Neurol* 9:3, 1987.
13. Bogdanoff BM, Stafford CR, Green L et al: Computerized transaxial tomography in the evaluation of patients with focal epilepsy, *Neurology* 25:1013, 1975.
14. Ramirez-Lassepas M, Cipolle RJ, Morillo LR et al: Value of computed tomographic scan in the evaluation of adult patients after their first seizure, *Ann Neurol* 15:536, 1984.
15. Schwartz HS, Yarnell PR, and Vanderark G: Focal motor seizures in patients with alcoholism, *J Am Coll Emerg Physicians* 3:394, 1974.
16. Camp JD: Pathologic non-neoplastic intracranial calcification, *JAMA* 137:1023, 1948.
17. Camp JD: Significance of intracranial calcification in roentgenologic diagnosis of intracranial neoplasms, *Radiology* 55:659, 1950.
18. Tyson GW: *Head injury management for providers of emergency care,* Baltimore, 1987, Williams & Wilkins.
19. Weisberg LA, Nice C, and Katz M: *Cerebral computed tomography: a text-atlas,* Philadelphia, 1978, WB Saunders.
20. Gastaut H, Gastaut JL: Computerized transverse axial tomography in epilepsy, *Epilepsia* 17:325, 1976.
21. Caille JM, Cohadon F, Loiseau P et al: Summary: computerized transverse axial tomography in epilepsy, *Epilepsia* 17:341, 1976 (abstract).
22. Bachman DS, Hodges FJ, and Freeman JM: Computerized axial tomography in chronic seizure disorders of childhood, *Pediatrics* 58:828, 1976.
23. Janz D: Morphological diagnosis in epilepsy by computer assisted brain tomography. In Meinardi H, Rowan AJ, eds: *Advances in epileptology—1977,* Amsterdam, 1978, Swets & Zeitlinger.
24. Gastaut H, Gastaut JL: Computerized axial tomography in epilepsy. In Penry JK, ed: *Epilepsy: the Eighth International Symposium,* New York, 1977, Raven.
25. Scollo-Lavizzari G, Eichhorn K, and Wüthrich R: Computerized transverse axial tomography in the diagnosis of epilepsy, *Eur Neurol* 15:5, 1977.
26. Zimmerman AW, Neidermeyer E, and Hodges FJ: Lennox-Gastaut syndrome and computerized axial tomography findings, *Epilepsia* 18:463, 1977.
27. Carrera GF, Gerson DE, and Schnur J: Computed tomography of the brain in patients with headache or temporal lobe epilepsy: findings and cost effectiveness, *J Comput Assist Tomogr* 1:200, 1977.
28. Ghazy A, Slettnes O, and Lundervold A: Electroencephalography and computerized transaxial tomography in epilepsy diagnosis, *Clin Electroencephalogr* 9:159, 1978.
29. Reisner T, Zeiler K, and Dal Bianco P: Computertomographische Ergebnisse bei Kindern mit Cerebralen Anfällen, *Neuroradiology* 16:20, 1978.
30. Ratzka M, Glötzner F, Nadjmi M et al: CT-Ergebnisse bei patienten mit Epilepsie, eine prospektive Studie, *Neuroradiology* 16:332, 1978.
31. McGahan JP, Dublin AB, and Hill RP: The evaluation of seizure disorders by computerized tomography, *J Neurosurg* 50:328, 1979.
32. Lagenstein I, Kühne D, and Sternowsky HJ: Computerized cranial transverse axial tomography (CTAT) in 145 patients with primary and secondary generalized epilepsies—West syndrome, myoclonic-astatic petit mal, absence epilepsy, *Neuropaediatrie* 10:15, 1979.
33. Ladurmer G, Sager WD, Dusik B et al: Die Bedeutung der Computertomographie in der Diagnose der Epilepsie, *Fortschr Neurol Psychiatr* 47:264, 1979.
34. Davis KR, Taveras JM, Roberson GH et al: Some limitations of

computed tomography in the diagnosis of neurological diseases, *AJR* 127:111, 1976.

35. Kent DL, Larson EB: Magnetic resonance imaging of the brain and spine: is clinical efficacy established after the first decade? *Ann Int Med* 108:402, 1988.

36. Ormson MJ, Kispert DB, Sharbrough FW et al: Cryptic structural lesions in refractory partial epilepsy: MR imaging and CT studies, *Radiology* 160:215, 1986.

37. Latack JT, Abou-Khalil BW, Siegel GJ et al: Patients with partial seizures: evaluation by MR, CT, and PET imaging, *Radiology* 159:159, 1986.

37a. Ramsey RG: Angiographic technique and applied cerebrovascular embryology and normal anatomy. In Ramsey RG: *Neuroradiology,* ed 2, Philadelphia, 1987, WB Saunders.

38. Jabbari B, Gunderson CH, Wippold F et al: Magnetic resonance imaging in partial complex epilepsy, *Arch Neurol* 43:869, 1986.

39. Sperling MR, Wilson G, Engel J Jr et al: Magnetic resonance imaging in intractable partial epilepsy: correlative studies, *Ann Neurol* 20:57, 1986.

40. Lesser RP, Modic MT, Weinstein MA et al: Magnetic resonance imaging (1.5 tesla) in patients with intractable focal seizures, *Arch Neurol* 43:367, 1986.

41. Theodore WH, Dorwart R, Holmes M et al: Neuroimaging in refractory partial seizures: comparison of PET, CT, and MRI, *Neurology* 36:750, 1986.

42. Baker HL Jr, Berquist TH, Kispert DB et al: Magnetic resonance imaging in a routine clinical setting, *Mayo Clin Proc* 60:75, 1985.

43. McLachlan RS, Nicholson RL, Black S et al: Nuclear magnetic resonance imaging: a new approach to the investigation of refractory temporal lobe epilepsy, *Epilepsia* 26:555, 1985.

44. Guberman A: The role of computed cranial tomography (CT) in epilepsy, *Can J Neurol Sci* 10:16, 1983.

45. Young AC, Mohr PD, Borg-Costanzi J et al: Is routine computerized axial tomography in epilepsy worthwhile? Lancet, 1982, p 1446.

46. McCrea ES, Rao KC, and Diaconis JN: Roentgenographic changes during long-term diphenylhydantoin therapy, *South Med J* 73:310, 1980.

47. Sheldon JJ, Siddharthan R, Tobias J et al: MR imaging of multiple sclerosis: comparison with clinical CT exam in 74 patients, *Am J Neuroradiol* 6:683, 1985.

48. Leo JS et al: CT in herpes simplex encephalitis, *Surg Neurol* 10:313, 1978.

49. Levy RM, Rosenbloom S, and Perrett LV: Neuroradiologic findings in AIDS: a review of 200 cases, *Am J Neuroradiol* 7:833, 1986.

50. Elkin CM, Leon E, Grenell SL et al: Intracranial lesions in AIDS: radiologic (CT) features, *JAMA* 253:393, 1988.

51. Rosenthal RH, Heim ML, and Waeckerle JF: First time major motor seizure in an ED, *Ann Emerg Med* 9(5):242, 1980.

52. DeReuck JL, Vander Eecken HM: Periventricular leckomalasia in adults, *Arch Neurol* 35:517, 1978.

53. Miura T, Mitomo M, Kawai R et al: CT of the brain in acute carbon monoxide intoxication: characteristic features and prognosis, *Am J Neuroradiol* 6:739, 1985.

54. Jabbari B, Huott AD, DiChiro G et al: Surgically correctable lesions solely detected by CT scan in adult onset chronic epilepsy, *Ann Neurol* 7:344, 1980.

55. LeBlanc FE, Rasmussen T: Cerebral seizures and brain tumors. In Vinken BJ, Bruyn GW, eds: *Handbook of clinical neurology,* vol 15, *The epilepsies,* Amsterdam, 1974, Elsevier North Holland.

56. Lee YY, Glass JP, Geoffray A et al: Cranial computed tomographic abnormalities in leptomeningeal metastasis, *Am J Neuroradiol* 5:559, 1984.

56a. Holmes RA, Staab EV: The central nervous system. In Freeman LM, Johnson PM: *Clinical scintillation imaging,* ed 2, New York, Grune & Stratton.

57. LaHaye PA, Gade GF, and Becker DP: Injury to the cranium. In Mattox KL, ed: *Trauma,* Norwalk, CT, 1988, Appleton Lange.

58. Roberts F, Shopfner CE: Plain skull roentgenograms in children with head trauma, *AJR* 114:230, 1972.

59. Hadley DM, Teasdale GM, Jenkins A et al: MRI in magnetic resonance imaging in acute head injury, *Clin Radiol* 39:131, 1988.

60. Caveness WF: Epilepsy: a product of trauma in our time, *Epilepsia* 17(2):207, 1976.

61. Kishore PRS, Lipper MH, Becker DP et al: The significance of CT in the management of patients with severe head injury: correlation with CT, *Am J Neuroradiol* 2:307, 1981.

62. Jamieson KG, Yelland JDN: Extradural hematoma: report of 107 cases, *J Neurol* 29:13, 1968.

63. Earnest MP, Feldman H, Marx JA et al: Intracranial lesions shown by CT scans in 259 cases of first alcohol related seizures, *Neurology* 38:1561, 1988.

64. Moon KL, Brant-Zwadzki M, Pitts LH et al: NMR imaging of CT isodense subdural hematomas, *Am J Neuroradiol* 5:319, 1984.

65. Kramer RA, Wing SD: Computed tomography of angiographically occult cerebral vascular malformations, *Radiology* 123:649, 1977.

66. Ramina R, Ingunza W, and Vonofakos D: Cystic cerebral cavernous angioma with dense calcification, *J Neurosurg* 52:259, 1980.

67. LeBlanc R, Ethier R, and Little JR: CT findings in AVM of the brain, *J Neurosurg* 51:765, 1979.

68. Terbrugge KG, Scotti G, Ethier R et al: CT in AVM, *Radiology* 122:703, 1977.

69. Rothfus WE, Albright AL, Casey KF et al: Cerebellar venous angioma: "benign" entity? *Am J Neuroradiol* 5:61, 1984.

70. Inoue Y, Takemota K, Miyamoto T et al: Sequential CT scan in acute cerebral infarction, *Radiology* 135:655, 1980.

71. Fitz CR, Harwood-Nash DC, and Thompson JR: Neuroradiology of tuberous sclerosis in children, *Radiology* 116:635, 1974.

72. Dieker H, Edwards RH, ZuRhein G et al: The lissencephaly syndrome, *Birth Defects* 5:53, 1969.

73. Daube JR, Chou SM: Lissencephaly: two cases, *Neurology* 16:179, 1966.

Headache

Neal Little
Elizabeth A. Eelkema

Headache is an extremely common symptom in the general population, and patients with headache present to the emergency department with moderate frequency. Although many headaches do not represent a life threat, some patients with headache do, in fact, have a life-threatening medical or surgical problem. It is the task of the emergency physician to try to differentiate those causes of headache that pose a serious threat to the patient's life or health from those that present a painful nuisance.

In a general population study, 57% of men and 76% of women reported a headache in the month before the survey. In that month, 3% of men and 7% of women reported a migraine.[1] It is estimated that 19% of men and 29% of women will experience a migraine during their lifetime.[2] In emergency department studies, headache occurs as a presenting complaint in 1.3%[3] to 1.6%[4] of patients: serious neurologic causes are involved in 1.2% to 5% of these headache patients. Of the 12 million patients who present annually to emergency departments with the complaint of headache, 25,000 to 33,000 have subarachnoid hemorrhage and a similar number have bacterial meningitis.[2]

TREATING HEADACHE IN THE EMERGENCY DEPARTMENT

The general approach to the patient who presents to the emergency department with a headache is one that should enable the physician to rapidly sort patients into two broad categories: those whose headaches represent a serious threat to their life or health and those who have headaches as a nuisance-creating but not life-threatening medical problem. The first group require further diagnostic testing on an emergent basis; the second group may require such testing on a more elective basis. This process of sorting patients is not necessarily an easy one; some general guidelines serve to help.

Two kinds of clues can indicate that a patient's headache may represent a serious threat to life or health: abnormal mental status and abnormal vital signs. For example, fever in the presence of headache makes one immediately suspect an intracranial infectious problem such as meningitis.

Physical examination

The general *physical examination* of the patient with headache should focus on the head for potential signs of trauma or areas of tenderness; palpation or percussion should be performed over the maxillary and frontal sinuses; the scalp arteries should be palpated either for relief of headaches, such as with vascular headaches, or for the production of headache in the elderly patient, such as occurs with temporal arteritis; and the ears and throat should be examined for signs of infection.

An important physical examination finding is neck stiffness in the nontraumatized patient. To elicit this finding accurately may require great skill, and it can be a very subtle finding. The test for neck stiffness should be performed with the patient lying supine with the head flexed so that the chin is directed to the chest. The test should not be performed in the sitting position and it should not be done voluntarily by the patient; the finding to elicit is involuntary resistance to flexion, not other movements, and a report of pain is not the end point. Other "meningeal signs," such as Kernig and Brudzinski signs, are usually only present in advanced cases of meningeal irritation and are not as sensitive as the test for neck stiffness.

The *neurologic examination* should focus on high-yield tests, which consist of evaluation of mental status and examination of the cranial nerves with specific attention to extra-ocular movements, the pupils, and the fundus. However, it is rare for tests of cranial nerves I or IX through XII to have a very significant yield in the patient with headache.

In the *motor examination* the component with the highest yield (in the absence of motor symptoms) is a test for drift of the outstretched upper extremities and an examination of the patient's gait. The presence of abnormalities in either one of these or the presence of motor symptoms should prompt a more detailed and focused examination.

A *sensory examination* (in the absence of sensory symptoms) is unlikely to be helpful. A quick screening with a light touch and perhaps double-simultaneous stimulation is all that is likely to be helpful. A reflex examination—other than checking for asymmetry or pathologic signs—is also seldom revealing.

An elevation of *blood pressure* is in general a nonspecific sign. Elevated blood pressure may be a reflection of a painful condition, whether it is located in the head or elsewhere. It is rare for blood pressure elevation alone to be a cause for headache. Headache is actually no more common in patients with elevated blood pressures than in those without. However, there is a certain subset of patients who do experience typically suboccipitally located headaches when their blood pressure is elevated. Headache cannot be attributed to uniformly elevated blood pressure, but many authors believe that the range of 120 to 140 diastolic is

significant.[5] Nevertheless, greatly elevated blood pressure in the patient with headache may be the first clue that the patient may have experienced a subarachnoid hemorrhage. Many patients who have a subarachnoid hemorrhage (32%) have an elevated blood pressure, either as a result of the hemorrhage or as one of the contributing causes.[10] Although subarachnoid hemorrhage can occur without evidence of hypertension at the time of presentation, significant hypertension on evaluation enhances the clinical possibility of subarachnoid hemorrhage.

An elevated *pulse rate* is a very nonspecific finding in patients with pain of any kind, including headache, and its presence alone is not sufficiently sensitive to assist in determining a particular cause. However, pulse may be elevated in patients who have significant toxicity from an infectious process or who are extremely ill for other reasons.

Bradycardia, although at times a component of the so-called Cushing response, is not invariably present with elevated intracranial pressure. When present, it is usually a late finding and not one that is useful in suggesting a severe intracranial process that is not obvious by other observations.

Respiratory rate is a relatively nonspecific sign. Only at its greatest extremes—either very slow or very fast—is it useful in suggesting a significant intracranial process, and in that setting, other factors are more likely to be the first clues to the physician.

Patients with a headache and altered *mental status* should be considered to have a medically significant cause for their headache and should be investigated with that in mind. Clinical entities such as subdural hematoma, subarachnoid hemorrhage, intracerebral bleeding, meningitis, and carbon monoxide poisoning come to mind and should be further pursued initially with a directed history and physical examination.

History

Perhaps the most important historical fact to be noted is the time course from the onset of a headache. Those headaches that begin and reach their maximal intensity instantaneously should cause one to seriously consider the diagnosis of subarachnoid hemorrhage. It is rare for other entities to present with such suddenness. Most findings that develop over seconds to minutes in the nervous system are vascular in nature. The time course of a headache that builds and progresses over weeks to months is consistent with an intracranial expanding lesion and is a rare cause of headache in the emergency department.

The quality of the pain may likewise be helpful in distinguishing several common causes of headache. The pounding or throbbing quality of vascular headaches, which are usually worsened by exertion, characteristically occur in patients with vascular headaches of any cause, including migraine.

Associated symptoms such as nausea and particularly vomiting, although present in medically benign conditions such as migraine, are also frequently present in severe intracranial pathologic states, such as subarachnoid hemorrhage and meningitis. The presence of significant vomiting should initiate the consideration of serious causes. Any history of trauma in the recent past should suggest a post-traumatic condition. Fever raises the possibilities of either an intracranial or systemic infectious process. However, patients with a brain abscess are often afebrile at the time of presentation. The box above lists other factors that are important in the history of the patient with headache.

The location of pain may provide important clues to the diagnosis. Pain located specifically over the maxillary or frontal sinuses, especially if exacerbated by bending forward, suggests sinusitis.[6]

Ancillary data

Ancillary studies that may be particularly useful include assessment for infection or metabolic causes and analyses of cerebrospinal fluid (CSF). Radiographic examination including a sinus radiographic series; CT scans for cerebral edema, hemorrhage, or masses; and magnetic resonance imaging (MRI) are important in diagnosing a specific condition or excluding serious causes.

In summary, the high-yield differentiating criteria of headache evaluation include details of the time course at the onset of the headache, associated findings such as loss of consciousness or fever, the presence of abnormal vital signs, a physical examination directed at the head and neck, and a focused screening neurologic examination. Once these have been accomplished, the patient can usually be placed into one of the two categories previously described: those whose headaches are suspected to be caused by serious medical problems or those whose headaches are suspected to be caused by noncritical medical illness (see box above on the right).

Anatomic and physiologic considerations

A limited number of intracranial and extracranial structures in and around the head are capable of initiating pain, including the scalp and scalp appendages, such as hair follicles, the scalp muscles themselves, and the periosteum of the skull. Intracranially, the dura, the large blood vessels at the base of the brain, and cranial nerves V, IX, XI, and the upper cervical nerves are capable of transmitting painful stimuli.

The parenchyma of the brain itself is insensitive to pain. Pain, therefore, is produced by stimulation of one of the previously discussed pain-sensitive structures either by direct pressure, displacement, stretching, or by actual inflammation or infection of that structure. It is for this reason that primary brain tumors rarely cause headache without concomitant neurologic findings. Tumors, such as a meningioma, that originate in pain-sensitive structures are an obvious exception.

The skull bones are not sensitive to pain; however, the periosteum and dural lining are sensitive. It is for this and other reasons that plain radiographs of the skull are seldom, if ever, helpful in patient evaluation. The only indirect radiographic evidence for an intracranial process causing headache, such as intracranial shift of the pineal gland, is so rare as to be virtually useless in the evaluation of the patient with headache. Only if specific bony abnormalities, such as a bony tumor, are suspected are plain radiographs of any use; the CT scan is superior and has largely replaced plain film radiography. The paranasal sinuses, however, are discussed separately in this chapter because they may represent an important and medically treatable cause for headache that can be determined by specific radiographic studies.

BASIC CONSIDERATIONS IN COMPUTED TOMOGRAPHY

Computed tomography (CT scan) of the head is a rapid, safe, widely available, and fairly sensitive method to detect acute intracranial hemorrhage, cerebral masses, hydrocephalus, and abnormalities of the sinuses, skull base, and cranial vault. Because the CT scan is currently more widely available and less expensive than MRI, it is emphasized in this chapter. It should be acknowledged, however, that MRI is much more sensitive than the CT scan for detecting certain intracranial pathologic conditions, such as multiple sclerosis, meningeal infections, tumors, acute stroke, and brain stem or posterior fossa pathologic states. The use of a CT scan or MRI as the initial imaging technique should be guided by the clinical setting and by the availability of the different modalities. For those patients with headache severe or acute enough to warrant immediate imaging, a CT scan is appropriate because it is more sensitive than MRI for acute hemorrhage and can detect hydrocephalus or intracranial masses that preclude lumbar puncture. If a more elective workup is indicated, MRI should be considered.

Once the decision has been made to use the CT scan, the next issue is whether or not intravenous contrast material should be used. A nonenhanced CT scan is appropriate to evaluate post-trauma patients and those with suspected acute cerebral vascular accident or recurrent hydrocephalus caused by shunt malfunction. For patients with a suspected aneurysm, vascular malformation, meningitis, abscess, and primary or secondary neoplasm, an enhanced CT scan is recommended. Patients with suspected intracranial hemorrhage, particularly subarachnoid hemorrhage, should undergo both enhanced and nonenhanced CT scans.

The CT scan image is composed of a matrix of discrete pixels (picture elements), whose brightness depends both on the amount of x-rays absorbed (or attenuated) by the represented volume of tissue and on the display settings. Those structures that absorb x-rays well (bone, contrast material) are of higher densities and appear "whiter" than substances that attenuate fewer of the x-rays. The "window width" and "window level" settings are parameters that determine how the shades of gray are distributed in the image. For most CT scans of the brain, relatively narrow window widths (80 to 150 Hounsfield units) are usually used. Wider windows (250 Hounsfield units) help differentiate small amounts of subdural or subarachnoid hemorrhage from adjacent bone. Much wider windows (2000 to 4000 Hounsfield units) are necessary to inspect the details of the bones. Viewing the CT scan image of the head at the console with multiple window settings or filming the

study with multiple settings is mandatory to maximize the information gained from each CT scan.

Normal anatomy

A normal, contrast-enhanced head CT scan of an adult patient is shown in Fig. 17-1. The cortical gray matter is of slightly higher density and is well differentiated from the subjacent, lower-density white matter. The basal ganglia (caudate, putamen, globus pallidus) are also composed of gray matter and are of a higher attenuation compared with the adjacent white matter of the internal capsule. The gray-white junction of the cerebral hemisphere curves gently and conforms to the contour of the inner table of the skull. The frontal, occipital, and temporal horns of the lateral ventricles are symmetric. The midline third and fourth ventricles are easily seen. Low-density CSF fills the ventricular system and is usually seen in normal-sized sulci over the cerebral hemispheres and cerebellar vermis and in the sylvian fissures and basal cisterns. There is marked enhancement of the intracranial vascular structures. However, even on this high-quality CT scan obtained with a current generation scanner, there are considerable streaking artifacts from the dense bones of the skull base that obscure the detail of the posterior fossa.

Indications for diagnostic imaging

In general, the radiographic considerations for the emergency physician who is evaluating the patient with headache are:

- Does the patient present clinically with sinusitis so that plain radiographs of the sinuses might be useful in further patient care?
- Or does this patient require a CT scan?

Specific indications for diagnostic imaging in the patient with headache include suspected subarachnoid hemorrhage, epidural hematoma, acute subdural hematoma, chronic subdural hematoma, fractures, intracerebral and intracranial hemorrhage, tumors, brain abscess, hydrocephalus, posterior fossa mass, sinusitis, and bone lesions.

SUSPECTED SUBARACHNOID HEMORRHAGE
Clinical findings

Subarachnoid hemorrhage (SAH) is probably one of the most important diagnostic considerations in evaluating the patient with headache in the emergency department. Although approximately one third of all patients sustaining SAH die either before or immediately after presentation to the emergency department, the remaining two thirds may represent a diagnostic challenge to the clinician. Those patients with obvious neurologic deficits, such as significant alteration of consciousness or focal findings, usually do not represent a diagnostic challenge because the suspected diagnosis is fairly obvious, and they require an immediate CT scan after clinical stabilization. The patient with a SAH who represents the greater diagnostic challenge is the one with a normal mental status and normal neurologic examination findings. Without treatment, 40% of patients

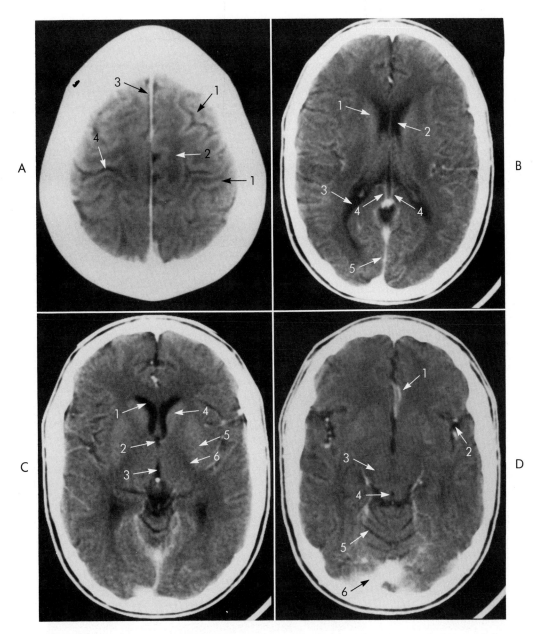

Fig. 17-1. Normal enhanced head CT scan of an adult. Axial sections, progressively more inferior (**A** to **F,** 10 mm thick; **G** to **H,** 5 mm thick). **A,** *1,* Cortical gray matter; *2,* white matter; *3,* falx cerebri; *4,* cerebrospinal fluid (CSF) in cortical sulci. **B,** *1,* Caudate nucleus; *2,* frontal horn of lateral ventricle; *3,* occipital horn of lateral ventricle; *4,* internal cerebral veins; *5,* falx cerebri. **C,** *1,* Frontal horn of lateral ventricle; *2,* foramen of Monro; *3,* third ventricle; *4,* caudate nucleus; *5,* lentiform nucleus; *6,* internal capsule. **D,** *1,* Pericallosal arteries; *2,* sylvian fissure; *3,* midbrain; *4,* cerebral aqueduct; *5,* cerebellar sulci; *6,* right transverse sinus.   *Continued.*

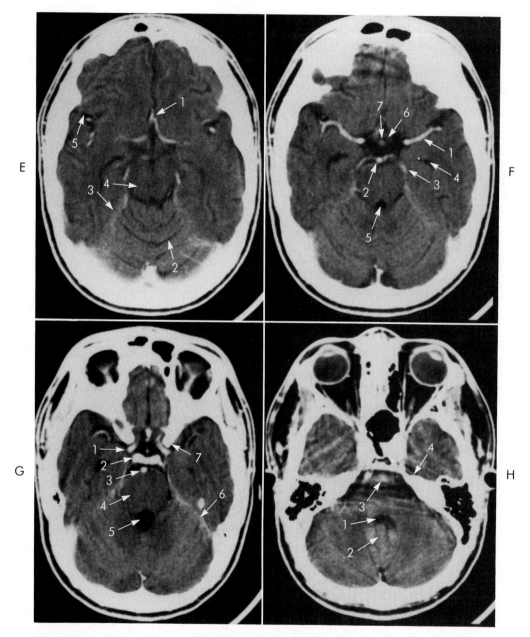

Fig. 17-1, cont'd. E, *1,* Anterior cerebral artery; *2,* cerebellar sulci; *3,* tentorium; *4,* midbrain; *5,* sylvian fissure. **F,** *1,* Middle cerebral artery; *2,* basilar artery; *3,* posterior cerebral artery; *4,* temporal horn of lateral ventricle; *5,* fourth ventricle; *6,* optic chiasm; *7,* infundibulum. **G,** *1,* Internal carotid artery; *2,* dorsum sella; *3,* basilar artery; *4,* pons; *5,* fourth ventricle; *6,* tentorium; *7,* anterior clinoid processes. **H,** *1,* Fourth ventricle; *2,* cerebellar vermis; *3,* basilar artery; *4,* petrous apex.

with aneurysms experience recurrent SAH within 8 weeks, and 60% of these recurrent hemorrhages are fatal.[7]

SAH is due to aneurysm rupture in 60% to 75% of cases, although some studies report an incidence as low as 50%[8] or as high as 90%.[10] Arteriovenous malformations (AVMs) account for 3% to 6% of SAHs.[66] If the hemorrhage is due to an AVM, neurologic deficit tends to be much more common because these commonly rupture both within and outside the substance of the brain. These hemorrhages tend to occur in patients younger than the typical patient with an aneurysm.

"Spontaneous" SAH, a hemorrhage in which no particular vascular abnormality can be found, occurs in 15% to 40% of patients.[9] This is obviously a diagnosis of exclusion and is made once a thorough investigation—including cerebral angiography and usually repeated angiography at a later date—has failed to reveal a source for hemorrhage. Other causes of nontraumatic SAH include primary and metastatic tumors, blood dyscrasias, meningoencephalitis, anticoagulation disorders, and cerebral vasculitis.

The patient with a SAH typically reports that the headache began suddenly and was unusually intense. SAH may occur during strenuous activity, sexual intercourse, or defecation: however, one third may occur during sleep. The pain initially may be localized but subsequently becomes generalized as a result of the spread of blood throughout the subarachnoid space. The blood may spread to the lumbar subarachnoid space and cause sciatica. Although many patients describe the headache as "the worst headache in my life" or "like something popped in my head," many patients will not use such phrases. However, on further questioning, it is clear that the headache was of sudden onset and was significantly painful. Diagnostically, perhaps the most difficult patient is the one who has an ongoing headache problem, such as migraine, who presents with a change in the pattern of headache.

Neurologic findings are frequently normal in the patient with suspected SAH, excluding those who present with obvious and profound depression of consciousness or focal neurologic findings. The most common neurologic finding, when one is present, is alteration of consciousness. In one study the state of consciousness was normal in one third of patients, confused or lethargic in one fifth, and responsive only to pain or unresponsive in the rest.[10] The blood in SAH travels through the subarachnoid space and rarely directly impinges on intracranial structures; focal neurologic findings are rare. Occasionally, the jet of blood released from the burst of the aneurysm penetrates the brain substance itself, resulting in intracerebral hematoma and related neurologic deficit. Unruptured aneurysms rarely cause symptoms. Occasionally, an aneurysm of the posterior communicating artery, when subjected to acute expansion or rupture, impinges on cranial nerve III, creating an isolated cranial nerve III palsy with dilated pupil. Rarely,

an unruptured aneurysm of the anterior communicating artery may cause visual field defects.

Other clinical signs associated with SAH include seizures in up to 25% of patients,[11] cardiac dysrhythmias in 50% to 100%,[12] and fever in up to 50%.[10] Photophobia, nausea and vomiting (75%), and nuchal rigidity (35%) are common. Neck pain (24%), back pain, and syncope (53%) may occur. Preretinal (subhyaloid) hemorrhages also may occur (5%) and when found in the appropriate clinical setting are pathognomonic.[10]

CT scan findings

The initial diagnostic modality of choice for the detection of subarachnoid hemorrhage is the nonenhanced CT scan with thin slices (5 mm or less) through the circle of Willis and posterior fossa. However, one must be aware of the limitations of the technique, specifically of false-negative CT scan results. The ability to detect blood in the subarachnoid space by a CT scan depends on the presence of a localized collection of clotted blood with sufficient density to make it radiographically visible. If one considers all patients with SAH, including those with profound alterations of consciousness and severe neurologic deficits, the sensitivity of a CT scan for detecting the hemorrhage is reported to be 74% to 84%.[13,14] However, in the patient with minor bleeding and a clinically unremarkable presentation, the sensitivity may be as low as 45%, especially for so-called sentinel bleeding.[13] The so-called "sentinel leak," causing the "warning headache" before a major SAH is very difficult to detect prospectively. Retrospectively, it is reported in 39% to 43% of patients with SAH.[15] Consideration of SAH should be entertained in all patients with severe headaches of sudden onset and with headaches that are unusual in nature.

With these considerations in mind, if the patient has the appropriate clinical presentation just described and there is no CT scan evidence of hemorrhage, a lumbar puncture should be performed, unless there is an intracranial mass lesion or significant midline shift. Results of the CT scan are falsely negative in 55% of these patients; however, a lumbar puncture may reveal the presence of blood or xanthochromic fluid.

In the patient in whom the clinical presentation suggests infection, a lumbar puncture is the initial study. In the less clear case, the patient can be started on antibiotic therapy while the CT scan is obtained, with the lumbar puncture performed after the CT scan shows no mass lesion.

For patients presenting more than 72 hours after an SAH, the diagnostic accuracy of the CT scan is very low (27%) as a result of breakdown of blood products.[16] Reasons for a false-negative CT scan include small hemorrhage, hemorrhage with a low hemoglobin content, hemorrhage very close to bone, remote hemorrhage in which sufficient blood has been absorbed to make the area isodense (5 to 7 days), or patient motion artifact significantly obscuring relatively subtle findings of subarachnoid blood.

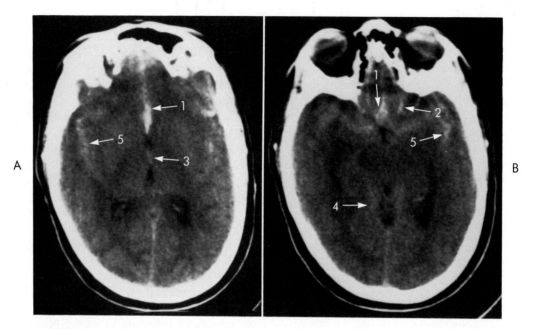

Fig. 17-2. Nonenhanced CT scans (**A** and **B**) demonstrate a high-density subarachnoid hemorrhage in the anterior interhemispheric fissure *(arrow 1)*, inferior frontal sulci *(arrow 2)*, third ventricle *(arrow 3)*, ambient cistern *(arrow 4)*, and sylvian fissure *(arrow 5)* caused by a ruptured anterior communicating artery aneurysm.

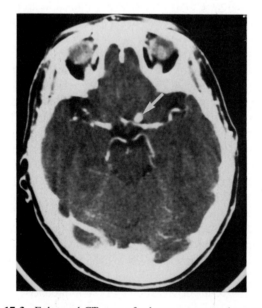

Fig. 17-3. Enhanced CT scan of a berry aneurysm demonstrates an 8 mm left ophthalmic artery aneurysm *(arrow)*.

The CT scan is not extremely sensitive to the presence of small amounts of blood in the subarachnoid space. Unless 70% of the CSF is replaced with blood, the CSF/blood mixture will be of low density or isodense in contrast to adjacent brain tissue.[16] Nevertheless, a positive nonenhanced CT scan result can confirm the presence of SAH and provide clues to the cause of the bleeding. A localized clot in the cisternal subarachnoid space usually indicates an aneurysm, whereas a peripheral parenchymal hematoma suggests an AVM or mycotic peripheral aneurysm.[17] A negative CT scan result does not exclude SAH nor preclude a lumbar puncture. SAH that is evident by a CT scan is displayed as high-density material in the basal cisterns, sulci, or sylvian fissures, replacing the low-density CSF (Fig. 17-2).

Trauma is a very common cause of SAH. Contrast enhancement is not necessary for a CT scan done to evaluate patients after known head trauma. However, in patients without a history of trauma and with known or suspected SAH, an enhanced CT scan is helpful in demonstrating lesions that may have bled (Fig. 17-3). If a berry aneurysm is suspected, thin (less than 5 mm thick) sections through the circle of Willis should be obtained after infusion of intravenous contrast material. The CT scan performed with this technique will detect most aneurysms larger than 5 mm.[18] Smaller aneurysms can only be excluded by angiography. MRI, because of its multiplanar capability and lack of signal from the complex, dense bone at the skull base, may well be better than the CT scan in the diagnosis

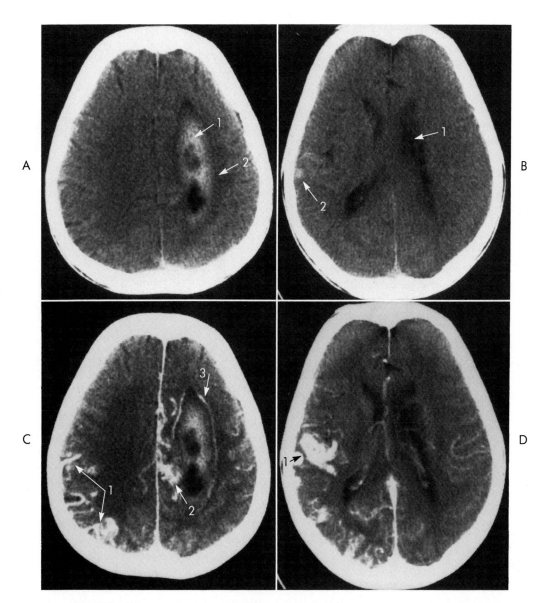

Fig. 17-4. Nonenhanced CT scans (**A** and **B**) and enhanced CT scans (**C** and **D**) of bilateral arteriovenous malformations. **A,** Left-sided malformation had bled previously, resulting in an intraparenchymal hematoma. The subacute hematoma has a high-density center *(arrow 1)* and surrounding low attenuation caused by edema and resolving hemorrhage *(arrow 2)*. **B,** On a more caudad section, part of the low-density periphery is seen *(arrow 1)*. Enlarged, faintly apparent, high-density vessels are demonstrated on the right *(arrow 2)*. **C** and **D,** With intravenous contrast enhancement, the right *(arrow 1)* and left *(arrow 2)* arteriovenous malformations undergo dense enhancement. There is rim enhancement of the hematoma *(arrow 3)*.

or exclusion of small aneurysms, but its role has not yet been fully defined.

Arteriovenous malformation as cause

Arteriovenous malformation (AVM) is a less common cause of SAH but is relatively more frequent in younger age groups.[17] A nonenhanced CT scan may display subarachnoid, intraventricular, and intraparenchymal hematomas caused by bleeding from an AVM. However, the malformation itself is not typically evident on nonenhanced studies. Occasionally, cavernous hemangiomas or large

feeding or draining vessels are evident on the nonenhanced CT scan as high-density structures caused by the blood's pooling effect. After contrast material is given, vascular malformations are displayed as densely enhancing, curving, superficial, tubular structures in and on the surface of the brain (Fig. 17-4).

Angiography for subarachnoid hemorrhage

If a cause for nontraumatic SAH is not demonstrated on a CT scan or if greater delineation of a detected aneurysm or vascular malformation is needed before surgery, angiography is performed. The recommended timing of angiography has varied over the years, depending on the surgical philosophy for early intervention. In 13% to 15% of patients with acute, nontraumatic SAH documented by CT scan or lumbar puncture, four-vessel cerebral angiography fails to demonstrate the site of bleeding.[9,19] Thrombosis of an aneurysm or spasm of the aneurysm or parent vessel may be causes for false-negative angiography findings. In one study, 16.5% of second angiograms performed 10 to 14 days later subsequently demonstrated an aneurysm.[20] On repeat angiography, some neuroradiologists also advocate selective injection of the external carotid vessels to detect dural AVMs.[21]

EPIDURAL HEMATOMA

The patient with an epidural hematoma following trauma usually presents to the emergency department with a chief complaint of headache. This clinical and radiographic entity is covered further in Chapters 3 and 15.

ACUTE SUBDURAL HEMATOMA

Acute subdural hematoma is almost universally associated with recent significant head trauma; its clinical and radiographic features are covered in Chapters 3 and 15.

FRACTURES

The patient with a skull fracture may present to the emergency department with a chief complaint of headache. There is usually a history of recent significant trauma, unless the patient's mental status is such that the history is unobtainable or unreliable. Chapters 3 and 15 detail the clinical and radiographic features of skull fracture.

CHRONIC SUBDURAL HEMATOMA
Clinical findings

The patient with a chronic subdural hematoma who presents to the emergency room with a chief complaint of headache usually has a history of trauma so remote that it is not remembered, either because of brief loss of consciousness at the time or because of the patient's abnormal mental status.

Patients with alcoholism are at great risk for chronic subdural hematoma. They experience brain atrophy, which thereby creates an enlargement of the subarachnoid space and a longer course for the bridging veins from the cerebral cortex to the dural venous sinuses. These veins are then more easily torn as the result of even minor trauma. The great capacity of the subarachnoid space requires that the hematoma become sufficiently large to exert pressure either locally or generally to cause significant symptoms. The multifactorial coagulopathy in persons with alcoholism also enhances a bleeding tendency. The propensity for frequent minor and major head trauma in such persons further increases the risk. For all these reasons, persons with alcoholism, brain atrophies, or coagulopathies, such as hemophilia, who experience new headache should be sus-

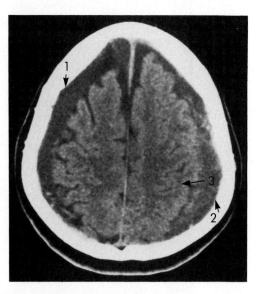

Fig. 17-5. Nonenhanced CT scan demonstrates a chronic bilateral subdural hematoma *(arrow 1)* with typical appearance of a low-density crescent of fluid interposed between the skull and slightly compressed cerebral cortex. On the left, the subdural fluid *(arrow 2)* is of higher attenuation than on the right; the latter is nearly isodense to the adjacent gray matter *(arrow 3)*.

pected of having a chronic subdural hematoma if there is a remote history of trauma and of progressing or fluctuating headache following minor trauma.

The timing of the radiographic evaluation depends on the patient's clinical presentation. The clinical presentation of chronic subdural hematoma is usually that of remote trauma, which may, in fact, have been fairly trivial. There may or may not have been loss of consciousness and headache at the time, but there is usually a history of a headache that has become progressively worse or one that fluctuates in severity. The patient may have a coagulopathy. There may be symptoms of increased intracranial pressure, such as worsening headache in the morning, nausea and vomiting, papilledema, neurologic deficits, disturbances of consciousness (ranging from mild to profound), or dementia. The CT scan is usually diagnostic.

CT scan findings

Acute subdural hematomas (see Chapters 3 and 15) are typically of high density on CT scans. As an intracranial hemorrhage ages, its density fades, becoming isodense in contrast to the brain in 2 to 3 weeks. After this time, most subdural hematomas are of low density in comparison with adjacent brain tissue.

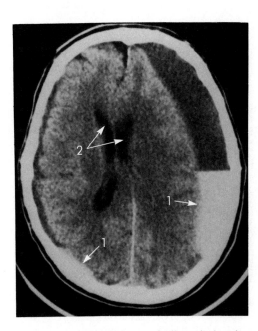

Fig. 17-6. Nonenhanced CT scan of bilateral chronic subdural hematomas with rebleeding demonstrates bilateral, nonuniform subdural fluid collections. There is dependent, high-density material *(arrow 1)* caused by layering of fresher blood elements from rebleeding into the chronic low-density hematomas. Collection on the left side is much larger, as is evident by shift of midline structures to the right. Lateral ventricles *(arrow 2)* have a characteristic narrow, compressed configuration.

If chronic subdural hematoma is suspected, a high-quality nonenhanced CT scan often is sufficient for diagnosis. Chronic subdural hematomas are typically of low density in relation to cortical gray matter and are, therefore, evident as a crescent-shaped, low-density fluid collection that displaces the brain from the inner surface of the skull (Figs. 17-5 and 17-6). The mass effect of the subdural fluid causes effacement of the underlying cortical sulci. This can be a helpful feature in differentiating extra-axial fluid from dilated subarachnoid spaces around atrophic brain. In elderly patients or others with marked volume loss, large subdural hematomas can be accommodated with little midline shift. From 11% to 14% of chronic subdural hematomas are bilateral.[22,23] In these patients the brain is compressed from both sides, and the lateral ventricles assume a narrow, parallel configuration (Fig. 17-6). The mechanism of enlargement of chronic subdural hematomas is bleeding from the surrounding vascular membrane.[24] Rebleeding may result in nonuniform layering of different densities or a collection that is isodense in contrast to brain tissue as a result of mixing of fresh, dense blood with older, low-density fluid.

Chronic subdural hematomas that are in an isodense phase caused by their normal aging process or by rebleeding of fresh dense blood into a chronic low-density collection may be difficult to detect on a nonenhanced CT scan (Fig. 17-7). Although the fluid collection itself may not be well displayed, there are several abnormalities on the CT scan that should suggest the presence of an isodense subdural hematoma. The compressed appearance of the ventricular system is characteristic. In addition, displacement

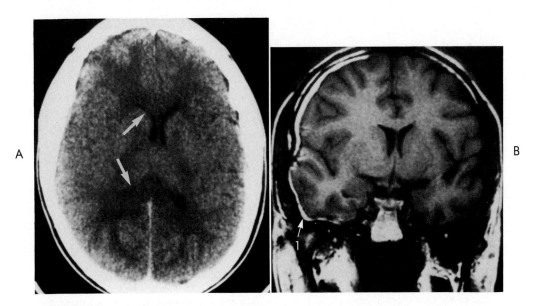

Fig. 17-7. Isodense subdural hematoma in 28-year-old patient experiencing worsening headaches 3 weeks after closed head injury. **A,** Nonenhanced CT scan demonstrates diffuse mass effect on the right cerebral hemisphere with shift of midline structures to the left. Right lateral ventricle is effaced *(arrows)*. **B,** Coronal T$_1$-weighted MRI image shows high-intensity subacute subdural hematoma *(arrow 1)* surrounding the right cerebral hemisphere.   *Continued.*

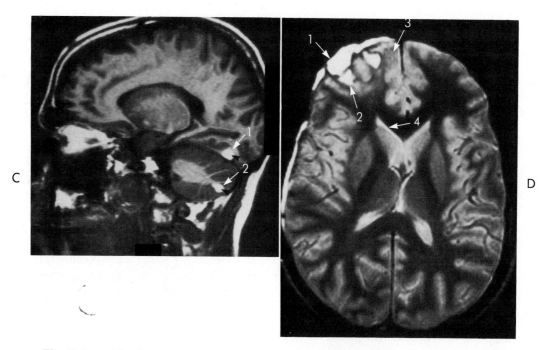

Fig. 17-7 cont'd. C, Sagittal T$_1$-weighted MRI image shows high-intensity intraparenchymal hematomas within left occipital lobe *(arrow 1)* and cerebellum *(arrow 2)*. **D,** Axial proton-weighted MRI image demonstrates right subdural hematoma *(arrow 1)* and right frontal hemorrhagic contusions *(arrow 2)* that exhibit marked high density in comparison with the cerebral cortex *(arrow 3)* but are isodense in comparison with the CSF *(arrow 4)*. (Courtesy HH Eelkema, MD.)

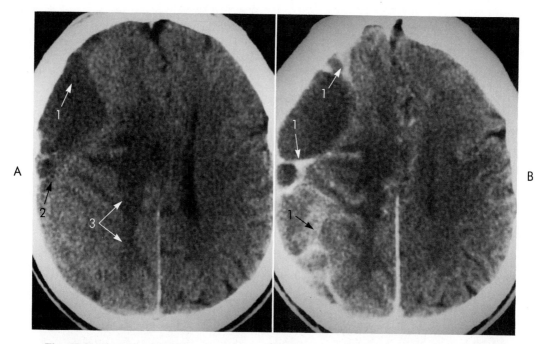

Fig. 17-8. Chronic subdural hematoma with membrane enhancement in an elderly man referred for CT scan because of possible stroke. **A,** Nonenhanced CT scan demonstrates extra-axial mass effect in the right cerebral hemisphere caused by fluid collection with a very unusual shape and nonuniform density. Anterior portion of the collection *(arrow 1)* is of low density, whereas posterior portion *(arrow 2)* is isodense in comparison with adjacent brain. Note inward buckling of the gray-white junction *(arrow 3)*. **B,** Enhanced CT scan demonstrates irregular membrane surrounding chronic subdural hematoma *(arrow 1)*. As is typical of an old subdural hematoma, this collection is biconvex or lens-shaped with a straightened medial margin.

of the gray-white junction from the inner table of the skull offers a clue to the presence of an extra-axial fluid collection. In equivocal cases the administration of intravenous contrast material highlights the cortical gray matter and increases the density of the brain relative to the subdural fluid. The vascular membrane that surrounds chronic subdural hematomas also enhances with intravenous contrast material (Fig. 17-8). MRI is also very helpful in demonstrating subdural hematomas that are isodense in comparison with brain tissue on CT scans (see Fig. 17-7).

CENTRAL NERVOUS SYSTEM MASS LESIONS
Intracerebral hemorrhage

The patient with an intracerebral hemorrhage may, in fact, not complain of headache. The parenchyma of the brain is not sensitive to pain, and, therefore, a hemorrhage must be of sufficient size to create pressure on adjacent pain-sensitive structures or to raise intracranial pressure before pain is perceived. Usually by that stage, the focal neurologic deficits overshadow the pain. The patient may, in fact, have no more headache than the patient with a thrombotic stroke, who is also frequently prone to a headache of a mild nature. However, as these patients invariably present with focal neurologic deficits, the decision to proceed with CT scan is usually obvious.

Intracranial hemorrhage

There are multiple causes of intracranial bleeding, including trauma (see Fig. 17-7), hypertension (Fig. 17-9), amyloid angiopathy, vascular malformation (see Fig. 17-4), aneurysm (see Figs. 17-2 and 17-3), and primary or secondary neoplasm. The location of a hematoma may provide clues in defining the cause of the hemorrhage. For example, hypertensive bleeding usually occurs in the basal ganglia or thalamus, whereas bleeding caused by an AVM or amyloid angiopathy is typically peripheral. If acute hemorrhage is suspected, a nonenhanced CT scan should be obtained to avoid the potential confusion of equating enhanced normal structures with high-density hemorrhage. If hemorrhage is detected and an underlying aneurysm or vascular malformation is suspected, intravenous contrast material may be helpful (see Fig. 17-4).

Tumors

Primary central nervous system tumors. Patients with primary tumors of the central nervous system (CNS) rarely present to the emergency department with the chief complaint of headache. In general, by the time a primary CNS tumor is of sufficient size to cause headache, it has usually displaced intracranial structures and neurologic findings are present. One exception to this is the meningioma, which, by originating on the meninges, can produce pain long before a sufficient size is obtained to cause focal neurologic deficits. Another very rare condition, intraventricular colloid cyst, may cause headache (often positional) by temporarily occluding the ventricular system. The

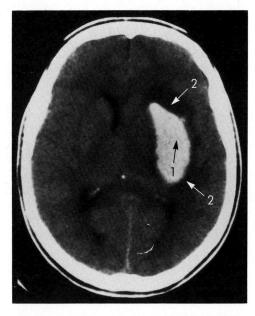

Fig. 17-9. CT scan of hypertensive hemorrhage demonstrates a large high-density hematoma *(arrow 1)* in the left basal ganglia. This hemorrhage is a few days old and is surrounded by a rim of low attenuation, representing edema *(arrow 2)*.

worry of brain tumor, however, is one that is paramount in the mind of many patients who present to the emergency room with headache. It is also rare that the discovery of a brain tumor should present an emergent problem for the emergency physician; rather, it presents more as an urgent problem for which an adequate diagnosis must be achieved so that timely therapeutic plans can proceed.

The typical history for brain tumor includes symptoms of an expanding intracranial lesion, which include headache that is variable in location, typically worse in the morning, and relieved by vomiting. Nausea and papilledema, although uncommon, may also occur. Typically, neurologic deficits are found by the time a headache is present.

CT scan findings. If a mass lesion is suspected, both enhanced and nonenhanced CT scans should be obtained. Most intracranial neoplasms are evident on CT scans using contrast material by virtue of their abnormal enhancement or mass effect on adjacent structures. Tumor enhancement may appear as a discrete mass or as infiltrating regions of enhancement or low attenuation. Biopsy correlation has shown that the tumor boundaries do not correspond to the interfaces of enhanced and nonenhanced areas.[25] Most metastatic lesions and high-grade gliomas enhance with intravenous contrast material (Fig. 17-10). Low-grade gliomas may not enhance; CT scan findings are evident pri-

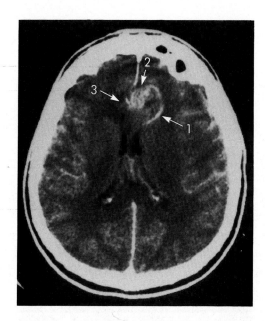

Fig. 17-10. Enhanced CT scan of glioma shows abnormal enhancement in the left frontal lobe *(arrow 1)* and corpus callosum *(arrow 2)*. Abnormal low density, caused by tumor extension or edema, crosses to the right corpus callosum *(arrow 3)*.

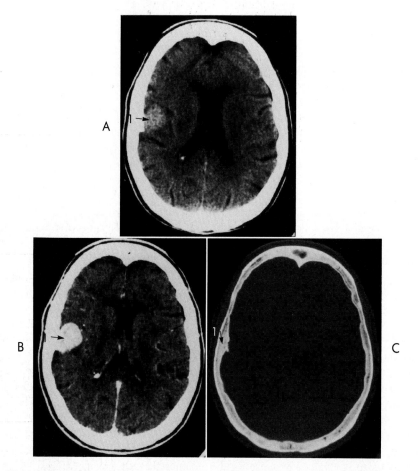

Fig. 17-11. Meningioma. **A,** Nonenhanced CT scan demonstrates small, approximately 2 cm, high-density nodular area *(arrow 1)* adjacent to the inner table of the skull. **B,** Enhanced CT scan demonstrates marked enhancement of the mass. **C,** Enhanced CT scan with widened window demonstrates hyperostosis of the inner table of the skull.

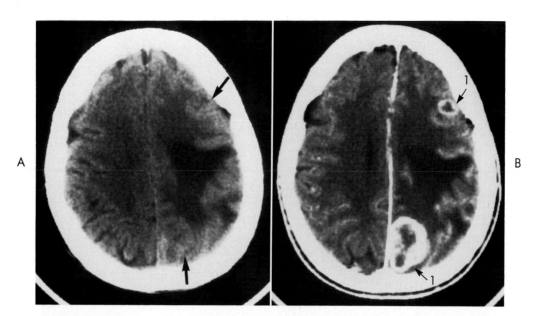

Fig. 17-12. Multiple metastatic lesions. **A,** Nonenhanced CT scan demonstrates only low attenuation and mass effect in the left cerebral convexity *(arrows)*. Mass effect is demonstrated by effacement of the overlying sulci. Sulci on the right are normal. **B,** Enhanced CT scan demonstrates multiple metastatic masses *(arrow 1)*.

marily by their mass effect. The mass effect of malignant neoplasms is evident by displacement of adjacent structures, herniation, and obstructive hydrocephalus.

Meningiomas are very common benign intracranial neoplasms. Meningiomas are usually of high density in comparison with brain tissue before contrast material is given, are markedly enhanced after contrast material administration, and cause hyperostosis of the underlying bone (Fig. 17-11).

Metastatic central nervous system tumors. These tumors are much more common than primary CNS tumors, and patients with metastatic CNS tumors present more commonly to the emergency department. The usual clinical presentation is that of mental confusion or neurologic deficits that may be multifocal. By the time a single intracranial metastasis has become clinically symptomatic, other silent metastases may be present. Usually, but not invariably, there is a history of the primary neoplasm. Sometimes, however, the first clinical manifestation of distant tumors may be symptoms caused by the intracranial metastases. Seizures may also be part of the clinical presentation in patients with metastatic CNS tumors. Otherwise, the clinical history is similar to that of primary CNS tumor.

CT scan findings. Enhanced CT scans are more sensitive than nonenhanced CT scans in detecting intracranial metastases (Fig. 17-12). The "scout view" provides a relatively diagnostic lateral radiographic view of the skull and should always be inspected for bony lesions. Filming or viewing the axial images with wide "bone" windows should be routine in any patient with suspected metastatic disease (Fig. 17-13).

BRAIN ABSCESS
Clinical findings

Brain abscess typically occurs in patients who have extension of an infection from an adjacent cranial structure, such as a paranasal sinus, or a metastatic infection from a remote source, such as endocarditis or systemic bacteremia. Patients with right-to-left intracardiac shunts are at greater risk for brain abscesses. Therefore patients in whom abscesses should be clinically suspected are those with longstanding or possibly untreated or unresolved sinusitis or otitis media, those with endocarditis, intravenous drug abuse, and those with other causes for systemic bacteremia and sepsis. Patients may not be febrile at the time of clinical presentation, and some studies report fever in fewer than 50% of patients with brain abscess at the time of clinical presentation.[26] Patients may experience a seizure at the onset of the cerebritis, which precedes the actual development of a focal collection of pus. The spontaneous rupture of a brain abscess into the subarachnoid or intraventricular space is frequently a catastrophic event and is almost universally fatal. Patients with intracranial abscess and those with brain tumor may present to the emergency department with similar signs and symptoms because both are expanding intracranial lesions.

CT scan findings

Infections of the cerebral parenchyma occur in a pathologic continuum, from cerebritis to frank abscess. The CT scan appearance depends on the stage of the infection. In cerebritis the CT scan may be normal or may demonstrate an irregular, poorly defined area of low attenuation or faint

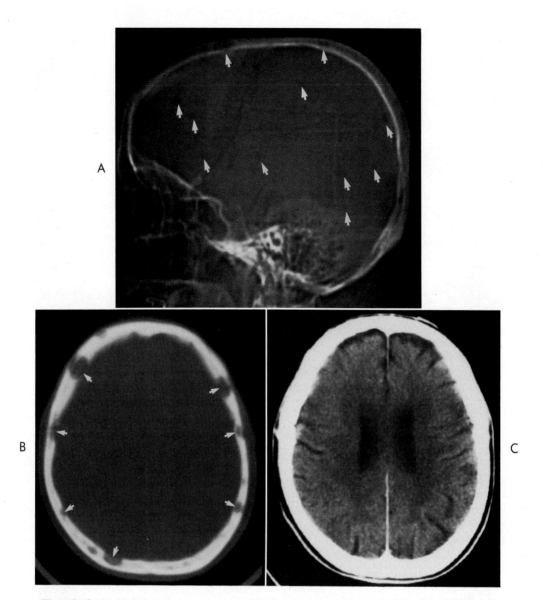

Fig. 17-13. Multiple bone metastases caused by breast cancer. **A,** Scout view demonstrates multiple metastatic lesions *(arrows)*. **B,** CT scan with wide window widths demonstrates multiple metastatic lesions *(arrows)*. **C,** CT scan with narrow window width, usually used in brain imaging, does not demonstrate bone lesions.

contrast material enhancement.[27] Abscesses are more apparent. On nonenhanced CT scans, the isodense rim of the abscess is usually well demonstrated (Fig. 17-14). The rim is evident as a result of low-density pus and necrotic material within and low-density edema surrounding the wall[28] (Fig. 17-14). After intravenous contrast material is given, the rim of the abscess enhances. The CT scan appearance, although typical, is nonspecific. A ring-enhancing lesion may also be demonstrated with resolving hematoma, infarction, or neoplasm.

The CT scan is not sensitive to the presence of meningitis. Occasionally in meningitis, the CT scan shows thickened, densely enhancing meninges (Fig. 17-15); however, it cannot differentiate bacterial meningitis from carcinoma-

tous meningitis. MRI especially with gadolinium enhancement is much more sensitive for detecting meningeal pathologic states, but it is also nonspecific.[26] Rarely, enhancement of the pial surface is shown in meningitis (Fig. 17-16).

HYDROCEPHALUS
Previously shunted hydrocephalus

Patients with previously shunted hydrocephalus may present to the emergency department with a chief complaint of headache. Almost invariably a history or physical evidence of the shunt can be obtained or found on palpation of the scalp, usually behind the ear. One may find surgical scars from placement of catheters. When the shunt malfunctions and CSF can no longer drain from the intra-

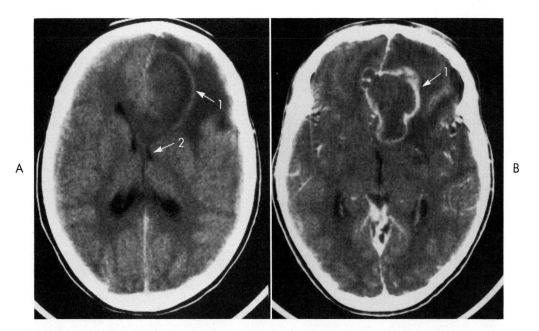

Fig. 17-14. A, Nonenhanced CT scan shows thin abscess rim *(arrow 1)* that is isodense in comparison with the brain. There is a large surrounding area of low density and mass effect. Left frontal horn *(arrow 2)* is compressed and displaced. **B,** With contrast material, the irregular abscess rim enhances *(arrow 1)*.

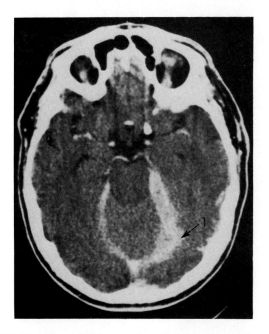

Fig. 17-15. Enhanced CT scan of an adult woman with bacterial meningitis documented by lumbar puncture. There is dense enhancement and thickening of the tentorium *(arrow 1)*.

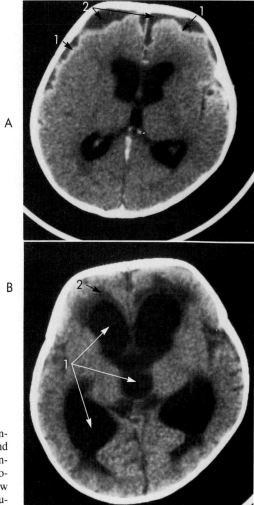

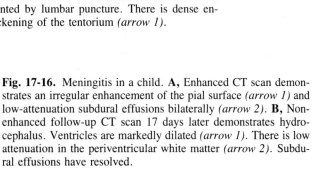

Fig. 17-16. Meningitis in a child. **A,** Enhanced CT scan demonstrates an irregular enhancement of the pial surface *(arrow 1)* and low-attenuation subdural effusions bilaterally *(arrow 2)*. **B,** Nonenhanced follow-up CT scan 17 days later demonstrates hydrocephalus. Ventricles are markedly dilated *(arrow 1)*. There is low attenuation in the periventricular white matter *(arrow 2)*. Subdural effusions have resolved.

ventricular system, the buildup of pressure creates symptoms of increased intracranial pressure with headache, nausea, vomiting, and obtundation. Fever may be present. Infrequently, focal neurologic findings are present. Incontinence of urine and difficulty with gait may occur. CT scan is the diagnostic modality of choice in evaluating the patient for shunt malfunction, but it may not be diagnostic, especially without previous CT scans done after shunt placement for comparison.

Newly developed hydrocephalus

Clinical findings. Hydrocephalus may develop in a number of clinical situations. The patient who has sustained head trauma and a traumatic SAH may experience the delayed onset of obstruction of the CSF absorption pathways and therefore the development of communicating hydrocephalus. Spontaneous SAH may also produce this. The patient then develops the clinical presentation of increased intracranial pressure with headache (typically

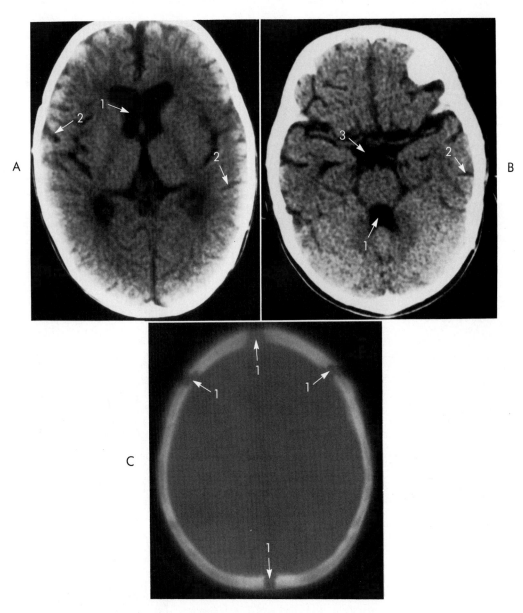

Fig. 17-17. Hydrocephalus. **A** and **B,** Nonenhanced CT scans in young child demonstrate diffuse prominence of the CSF spaces, including the ventricular system *(arrow 1),* sulci *(arrow 2),* and basal cisterns *(arrow 3).* Appearance could be due to hydrocephalus or cerebral volume loss. **C,** Widened window in nonenhanced CT scan demonstrates spreading of sutures *(arrow 1).* Patient was macrocephalic, indicating communicating hydrocephalus.

worse in the morning), nausea, vomiting, gait disturbance, and urinary incontinence without focal neurologic findings. Patients who have previously had meningitis may also develop hydrocephalus, although this is not usually a diagnostic dilemma.

CT scan findings. The diagnosis of hydrocephalus can be a very easy one to make or a very difficult one to exclude on a CT scan. The size and prominence of the ventricular system depends on the patient's age. Newborn infants have lateral ventricles and cortical sulci that are readily apparent, and these should not be mistaken for hydrocephalus. In young infants, it can occasionally be very difficult to distinguish diffuse cerebral atrophy or volume loss from communicating hydrocephalus with prominence of the ventricles and extraventricular CSF spaces. In these cases clinical correlation with head measurements is necessary (Fig. 17-17). In older infants and children, the maturing brain occupies relatively more of the intracranial space. In these patients the ventricles may normally appear somewhat effaced. In adolescents and adults the lateral, third, and fourth ventricles are again readily apparent. In normal adults CSF should also be readily visible in at least a few cortical sulci and in the basal, superior vermian, supracellar, prepontine, and ambient cisterns.

In hydrocephalus the ventricular system dilates in response to increased pressure. The temporal horns are the first to expand, and prominence of the temporal horns is therefore a clue to early hydrocephalus. Rounding of the frontal horns is another sign of ventricular dilatation (Fig. 17-16 and 17-18). Depending on the level of the obstruction, the remainder of the ventricles may be normal or dilated. Lesions at the foramen of Monro cause dilatation of the lateral ventricles only (see Fig. 17-8). Lesions at the level of the sylvian aqueduct cause dilatation of the third and lateral ventricles. Lesions distal to the fourth ventricle, including communicating hydrocephalus, should cause all the ventricles to expand. Practically, however, the fourth ventricle is rather resistant to dilatation, and therefore a normal-appearing fourth ventricle cannot help distinguish mild communicating hydrocephalus ("extraventricular obstructive hydrocephalus") from hydrocephalus caused by obstruction at the level of the sylvian aqueduct.

In addition to dilatation of the ventricles and effacement of the sulci on the brain surface in obstructive hydrocephalus, an abnormal, low attenuation of the periventricular white matter occurs as a result of blockage of the transependymal flow of fluid into the ventricles (see Fig. 17-16). Very prominent ventricles in patients with cerebral volume loss may mimic hydrocephalus, but in these patients the cortical sulci are also very prominent.

After shunting of obstructive hydrocephalus, the ventricles may return to normal size or residual dilatation of varying degrees may persist. Although dilated ventricles and periventricular low attenuation may suggest recurrent obstruction, comparison with previous CT scans is the only practical way to evaluate the ventricular system.

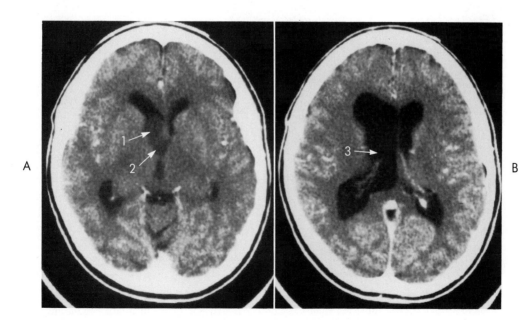

Fig. 17-18. Ependymoma with obstructive hydrocephalus. **A** and **B,** Enhanced CT scans of a young woman with intermittent headaches. Mass that is slightly denser than the CSF is demonstrated in the frontal horn of the right lateral ventricle *(arrow 1)* and the anterior third ventricle *(arrow 2)*. The mass, an ependymoma, obstructs the right foramen of Monro, causing dilatation of the right lateral ventricle *(arrow 3)*.

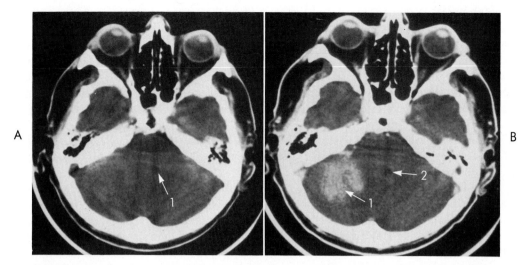

Fig. 17-19. Cerebellar metastases. **A,** Nonenhanced CT scan exhibits essentially normal findings. Fourth ventricle *(arrow 1)* may be located slightly to the left of midline but is obscured by streaking artifact. **B,** Contrast material demonstrates dense enhancement of metastatic deposit of squamous cell carcinoma in the right cerebellar hemisphere *(arrow 1)*. Mild deviation of the fourth ventricle to the left is more clearly shown *(arrow 2)*.

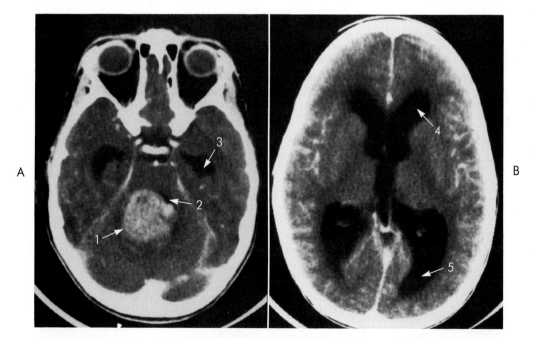

Fig. 17-20. Primary posterior fossa mass with obstructive hydrocephalus. **A** and **B,** Enhanced CT scans in a child demonstrate dense enhancement of primitive neuroectodermal tumor in the right cerebellar hemisphere *(arrow 1)*. Fourth ventricle is markedly displaced and compressed *(arrow 2)* with resultant obstructive hydrocephalus. Note prominence of the temporal horns *(arrow 3)*, rounding of the frontal *(arrow 4)* and occipital *(arrow 5)* horns, and effacement of the cortical sulci.

POSTERIOR FOSSA MASS
Clinical findings

Posterior fossa masses are described separately, primarily because they represent the highest risk if a spinal tap is performed. Herniation syndromes are more likely and more rapidly catastrophic with a posterior fossa mass; therefore one must be especially wary if a lumbar puncture is an indicated diagnostic procedure. Typical symptoms of a posterior fossa mass include headache; ataxia; an inability to walk, sit, or stand; diplopia; difficulty swallowing; or aspiration. In these circumstances, specific attention to the posterior fossa on CT scans is essential.

CT scan findings

If a posterior fossa mass is suspected, contrast material should be administered (Fig. 17-19). Because of streaking artifacts from the dense bones of the skull base, the CT scan displays the contents of the posterior fossa with much less detail and sensitivity than the structures of the supratentorial compartment (see Fig. 17-1). However, the fourth ventricle should be visible as a midline structure in all patients. Posterior fossa masses and swelling of the cerebellar hemisphere after stroke may cause hydrocephalus as a result of obstruction of the fourth ventricle or its outlets (Fig. 17-20).

PARANASAL SINUSITIS
Clinical findings

The clinical diagnosis of sinusitis in the emergency department is one that the physician should be especially careful in making. Patients frequently give a self-diagnosis of sinusitis when asked about the character of their headaches, but physicians should not be misled by these volunteered diagnoses and should instead pursue the typical findings for purulent paranasal sinusitis more closely. Patients typically develop acute sinusitis on recovery from an upper respiratory infection or in association with allergic vasomotor changes, atmospheric pressure changes, irritants, or mechanical obstruction.[9] They usually experience purulent discharge and typically exhibit fever and localized tenderness over the sinuses that produces some or many symptoms. They may have pain referred to the upper teeth if the maxillary sinuses are involved or referral of pain to the ear or behind the eye. There may be pain referred to the occiput or vertex.[29] The pain is typically steady and dull in nature, but it may be throbbing and severe. There may be swelling of the soft tissues overlying the involved sinus or around the eye on the involved side.

Sinusitis in children may be more difficult to recognize than in adults. The maxillary antra and ethmoid sinuses are present from infancy, but the frontal sinuses are rarely a site of infection before the ages of 6 to 10 years. The sphenoid sinus is rarely developed before ages 3 to 5 years.

Ethmoidal sinusitis, which is rare in adults, may occur in young children. Pain may be referred to the temples, behind the eyes, or to the mastoid region.[30]

One must be particularly wary about accepting a diagnosis of sinusitis based purely on radiographic findings. Mild clouding of the sinuses is a common and nonspecific finding, as is some evidence of inflammation of the sinuses on a CT scan. The clinical presentation and radiographic pictures must be carefully correlated to arrive at a clinically compatible diagnosis before proceeding with management.

Chronic sinusitis presents a different clinical picture. Typically, the symptoms are nonspecific, but usually they are associated with purulent nasal discharge.

Plain radiographs and CT scan findings

Plain radiographic evaluation of the paired but usually asymmetric paranasal sinuses includes at least four views: lateral, submentovertex, posteroanterior (PA), and Waters' views (Fig. 17-21). A normal sinus has a smooth and well-defined, gently curving or scalloped bony wall and is filled with air. Because of the complex and variable configuration of the sinuses and superimposed structures, only limited aspects of each sinus are well demonstrated on any single radiograph. A composite assessment of the different radiographs is required for complete evaluation of the sinuses. For example, the anterolateral and posterior maxillary sinus walls are best seen on Waters' and lateral views, respectively.

If acute bacterial sinusitis is suspected, plain radiographs of the sinuses are usually sufficient to document or exclude fluid. The air-fluid interface is shown as a crisp, straight border on radiographs obtained with a horizontal beam (Fig. 17-22). If the patient cannot sit or stand, a cross-table lateral radiograph should be obtained with a horizontal beam view.

Retention cysts or polyps are common and appear as rounded soft tissue densities, most commonly found in the maxillary sinuses (Fig. 17-23). A retention cyst in the floor of the maxillary sinus may simulate fluid on Waters' or PA views, but the lateral radiograph shows the cyst's rounded contour. On the lateral view, the coronoid processes of the mandible are projected over the maxillary sinuses and are often misdiagnosed as cysts.

Mucosal thickening in the paranasal sinuses is very common. Mucosal thickening can cause on overall increased density or "clouding" of the sinus (Fig. 17-24). Thickening mucosa is also commonly shown as an irregular soft tissue density that lines the sinus and obscures the normally crisp mucoperiosteal line. CT scans show the complex bony anatomy of the sinuses in exquisite detail (Fig. 17-25 to 17-27), but they are not indicated in uncomplicated acute sinusitis. If sinus radiographs show bone destruction suggesting malignancy or bone remodeling suggesting mucocele, these patients should be further evaluated by a CT scan. The clinical setting determines the urgency for performing the CT scan.

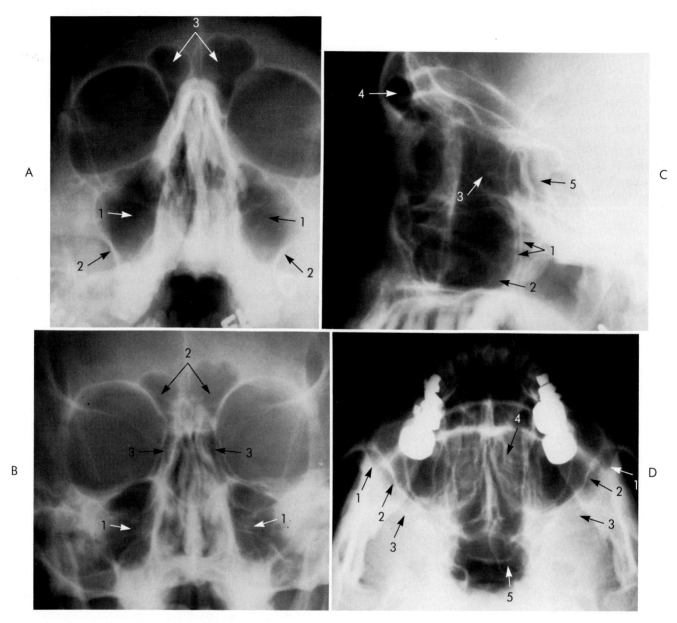

Fig. 17-21. Paranasal sinuses. Normal sinus, plain radiographic series. **A,** Waters' view. *1,* Maxillary sinuses; *2,* crisp mucoperiosteal line of anterolateral wall; *3,* frontal sinus. **B,** Posteroanterior (Caldwell) view. *1,* Maxillary sinuses (not as well seen as on the Waters' view because of superimposed structures); *2,* frontal sinuses; *3,* ethmoid sinuses. **C,** Lateral view. *1,* Maxillary sinus posterior walls; *2,* coronoid processes of mandible; *3,* ethmoid sinuses; *4,* frontal sinus; *5,* sphenoid sinus. **D,** Submentovertex view. *1,* Lateral wall of orbit; *2,* lateral wall of maxillary sinus; *3,* sphenoid wing; *4,* ethmoid sinus; *5,* sphenoid sinus.

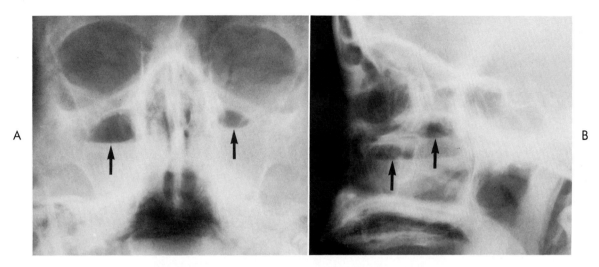

Fig. 17-22. Acute bacterial sinusitis. Waters' **(A)** and lateral **(B)** views demonstrate fluid levels *(arrows)* in the maxillary sinuses.

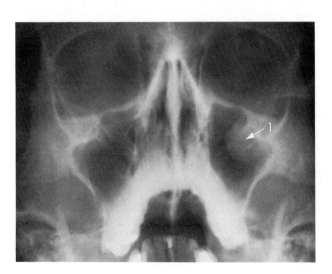

Fig. 17-23. Polyp. Waters' view shows a retention cyst or polyp *(arrow 1)* in left maxillary antrum.

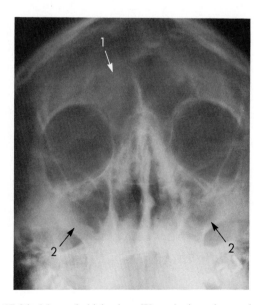

Fig. 17-24. Mucosal thickening. Waters' view shows clouding of right frontal sinus *(arrow 1)* and soft tissue thickening lining both maxillary sinuses *(arrow 2)*.

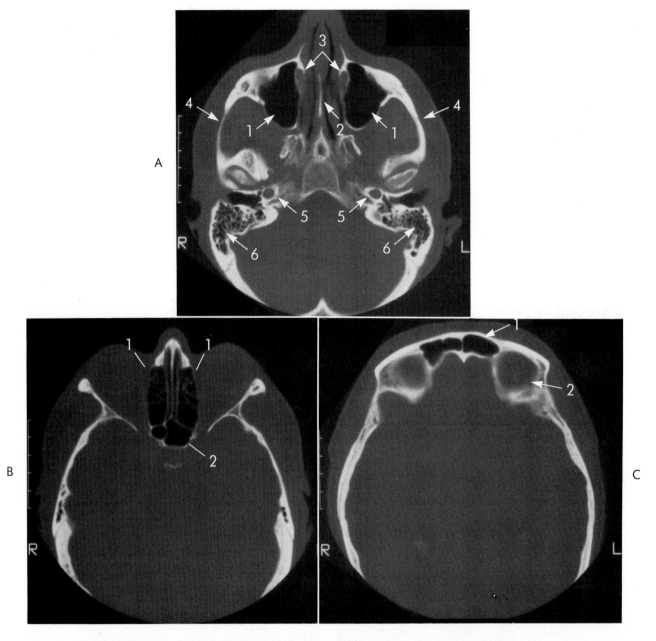

Fig. 17-25. Nonenhanced CT scans demonstrate normal sinus edge enhancement or "bone" algorithm. **A,** *1,* Maxillary sinuses; *2,* nasal septum; *3,* nasolacrimal duct; *4,* zygomatic arch; *5,* carotid canal; *6,* mastoid air cells. **B,** *1,* Ethmoid sinuses with multiple septations. *2,* sphenoid sinus. **C,** *1,* Frontal sinus; *2,* superior orbit.

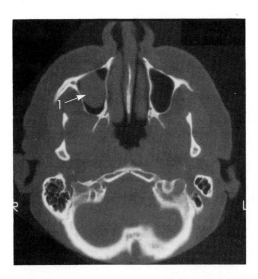

Fig. 17-26. Nonenhanced CT scan of retention cyst *(arrow 1)* in the right maxillary sinus demonstrates a rounded soft tissue structure in the otherwise normally aerated sinus.

BONE LESIONS

The CT scan is capable of displaying exquisite bony detail. However, the scan must be obtained and viewed properly to maximize information regarding the bony structures. For the face and sinuses, 4 to 5 mm thick sections should be obtained. For the cranial vault 8 to 10 mm thick sections are sufficient. Bony detail is best shown at very wide window widths (2000 to 4000 Hounsfield units). Normal cortical bone is a smooth, thin, continuous white structure. Medullary bone is less dense with a variable, but usually fairly uniform, appearance.

The "scout" view, or scanogram, provides a good lateral view of the skull and should always be inspected for bony abnormalities such as fractures or metastases. Abnormalities evident on the scout view often are not demonstrated on axial CT scans if they are filmed or viewed only at narrow "brain" windows (see Fig. 17-13).

ROLE OF MAGNETIC RESONANCE IMAGING

Because of their greater availability and much greater sensitivity to acute hemorrhage, CT scans continue to be the mainstay of neuroimaging in the emergency department. However, MRI is especially useful in evaluating the posterior fossa and is more sensitive than the CT scan in detecting several kinds of intracranial pathologic conditions. In particular, white matter abnormalities such as demyelination in multiple sclerosis[31] or shearing injury[32] and meningeal infections[33,34] are better demonstrated by MRI than CT scan. If acute hemorrhage is not suspected, MRI may be used as the initial and only imaging method to evaluate the patient with headache.

SUMMARY

Patients with headaches frequently present to the emergency department. Careful history and physical examination usually differentiates those patients whose headaches represent a serious threat to their life or health from those whose headaches are caused by noncritical medical conditions. Only those patients whose headaches are life-threatening require emergent CT scan evaluation. The exception is the patient with acute sinusitis whose diagnosis can be confirmed by plain radiographs. The role of MRI is rapidly expanding and in patients where acute hemorrhage is not suspected, MRI may be the initial and only imaging method used to evaluate the patient with headache.

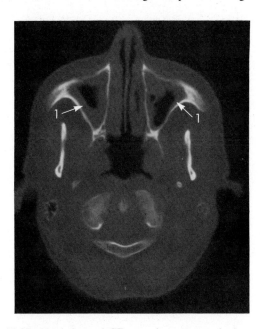

Fig. 17-27. Nonenhanced CT scan demonstrates both maxillary sinuses lined with soft tissue density, representing thickened mucosa *(arrow 1).*

REFERENCES

1. Linet M, Stewart W, Celentano D, and Sprecher M: An epidemiological study of headache among adolescents and young adults, *JAMA* 261(15):2211, 1989.
2. Saper J: Migraine. I: classification and pathogenesis, *JAMA* 239(22):2380, 1978.
3. Dickman R et al: The management of non-traumatic headache in a university hospital emergency room, *Headache* 19(7):391, 1979.
4. Leicht MJ: Non-traumatic headache in the emergency department, *Ann Emerg Med* 9(8):404, 1980.
5. McConnell RY: *Audio Digest Emerg Med* 3(12), 1986.
6. Slay R: Sinusitis. In Rosen P, Baker FJ II, Barkin R et al, eds: *Emergency medicine: concepts and clinical practice,* ed 2, St Louis, 1988, Mosby–Year Book.
7. Knaus W, Wagner D, and Davis D: CT for headache: cost/benefit for subarachnoid hemorrhage, *AJNR* 1:567, 1980.
8. Youmans JR: *Neurological surgery,* ed 3, Philadelphia, 1990, WB Saunders.
9. Alexander MS, Dias PS, and Uttley D: Spontaneous subarachnoid hemorrhage and negative cerebral panangiography: review of 140 cases, *J Neurosurg* 64(4):537, 1986.
10. Fontanarosa P: Recognition of subarachnoid hemorrhage, *Ann Emerg Med* 18(11):1199, 1989.
11. Hart RG, Byer JA et al: Occurrence and implications of seizures in subarachnoid hemorrhage due to ruptured intracranial aneurysms, *Neurosurgery* 8(4):417, 1981.
12. Andreoli A: Subarachnoid hemorrhage: frequency and severity of

cardiac arrhythmias—a survey of 70 cases in the acute phase, *Stroke* 18(3):558, 1987.

13. Liliequist B, Lindquist M: Computer tomography in the evaluation of subarachnoid hemorrhage, Acta Radiol Diagn 21(3):327, 1980.

14. Davis JM, Ploetz J et al: Cranial computed tomography in subarachnoid hemorrhage: relationship between blood detected by CT and lumbar puncture, *J Comput Assist Tomogr* 4(6):794, 1980.

15. Leblanc R: The minor leak preceding subarachnoid hemorrhage, *J Neurosurg* 66(1):35, 1987.

16. Chakeres DW, Bryan RN: Acute subarachnoid hemorrhage: in vitro comparison of magnetic resonance and computed tomography, *AJNR* 7:223, 1986.

17. Rothfus WE: Headache. In Straub WH, ed: Manual of diagnostic imaging: a clinician's guide to clinical problem solving, ed 2, Boston, 1989, Little, Brown.

18. Goshhajra K, Scott I, Marasco J et al: CT detection of intracranial aneurysms in subarachnoid hemorrhage, *AJR* 132:613, 1979.

19. Lokesly HB: Report on the cooperative study of intracranial aneurysms and subarachnoid hemorrhage. I. Natural history of subarachnoid hemorrhage, intracranial aneurysms and arteriovenous malformations, *J Neurosurg* 64:537, 1986.

20. AF Bjorksten G, Halonen V: Incidence of intracranial vascular lesions in patients with subarachnoid hemorrhage investigated by four-vessel angiography, *J Neurosurg* 23:29, 1965.

21. Perret G, Nishioka H: Report on the cooperative study of intracranial aneurysms and subarachnoid hemorrhage. IV. Cerebral angiography, *J Neurosurg* 25:98, 1966.

22. Horton JA: Personal communication.

23. Moller A, Ericson K: Computed tomography of isoattenuating subdural hematomas, *Radiology* 130:149, 1979.

24. Cameron MM: Chronic subdural hematoma: a review of 114 cases, *J Neurol Neurosurg Psychiatry* 41:834, 1978.

25. Weir BKA: The osmolality of subdural hematoma fluid, *J Neurosurg* 34:528, 1971.

26. Harrison MSG: The clinical presentation of intracranial abscess, *Q J Med* 51(204):461, 1992.

27. Earnest F IV, Kelly PJ et al. Cerebral astrocytomas: histopathologic correlation of MR and CT contrast enhancement with stereotactic biopsy *Radiology* 166:823, 1988.

28. Williams AL, Haughton VM, eds: Infectious diseases in cranial computed tomography: a comprehensive text, St Louis, 1985, Mosby–Year Book.

29. Sze G, Soletsky S, Bronew R et al: MR imaging of the cranial meninges with emphasis on contrast enhancement and meningeal carcinomatosis.

30. Jacobs E, Kaban L: Acute nontraumatic disorders of the ear, facial structures and upper airway. In May H, ed: *Emergency medicine*, New York, 1984, John Wiley & Sons.

31. Boat T, Doershuk C, Stern R et al: The respiratory system: sinusitis. In Behrman, Vaughn, eds: *Nelson's textbook of pediatrics*, ed 13, Philadelphia, 1987, WB Saunders.

32. Sheldon JJ, Siddharthan R, Tobias J et al: MR imaging of multiple sclerosis: comparison with clinical aspects and CT examinations in 74 patients, *AJNR* 6:683, 1985.

33. Kelly AB, Zimmerman RD, Snow RB et al: Head trauma: comparison of MR and CT experience with 100 patients, *AJNR* 9:699, 1988.

34. Chang K, Han MH, Roh JK et al: Gd-DTPA enhanced MR images of the brain in patients with meningitis: comparison with CT, *AJNR* 11:69, 1990.

Nontraumatic Neck and Back Pain

James J. Walter

Thomas Falvo

Vesna Martich

David Cohen

Nontraumatic neck and back pain are very common complaints among patients presenting for acute outpatient care in the emergency department.[1] The vast majority of these patients have a benign mechanical etiology for their pain, do not need extensive diagnostic studies, and will improve within several weeks with conservative care. The challenge for the emergency physician is to identify those few patients who are at risk for progressive neurologic compromise or who have a serious underlying pathology such as malignancy, infection, or visceral disease.

In order for the emergency department evaluation of patients with neck and back pain to be both timely and cost-effective, a focused and well-informed approach is essential. Fortunately, a directed history and physical examination, supplemented when appropriate, by simple laboratory testing have proved sufficient in identifying patients at risk for serious disease. For those patients who require further testing, the emergency physician must be knowledgeable about the role of the various imaging studies given the rapidly developing technology and the expanding number of options available.

This chapter emphasizes the clinical presentation of patients with neck and back pain and discusses how to identify those at risk for serious illness. The imaging modalities available and the advantages and limitations of each are described and an approach is recommended for the rational use of these studies. Finally, this chapter highlights clinical and radiographic features of the most important disease entities causing neck and back pain. Acute traumatic causes of neck and back pain are discussed in Chapter 9 whereas spinal cord and vertebral column diseases that can cause neurologic compromise are discussed in Chapter 20.

ANATOMY AND PHYSIOLOGY

A brief review of some aspects of spinal anatomy, physiology, and pathophysiology is essential in understanding the clinical presentation of patients with neck and back pain and in interpreting the results of diagnostic imaging studies.

The vertebral bodies, separated by fibrocartilaginous disks, make up the weight-bearing anterior portion of the spine. The intervertebral disks, the largest avascular structures in the body, are composed of a gelatinous nucleus pulposus encapsulated within the interwoven fibers of the annulus fibrosus. The annulus fibrosus, which gives shape and support to the disk, is somewhat thinner in its posterior and posterolateral aspects. The outer fibers of the annulus are pain sensitive, as is the periosteum of the vertebral body.

The posterior portion of the spine, composed of the vertebral arches, the paired facet joints, and the transverse and spinous processes, serves primarily to protect the cord and its nerve roots and to allow extension and rotation of the spine. The cervical and lower lumbar spine are the most mobile portions and are thus particularly susceptible to mechanical lesions (e.g., muscle/ligamentous injury, herniated disk, facet joint deterioration). The facet joints, formed by the superior and inferior articulating processes on either side of the arch, help to stabilize the disk joints against torsional strain. In turn, the disk joints, spinal ligaments, and muscles prevent excess motion of the facets. The capsule of the facet joint is poorly reinforced and is pain sensitive.

A network of spinal ligaments interconnects the vertebrae. The anterior longitudinal ligament, a strong fibrous band, and the weaker posterior longitudinal ligament run along the anterior and posterior surfaces of the vertebral bodies. The ligamentum flavum (yellow ligament) interconnects the thick lamina, and the interspinal and supraspinal ligaments connect the spinous processes. The spinal ligaments are pain sensitive, as are the paravertebral muscles. In fact, paravertebral muscle pain is probably the most frequent cause of both acute and chronic neck and back pain, although this theory continues to be debated.[2]

The canal formed by the neural arches contains the spinal cord, nerve roots, and the areolar tissue and vascular structures of the epidural space. The spinal cord extends from the occiput to the second lumbar vertebra (L2), where it terminates at the conus medullaris. Lumbar and sacral nerve roots, enveloped by the arachnoid and dural membranes, continue caudally as hairlike strands of the cauda equina to the termination of the dural sac at the second sacral vertebra (S2).

The nerve roots from each spinal segment exit the vertebral canal through the intervertebral foramina, which are paired openings formed by the pedicles of adjacent vertebrae. Although the pain-sensitive nerve root only occupies a small portion of the foramen as it exits, it is susceptible to compression if the foraminal opening becomes compromised (e.g., from osteoarthritis or spondylolisthesis). The pain from a nerve root compressed within a foramen is typically exacerbated by extension of the spine, which narrows the foraminal diameter.

For the purposes of clinical presentation, it is important to define the various types of back pain syndromes since the nature of a patient's pain will influence both the pace and the extent of diagnostic evaluation in the emergency department. Pain from other than the spinal cord and nerve roots can be felt locally at the site of the pathologic process and can be derived from any of those pain-sensitive structures discussed previously, including the vertebral body periosteum, annulus fibrosus, facet joints, ligaments, and muscles. By a poorly understood mechanism, such pain may also be felt at a distance from the local lesion in a nondermatomal distribution, for example, pain from the cervical spine is referred to the medial aspect of the scapula or the lateral aspect of the arm or pain from the lumbar area is referred to the flank, gluteal area, or thigh. *Referred pain* is typically dull, may cross the midline, and, if from the lower back, is noted below the knee in rare cases.

Referred pain syndromes occur often and may mimic the clinical presentation of nerve root compression syndromes.[3] Pain also can be referred to the back from visceral disease (e.g., aortic dissection, pelvic disease, pancreatitis).

It is crucial to assess whether local or referred pain is mechanical or nonmechanical. Most pain is mechanical, derived from injury or degeneration of muscles, ligaments, disks, or facet joints. Mechanical pain typically varies in intensity, is worse with movement, is relieved with rest or recumbency, and improves at night. Nonmechanical pain, on the other hand, is more often steady and unremitting, unrelated to activity, not relieved by recumbency, and worse at night and may be accompanied by fever or other systemic symptoms caused by an underlying disease process. Nonmechanical pain suggests a visceral, infectious, neoplastic, or metabolic etiology and demands further diagnostic evaluation in the emergency department.

Radicular pain is a symptom of nerve root compression. The pain is experienced in a dermatomal distribution, is usually sharp, often accompanied by paresthesias, and may be exacerbated by coughing or straining and by positions that stretch the involved nerve root. Motor, sensory, and reflex disturbances may be noted in a dermatomal and myotomal distribution, especially if the compressive lesion is chronic.

IMAGING MODALITIES

Plain film radiography of the cervical (C), thoracic (T), and lumbar (L) spine is often the first step in a conventional diagnostic workup because it is relatively inexpensive, easily and rapidly obtained, and can clarify basic questions concerning gross anatomy, degenerative changes, pathologic fractures, and extensive metastatic or infectious lesions.

The standard cervical spine series includes five views: anteroposterior (AP), lateral, open-mouth odontoid, and both obliques. The thoracic spine series includes only two views: AP and lateral. The standard lumbar series includes five views: AP, lateral, both obliques, and a coned-down lateral at L5/S1. The gonadal radiation dose for a five-view lumbosacral series is significant (80 mrad in the male, 390 mrad in the female), equivalent to 3500 times as much gonadal radiation in the female as a posteroanterior (PA) and lateral chest radiographic series. Current recommendations advise limiting the lumbosacral series to an AP and lateral view since the coned-down lateral and oblique views add little information but contribute significantly to gonadal radiation. The two-view lumbosacral series involves only one third as much gonadal radiation as the standard five-view series.[4-6] An exception to doing only a two-view series occurs in evaluating degenerative diseases of the spine, in which the oblique views are helpful in visualizing the posterior elements and facet joints.

Plain film radiography is most useful for (1) evaluating acute trauma, (2) ruling out a pathologic compression fracture, (3) visualizing degenerative changes, (4) demonstrating lytic or blastic changes of metastatic cancer, and (5) diagnosing inflammatory sacroiliitis. The major drawback of plain film radiography is its inability to diagnose early bone destruction or soft tissue lesions.

Computed tomography (CT scan) provides axial images with good visualization of bony structures, intervertebral disks, the spinal canal, and adjacent soft tissues. In most emergency departments, a CT scan may be obtained on a 24-hour basis at a cost four to five times that for conventional plain radiographs. The radiation dose delivered to the female reproductive organs by a lumbar CT scan is only one fourth that of conventional plain radiographs.[6]

The CT scan is excellent for a detailed study of bony elements—for example, in evaluating degenerative disease, subtle fractures, spinal stenosis, and neoplastic changes. Its sensitivity is greater than 90% in the diagnosis of a herniated disk.[5] The CT scan is also useful in the diagnosis of infectious and neoplastic mass lesions, although magnetic resonance imaging (MRI) is increasingly favored for these clinical entities. The major disadvantages of the CT scan are the relatively high radiation dose and the limited field of view since usually only short spinal segments are examined.

Myelography, described in Chapter 20, involves the introduction of contrast material directly into the thecal sac via a lumbar or cervical puncture. A myelogram delineates the thecal sac, spinal cord, and exiting nerve roots and can localize lesions in the extradural, intradural, or intramedullary compartments. Cerebrospinal fluid (CSF) can also be obtained for laboratory evaluation. In current practice, myelography is immediately followed by a CT scan to increase both the sensitivity and the specificity of spinal canal and bony vertebral imaging. A CT scan and myelography are as effective as MRI for diagnosing herniated disks or for demonstrating spinal epidural infections and neoplastic mass lesions. Myelography, however, is an invasive procedure with potential complications and is being increasingly replaced by MRI or a CT scan alone.

Magnetic resonance imaging (MRI) is rapidly becoming the examination of choice in spinal imaging. MRI allows direct imaging in the axial, sagittal, and coronal planes and visualizes the entire spinal axis if necessary. MRI provides the best resolution for lesions in the spinal canal as well as lesions within the cord, accurately identifies neoplastic and infectious processes, provides excellent visualization of disk disease, and can identify lesions within the bone marrow before any cortical destruction has occurred. The CT scan remains superior in evaluating bony detail, particularly of the facet joints and posterior elements, and it has the ability to be used in conjunction with myelography. MRI alone, however, competes favorably with the CT scan and the CT scan with myelography and is increasingly used as the definitive imaging procedure for evaluation of the spine. MRI does not use ionizing radiation and is the procedure of choice if spinal imaging is required during pregnancy.

Relative drawbacks to the extensive use of MRI include the expense (more expensive than a comparable CT scan) and its limited availability. Emergent 24-hour access to MRI scanning is not currently available at many institutions. Another potential difficulty is patient claustrophobia and lack of cooperation since the examination requires long periods of motionless scanning (30 to 120 minutes) within the narrow bore of the magnet although research to significantly reduce the scan time holds great promise. Monitoring of the critically ill patient is also difficult within such narrow confines. MRI is contraindicated in patients with pacemakers and certain metallic foreign bodies (e.g., intraocular fragments, aneurysm clips, metallic heart valves), which may migrate within the magnetic field.

Radionuclide imaging of the spine, although potentially useful, is not frequently used in the emergency department. A three-phase bone scan involves the use of technetium-99m (Tc 99m) diphosphonate, with images taken immediately (angiographic phase), within 15 minutes (blood pool phase), and at 2 to 3 hours (static phase). A bone scan is a very sensitive examination for the detection of metastatic lesions and early osteomyelitis. When combined with gallium 67 citrate imaging, the sensitivity for detecting osteomyelitis approaches 95%.[7] Further utility of the bone scan, however, is diminished by poor spatial resolution and low specificity. Use in the emergency department setting is also limited by the length of time required for radionuclide studies: 4 to 6 hours for a Tc 99m scan and up to 72 hours for a gallium 67 citrate scan. In addition, many institutions do not have 24-hour access to a trained nuclear medicine technician.

A recent nuclear medicine advance involves SPECT imaging. SPECT (single photon emission computed tomography) is a radionuclide study that images the spine in a series of 6 to 8 mm axial slices, coupling the sensitivity of nuclear medicine imaging with cross-sectional anatomic detail.[8] The role of SPECT imaging in disorders of the spine is still being defined.

APPROACH TO THE PATIENT WITH NECK AND BACK PAIN

In the pediatric and adolescent patient, complaints of neck or back pain should be regarded as significant and potentially serious in all cases.[9] In small children who cannot verbalize specific complaints, the physician should be alert to physical examination signs, such as obvious deformities, decreased spine mobility, point tenderness, abnormal gait, or a neurologic deficit that might suggest pathology of the spinal column.

The pediatric and adolescent patient with a complaint of back pain should have AP and lateral radiographs of the area in question. Oblique radiographs of the lumbosacral area rarely add clinically useful information, except for occasional demonstration of lumbar spondylolysis.[10] If plain radiographs are nondiagnostic but the possibility exists of an underlying infectious or neoplastic process or occult fracture, then a Tc 99m bone scan should be obtained. A CT scan or MRI of the symptomatic area is also a reasonable alternative, depending on the severity of the symptoms. In the evaluation of a child with back pain and an abnormal neurologic examination, a CT scan or MRI is the procedure of choice after consultation with a neurosurgeon.

In the emergency department evaluation of the adult patient with neck or back pain, a systematic approach and selective criteria should be used in determining whether imaging studies are indicated. The concern is primarily with the patient complaining of low back pain since it is so often encountered and leads to approximately 10 million lumbar spine series/year performed in the United States alone.[6] These lumbar spine radiographs constitute one of the largest sources of gonadal radiation and are unnecessary in most patients. For the 90% of patients who will improve spontaneously in 4 to 6 weeks, education and simple therapeutic measures are all that is required.[11] The role of plain radiographs is to assist in the detection of infection, neoplasia, inflammatory spondyloarthropathy, or an acute fracture. Fortunately, available data suggest that clinical criteria can reliably identify the 5% of patients at risk.[12,13]

Although proposed clinical criteria for identifying patients at risk for serious lumbosacral pathology have not been validated in large prospective trials and, when used, may not decrease the number of lumbosacral radiographs ordered in ambulatory settings,[14,15] we believe that such criteria are appropriate for use by emergency physicians. Although proposed as criteria to guide the evaluation of lumbosacral pain, they are also relevant for patients with cervical and thoracic spinal pain. Patients meeting the clinical criteria outlined in the box above warrant imaging studies performed as part of the acute evaluation in the emergency department.[6,13,15]

We recommend that the initial imaging study in patients with any of the these criteria should be a plain radiographic series, except in patients with a significant neurologic deficit, for whom the initial procedure of choice is a CT scan or MRI. It should be noted that the CT scan and particularly MRI are being increasingly used as primary imaging modalities in evaluating the spine, often without prior plain film radiography. Future studies are necessary to clarify optimal use and the sequence of these tests for many of the pathologic entities discussed in this chapter.

In the diagnostic evaluation of patients with suspected vertebral osteomyelitis or epidural abscess, a complete blood count (CBC) and erythrocyte sedimentation rate (ESR) should be obtained in addition to plain radiographs since elevation of the ESR is almost always present with vertebral infection.[16] If plain radiographs are negative (as they usually are during the first several weeks), but the clinical possibility of infection is high, the emergency physician may choose to obtain an MRI or a CT scan of the symptomatic area or a Tc 99m bone scan to identify and localize the infection. Although sensitive in identifying the presence of an inflammatory process,[17] a radionuclide

---

High-risk criteria in patients presenting with neck and back pain

Age less than 20 or greater than 50 years
Nonmechanical pain (i.e., pain that is progressive, unremitting, unrelated to activity, and unrelieved by recumbency)
History or suspicion of cancer
Pain persisting for longer than 1 month and not improved with treatment
Recent spinal surgery
History of alcohol or intravenous drug abuse
Immunosuppression
Chronic steroid therapy
History or suspicion of metabolic bone disease
Thoracic pain
Suspicion of sacroiliitis
History of significant trauma
Evidence of systemic illness
Fever
Localized vertebral tenderness or overlying erythema
Significant neurologic deficit

---

bone scan is not usually practical in the emergency department setting. Positive findings on plain radiographs or radionuclide bone scan should lead to further evaluation of the affected area by MRI or a CT scan. Although the two modalities are of nearly equal effectiveness, MRI, if available, appears to be the procedure of choice because of its multiplanar capabilities, extensive field of view, and superior soft tissue contrast resolution.[18] The patient with presumptive spinal infection and a neurologic deficit should be evaluated and treated as a neurosurgical emergency.

In patients with back pain and a history or suspicion of cancer, an ESR can be a helpful test because it is frequently elevated in patients with underlying cancer. In the patient with a suggestive history and an elevated ESR, a "negative" radiograph of the spine should be interpreted with caution. If plain radiographs are negative, but the clinical possibility of an underlying malignancy is strong (e.g., systemic manifestations, risk factors, nonmechanical pain, elevated ESR), a Tc 99m bone scan may be helpful as a particularly sensitive screening tool for metastatic lesions with a blastic component. Positive radionuclide bone scans may precede findings on plain radiographs by 3 to 18 months.[19] Alternatively, an MRI or CT scan of the symptomatic area may be ordered. Positive findings on plain radiographs, which are found in more than 80% of patients with epidural metastatic disease,[20,21] should be followed by an MRI or a CT scan. MRI appears equal or superior to the CT scan or the CT scan with myelography in evaluating suspected spinal epidural metastases and cord compression and has become the imaging modality of choice,[22-25] although as alluded to before the length of examination time can be problematic.[26] If MRI is not available, the CT scan is an effective alternative, with its principal limitation being the potential for missing sites of metastases and cord compression outside the area scanned (present in up to 10% of patients).[27,28] If epidural metastatic disease is diagnosed by the CT scan, a CT scan with myelography may then be ordered to define the presence and extent of spinal cord compression and to identify the presence of asymptomatic epidural lesions.[28] In the patient with a new neurologic deficit and presumed epidural spinal cord compression, neurosurgical consultation should by obtained immediately, high-dose dexamethasone given, and an emergency MRI or CT scan with myelography performed.

In the evaluation of suspected disk disease, we recommend imaging in the emergency department only if the patient has a significant neurologic deficit, multiple nerve root involvement, or clinical suspicion of tumor, infection, or fracture (see the high-risk criteria listed in the box on p. 478). The current approach to disk disease is to emphasize simple conservative measures and avoid surgical intervention unless patients develop intolerable pain, severe or progressive neurologic deficits, or evidence of myelopathy. Thus the focus of the emergency department evaluation is not to confirm the diagnosis of a herniated disk but rather to exclude other pathology.[2,4,13] The approach, therefore, should include plain radiographs, followed by a CT scan or MRI as needed. If the emergency physician wants to make a definitive diagnosis of a herniated disk, the CT scan alone is often the only imaging study required. Complicated cases may require the additional information that can be obtained from a CT scan with myelography.[29] Not surprisingly, MRI, which can assess the entire spine noninvasively and in multiple planes, appears to be the ideal test for evaluating disk disease and, if available, is the procedure of choice.[5,30,31]

Degenerative disease of the spine does not usually require identification in the emergency department, but imaging studies may be necessary to exclude other processes. If the emergency physician wants to confirm the diagnosis of degenerative disease, plain radiographs are adequate in demonstrating *spondylosis* (degenerative osteoarthropathy of the spine) involving the vertebral bodies, neural foramina, and facet joints. In defining the extent of degenerative disease, the lateral radiograph accurately demonstrates bony and disk space changes as well as *spondylolisthesis* (the anterior slippage of one vertebral body on another), whereas the oblique radiograph is helpful in demonstrating arthritic changes of the facets and *spondylolysis* (a defect in the pars interarticularis). The CT scan is the imaging modality of choice in the definitive evaluation of degenerative disease of the spine and in this area has proved superior to MRI. A CT scan clearly delineates bony abnormalities of the anterior and posterior elements, ligamentous hypertrophy, and disk herniation. Bony detail is better vi-

sualized with the CT scan than with MRI, although MRI remains an excellent test for demonstrating nerve root and cord compression associated with spondylosis. However, the use of a CT scan or MRI to provide detailed imaging of degenerative disease of the spine would not ordinarily be ordered as part of an evaluation in the emergency department. Tc 99m bone scan or SPECT radionuclide imaging can play a role in the evaluation of spondylolysis, spondylolisthesis, and facet osteoarthritis,[32] but this testing is not usually conducted in an emergency setting.

In the evaluation of suspected inflammatory sacroiliitis, an ESR is helpful because it will be elevated in most patients with seronegative spondyloarthropathy. Plain film radiography of the lumbosacral spine is the imaging study of choice. On plain radiographs of the lumbosacral spine, the sacroiliac joints should always be carefully evaluated.

Finally, a special approach to patients with cord compression or cauda equina syndrome, which are true neurosurgical emergencies, deserves emphasis. Whether caused by a neoplastic or infectious mass lesion, hematoma, or massive disk herniation, these entities require emergent evaluation, consultation, and intervention. Delay in diagnosis and treatment can cause irreversible loss of neurologic function.

SELECTED DISEASES ASSOCIATED WITH NECK AND BACK PAIN
Mechanical disorders

Spondylosis. Spondylosis refers to degenerative changes of the disks, vertebral bodies, and facet joints that develop as a result of the aging process. By age 50, more than 80% of adults demonstrate radiographic evidence of such changes.[33] The process primarily affects the cervical and lower lumbar regions because, as noted, these are the areas most exposed to mechanical stress and repetitive injury.

The nature and progression of spondylosis has been well characterized and is usually initiated by deterioration of the intervertebral disks with age.[34] Disk degeneration leads to disk space narrowing, end-plate sclerosis, and reactive new bone formation with the development of osteophytes around the periphery of the vertebral bodies. Osteophytic development ranges from small traction spurs to exuberant overgrowth with bridging of vertebrae and bony encroachment on the cord and neural foramina.

Disk degeneration may also be evidenced by other radiographic signs. Schmorl's nodes may be noted, which are seen as defects in the vertebral body end-plates caused by herniation of nuclear material[35] (Figs. 18-1 and 18-2). Nitrogen gas may collect in the clefts of the degenerating disk and be seen as linear, radiolucent shadows in the intervertebral space ("vacuum sign").

In addition to degenerative disk disease, the other important component of spondylosis is the development of

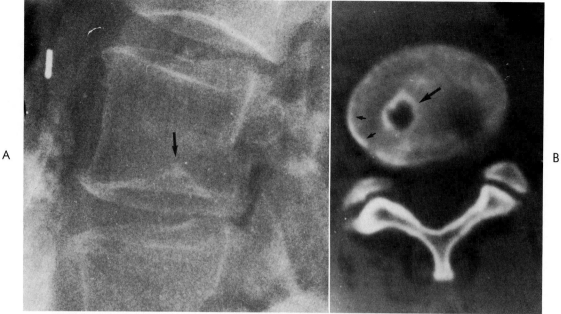

Fig. 18-1. Schmorl's node. **A,** Lateral view of L3 reveals a Schmorl's node seen as a well-defined invagination of the inferior end-plate *(arrow)*. Such defects, caused by herniation of disk material through the end-plate, are commonly seen and occur most often in the lumbar spine. **B,** On CT scan, a Schmorl's node *(large arrow)* is seen as a lucent area surrounded by sclerotic borders. Note the adjacent end-plate seen along the right lateral border of the vertebral body *(small arrows)*. (Courtesy Larry Dixon, MD.)

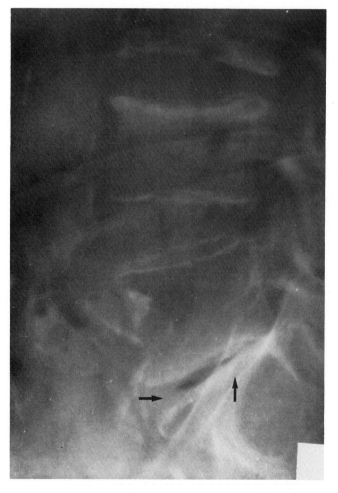

Fig. 18-2. Degenerative disk disease. Lateral radiograph of the lower lumbar spine demonstrates disk space narrowing and adjacent end-plate sclerosis at the L5/S1 level *(vertical arrow)*. A "vacuum sign" of a degenerating disk at the same level is evidenced by the linear lucencies within the disk space *(horizontal arrow)*. (Courtesy American College of Radiology.)

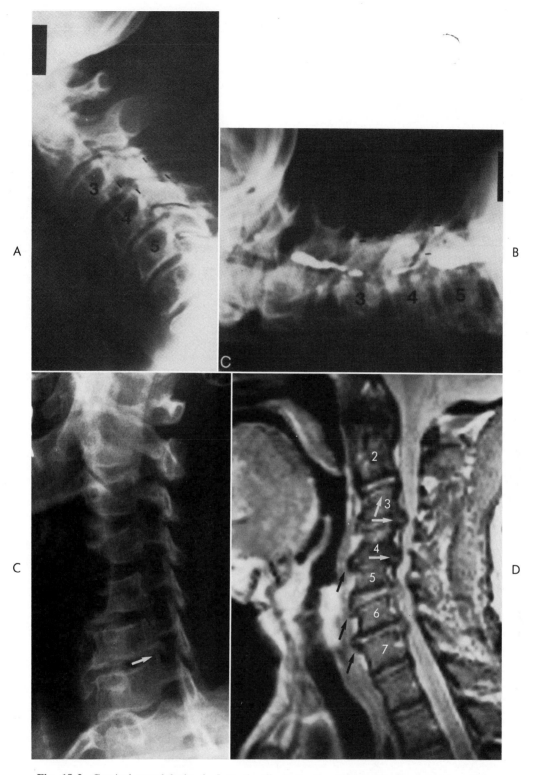

Fig. 18-3. Cervical spondylosis. **A,** Lateral radiograph of a patient with compensatory subluxation of the third or the fourth cervical vertebra. **B,** Lateral cervical myelogram demonstrating cervical spinal canal impingement at C3/C4 as well as at C4/C5. The spinal canal measured 10 mm in the AP diameter at the fourth and fifth cervical levels. **C,** Oblique radiograph of the cervical spine reveals normal neural foramina from the C2/C5 level. At the C6/C7 level a posterior osteophyte is present that could cause impingement on the exiting nerve root and be associated with radicular symptoms *(arrow)*. **D,** Sagittal T$_2$-weighted image of the cervical spine demonstrates diffuse spondylosis particularly evident at the C3/C4 and C4/C5 levels. The degenerating disks at these levels reveal loss of signal with posterior bulging and herniation *(horizontal arrows)*. Reactive bone formation has produced prominent anterior *(vertical arrows)* and posterior osteophytes seen from C3/C6. (**A** and **B** reproduced from Bohlman HH: Degenerative arthritis of the lower cervical spine. In Evarts CM, ed: *Surgery of the musculoskeletal system,* ed 2, New York, 1990, Churchill-Livingstone.)

degenerative osteoarthritis of the facet joints, characterized by sclerosis, osteophyte formation, and subluxation. The inflammation and subsequent deterioration of the facet joints in spondylosis is believed to be one of the most common causes of referred back pain.[3]

Cervical spondylosis is a disease of older patients and is one of the most common causes of neck pain in this population.[36] The disorder usually presents with local or referred pain. Myelopathic or radicular symptoms are seen less often and are caused by encroachment on the cord or nerve roots (central or lateral spinal stenosis). Cord encroachment is more likely to occur as the sagittal diameter of the cord is reduced to less than 11 mm. Degenerative changes are usually most pronounced at C5/C6 and C6/C7 (Fig. 18-3).

Radiographic evidence of lumbar spondylosis, such as traction spurs, "claw" osteophytes, and lower lumbar disk space narrowing, may be associated with an increased incidence of low back pain[37] (Fig. 18-4). However, since such changes are seen so frequently in the older adult, these findings are not usually very helpful in determining the cause of a patient's pain. Severe disease in the lumbosacral area may lead to the development of spinal stenosis, with encroachment on the cord, the cauda equina, or the nerve roots.

Spondylolysis and spondylolisthesis. Spondylolysis and spondylolisthesis are seen in 2% to 5% of adults, with spondylolysis being slightly more common.[2,38] Although rarely the cause of acute back pain, such changes do appear more frequently in patients with recurrent back complaints.[39]

Spondylolysis is defined as a defect through the pars interarticularis, acquired as a result of acute trauma or repetitive stress. The defect may be unilateral or bilateral and is most frequently seen in the lower lumbar region. Oblique plain radiographs will demonstrate the lesion as a defect in the neck of the "Scotty dog" (Fig. 18-5). If there is suspicion that such a defect may be acute, as in the young athlete, a radionuclide bone scan demonstrating positive uptake suggests a recent fracture capable of healing.

Spondylolisthesis is the anterior slippage of one vertebral body on another, most often occurring at L4/L5 and L5/LS1. It is best demonstrated on lateral plain radiographs and is graded according to the amount of slippage of the upper on the lower vertebra (grade I = 25% to grade IV = 100%) (Fig. 18-6). In most cases the slippage occurs in association with bilateral defects in the pars interarticularis (degenerative spondylolysis). Spondylolisthesis in the older adult can be viewed as part of the spectrum of changes seen with lumbar spondylosis. Degenerative spondylolisthesis is almost always accompanied by disk space narrowing and bony overgrowth of the facet joints and, occasionally, may produce symptomatic narrowing of the spinal canal and lateral recesses.

Spinal stenosis. The same pathologic processes occurring in spondylosis can also combine to produce the structural and clinical disorder known as spinal stenosis.[40] Spinal stenosis is seen most often in the lumbar region, where

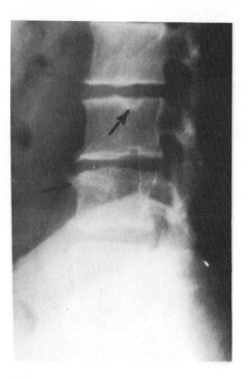

Fig. 18-4. Lumbar spondylosis. Lateral radiograph of the lumbar spine demonstrates degenerative changes at the L2/L3, L3/L4, and L4/L5 levels with disk space narrowing and osteophyte formation *(arrow)*. (From Floman V: *Disorders of the lumbar spine*, Rockville, Md, 1990, Aspen Publishers. Reproduced with permission.)

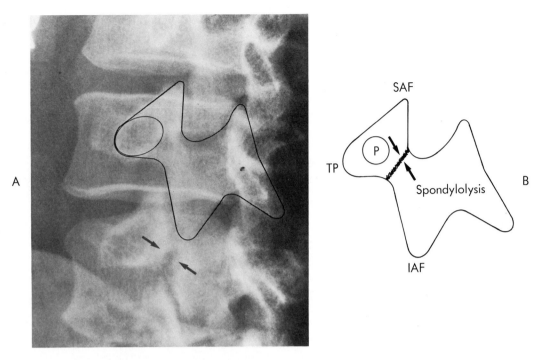

Fig. 18-5. Spondylolysis. **A,** Oblique radiograph of the lumbar spine demonstrates a lucency *(arrows)* through the pars interarticularis indicative of spondylolysis at the L4 level. **B,** On a properly positioned oblique radiograph the area of the pedicle *(P)* transverse process *(TP)* and the superior *(SAF)* and inferior *(IAF)* articulating facets takes on the appearance of a "Scotty dog." A lucency through the neck of the "Scotty dog" signals spondylolysis.

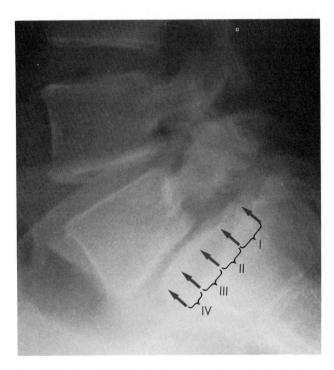

Fig. 18-6. Spondylolisthesis. Lateral radiograph of the lower lumbar spine shows 25% to 50% displacement of the L5 vertebral body on S1 consistent with a grade II spondylolisthesis (Meyerding classification).

it presents with radiculopathy and pseudoclaudication; however, it can also occur in the cervical spine, where it is associated with both radiculopathy and myelopathy. This disorder is usually caused by a combination of degenerative disk disease, with bulging or herniation of disk material, osteophytic growth on the dorsal aspects of the vertebral bodies, osteophytic enlargement and subluxation of the facet joints, and hypertrophy and buckling of the ligamentum flavum. Such changes can lead to a critical reduction in the diameter of the vertebral canal (central stenosis) or a narrowing of the lateral recesses (lateral stenosis), causing compression of the spinal cord, cauda equina, or nerve roots.[34] Lateral stenosis is the cause of radicular symptoms almost as often as is disk herniation.[3]

As a manifestation of advanced degenerative disease, spinal stenosis is a disorder of older patients, with symptoms beginning in the sixth decade of life.[2] Patients with lumbosacral spinal stenosis typically present with a subacute or chronic history of lumbosacral back pain or sciatica. The symptoms of back, buttock, or leg pain are often associated with paresthesia or weakness; these symptoms increase during the day and are especially aggravated by standing or walking. This worsening of symptoms with walking is referred to as *neurogenic claudication* or *pseudoclaudication*. Symptoms are relieved by sitting or bending forward, positions that flex the spine and increase

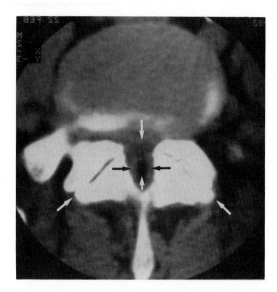

Fig. 18-7. Spinal stenosis. CT scan of a lumbar vertebral body demonstrates spinal stenosis caused by degenerative changes that include hypertrophy of the ligamentum flavum *(horizontal arrows)*, bony hypertrophy of the facet joints *(diagonal arrows)*, and bulging of the disk *(down vertical arrow)*. It is difficult to delineate the anterior extent of the thecal sac, but the posterior border is well outlined by low-density epidural fat *(small arrow)*. *(Courtesy American College of Radiology.)*

the diameter of the spinal canal and lateral recesses. The compressive symptoms may take several minutes to resolve.

Plain radiographs will reveal osteophytes at many levels and other signs of spondylosis. A CT scan or MRI can delineate narrowing of the spinal canal and lateral recesses and can visualize compression of the cord and nerve roots (Fig. 18-7).

Degenerative disk disease and herniated nucleus pulposus. As noted, degenerative disk disease is an essential feature of spondylosis and is characterized by deterioration of the nucleus pulposus and weakening of the annulus fibrosus. The consequences of such degeneration are seen radiographically as disk space narrowing, the "vacuum" sign, end-plate sclerosis, Schmorl's nodes, and spur formation.[41] On a CT scan or MRI, bulging of the annulus is often noted, which may produce cord or nerve root compression, especially in the presence of extensive osteophytosis. Disk protrusion is a common finding even in asymptomatic individuals. In the cervical spine, for example, disk protrusion diagnosed by MRI has been found in 20% of asymptomatic patients over 45 years old and in 60% of those over 65.[42]

Disk disease can also present as herniation of the nucleus pulposus. Although it may occur in association with chronic degenerative disk disease, disk herniation is best viewed as a distinct entity, typically occurring in a somewhat younger population and often not in association with advanced spondylosis or evidence of disk disease on plain radiographs.

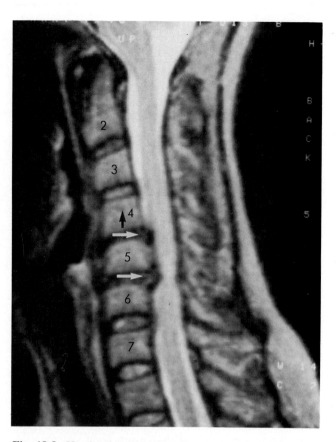

Fig. 18-8. Herniated cervical disk. Herniated disk material at the C4/C5 and C5/C6 level is visible on this sagittal T$_2$-weighted image of the cervical spine *(horizontal arrows)* with potential compromise of the spinal cord and exiting nerve roots. Note the dark appearance of the degenerating, dessicated disks at the C4/C5 and C5/C6 levels.

Disk herniation is initiated by weakening and circumferential tears in the annulus fibrosus as a result of repetitive stress. The circumferential tears then predispose to the development of radial tears through which nuclear material may herniate. The radial tearing occurs most often in the weaker posterolateral aspect of the annulus. Approximately 60% of herniations are posterolateral, 30% posterior (central), and 10% lateral (foraminal).[30] Symptomatic herniation of the nucleus pulposus occurs most often in patients 20 to 50 years of age, with the highest incidence in the fourth decade.[2,13]

Disk herniations in the cervical spine most often involve C5/C6 and C6/C7. More than 90% of patients have no history of trauma.[43] The patient may have classic radicular symptoms with or without accompanying neurologic deficit or myelopathic symptoms and signs that may present more of a diagnostic dilemma[44] (Fig. 18-8).

Thoracic disk herniation is rare. There is usually no precipitating event, pain is seldom a major component, and myelopathic features may predominate. A herniated disk in the cervical or thoracic region should be considered

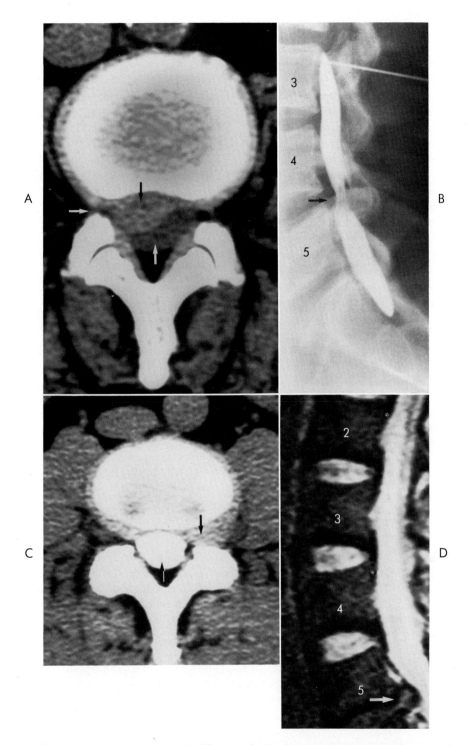

Fig. 18-9. Herniated lumbar disk. **A,** CT scan of a lumbar vertebral body demonstrates right-sided disk herniation *(white vertical arrow)* that compresses the thecal sac *(black vertical arrow)* and obliterates the right neural foramen *(horizontal arrow)*. **B,** Myelogram of the lumbar spine demonstrates contrast opacification of the thecal sac following L2/L3 puncture (needle still in place). An anterior epidural defect *(arrow)* is visualized at the L4/L5 level consistent with external compression of the thecal sac by the herniated disk material. **C,** CT scan was performed following the myelogram. Note the dense contrast outlining the thecal sac *(large vertical arrow)*. Herniation of disk material is seen obliterating the left neural foramen *(small vertical arrow)*. **D,** sagittal T_2-weighted image of the lower lumbar spine clearly shows herniation of the L5/S1 disk *(arrow)*. Note the lack of signal in the degenerating herniated disk. (**B,** Courtesy American College of Radiology.)

in patients with obscure neurologic symptoms in the lower extremities.

Disk herniation occurs most often in the lumbar region, where it is six times more likely to occur than in the cervical spine.[43] Of the herniated disks in the lumbar region causing back pain and compressive nerve root symptoms, more than 95% involve L4/L5 and L5/S1. A herniated nucleus pulposus in the lower lumbar region is the most common cause of back pain with radiculopathy (lateral stenosis, as mentioned, is the second most likely etiologic factor).[3,13]

Patients with a herniated lumbar disk usually complain of a dull, aching pain in the lower back, with associated pain and paresthesia in a specific dermatomal distribution. Radicular pain is often exacerbated by coughing or bearing down and is relieved by rest. Motor and reflex changes corresponding to the involved nerve root are often noted. Most patients with a lumbar herniated disk manifest some foot weakness or impairment of the ankle reflex. Straight leg raising causing nerve root pain at less than 60 degrees of elevation is found in more than 90% of these patients.[13] A CT scan or MRI must be interpreted carefully and in conjunction with physical findings since herniated lumbar disks are found in approximately 20% of asymptomatic adults[4,13] (Fig. 18-9).

Herniated disks are treated conservatively, with surgical intervention only considered for patients with intractable pain, severe or progressive neurologic deficit, or failure to respond to 6 to 12 weeks of conservative care. The cauda equina syndrome, which can be caused by a massive central disk herniation, is a neurosurgical emergency that requires prompt diagnosis and surgical intervention.

Diffuse idiopathic skeletal hyperostosis. Diffuse idiopathic skeletal hyperostosis (DISH) is a disease of the spine predominantly affecting elderly men. The disease is characterized by calcification and ossification of the anterior longitudinal ligament, primarily in the cervical and thoracic spine. Clinically, patients usually note mild back pain, stiffness, and restricted motion. Symptoms of spinal stenosis can occur.[2]

On plain radiographs, bulky syndesmophytes are seen bridging the anterolateral aspects of adjacent vertebrae (Fig. 18-10).

Infectious disorders

For further discussion of infectious disorders, see Chapter 19.

Vertebral osteomyelitis. Hematogenous pyogenic vertebral osteomyelitis is a disease of increasing importance, with a growing number of patients at high risk. Despite an increased recognition of this disorder, the insidious onset and clinical course characteristic of spinal infections often lead to the diagnosis being delayed for several weeks.

The vertebral bodies are currently the most frequent sites of hematogenous osteomyelitis in adults. The lumbar spine is affected more frequently than the thoracic area,

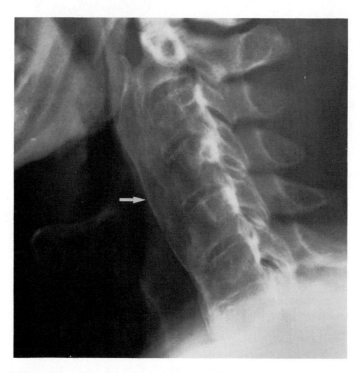

Fig. 18-10. Diffuse idiopathic skeletal hyperostosis (DISH). Thick paravertebral ossification is seen diffusely throughout the cervical spine on this lateral radiograph *(arrow).* The bulky ossification seen in DISH is unlike the thin, flowing syndesmophytes characteristic of ankylosing spondylitis (see Fig. 18-27). (Courtesy Larry Dixon, MD.)

and cervical involvement is rare. The initial site of infection is in the subchondral bone of the vertebral body,[45] with the infection characteristically spreading to involve the intervertebral disk and adjacent vertebral body.[46] Suppurative arthritis of the sacroiliac joints is being seen with increasing frequency, especially in intravenous drug abuse.[47]

The following disorders place patients at high risk for pyogenic vertebral osteomyelitis:

- Recent urinary tract infection or instrumentation.
- Pelvic infection or surgery.
- Soft tissue infection.
- Intravenous drug abuse.
- Chronic hemodialysis.
- Diabetes.
- Sickle cell disease.
- Immunosuppression.

Staphylococcus and gram-negative coliforms are the organisms most frequently involved in osteomyelitis. Tuberculosis is seen infrequently.

Patients with vertebral osteomyelitis typically complain of dull, slowly progressive, nonmechanical back pain and may note malaise and weight loss. Fever occurs in only 50% of patients and is usually low grade.[48] On physical examination, careful palpation of the spinous processes almost always elicits pain. Paravertebral muscle spasm may be noted. Evidence of radiculopathy suggests an epidural abscess. The white blood cell count (WBC) is normal in more than 50% of these patients, and blood cultures are positive in only 25%. The ESR, fortunately, remains a very useful screening test and is elevated in more than 90% of patients with vertebral osteomyelitis.[48]

Evidence of positive findings for vertebral osteomyelitis on plain radiographs may not be demonstrable for 2 to 8 weeks, appearing in 90% of patients by 4 weeks.[49] The earliest findings are disk space narrowing and erosions of the involved vertebral body end-plates.[50] The end-plates become poorly defined, frayed, and irregular (Figs. 18-11 and 18-12). Progressive vertebral body destruction follows, often associated with the development of a paraver-

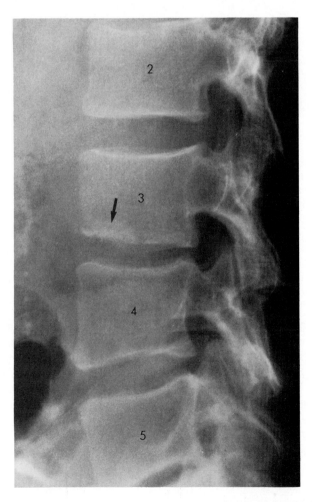

Fig. 18-11. Vertebral osteomyelitis. Radiographic evidence of osteomyelitis of the spine is often subtle early in the course of the disease. Note the ill-defined, irregular destruction of the anterior aspect of the inferior end-plate of L3 *(arrow)* in this case of early vertebral osteomyelitis. (Courtesy A Melinda Liller, MD.)

A   B   C

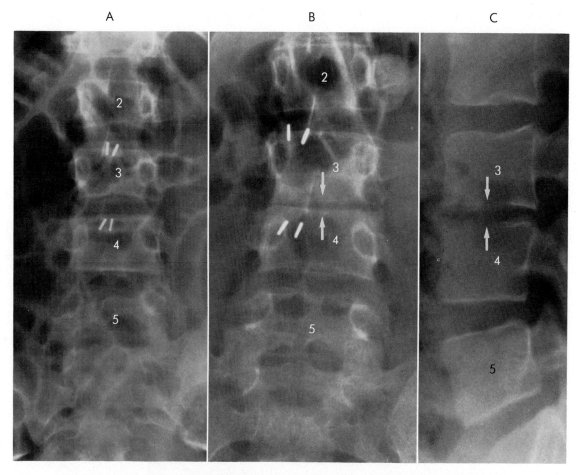

Fig. 18-12. Vertebral osteomyelitis. **A,** Normal AP radiograph of the lumbar spine. **B,** AP radiograph in the same patient several months later during an episode of vertebral osteomyelitis demonstrates severe disk space narrowing at L3/L4 with loss of definition of the inferior and superior end-plates *(vertical arrows)*. Note the sharp cortical lines of the end-plates of L2/L3 in comparison. **C,** Lateral radiograph of the lumbar spine in the same patient also demonstrates the L3/L4 disk space narrowing and the cortical bony destruction of the vertebral end-plates *(vertical arrows)*.

tebral soft tissue mass. Reactive sclerosis, new bone formation, and fusion of vertebrae are late findings (Fig. 18-13). Tubercular spondylitis, now rarely seen in the United States, progresses more slowly than pyogenic disease and is characterized by decreased vertebral body density, disk space narrowing, end-plate erosions, paravertebral abscesses dissecting along fascial planes, and late vertebral body collapse, producing the kyphotic gibbus deformity (Fig. 18-14).

Combined radionuclide bone and gallium 67 scans are a very sensitive screening examination for the early detection of vertebral osteomyelitis[49] (Fig. 18-15). A CT scan is useful for demonstrating subchondral bony destruction, cortical erosions, disk space involvement, soft tissue mass, and extension into the spinal canal[51] (Fig. 18-16). MRI is as sensitive as combined Tc 99m and gallium 67 scans in detecting vertebral osteomyelitis and is also the study of choice if an epidural abscess is suspected[50] (Fig. 18-17). Vertebral osteomyelitis is complicated by the development

of an epidural abscess in up to 20% of patients.[16]

Epidural abscess. Epidural abscess is occurring with increasing frequency over recent years.[52] This is a devastating disease that can rapidly lead to paralysis or death. Expeditious evaluation and treatment are essential.

Risk factors are essentially the same as for vertebral osteomyelitis. Approximately 40% of spinal epidural abscesses are secondary to a spread of infection from an adjacent vertebral osteomyelitis; the remainder are caused by bacteremic seeding, extension from other contiguous infection, or direct inoculation.[48] Intravenous drug abuse has become an increasingly important risk factor.[53]

In those cases associated with vertebral osteomyelitis, weeks or even months of low-grade symptoms may occur before the infection extends into the epidural space. With hematogenous seeding of the epidural space, the disease progression is usually rapid. The clinical presentation of epidural abscess is characterized by fever, back pain, and spinal tenderness. Radiculopathy and other neurologic def-

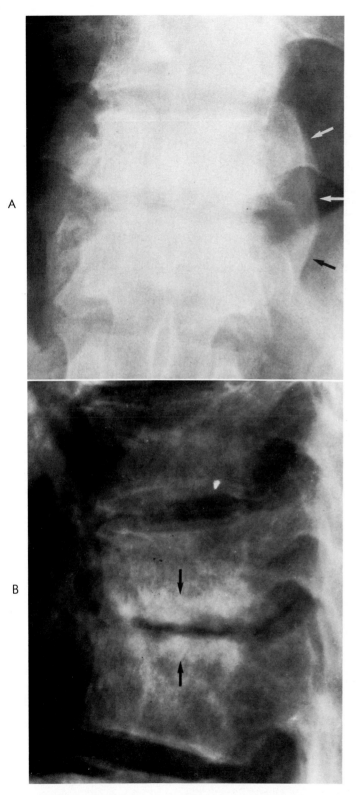

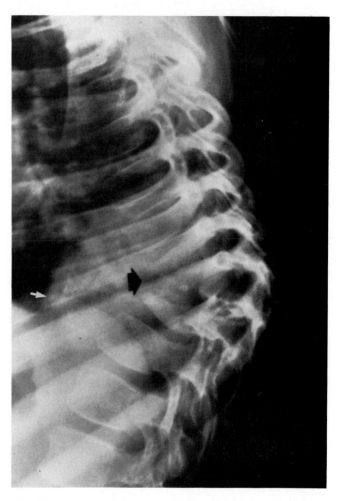

Fig. 18-14. Gibbus deformity results from collapse of multiple mid-thoracic vertebral bodies, a finding classically described in tuberculous osteomyelitis *(arrowhead)*. The extent of an associated paravertebral abscess is demarcated *(arrow)*. (Courtesy American College of Radiology.)

Fig. 18-13. Vertebral osteomyelitis. **A,** In addition to the disk space narrowing and bony destruction, osteomyelitis of the spine can also produce a paraspinal mass, occasionally visible on plain radiographs *(arrows)*. **B,** Late findings of vertebral osteomyelitis include disk space narrowing, loss of height of the involved vertebral bodies, and sclerotic, irregular end-plates *(vertical arrows)*. (Courtesy American College of Radiology.)

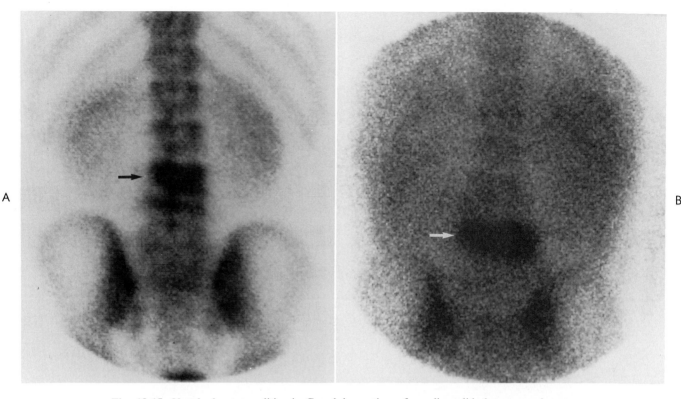

Fig. 18-15. Vertebral osteomyelitis. **A,** Coned-down view of a radionuclide bone scan demonstrates intense uptake of the L3 vertebral body in this patient with osteomyelitis *(arrow)* (see Fig. 18-11 for plain radiograph findings). Note the normal uptake seen in the rest of the spine, kidneys, and sacroiliac joints bilaterally. Tc 99m bone scan is a sensitive test for the diagnosis of osteomyelitis but lacks specificity. **B,** Gallium 67 citrate scan of the same patient. Intense uptake is demonstrated in the region of L3, which correlates with the uptake on the Tc 99m bone scan. Note the normal vague bony and soft tissue uptake as well as the normal increased uptake in the sacroiliac joints bilaterally. Compared with the Tc 99m bone scan, the gallium scan has higher specificity in the diagnosis of osteomyelitis but suffers from poor anatomic resolution. Tc 99m bone scan and the gallium scan should be used together in the evaluation of suspected osteomyelitis. (Courtesy A Melinda Liller, MD.)

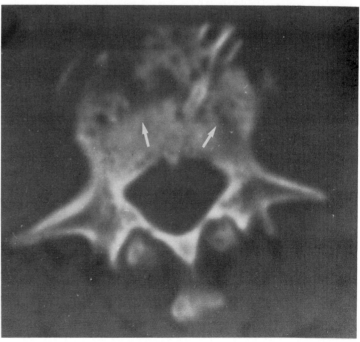

Fig. 18-16. Vertebral osteomyelitis. CT scan will often reveal frank bony destruction involving predominantly the anterior vertebral body *(arrows).*

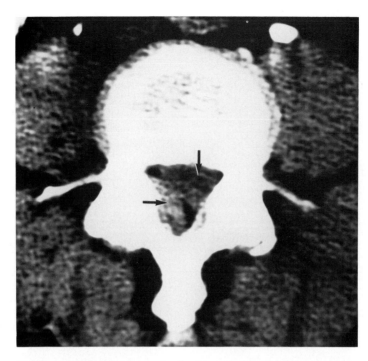

Fig. 18-17. Epidural abscess. CT scan of a lumbar vertebral body shows an epidural abscess *(horizontal arrow)* encroaching on the spinal canal with leftward displacement of the thecal sac *(vertical arrow)*. Note the enhancement of the epidural abscess on this enhanced CT scan.

icits may also be present. Unfortunately, patients with epidural abscess may present without fever or other signs of sepsis, and misdiagnosis may occur.[54]

The emergency physician must be aware that, regardless of the apparent tempo of the epidural abscess progression, weakness and paralysis can develop suddenly and unpredictably. The interval from the onset of any weakness to the development of complete paralysis rarely exceeds 24 hours.[16,52] Multiple factors appear to contribute to the development of paralysis since the damage to the cord often appears out of proportion to the observed degree of compression.[16] Treatment consists of intravenous antibiotics and rapid decompression and drainage.

Plain radiographs of the spine may show an associated vertebral osteomyelitis or paraspinal mass but often are negative. Patients with a neurologic deficit and suspected spinal epidural sepsis should immediately have a CT scan with myelography or an MRI performed after neurosurgical consultation is obtained.[55]

Neoplastic disorders

For further discussion of neoplastic disorders, see Chapter 20.

Primary lesions. The most common "primary" tumor of the spinal column is *multiple myeloma,* a neoplastic disease of plasma cells with a predilection for male patients over 40 years old. The patient typically presents with low back pain of more than a month's duration with associated weakness and fatigue. Anemia, rouleaux formation of red

blood cells, and an elevated ESR rate are noted on laboratory testing. Plain radiographs demonstrate diffuse osteopenia or focal punched-out lytic lesions (Fig. 18-18). The osteolytic process frequently leads to loss of vertebral height and painful compression fractures.[56] A CT scan or MRI will reveal replacement of the vertebral body spongiosa by tumor. Radionuclide bone scan is not helpful since these lesions lack an osteoblastic component.

Metastatic lesions. Metastatic disease of the spine occurs in 10% of patients with cancer and accounts for 40% of all metastatic bone disease.[57,58] Back pain from metastatic spinal disease can be the presenting symptom of a previously unrecognized malignancy or can warn of impending epidural spinal cord compression.

Metastatic disease of the spine often occurs with nonmechanical pain that has been present for several weeks or more. Osteolytic metastases tend to cause symptoms earlier than osteoblastic metastases because of the more frequent occurrence of pathologic fractures. Metastatic disease most often involves the pedicles and vertebral bodies, and these bony areas should be carefully assessed on plain radiographs. A plain radiographic series may reveal the following findings[56] (Fig. 18-19):

- Osteolytic, osteoblastic, or mixed lesions of the vertebral bodies.
- Destruction of vertebral body cortical edges.
- Vertebral body compression fractures.
- Pedicle destruction ("winking owl sign").
- Paraspinal soft tissue mass.

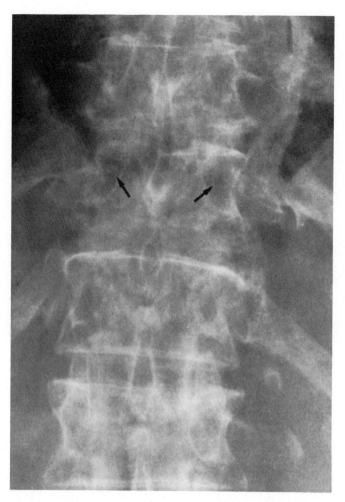

Fig. 18-18. Multiple myeloma, the most common malignancy of bone, most frequently affects the axial skeleton. On this AP radiograph of the lower thoracic spine, lytic lesions are seen throughout the vertebral bodies and adjacent ribs. Note the characteristic sparing of the vertebral pedicles *(arrows)* (a differentiating characteristic between multiple myeloma and widespread metastatic disease). The lack of pedicular involvement in multiple myeloma is secondary to the lack of red marrow in this location.

Fig. 18-19. Metastatic disease. **A,** Diffuse sclerosis of a single vertebral body *(arrow)* is referred to as an "ivory vertebra." Although consistent with metastatic disease, an "ivory vertebra" is also seen in lymphoma, leukemia, and Paget's disease. **B,** Metastatic lesions have a strong predilection for the spinal pedicle, manifested as either a sclerotic or destroyed pedicle. Note the sclerosis of the right tenth pedicle *(large arrow)* with an associated paravertebral soft tissue mass *(small arrows)* in this patient with metastatic prostatic cancer. **C,** This radiograph demonstrates destruction of multiple thoracic pedicles due to widespread metastatic disease *(diagonal arrows)*. Also note the loss of cortical detail in the end-plates of T11 and T12. Regions of increased lucency, especially with loss of clear bony cortical margins, are suspicious for metastatic bony lesions. **D,** Collapse of a mid-thoracic vertebral body due to metastatic breast carcinoma *(large arrow)*. Note the adjacent paravertebral soft tissue mass *(small arrow)*.   *Continued.*

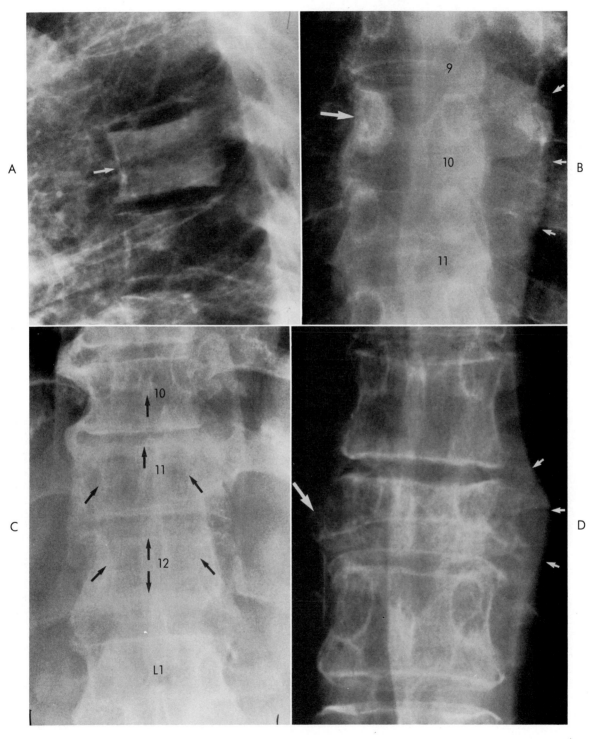

Fig. 18-19. For legend see opposite page.

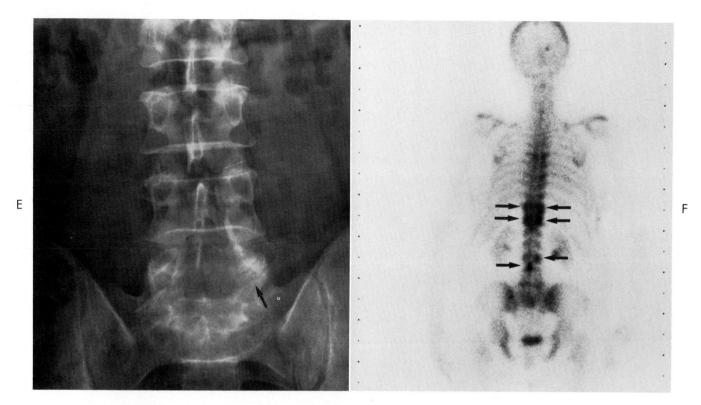

Fig 18-19, cont'd. E, Note the destruction of the left pedicle at L5 secondary to metastatic involvement, resulting in the radiographic appearance of a "winking owl" *(arrow)*. **F,** Plain radiographs are an insensitive test in the diagnosis of primary and metastatic cancer involving the spine. This patient had normal bones on plain radiography, but a radionuclide bone scan reveals metastatic involvement of numerous thoracic and lumbar vertebral pedicles *(arrows)* demonstrating the utility of a bone scan in the evaluation of patients with suspected malignancy when plain radiographs are nondiagnostic. (**E,** Courtesy Walter S Tan, MD; **F,** Courtesy A Melinda Liller, MD.)

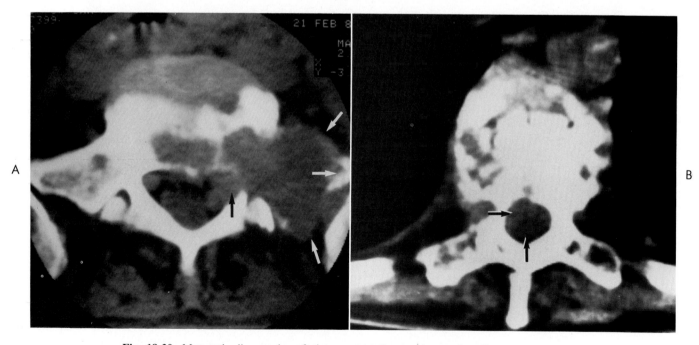

Fig. 18-20. Metastatic disease. **A,** soft tissue metastatic mass is seen invading, destroying, and completely replacing the left bony pedicle of this lumbar vertebral body *(white arrows)*. In addition, this soft tissue mass is seen extending into the left neural foramen, completely engulfing the exiting lumbar nerve root *(black arrow)*. Comparison can be made to the relatively uninvolved right nerve root surrounded by normal low-density epidural fat. Impingement upon the thecal sac is also seen. **B,** CT scan demonstrates lytic destruction of the vertebral body and posterior elements, especially the pedicles. A mass is also seen extending into the spinal canal *(horizontal arrow)* compressing the thecal sac *(vertical arrow)*. (**A,** Courtesy American College of Radiology.)

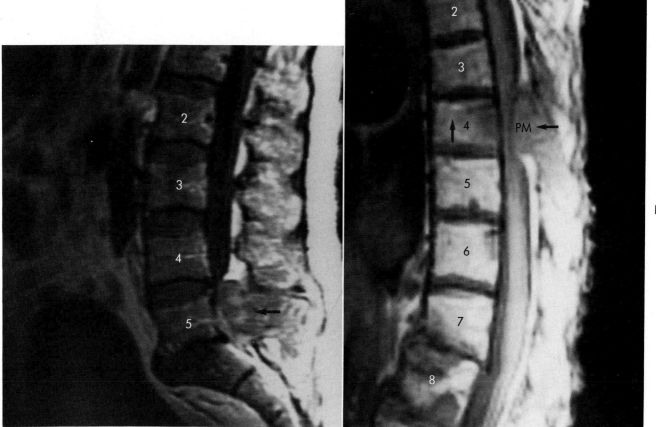

Fig. 18-21. Metastatic disease. **A,** Sagittal T_2-weighted image of the lower lumbar spine demonstrates extensive, bulky metastatic involvement of the L5 pedicle *(arrow)* with resulting compromise of the thecal sac at this level. Clinically, this patient presented with cauda equina syndrome. **B,** Sagittal T_2-weighted image of the thoracic spine reveals a large metastatic lesion engulfing the T4 pedicle *(arrow)* with associated compression of the spinal cord at this level. Note the additional metastatic bony vertebral involvement, particularly affecting vertebral bodies T5, T7, and T8. *PM,* pedicle mass. (**A,** Courtesy Walter S Tan, MD.)

Studies have shown that more than 30% of the bony matrix needs to be replaced by tumor before the metastatic process can be seen on plain radiographs. More than 25% of metastatic bone lesions of the spine are not visible on plain radiographs.[59]

On a CT scan or MRI, destruction of cortical bone, replacement of normal spongiosa by tumor, and extension of the tumor into the paravertebral or epidural space may be seen. Involvement of the posterior elements, osteoblastic changes, and minimal prevertebral soft tissue swelling indicate neoplasia rather than infection.[60]

Metastatic epidural spinal cord compression is a process that should be well understood by the emergency physician (Fig. 18-20). The most common symptoms on presentation are back pain, leg weakness or numbness, and urinary retention.[61] Occasionally, patients may have only ataxia or other neurologic symptoms without back pain, and such atypical presentations may be associated with significant delays in diagnosis.[62] Once spinal cord symptoms appear

in this process, paraplegia can develop within hours. A delay in diagnosis and treatment can be catastrophic since fewer than 5% of patients who become paraplegic before treatment will regain function.[23] In general, patients with rapidly progressive lesions causing neurologic compromise respond poorly to treatment once a neurologic deficit is established.

In more than 80% of patients with epidural spinal cord compression, bone lesions at the site of compression can be seen on plain radiography[20] (Fig. 18-21). The corollary, however, is that normal plain radiographs do not exclude epidural metastatic disease.[28] A radionuclide bone scan, a CT scan, or an MRI should follow if suspicion remains high. A CT scan with myelography or MRI, after neurosurgical consultation, is required in the patient with a neurologic deficit when neoplastic spinal cord compression is suspected. High-dose steroids are used before confirming the diagnosis.

Patients with the *cauda equina syndrome* present with

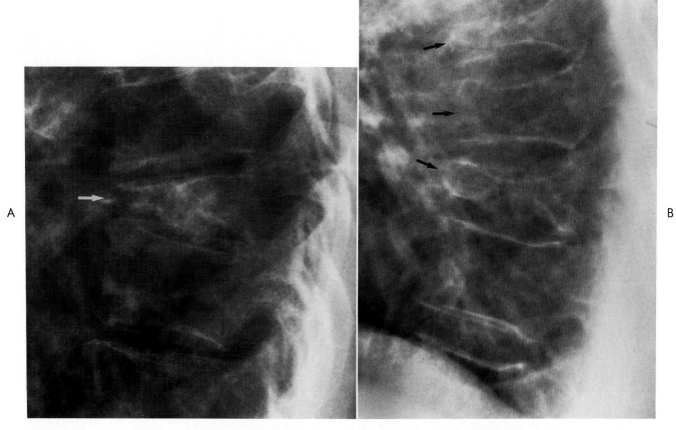

Fig. 18-22. Osteoporosis. **A,** Osteoporosis with associated compression fracture *(arrow)* seen on a lateral radiograph of the thoracic spine. This is the typical appearance of such a fracture, and does not allow for a distinction between osteoporosis or metastatic disease as the underlying cause. Further testing is often necessary. **B,** Osteoporotic compression fractures *(arrows)* with varying degrees of vertebral body collapse. Note the anterior wedging and relative sparing of the vertebral end-plates. "Cupping deformity" of the vertebral body end-plates is also present.

asymmetric lower extremity weakness and hyporeflexia and bilateral lumbosacral nerve root abnormalities including saddle anesthesia, urinary or fecal retention or incontinence and diminished rectal tone. This syndrome is a neurosurgical emergency and must be recognized in its early stages. If the syndrome develops subacutely, the diagnosis is more likely malignancy, whereas acute onset is most consistent with central disk herniation. Epidural abscess and epidural hemorrhage can also cause this syndrome.

Metabolic disorders

Osteoporosis. Osteoporosis is the most common of the metabolic bone disorders, occurring primarily in postmenopausal women and the elderly.[58] It is characterized by a thinning of bony trabeculae and a subsequent decrease in bone density. The vertebral bodies, made up of cancellous bone, are often the first bones to reflect osteoporotic changes. Patients may remain asymptomatic despite considerable loss of bone substance until a wedge or crush fracture of a vertebral body occurs, often during routine activity[63] (Fig. 18-22). These vertebral body compres-

sion fractures may produce pain that can be persistent or subside after several weeks. In some patients the fractures occur gradually and with minimal symptoms. The typical patient notes a decrease in height and development of a thoracic kyphosis and complains of dull, nagging back pain interpersed with episodes of acute pain. Laboratory data that may be helpful include an ESR; calcium, phosphorus, and alkaline and acid phosphatase levels; and serum protein electrophoresis.

Plain radiographs of the thoracic and lumbar spine reveal:

- Diffuse osteopenia (visible after bone density is decreased by more than 30%).
- Prominence of the vertical trabeculae.
- Relative accentuation of vertebral body end-plates.
- Vertebral body compression fractures.
- Anterior wedging of vertebral bodies in the thoracic spine.

Pressure from the adjacent nucleus pulposus on the weakened vertebral bodies may produce a cuplike deformity as the disk bulges through the cortical end-plates. This bicon-

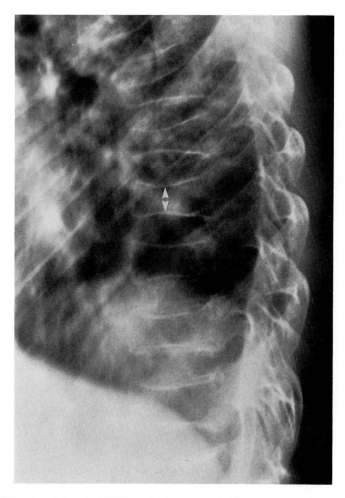

Fig. 18-23. "Cupping deformity" Diffuse, fairly symmetric bi-concave deformity of the vertebral bodies can be seen, secondary to chronic steroid therapy. Note the "washed-out" appearance of the bones with sparing of the end-plates, characteristic of generalized osteoporosis *(arrowheads)*. (Courtesy American College of Radiology.)

cave "fish-mouth" appearance of the vertebral bodies can occur in many of the metabolic bone diseases (Fig. 18-23). Schmorl's nodes may also be seen.

The differential diagnosis of osteoporosis includes osteomalacia, hyperparathyroidism, hyperthyroidism, and glucocorticoid excess. The major concern, however, is to exclude multiple myeloma and metastatic cancer. Laboratory tests, radionuclide bone scan, and the CT scan can be helpful in determining the correct diagnosis.

Paget's disease. Paget's disease is a metabolic bone disorder of unknown etiology most frequently seen in white males over 50 years of age. The disease is characterized by an acceleration of both bone resorption (lytic phase) and bone formation (sclerotic phase). In the sclerotic phase, dense and disorganized bone is formed that is typically enlarged, weak, and susceptible to injury.

Paget's disease occurs most often in the pelvis, lumbosacral spine, skull, humerus, and femur. Up to 90% of patients with Paget's disease are asymptomatic, with the

diagnosis first suggested by an elevated alkaline phosphatase level or abnormalities found unexpectedly on routine radiographs.[64] In symptomatic patients with Paget's disease of the spine, the most common complaint is nonspecific back pain. A clinical picture of spinal stenosis with radiculopathy, neurogenic claudication, or myelopathy may occasionally be seen; this is caused by pagetic bony hypertrophy and concomitant degenerative changes encroaching on the spinal canal and neural foramina. Fractures and subluxations can occur. It is often difficult to determine the etiology of a patient's symptoms since Paget's disease and osteoarthritis often co-exist.[65]

On plain radiographs the bony structures have an abnormal mosaic appearance with a coarse and irregular trabecular pattern. Radiolucent areas surrounded by sclerosis may be seen, especially early in the disease. Cortical thickening may give rise to a "picture frame" appearance of the vertebral bodies (Fig. 18-24). Bony elements are often enlarged and prone to fractures and encroachment.

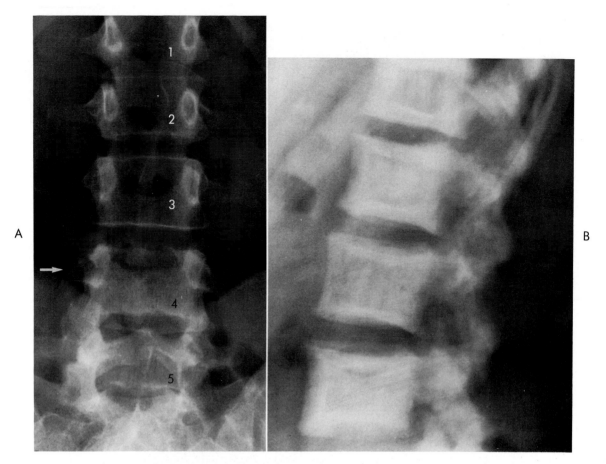

Fig. 18-24. Paget's disease. **A,** Isolated, early Paget's disease of the spine is seen in this plain radiograph. There is vertebral expansion and coarsening of the bony trabecular pattern involving L4 *(arrow).* The posterior elements of the spine are often involved with cortical thickening of the lamina, pedicles, and spinous processes. **B,** Lateral radiograph of the lumbar spine demonstrates the sclerosis and cortical thickening that produce the classic "picture frame" appearance of vertebral bodies in advanced Paget's disease. (**A,** Courtesy A Melinda Liller, MD; **B,** Courtesy Larry Dixon, MD.)

With disease progression a dense, disordered, and homogeneous sclerosis of the vertebral bodies may be seen ("ivory vertebra").[64,66]

Pagetic bony expansion of the vertebral bodies and neural arch can lead to central or lateral spinal stenosis and is well delineated on a CT scan.[65]

Sickle cell disease. In many patients with sickle cell disease, a characteristic "H-type" deformity of the vertebral body end-plates develops. This deformity represents a focal abnormality in bone growth and is manifest by late adolescence.[67] The appearance of the deformity is based on the perfusion characteristics of the vertebral body, which has an anterior and posterior vascular supply, leaving the central region of the cartilaginous end-plate as an anastomotic "watershed" region susceptible to repeated episodes of infarction.[38] Unlike the smoothly concave, fishmouth vertebrae of osteoporosis, the "cupping deformity" seen in sickle cell disease primarily involves the central portion of the end-plate, whereas the peripheral aspects retain their normal flat surfaces. These "H-type" vertebrae

are often seen most clearly in the thoracic spine (Fig. 18-25).

Another bony abnormality that may involve the spine in patients with sickle cell disease is osteomyelitis, with an incidence several hundred times greater than in the normal population.[49] It may be difficult to distinguish bony infarction from osteomyelitis on clinical grounds. Infarction is perhaps 50 times more likely to occur, but infection must often be excluded. Combined Tc 99m and gallium 67 scans have been shown to reliably distinguish between these two processes.[68]

Inflammatory disorders

Rheumatoid arthritis. Rheumatoid arthritis is a multisystem inflammatory disease of unknown etiology, primarily affecting synovial membranes. Females are affected three times more often than males. The usual age of onset is 20 to 40 years. The joints of the cervical spine are frequently involved in the inflammatory process, which is characterized by synovitis, weakening and destruction of

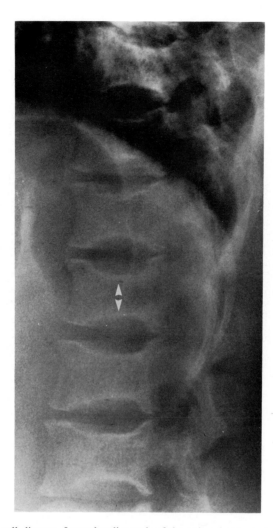

Fig. 18-25. Sickle cell disease. Lateral radiograph of the spine demonstrates the pathognomonic "H-type" vertebral bodies of sickle cell disease with "cupping deformity" only involving the central portion of the end-plate *(arrowheads)*. (Courtesy Larry Dixon, MD.)

cartilage and ligaments, and bony erosions.[69] The cervical spine has been reported to be involved in up to 80% of these patients.[70]

Three major types of subluxation involving the cervical spine have been described in rheumatoid arthritis.[71] *Atlanto-axial subluxation* is found in approximately 25% of patients; its occurrence correlates with disease duration and severity. *Subluxation of other cervical vertebrae* also occurs, secondary to destruction of facets, ligaments, and disks, and is typically seen at multiple levels. Finally, *atlanto-axial impaction,* also termed *cranial settling,* can occur in advanced disease. This is caused by erosion of the lateral masses and occipitocervical joints, which allows settling of the skull downward onto the atlas, with potential upward migration of the odontoid process into the foramen magnum.[72]

Clinically, patients frequently complain of neck pain and stiffness. Occipital headache may be noted. Severe subluxations can result in symptoms of spinal cord com-

pression and occasionally cranial nerve abnormalities and vertebrobasilar insufficiency. Localized tenderness, muscle spasm, and limitation of motion may be noted on physical examination.

Plain radiographs of the cervical spine may demonstrate erosions of the odontoid process, vertebral bodies, and facets; narrowing of disk spaces; or any of the subluxations previously noted.[70] Lateral radiographs with the patient in flexion and extension, performed cautiously, are helpful. With anterior atlanto-axial subluxation, the distance between the odontoid process and the anterior arch of the atlas increases to greater than 3 mm with flexion (Fig. 18-26).

If further imaging is required, MRI is the most precise method of assessing the status of the spinal cord and brain stem.[73,74]

In general, conservative therapy is advised for the cervical subluxations seen with rheumatoid arthritis. Cervical fusion is only rarely indicated.[75]

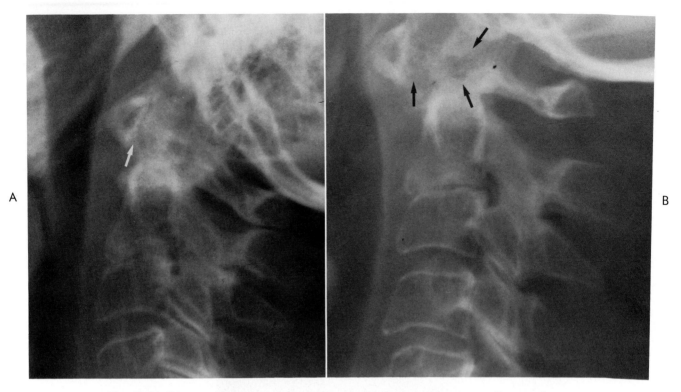

Fig. 18-26. Rheumatoid arthritis. **A,** Lateral cervical radiograph demonstrates the normal predental joint between C1 and C2 in this patient with rheumatoid arthritis *(vertical arrow)*. Normal C1/C2 distance in adults should be less than 2.5 mm. **B,** In this same patient, a flexion view demonstrates atlanto-axial subluxation secondary to destruction of the stabilizing ligaments *(vertical arrow)*. Note also the extensive erosion of the anterior and superior aspects of the odontoid process, which can occur in patients with rheumatoid arthritis *(oblique arrows)*. (**A,** Courtesy Larry Dixon, MD.)

Inflammatory spondyloarthropathies. The inflammatory spondyloarthropathies, including ankylosing spondylitis, psoriatic arthritis, Reiter's syndrome, and enteropathic arthritis, are a group of diverse disorders associated with a high frequency of the HLA-B27 antigen and with the development of sacroiliitis and spondylitis.

Ankylosing spondylitis is an inflammatory disorder of unknown cause that primarily involves the joints of the axial skeleton. The disease most often affects males, with onset in the second and third decades of life. Patients typically present with gradual onset of pain (longer than a 3 month duration), morning stiffness, and progressive limitation of movement. The ESR is elevated in most patients, and a positive HLA-B27 antigen is found in 90%.

Destruction and eventual obliteration of the sacroiliac joints; development of syndesmophytes (ossified ligaments) that bridge adjacent vertebrae; and ascending involvement are the radiographic hallmarks of ankylosing spondylitis. The involvement of the sacroiliac joints begins with blurring of the joint margins, irregular subchondral erosions, and patchy sclerosis and progresses to osseous fusion of the joint space.[38] Subsequent involvement of the spine is characterized by ossification of the anterior longitudinal ligament and peripheral portions of the annulus fi-

brosus, along with squaring and demineralization of the vertebral bodies. Widespread bridging of vertebrae by syndesmophytes produces a radiographic picture referred to as "bamboo spine" (Fig. 18-27). Motion is further restricted by fusion of the facet joints. Ankylosis of the lumbar spine, and eventually the thoracic and cervical spine, generally progresses for 10 to 20 years, leading to spinal rigidity and kyphosis.

The sacroiliitis and spondylitis associated with *psoriatic arthritis* is usually only seen in patients with a severe form of the disease. Although the radiographic changes in the sacroiliac joints are similar to those seen with ankylosing spondylitis, psoriatic spondylitis can be distinguished by the coarseness and asymmetry of the syndesmophytes (Fig. 18-28).

Reiter's syndrome is a disorder characterized by arthritis, conjunctivitis, mucocutaneous lesions, and urethritis that primarily affects males less than 30 years of age. The disease follows in days to weeks after infection with *Chlamydia, Shigella, Salmonella, Campylobacter,* or *Yersinia* organisms. Sacroiliitis and ankylosing spondylitis is found in 20% of patients. The clinical presentation is similar to that of ankylosing spondylitis, with patients noting persistent back pain and stiffness that worsens in the

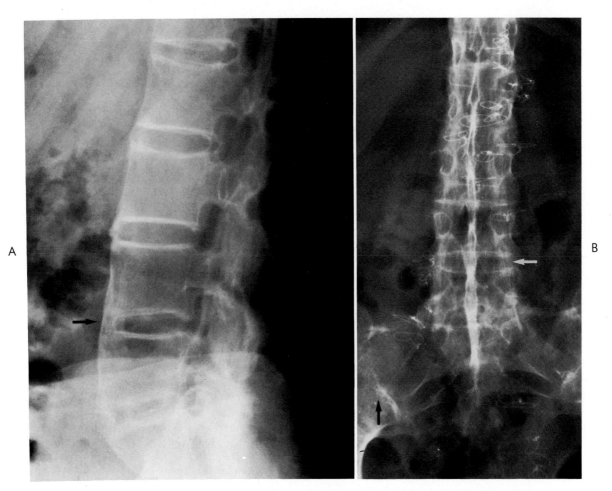

Fig. 18-27. Ankylosing spondylitis. **A,** Lateral radiograph of the lumbar spine clearly shows the slender, flowing syndesmophytes characteristic of ankylosing spondylitis *(arrow)*. The syndesmophytes are formed by ossification of the anterior longitudinal ligament and peripheral portions of the annulus fibrosus. **B,** AP radiograph of the lumbar spine best demonstrates the "bamboo spine" that results from the flowing syndesmophyte formation. Note the fused sacroiliac joints characteristic of ankylosing spondylitis *(vertical arrow)*. Extensive ankylosis of the facet joints is also seen, further compromising motion of the spine *(horizontal arrow)*. (**A,** Courtesy Larry Dixon, MD; **B,** Courtesy Fawn Cohen, MD.)

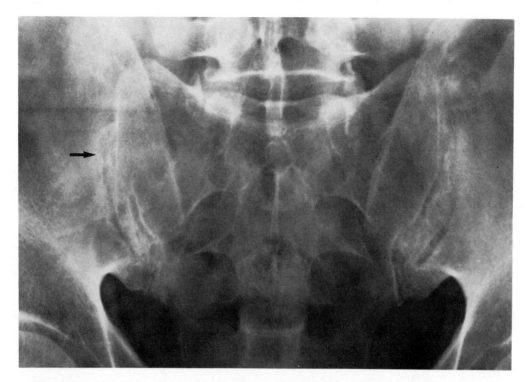

Fig. 18-28. Sacroiliitis as seen with seronegative spondyloarthropathies. Seronegative spondyloarthropathies such as Reiter syndrome and psoriatic arthritis can present with an asymmetric sacroiliitis, evidenced radiographically by joint space narrowing and cortical sclerosis and erosions, seen involving the right sacroiliac joint *(arrow)*. (Courtesy American College of Radiology.)

morning and is relieved with exercise. The sacroiliitis is often asymmetric, and the syndesmophytes are typically large and asymmetric, as in psoriatic disease.

Enteropathic arthritis refers to the joint disease occasionally seen in association with inflammatory bowel disease. The ankylosing sacroiliitis and spondylitis that can occur as part of this disorder are indistinguishable from idiopathic ankylosing spondylitis and tend to progress in a manner unrelated to the activity of the underlying bowel disease.

PEDIATRIC CONSIDERATIONS

Complaints of neck or back pain in children and adolescents are significant and require evaluation by diagnostic imaging as well as appropriate blood tests. This caveat recognizes that the underlying cause of back pain may be infection or malignancy in 20% to 30% of these patients.[10] In patients less than 10 years of age, infections and malignancy are the major concerns in the differential diagnosis. In patients older than 10 years of age, spondylolysis, spondylolisthesis, Scheuermann's disease, overuse syndromes, and herniated disk are additional considerations.[9]

In diagnosing spinal column disorders in children, the clinician should be aware of symptoms and signs that may reflect a potentially serious underlying disorder. Attention should be paid particularly to overlying skin lesions, ab-

normal posture (kyphosis, lordosis, scoliosis, torticollis), decreased mobility, gait disturbance, bowel or bladder dysfunction, muscle spasm, hamstring tightness, spinal tenderness on palpation, neurologic deficits, and an abnormal straight-leg-raising test.

Some of the more important disorders causing pediatric neck and back pain are discussed in the following sections.

Mechanical disorders

Spondylolysis and spondylolisthesis. Spondylolysis (a defect in the pars interarticularis) and spondylolisthesis (anterior subluxation of a vertebral body) can occasionally be noted in children ages 5 years and older. The incidence of these lesions increases until age 20 years and then remains constant at 2% to 5% of the population.[76] Approximately 90% of these lesions occur at L5/S1, with most of the remainder at L4/L5. In most patients, spondylolisthesis is associated with bilateral spondylolysis.

Symptoms occur infrequently in children less than 10 years of age. The onset of symptoms typically coincides with the adolescent growth spurt, which is also a time when increasing anterior slippage of the involved vertebral body is likely to occur.[9,77] Spondylolysis and spondylolisthesis are fairly common causes of low back pain in adolescents, but symptoms are typically mild and often do not prompt the individual to seek medical attention. More than

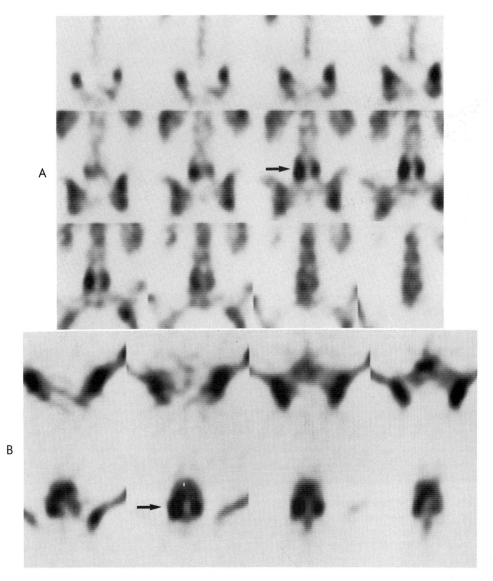

Fig. 18-29. SPECT. The multi-planar imaging (coronal in **A** and axial in **B**) reveals bilateral spondylolysis with greater involvement of the right *(arrow)* than left pars interarticularis in this adolescent gymnast with low back pain. (Courtesy A Melinda Liller, MD.)

half of patients with these lesions remain asymptomatic.[78]

The affected adolescent may complain of low back pain. A postural deformity or abnormal gait may be noted. Eighty percent of symptomatic patients also have hamstring tightness, contributing to the peculiar gait, which has been referred to as a "pelvic waddle."[76] On physical examination, lumbar offset, lumbar lordosis, and tenderness to palpation may be appreciated.

Spondylolysis is best visualized on oblique radiographs, whereas spondylolisthesis is diagnosed on a lateral radiograph of the lumbosacral spine (see Figs. 18-5 and 18-6). A radionuclide bone scan can distinguish a relatively acute stress fracture of the pars interarticularis from established nonunion. Such a distinction may be useful because an

acute lesion may benefit from immobilization. SPECT has proved to be more sensitive than planar bone scans in the evaluation of these lesions[79] (Fig. 18-29).

Scheuermann's disease. Scheuermann's disease, also termed *juvenile kyphosis,* is a kyphotic deformity involving the thoracic spine that develops around the time of puberty. The kyphosis is secondary to vertebral body wedging of unclear etiology, perhaps related to avascular necrosis of bony growth centers. Diagnosis requires the vertebral body wedging to be greater than 5 degrees over three adjacent vertebrae and the thoracic kyphosis to exceed 35 degrees (Fig. 18-30).

These patients may be brought to medical attention because of the postural abnormality. Back pain is also a fre-

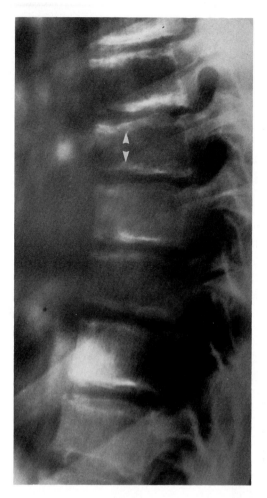

Fig. 18-30. Scheuermann's disease. Lateral radiograph demonstrates end-plate irregularity, sclerosis, and anterior wedging of multiple thoracic vertebral bodies leading to the characteristic kyphosis *(arrowheads)*. (Courtesy Larry Dixon, MD.)

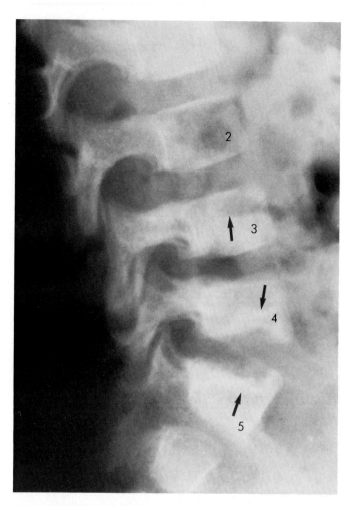

Fig. 18-31. Childhood diskitis. In this pediatric patient recovering from diskitis, note the intense sclerosis of the L4 and L5 vertebral bodies with irregularity and fraying of the end-plates *(arrows)*. Unusual in this case is the intensity of the vertebral body involvement and the amount of disk space recovery that has occurred. At times, a distinction cannot be made between childhood diskitis and vertebral osteomyelitis.

quent complaint, described as aching along the involved segment.[9] Physical examination reveals an increase in both thoracic kyphosis and lumbar lordosis.

The diagnosis of Scheuermann's disease is confirmed on a lateral radiograph of the thoracic spine, demonstrating vertebral body wedging over at least three adjacent vertebrae, and vertebral body end-plate irregularities. Schmorl's nodes may be present, representing protrusion of disk material into the vertebral body.

Herniated nucleus pulposus. Herniation of the nucleus pulposus occurs very rarely in children less than 10 years of age but should be considered in the differential diagnosis of back pain or sciatica in older children and adolescents.[9] Approximately 2% of all herniated disks occur in this age group.[80]

The clinical presentation may include scoliosis, gait disturbance, low back pain, and radicular pain. Physical examination is likely to reveal limitation of motion, muscle spasm, and a positive straight-leg-raising sign.[81,82]

A CT scan or MRI is necessary for definitive diagnosis of a herniated disk and to exclude the possibility of tumor or infection.

Infectious disorders

Childhood diskitis. Childhood diskitis is a self-limited inflammation of the intervertebral disk primarily affecting children 2 to 6 years old. The disorder almost always occurs in the lumbar spine and is confined to a single disk space. In considering the etiology of diskitis, it is important to note that the intervertebral disk in childhood is still a vascular structure, receiving its blood supply from vessels that traverse the vertebral body end-plates (the disk does not become avascular until the second or third decade of life). The current understanding is that this disorder represents a spectrum of diseases and may be caused by any of the following[83-85]:

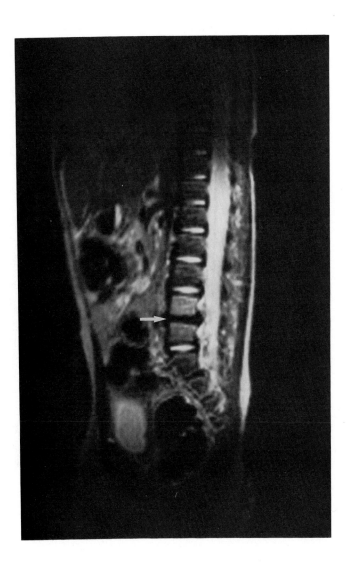

Fig. 18-32. Childhood diskitis. Sagittal T_2-weighted image of a pediatric patient demonstrates findings consistent with diskitis: loss of signal of the affected disk *(arrow)* with increased signal seen in the adjacent involved vertebral bodies. Narrowing of the disk space has not yet occurred.

- Transient disruption of blood flow to the disk.
- Bacterial seeding of the disk space during transient bacteremia.
- Low-grade vertebral osteomyelitis extending into the disk space.

On disk biopsy, cultures are positive in 25% of patients, with *Staphylococcus aureus* the primary pathogen.[85]

Children with diskitis most often present with irritability, malaise, low back pain, difficulty sitting up or walking, and a limp. In general, these children do not appear systemically ill.[86] Physical examination may reveal an exaggerated lumbar lordosis, gait disturbance, localized tenderness over the lumbar spine with paravertebral muscle spasm, and a positive straight-leg-raising sign.

A Tc 99m bone scan may be positive as early as 1 week after the onset of symptoms, when plain radiographs of the lumbar spine are still normal. However, false-negative bone scans may occur.[85] A characteristic progression of findings is seen on serial plain radiographs. Disk space narrowing,

the radiographic prerequisite of the disease, is usually apparent 2 to 4 weeks after the onset of symptoms.[85,87] This is followed by erosions and irregularities of the adjacent vertebral end-plates, which develop over the next several weeks (Fig. 18-31). The final phase is characterized by repair and reactive sclerosis of the vertebral end-plates and at least partial recovery of disk space height. The recovery process is usually complete by 3 months.[88]

A CT scan or MRI has shown that the inflammatory process of diskitis is often more extensive than suspected and may include the development of a paravertebral soft tissue mass and extension into the epidural space.[85] Recent studies suggest that MRI is highly sensitive and specific and is the imaging procedure of choice. MRI allows for early diagnoses, defines the extent of the inflammatory process, rules out a more serious pyogenic bone lesion, and avoids the need for further radiation exposure in these young children[89] (Fig. 18-32).

Patients with childhood diskitis are treated with rest, immobilization, and antibiotics. Biopsy of the disk space is usually not required if the clinical and radiographic presentation is characteristic. Symptoms resolve in 1 to 2 months, and long-term sequelae rarely occur.

Vertebral osteomyelitis. The clinical presentation of vertebral osteomyelitis in children may be similar to diskitis although it is likely to affect an older age group and be associated with more systemic symptoms.[9] The child with vertebral osteomyelitis usually presents with a period of low-grade fever, malaise, and the gradual onset of back pain. Findings on physical examination may include a postural or gait disturbance, pain on palpation of the involved area, and paravertebral muscle spasm. Since osteomyelitis and septic arthritis can also involve the iliac bone and sacroiliac joint, this area should also be carefully palpated.[90] The evaluation of the child with systemic symptoms should always include a thorough examination of the back.

The ESR is invariably elevated, leukocytosis typically occurs, and blood cultures are positive in approximately 50% of these patients.[80]

Plain radiographs are often unremarkable for the first 2 weeks. During this early phase, radionuclide bone scan is a sensitive and helpful test. MRI, if available, is the diagnostic procedure of choice for early detection and for accurately defining the site and extent of the infectious process.[91] As the infection progresses, plain radiographs eventually show narrowing of the disk space and erosions of the involved vertebral body. Reactive sclerosis, bridging of vertebrae, and vertebral body collapse may also occur. Para-

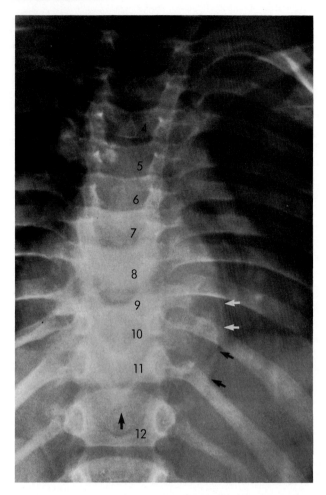

Fig. 18-33. Vertebral osteomyelitis. In this pediatric patient with tuberculous osteomyelitis, a large paravertebral soft tissue mass is present *(arrows)*. Loss of height of several vertebral bodies (T8/T10) can be seen. The involved vertebral bodies also demonstrate loss of bony cortical definition suggestive of extensive bony destruction from the infectious process. (Courtesy American College of Radiology.)

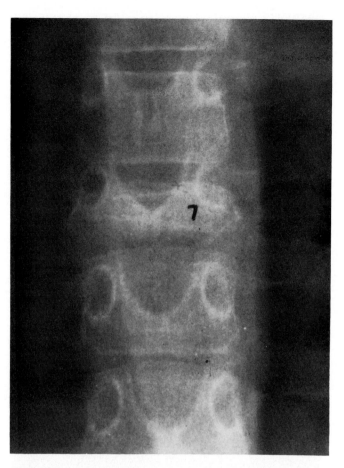

Fig. 18-34. Eosinophilic granuloma. Lateral radiograph demonstrates complete and uniform collapse of T7 vertebral body, termed "vertebra plana," in a pediatric patient with eosinophilic granuloma. (Courtesy Larry Dixon, MD.)

vertebral abscess formation may be noted in advanced cases (Fig. 18-33).

Neoplastic disorders

Back pain, especially nocturnal, is the most frequent presenting complaint of children with primary or metastatic tumors involving the spinal column.[9] Any of the following may also be noted: systemic symptoms, painful scoliosis, gait disturbance, foot deformity, and incontinence. A history of trauma may be obtained in children with an underlying neoplastic process and should not distract the physician from considering the possibility of tumor or infection. On physical examination, the physician should pay particular attention to point tenderness on palpation of the spine and neurologic deficits. As in adults, an ESR is a useful screening test.

Primary intraspinal tumors are rare and usually appear in the first 4 years of life. Plain radiographs often reveal interpedicular widening caused by an attempted accommodation of spinal growth around the expanding intraspinal mass. Erosion of the vertebral bodies and pedicles may also be noted.[80]

Metastatic disease to the spine may present radiographically with erosion or partial collapse of one or more vertebral bodies, as well as erosion of the pedicles and spinous and transverse processes.

Osteoid osteoma is a benign bone lesion that can involve the posterior elements of the spine in adolescent males and is almost invariably associated with scoliosis. Radiographically the lesion presents as a small lucent region (nidus) surrounded by reactive bone formation, which may be difficult to visualize on plain radiographs. A radionuclide bone scan or a CT scan can be used to confirm the diagnosis.

Occasionally, plain radiographs of the spine may reveal a single, greatly compressed, uniformly collapsed vertebral body. This entity is termed "vertebra plana" and is highly suggestive of *eosinophilic granuloma*, a nonaggressive lytic bone lesion (Fig. 18-34).

MRI has emerged as the imaging modality of choice when a spinal tumor is suspected. MRI is sensitive and noninvasive, accurately defines the extent of the lesion, and visualizes the entire spinal axis.

SUMMARY

The emergency department evaluation of patients with neck and back pain should focus on identifying those patients at risk for progressive neurologic compromise, malignancy, infection, or occult fracture. High-risk criteria, such as outlined in the box on p. 478, can be helpful in determining which patients warrant laboratory testing and diagnostic imaging in the emergency department. Until validated by further study, however, such criteria should be considered only as guidelines in the decision-making process and are not intended to override clinical judgment. The clinician must also be aware of the advantages and limitations of the various imaging modalities and indications for their use. Since there is still some lack of consensus regarding the appropriate sequence of testing, consultation with a radiologist can be helpful in difficult cases.

REFERENCES

1. Reuler J: Low back pain, *West J Med* 143:259, 1985.
2. Frymoyer J: Back pain and sciatica, *N Engl J Med* 318:291, 1988.
3. Bernard T, Kirkaldy-Willis W: Recognizing specific characteristics of non-specific low back pain, *Clin Orthop Relat Res* 217:266, 1987.
4. Deyo R, Bigos S, and Maravilla K: Diagnostic imaging procedures for the lumbar spine, *Ann Intern Med* 111:865, 1989.
5. Pelz D, Haddad R: Radiologic investigation of low back pain, *Can Med Assoc J* 140:289, 1989.
6. Kelen G, Noji E, and Doris P: Guidelines for use of lumbar spine radiography, *Ann Emerg Med* 15:245, 1986.
7. Modic M et al: Vertebral osteomyelitis: assessment using MR, *Radiology* 157:157, 1985.
8. Collier B, Hellman R, and Krasnow A: Bone SPECT, *Semin Nucl Med* 17:247, 1987.
9. King H: Back pain in children, *Pediatr Clin North Am* 31:1083, 1984.
10. King H: Evaluating the child with back pain, *Pediatr Clin North Am* 33:1489, 1986.
11. Deyo R, Diehl A, and Rosenthal M: Reducing roentgenography use: can patient expectations be altered? *Arch Intern Med* 147:141, 1987.
12. Deyo R: Plain roentgenography for low back pain: finding needles in a haystack, *Arch Intern Med* 149:27, 1989.
13. Deyo R, Loeser J, and Bigos S: Herniated lumbar intervertebral disk, *Ann Intern Med* 112:598, 1990.
14. Frazier L et al: Selective criteria may increase lumbosacral roentgenogram use in acute low back pain, *Arch Intern Med* 149:47, 1989.
15. Deyo R, Diehl A: Lumbar spine films in primary care: current use and effects of selective ordering criteria, *J Gen Intern Med* 1:20, 1986.
16. Verner E, Musher D: Spinal epidural abscess, *Med Clin North Am* 69:375, 1985.
17. Adatepe M et al: Hematogenous pyogenic vertebral osteomyelitis: diagnostic value of radionuclide bone imaging, *J Nucl Med* 27:1680, 1986.
18. Post M et al: Spinal infection: evaluation with MR imaging and intraoperative US, *Radiology* 169:765, 1988.
19. O'Rourke T et al: Spinal computed tomography and computed tomographic metrizamide myelography in the early diagnosis of metastatic disease, *J Clin Oncol* 4:576, 1986.
20. Posner J: Back pain and epidural spinal cord compression, *Med Clin North Am* 71:185, 1987.
21. Rodichok L et al: Early diagnosis of spinal epidural metastasis, *Am J Med* 70:1181, 1981.
22. Godersky J, Smoker W, and Knutzon R: Use of magnetic resonance imaging in the evaluation of metastatic spinal disease, *Neurosurgery* 21:676, 1987.
23. Colman L et al: Early diagnosis of spinal metastases by CT and MR studies, *J Comput Assist Tomogr* 12:423, 1988.
24. Karnaze M et al: Comparison of MR and CT myelography in imaging the cervical and thoracic spine, *AJNR* 8:983, 1988.
25. Williams M, Cherryman G, and Husband J: Magnetic resonance imaging in suspected metastatic spinal cord compression, *Clin Radiol* 40:286, 1989.
26. Miller G, Forbes G, and Onofrio B: Magnetic resonance imaging of the spine, *Mayo Clin Proc* 64:986, 1989.
27. Bernat J, Greenberg R, and Barrett J: Suspected epidural compression of the spinal cord and cauda equina by metastatic carcinoma, *Cancer* 51:1953, 1983.
28. Portenoy R, Lipton R, and Foley K: Back pain in the cancer patient: an algorithm for evaluation and management, *Neurology* 37:134, 1987.
29. Ketonen L, Gyldenstad C: Lumbar disc disease evaluated by myelography and postmyelography spinal computed tomography, *Neuroradiology* 28:144, 1986.
30. Lukin R, Gaskill M, and Wiot J: Lumbar herniated disk and related topics, *Semin Roentgenol* 23:100, 1988.
31. Lee S, Coleman P, and Hahn F: Magnetic resonance imaging of degenerative disk disease of the spine, *Radiol Clin North Am* 26:949, 1988.
32. Pochis W, Krasnow A, and Collier B: Diagnostic imaging of the lumbar spine (letter), *Ann Intern Med* 112:310, 1990.
33. Quinet R, Hadler N: Diagnosis and treatment of backache, *Semin Arthritis Rheum* 8:261, 1979.
34. Yong-Hing K, Kirkaldy-Willis W: The pathophysiology of degenerative disease of the spine, *Orthop Clin North Am* 14:491, 1983.
35. Hilton R, Ball J, and Benn R: Vertebral end-plate lesions (Schmorl's nodes) in the dorsolumbar spine, *Ann Rheum Dis* 35:127, 1976.
36. Moskovich R: Neck pain in the elderly: common causes and management, *Geriatrics* 43:65, 1988.
37. Frymoyer J et al: Spine radiographs in patients with low back pain: an epidemiological study in men, *J Bone Joint Surg* 66A:1048, 1984.
38. Resnick D: Roentgen signs of emergent spines, *Radiol Clin North Am* 16:65, 1978.
39. Torgerson W, Dotter W: Comparative roentgenographic study of the asymptomatic and symptomatic lumbar spine, *J Bone Joint Surg* 58A:850, 1976.
40. Moreland L, Lopez-Mendez A, and Alarcon G: Spinal stenosis: a comprehensive review of the literature, *Semin Arthritis Rheum* 19:127, 1989.
41. Modic M et al: Imaging of degenerative disk disease, *Radiology* 168:177, 1988.
42. Teresi L et al: Asymptomatic degenerative disk disease and spondylosis of the cervical spine: MR imaging, *Radiology* 164:83, 1987.
43. Heiss J, Tew J: Diskogenic diseases of the spine: clinical aspects, *Semin Roentgenol* 23:93, 1988.
44. Simon J, Lukin R: Diskogenic diseases of the cervical spine, *Semin Roentgenol* 23:118, 1988.
45. Abbey D, Hosea S: Diagnosis of vertebral osteomyelitis in a community hospital by using computed tomography, *Arch Intern Med* 149:2029, 1989.
46. Waldvogel F, Vasey H: Osteomyelitis: the past decade, *N Engl J Med* 303:360, 1980.

47. Hodgson B: Pyogenic sacroiliac joint infection, *Clin Orthop Relat Res* 246:146, 1989.

48. Sapico F, Montgomerie J: Pyogenic vertebral osteomyelitis: report of nine cases and review of the literature, *Rev Infect Dis* 1:754, 1979.

49. David R, Barron B, and Madewell J: Osteomyelitis, acute and chronic, *Radiol Clin North Am* 25:1171, 1987.

50. Osenbach R, Hitchon P, and Menezes A: Diagnosis and management of pyogenic vertebral osteomyelitis in adults, *Surg Neurol* 33:266, 1990.

51. Golimbu C, Firooz" H, and Rafir M: CT of osteomyelitis of the spine, *AJR* 142:156, 1984.

52. Danner R, Hartman B: Update of spinal epidural abscess: 35 cases and review of the literature, *Rev Infect Dis* 9:265, 1987.

53. Koppel B et al: Epidural spine infection in intravenous drug abusers, *Arch Neurol* 45:1331, 1988.

54. Siao P, Yagnik P: Spinal epidural abscess, *J Emerg Med* 6:391, 1988.

55. Angtuaco E et al: MR imaging of spinal epidural sepsis, *AJR* 149:1249, 1987.

56. Zimmerman R, Bilanuik L: Imaging of tumors of the spinal canal and cord, *Radiol Clin North Am* 26:965, 1988.

57. Sarpel S, et al: Early diagnosis of spinal epidural metastases by magnetic resonance imaging, *Cancer* 59:1112, 1987.

58. Gandy S, Payne R: Back pain in the elderly: updated diagnosis and management, *Geriatrics* 41:59, 1986.

59. Wong D, Fornasier V, and MacNab I: Spinal metastases: the obvious, the occult, and the imposters, *Spine* 15:1, 1990.

60. Von Lom K et al: Infection versus tumor in the spine: criteria for distinction with CT, *Radiology* 166:851, 1988.

61. Copeman M: Presenting symptoms of neoplastic spinal cord compression, *J Surg Oncol* 37:24, 1988.

62. Schaberg J, Gainor B: A profile of metastatic carcinoma of the spine, *Spine* 10:19, 1985.

63. Consensus conference: Osteoporosis, *JAMA* 252:799, 1984.

64. Dalinka M, Aronchik J, and Haddad J: Paget's disease, *Orthop Clin North Am* 14:3, 1983.

65. Zlatkin M et al: Paget disease of the spine: CT with clinical correlation, *Radiology* 160:155, 1986.

66. Merkow R, Lane J: Paget's disease of bone, *Orthop Clin North Am* 21:171, 1990.

67. Reynolds J: Radiologic manifestations of sickle cell hemoglobinopathy, *JAMA* 238:247, 1977.

68. Amundsen T, Siegel M, and Siegel B: Osteomyelitis and infarction in sickle cell hemoglobinopathies: differentiation by combined technetium and gallium scintigraphy, *Radiology* 153:807, 1984.

69. Moncur C, Williams H: Cervical spine management in patients with rheumatoid arthritis, *Phys Ther* 68:509, 1988.

70. Wolfe B et al: Rheumatoid arthritis of the cervical spine: early and progressive radiographic features, *Radiology* 165:145, 1987.

71. Lipson S: Rheumatoid arthritis in the cervical spine, *Clin Orthop Relat Res* 239:121, 1989.

72. Santavirta S et al: Evaluation of patients with rheumatoid cervical spine, *Scand J Rheum* 16:9, 1987.

73. Aisen A et al: Cervical spine involvement in rheumatoid arthritis: MR imaging, *Radiology* 165:159, 1987.

74. Halla J et al: Involvement of the cervical spine in rheumatoid arthritis, *Arthritis Rheum* 32:652, 1989.

75. Fehring T, Brooks A: Upper cervical instability in rheumatoid arthritis, *Clin Orthop Relat Res* 221:137, 1987.

76. Hensinger R: Spondylolysis and spondylolisthesis in children and adolescents, *J Bone Joint Surg* 71A:1098, 1989.

77. Blackburne J, Velikas E: Spondylolisthesis in children and adolescents, *J Bone Joint Surg* 59B:490, 1977.

78. McKee B, Alexander W, and Dunbar J: Spondylolysis and spondylolisthesis in children: a review, *J Can Assoc Radiol* 22:100, 1971.

79. Bodner R: The use of SPECT in the diagnosis of low back pain in young patients, *Spine* 13:1155, 1988.

80. Bunnell W: Back pain in children, *Orthop Clin North Am* 13:587, 1982.

81. Russworm H, Bjerkreim I, and Ronglan E: Lumbar intervertebral disc herniations in the young, *Acta Orthop Scand* 49:158, 1978.

82. Nelson C et al: Disk protrusions in the young, *Clin Orthop Relat Res* 88:142, 1972.

83. O'Brien T, McManus F: Discitis: the irritable back of childhood, *IJMS* 152:404, 1983.

84. Gabriel K, Crawford A: Magnetic resonance imaging in a child who had clinical signs of discitis, *J Bone Joint Surg* 70A:938, 1988.

85. Sartoris D et al: Childhood diskitis: computed tomographic findings, *Radiology* 149:701, 1983.

86. Hensey O et al: Juvenile discitis, *Arch Dis Child* 58:983, 1983.

87. Magera B, Klein S, and Derrick C: Radiological case of the month: diskitis, *Am J Dis Child* 143:1479, 1989.

88. Smith R, Taylor T: Inflammatory lesions of intervertebral discs in childhood, *J Bone Joint Surg* 49A:1508, 1967.

89. Heller R et al: Disc space infection in children: magnetic resonance imaging, *Radiol Clin North Am* 26:207, 1988.

90. Beaupre A et al: The three syndromes of iliac osteomyelitis in children, *J Bone Joint Surg* 61A:1087, 1979.

91. Fletcher B, Scoles P, and Nelson A: Osteomyelitis in children: detection by magnetic resonance, *Radiology* 150:57, 1984.

Limp and Altered Gait

Ron W. Lee
Terrence C. Demos

Patients with limp or altered gait commonly present to the emergency department. Most of these patients have had minor trauma and seldom represent a diagnostic dilemma. However, a small group of individuals with gait disturbance have no obvious etiology. A wide variety of diseases can produce altered gait, and in some patients this is the first manifestation of their disease (see the box on p. 510). Recognition of the significance of altered gait can lead to early diagnosis of the underlying disease. Failure to make the proper diagnosis may lead to delayed treatment and increased morbidity. This chapter focuses on clinical entities that may be occult even when they cause altered gait.

NORMAL GAIT

The human gait is composed of two major components: the stance and swing phases.[1,2,3] The *stance phase* begins when the foot initially contacts the floor. This initial contact is the heel strike and is followed by midstance and completed with push off. The *swing phase* is characterized by the foot *not* being in contact with the floor. The swing phase begins with the foot leaving the ground and ends when the forward swing motion ends. The three parts of the swing phase are acceleration, swing through, and deceleration.

Locomotion is accomplished through a combination of loss of balance followed by recovery of balance. The coordination of many muscles is needed to accomplish this interplay of loss and recovery with a minimal expenditure of energy. The center of gravity of the human body is thought to be located anterior to the second sacral vertebra (S2). This center traces a sinusoidal wave form as the human body moves through space. The wave form has both a vertical and a horizontal component.

The normal human gait avoids an exaggerated, stiff, "goose leg" vertical movement or an awkward sideward swagger by the interplay of several determinants. These determinants are pelvic rotation, pelvic tilt, knee flexion, knee extension, and foot and ankle motion. A disturbance of any of these determinants can result in an altered gait. The most common causes of such disturbances are contracture, loss of supporting structure, pain, paralysis, and a shortened extremity.[4] Disease processes that limit movement of the hip will impair pelvic rotation and tilt because these pelvic movements occur through the hip joint. Paralysis of the muscles controlling hip movement will similarly affect pelvic tilt and rotation.[5]

ABNORMAL GAIT

Patients with altered gait may present with abnormalities of one or more gait determinants. For this reason the clinician who evaluates the entire spectrum of the gait is better able to isolate the cause of the disease. Certain gait abnormalities are characteristic. Table 19-1 highlights several gaits and their associated disease entities.

The *Trendelenburg gait* is recognized by abnormal movement of the pelvis. A Trendelenburg lurch is seen

Causes of altered gait

Traumatic

Spondylosis
Spondylolisthesis
Osgood-Schlatter disease
Sinding-Larsen-Johansen
  syndrome
Myositis
Chondromalacia
Retained foreign body
Avulsion injury

Fractures

Complete
Incomplete
  Torus
  Greenstick
  Bowing
  Stress
  Fatigue
  Insufficiency

Infection

Osteomyelitis
Brodie abscess
Septic joint
Lyme disease
Cerebral abscess
Meningitis, encephalitis
Hepatitis
Brucellosis
Rat bite fever
Congenital syphilis
Kawasaki disease
Cellulitis
Tick paralysis
Retroperitoneal abscess
Tuberculosis

Congenital

Focal femoral deficiency
Hemiatrophy
Congenital absence or
  shortening of tibia
Tibia pseudoarthrosis
Tarsal coalition
Accessory navicular
Congenital hip dislocation
Calcaneus valgus
Congenital vertical talus
Metatarsus adductus
Pes cavus
Spina bifida and
  meningomyelocele
Scoliosis
Tibial torsion
Femoral anteversion

Inflammatory

Rheumatoid arthritis
Rubella
Rubella vaccination
Rheumatic fever
Caffey disease
Henoch-Schönlein purpura
Dermatomyositis
Appendicitis
Iliac adenitis
Thrombophlebitis
Reiter syndrome
Osteoarthritis
Sudek atrophy
Gout
Polymyalgia rheumatica
Systemic lupus erythematosus
Calcium pyrophosphate
  dihydrate deposition disease
Sjögren syndrome
Scleroderma
Polyarteritis nodosa
Transient synovitis
Giant cell arteritis
Ankylosing spondylitis
Pigmented villonodular
  synovitis
Tendinitis
Osteochondritis dessicans
Chondromalacia
Inflammatory bowel disease
Erythema nodosum
Baker cyst

Neoplastic

Leukemia
Osteosarcoma
Ewing sarcoma
Neuroblastoma
Osteoid osteoma
Rhabdomyosarcoma
Eosinophilic granuloma
Central nervous system tumors
Hemangioma
Lymphangioma
Lymphoma
Multiple exostoses
Enchondromatosis
Fibrous dysplasia
Giant cell tumor
Metastatic breast, lung, kidney,
  or prostate cancer
Unicameral (monolocular) bone
  cyst
Paget sarcoma (disease)
Chondrosarcoma
Multiple myeloma
Histiocytosis X
Adamantinoma

Metabolic

Rickets
Scurvy
Hypervitaminosis
Glycogen storage disease
Porphyria
Hyperparathyroidism
Renal osteodystrophy
Osteopetrosis
Diabetes mellitus
Morquio syndrome
Hurler syndrome

Neurologic

Hemiatrophy
Muscular dystrophy
Poliomyelitis
Peripheral nerve trauma
Normal pressure hydrocephalus
Cortical cerebellar degeneration
Cerebral palsy
Friedreich ataxia
Atypical polyneuritis
Acute transverse myelopathy
Guillain-Barré syndrome
Complicated migraine

Vascular

Legg-Calvé-Perthes disease
Köhler disease
Freiberg infarction (disease)
Ischemic contractures

Systemic

Hemophilia
Sickle cell anemia
Neurofibromatosis
Thalassemia
Gaucher disease
Mucopolysaccharoidosis
Larsen syndrome
Klippel-Trenaunay-Weber
  syndrome
Hypertrophic osteoarthrophy

Other

Leg length discrepancy
Blount disease
Scoliosis
Reflex sympathetic dystrophy
Steroid use
Charcot-Marie-Tooth disease
Refsum disease
Déjérine-Sottas disease
Roussy-Lévy disease
Appendicitis
Heavy metal intoxication
Malingering

Table 19-1. Syndromes associated with abnormal gait

Gait	Associated syndromes
Spastic	Cerebral palsy hemiplegia
Dyskinetic	Cerebral palsy
Ataxic	Multiple sclerosis
	Tabes dorsalis
	Chronic polyneuropathy
	Diabetic neuropathy
	Friedreich ataxia
Waddling (bilateral Trendelenburg)	Muscular dystrophies
Steppage	Charcot-Marie-Tooth disease
	Poliomyelitis
	Paralytic foot drop
Equinus	Cerebral palsy
	Charcot-Marie-Tooth disease
	Peripheral neuropathies
	Shortened extremity
Festinating	Parkinson disease
Antalgic	Osteomyelitis
	Septic joint
	Trauma
Trendelenburg	Paralysis of the gluteus medius muscle
	Congenital hip disease
	Slipped femoral capital epiphysis
	Coxa vara

when paralysis of the gluteus medius muscle occurs. This muscle is a major abductor of the hip and is essential in stabilizing the hip and pelvis during movement. A Trendelenburg sign is elicited by having the patient stand on the affected side while the pelvic tilt is noted. Normally the intact gluteus medius muscle maintains the pelvis in a horizontal position when a person stands on one foot. A positive Trendelenburg sign refers to a drop of the pelvis opposite the affected side because of ineffectiveness of the gluteus medius. The patient compensates for the inability to maintain the pelvis horizontal while walking by shifting the center of gravity toward the affected hip, thus reducing the work of the affected muscle group. The center of gravity is moved by lurching the trunk over the affected side.

The *antalgic gait* is frequently observed in the emergency department. The basic feature of this gait is the inability or reluctance to stand on the affected side. The pain produced by weight bearing causes the patient to shorten the stance phase of the gait on the affected side. This reduction in the stance phase causes the swing phase of the unaffected side to shorten. If the pain is localized to a specific joint, a compensatory mechanism also will exist that lessens the pain in the joint while altering the gait. The patient with a painful hip attempts to maximize the volume of the hip joint, holding the painful hip in abduction, external rotation, and slight flexion. The gait is modified to reduce pain by reducing the pull of muscle groups on the hip joint. Therefore, during the stance phase, the patient moves the center of gravity over the hip to reduce the work of the hip. The movement of the center of gravity is

accomplished by swaying the trunk over the hip, thereby reducing the amount of hip abduction and extension required. The patient attempts to avoid painful heel strike by increasing plantar flexion of the foot so that the impact of contacting the ground is absorbed by the ball of the foot and ankle joint. The resulting plantar flexion increases the length of the extremity, which is compensated for by flexion of the knee. If the knee joint is the source of discomfort, a similar antalgic limp develops, but the Trendelenburg lurch is absent and there is no drop of the opposite side of the pelvis.

EVALUATION

Once an abnormal gait is identified, patient history and physical examination provide important information. It is important to ascertain if the gait varies during the day. If the antalgic gait is worse in the morning and improves during the day, this suggests an inflammatory process such as rheumatoid arthritis. The antalgic gait that worsens during the day suggests muscle fatigue and may result from a mechanical problem such as femoral anteversion. The first procedure following patient history and physical examination is usually evaluation of the involved bone or joint with plain radiographs. Bones and joints can be screened for most congenital, traumatic, advanced infectious, and arthritic disease with these radiographs.

In the child or adult the pelvis and hips can be evaluated using anteroposterior (AP) and frog-leg AP radiographs. This also facilitates comparison of the hips. To identify subtle unilateral hip subluxation, the clinician must ensure that the pelvis is not rotated. The sacroiliac joints are better demonstrated by tilting the x-ray tube 30 degrees toward the head of the supine patient.[6] The lumbar (L) spine and sacrum (S) are evaluated with AP and lateral radiographs along with a lateral radiograph coned down to L5/S1. The knee, ankle, and foot joints are best demonstrated by three radiographs: AP, oblique, and lateral.[6]

Conventional tomography, ultrasonography, computed tomography (CT scan), magnetic resonance imaging (MRI), and nuclear medicine (radionuclide bone scan) are available for problem-solving in selected patients.

Young children suspected of having hip joint effusion based on clinical findings, radiographic signs, or both can have ultrasonography to confirm the presence of a joint effusion and ultrasonographically guided joint aspiration if indicated.[7,8] A three-phase radionuclide bone scan, employing a vascular phase immediately after the radionuclide injection, a blood pool phase a few minutes after injection, and static scans hours after injection, is a valuable means of evaluating some patients who have normal radiographs and persistent symptoms and are strongly suspected of having pathology (Fig. 19-1). Such radionuclide scanning is very sensitive and surveys the entire body but is nonspecific.[9] MRI is also sensitive but is confined to a small portion of the body and is expensive. MRI is used

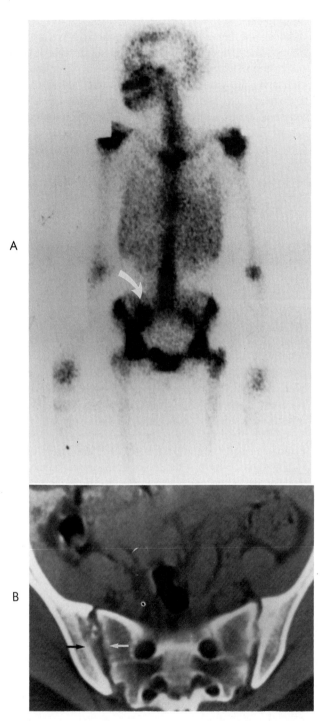

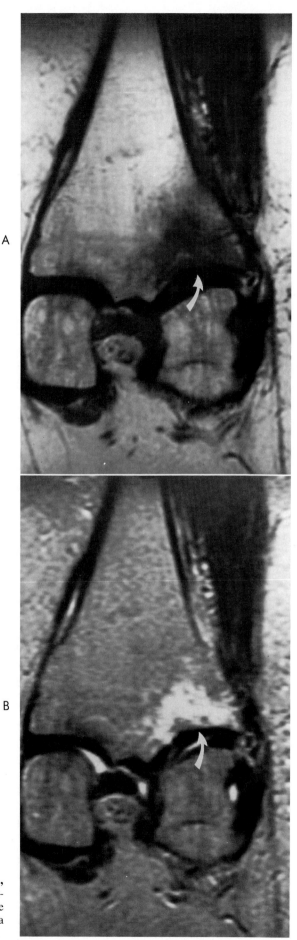

Fig. 19-1. Sacroiliitis. **A,** PA view of a Tc 99m–methylene-diphosphate (MDP) bone scan shows increased uptake *(arrow)* in the area of left sacroiliac joint. Radiographs were normal. **B,** CT scan shows widening and loss of the cortical margins of the left sacroiliac joint *(arrows)*.

Fig. 19-2. Traumatic bone bruise in a 47-year-old woman. **A,** Coronal T_1-weighted MRI image shows a low signal in the lateral tibial plateau *(arrow)*. **B,** Coronal T_2-weighted MRI image shows a high signal in the lateral tibial plateau indicating edema *(arrow)*. Radiographs were normal.

for solving specific problems rather than serving as a means of survey. MRI is the method of choice for evaluating soft tissue lesions of the joints and can identify traumatic lesions and bone bruises when radiographs are normal (Fig. 19-2). The CT scan is used in selected anatomic areas, including the sacroiliac joints, pelvis, and joints of the feet. Bone lesions in the sacrum may be clearly shown by a CT scan when they are subtle or not visible on radiographs[9,10] (Fig. 19-3).

CONGENITAL ABNORMALITIES
Congenital hip dislocation

Congenital hip dislocation (CHD) is a common abnormality of the lower extremity.[11] The interplay of genetic and environmental factors causes considerable variety in the incidence of CHD. Recent data suggest several in utero factors result in abnormalities of the acetabulum. Approximately 60% of patients are first born. It is postulated that the primigravida pelvis does not accommodate the fetus

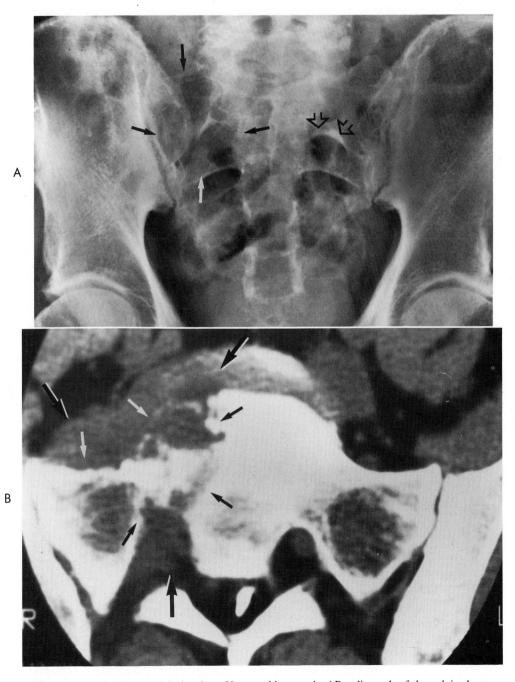

Fig. 19-3. Leukemic sacral lesion in a 58-year-old man. **A,** AP radiograph of the pelvis shows destruction of the right sacral foramen *(arrows)* compared to the intact left sacral foramen *(open arrows)*. **B,** CT scan shows destruction of the right side of the sacrum *(small arrows)* and an overlying soft tissue mass *(large arrows)*.

readily, which causes the hips to be extended rather than flexed. This is important because the acetabulum requires contact with the femoral head for adequate development. Since the extended hip does not provide an appropriate stimulus, acetabular dysplasia results. This hypothesis is further supported by the increased incidence of CHD following breech deliveries. There is a female-to-male ratio of 6:1; this female dominance is thought to result from the release of maternal hormone before birth. This hormone relaxes the maternal pelvic ligaments but also causes excess relaxation of the ligaments of the female fetus.

Most patients with CHD are discovered at birth during routine screening for the deformity. The neonate may have a gross dislocation, a subluxation, or an unstable hip that can be passively dislocated. Despite routine screening, some patients with CHD remain undiagnosed until they begin to walk. Barlow or Ortolani signs are important in detecting CHD in the newborn but rarely are helpful in the toddler. The toddler with a dislocated hip may have a piston or telescoping movement of the hip on physical examination; the femoral head can be displaced laterally and upward. Most children with late presentation have decreased mobility of the hip along with weak, shortened abductors of the hip. The adductors also contract, which further limits abduction. The child also may have a shortened extremity. The

Galeazzi sign can be observed when the child is supine with the hips and knees flexed 90 degrees. This sign is positive when the tip of the flexed knee on the abnormal side is not at the same level as the normal extremity. These children have a Trendelenburg gait if the extremity is greatly shortened. Bilateral CHD is distinguished by a waddling gait (bilateral Trendelenburg), a widened perineum, prominent trochanters, flattened buttocks, and an increased lordosis of the spine. The hyperlordosis occurs as the trunk shifts to move the center of gravity posteriorly to match the migration of the femoral heads posteriorly. Avascular necrosis can occur if the medial circumflex artery supplying the hip joint is compromised by the migration of the femoral head.

In CHD, the hip is usually dislocatable rather than dislocated in the newborn; radiographs are therefore usually normal. If there is questionable subluxation, the hip can be shown to be dislocatable on the Andren–von Rosen view: the hips are abducted 45 degrees, followed by extension and internal rotation. The hip is dislocatable if the long axis of the femur projects outside the acetabulum. This view should not be confused with the frog-leg lateral view, which may actually reduce a subluxed hip.[12]

When CHD is well established, usually in an older child, characteristic radiographic findings include subluxation of the femoral neck and ossification center, delayed or small ossification center, and an increase in the acetab-

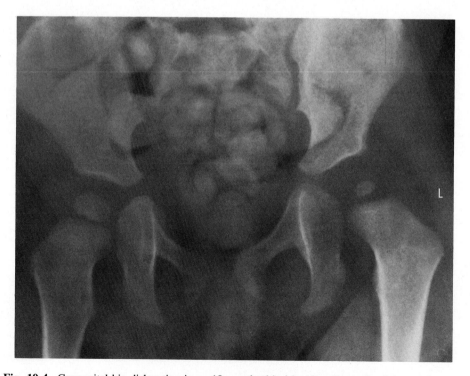

Fig. 19-4. Congenital hip dislocation in an 18-month-old girl. AP radiograph of the pelvis demonstrates that the left hip is subluxed laterally and the capital femoral epiphysis is smaller than the opposite hip. The angle of the left acetabular roof is greater than the opposite side also.

ular angle. The radiographic diagnosis is usually obvious at this time (Fig. 19-4).

Treatment depends on the severity and duration of dislocation. A child who has begun to walk usually has enough displacement to require surgical intervention.

Tarsal coalition

Tarsal coalition is an occult cause of foot pain. This fusion can be congenital or secondary to trauma, infection, or inflammatory arthritis. The congenital type is most common and occurs in up to 1% of children, but not all are symptomatic. Most frequently the calcaneus is united with the navicular and the middle (sustentacular) talocalcaneal joint is affected. Coalition can be fibrous, cartilaginous, or bony.

Congenital fusion becomes symptomatic at puberty, when progressive ossification increases rigidity and decreases joint mobility. Pain is episodic, brought on by prolonged activity or minor injury, and is relieved by rest. The foot is often flat, and midtarsal or subtalar motion is decreased. Anterior tibial muscle spasm may occur. The combination of this spasm and a flat foot has been called *peroneal spastic flat foot* and is characteristic of tarsal coalition.

If the diagnosis is made early before secondary changes occur, the coalition can be resected. Later, treatment is conservative. If wedges, supports, and casts are not successful, pain can be relieved with triple arthrodesis.

An important clue to the radiographic diagnosis of tarsal coalition is a talar beak (Fig. 19-5). This is a beaklike, bony projection extending superiorly from the most anterior margin of the talus. The beak results from abnormal subtalar joint motion. A calcaneonavicular coalition is usually visible on an oblique radiograph of the foot (Fig. 19-6). A subtalar coalition is more difficult to demonstrate with radiographs but usually is easily visible on a coronal CT scan of the foot[13,14] (Fig. 19-7).

Femoral anteversion and retroversion; tibial torsion; metatarsus adductus

Patients with these disorders present with a gait disturbance typically described as an excessive toe-in or toe-out gait.[15] Normal adults generally walk or stand such that the axis of the foot points 15 degrees lateral to the sagittal plane of the body. A child whose toes point medial to this orientation during gait or stance is termed as *toeing in*. Toeing in is usually caused by femoral anteversion, internal tibial torsion, or metatarsus adductus.[16] Toeing in during early childhood or a small degree of femoral anteversion and internal tibial torsion occur naturally, and there is spontaneous correction over time. Failure to correct by late childhood could represent a developmental delay, or an undiagnosed neuromuscular disorder. Metatarsus adductus is a developmental deformity, and spontaneous correction is rare. Toeing out is caused by femoral retroversion or external tibial torsion.

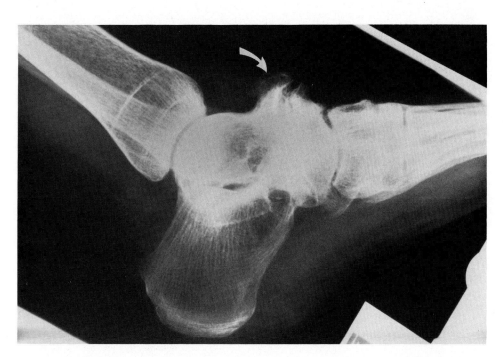

Fig. 19-5. Congenital tarsal coalition with a talar beak in an 18-year-old boy. Lateral radiograph of the left foot demonstrates a beaklike projection *(arrow)* from the talus, which is characteristic of a tarsal coalition. It is the result of fusion of the middle talocalcaneal joint. (Reprinted with permission from Demos TC: *Orthopedics* 4:200, 1981.)

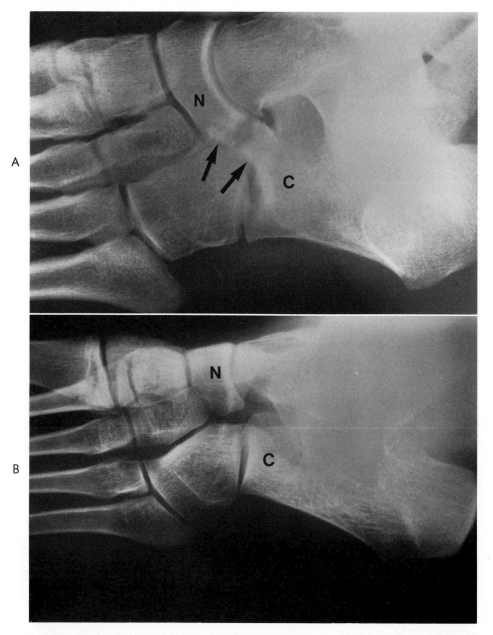

Fig. 19-6. Congenital tarsal (calcaneonavicular) coalition in a 14-year-old boy. **A,** Oblique radiograph of the right foot shows irregular bony projections *(arrows)* from the calcaneus *(C)* and the navicular *(N)*. **B,** Normal foot for comparison.

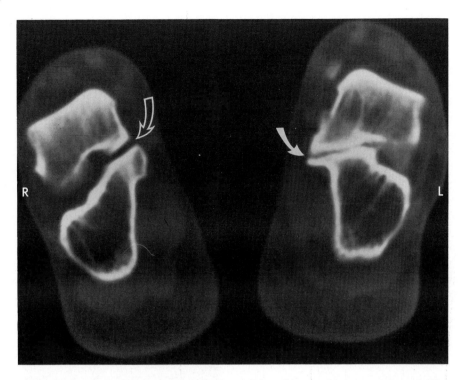

Fig. 19-7. Congenital tarsal coalition (talocalcaneal) in a 28-year-old woman. Coronal CT scan shows the normal right middle talocalcaneal joint *(open arrow)* and the tilted, narrowed joint of the left foot *(closed arrow).*

Children with femoral anteversion or retroversion will have the toe-in or toe-out gait associated with orientation of the patella inward or outward on gait. When the diagnosis is suspected, the ability of the femur to rotate internally and externally should be compared. The normal child demonstrates equal internal and external rotation. However, if there is femoral anteversion, internal rotation of the hip with the hip in extension is much greater than the external rotation. If the amount of excess internal rotation lessens when the hip is flexed, this is considered mild-to-moderate anteversion. If the rotation is severe enough, the toe impacts the opposite heel during gait, causing tripping. This may require the use of braces. Femoral osteotomy is advised for the most severe cases.

Tibial torsion is defined as a change in the axis of the tibia such that when the patella points forward, the orientation of the tibia and fibula causes the ankle midline axis to point medially. The prognosis and treatment is the same as for femoral anteversion.

In metatarsus adductus, deviation of the metatarsal bones away from the midline axis of the foot and heel occurs, such that the toes point inward. The exact cause of this deformity is unknown but it may be secondary to uterine packing. Metatarsus adductus differs from femoral anteversion and tibial torsion in that it is usually unilateral compared with the bilaterality of the other two disorders. Evaluation of the angle between the midline axis of the heel and the metatarsal heads will identify patients with metatarsus adductus. The deformity is considered severe when the midline axis of the heel, viewed from the anterior position, falls lateral to the second web space, and forceful abduction of the foot does not substantially reduce the deformity. If the midline axis of the heel falls medial to the second web space when forceful abduction is applied, the disease is considered moderate.

The angle of femoral anteversion can be determined trigonometrically using two radiographs at right angles to each other. A CT scan can provide a slightly more accurate determination.[17] Tibial torsion is often associated with developmental bowing of the lower extremities. The evaluation is clinical, and radiographs add little information. The CT scan has been used to quantify tibial torsion in adults with degenerative changes of the knee. Metatarsus adductus shows inversion of the foot in addition to adduction of the metatarsals on radiographs. In mild cases the hindfoot is normal, but in some severe cases the hindfoot is in valgus. Treatment includes braces, casting, or surgical repositioning in severe cases.

ARTHRITIS
Rheumatoid arthritis

Rheumatoid arthritis (RA) is a chronic inflammatory disease whose hallmark is deforming and often debilitating degeneration of the joints. RA can occur as a gait disturbance as a result of joint inflammation of the lower extremities. It is estimated that 3% of the general population have RA, with a 3:1 female-to-male ratio. Symptoms may begin at any age, but onset is usually between ages 25 and 50.

The cause of RA remains unknown, but the disease itself is probably an auto-immune response, which leads to serositis, nodules, and vasculitis.[18] The synovial tissue inflammation results in the formation of large villi (pannus) that spread over the articular cartilage. This pannus destroys the underlying cartilage and later the subchondral bone. Rheumatoid nodules are inflammatory processes of the subcutaneous tissue, generally occurring in areas known as pressure points.

The clinical picture of RA is extremely varied, but most patients present with joint symptoms. Approximately 75% of patients have multiarticular disease initially. The hands and feet are typically involved. About 25% of patients have involvement of only a single joint, usually in the lower extremity. This group generally has no systemic findings and often presents with antalgic gait and pain in the knee (50%), ankle, or hip. The antalgic gait may be worse in the morning and improve through the day. The onset of pain is described as insidious. When questioned, patients often describe fatigue, weakness, and joint stiffness several weeks before the onset of pain. There is an increase in warmth, tenderness, and swelling of the joint. Good range of motion is usually maintained initially, but as the disease progresses, flexion contractures can occur. The continued destruction of the joint can permanently alter the gait because of limb shortening and contracture of the surrounding support structures.

The systemic manifestations of RA can be devastating, with pulmonary involvement, pericarditis, valvular destruction, ocular disease, and Felty syndrome (splenomegaly with neutropenia).

Initially the bones are normal or show only periarticular osteoporosis on radiographs. A knee joint effusion may be visible as a distended suprapatellar bursa on lateral radio-

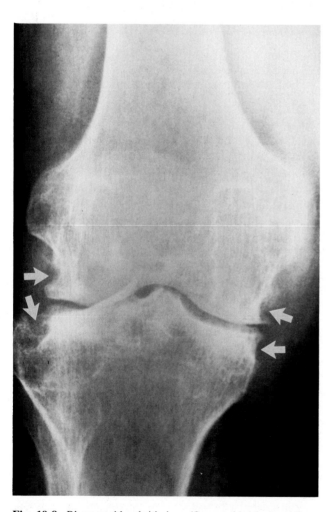

Fig. 19-8. Rheumatoid arthritis in a 49-year-old woman. AP radiograph of the right knee demonstrates a knee joint that is moderately and uniformly narrowed with multiple peripheral erosions *(arrows)*.

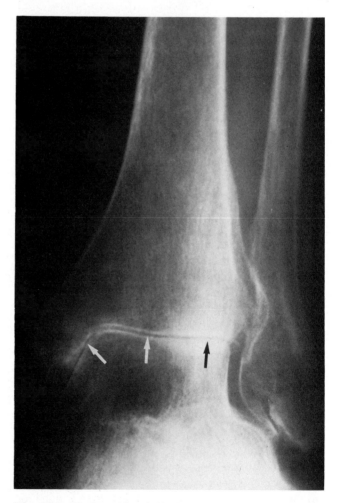

Fig. 19-9. Rheumatoid arthritis in a 38-year-old woman. Oblique radiograph of the left ankle demonstrates that the joint between the tibia and talus is uniformly narrowed *(arrows)*. This uniformity is characteristic of inflammatory arthritis.

graphs. Later, pannus erodes the articular cortex of the bone. The first erosions occur at sites where the bone is inside the joint capsule but not protected by overlying thick articular cartilage. These so-called bare areas are in the peripheral non-weight-bearing portions of the joint (Fig. 19-8). When joint space narrowing occurs in the knee, ankle, and foot, the narrowing is most often strikingly uniform across the joint (Fig. 19-9). This is in contrast to degenerative joint disease, in which joint space narrowing is almost always eccentric. Hip joint space narrowing caused by RA is central, that is, in the projection of a line through the femoral neck (Fig. 19-10). This contrasts with degenerative change, in which narrowing is isolated to the superior aspect or, less often, to the medial aspect of the joint space. The characteristic osteophytes of degenerative change are also absent in RA unless there are complicating degenerative changes.[19]

Patients with RA may have anemia, mild leukocytosis, and a moderately high erythrocyte sedimentation rate (ESR). Most patients have an elevated rheumatoid factor or antinuclear antibodies to native deoxyribonucleic acid (DNA). The synovial fluid analysis demonstrates inflammation, with white blood cell counts (WBCs) in the 10,000 to 50,000 range, a poor mucin clot, and often decreased glucose.

The prognosis in RA is often difficult to predict because many cases thought to represent early RA are, in fact, another disease. Most patients, however, progress to chronic illness, marked by remissions and relapses months to years apart. Patients with vasculitis, multiple nodules, and high-titer rheumatoid factor are most likely to have severe disease and a poor prognosis.

Treatment of patients with RA should focus on reducing joint inflammation with rest, splints, and anti-inflammatory drugs. Orthopedic surgery is reserved for the more severe chronic deformities.

Seronegative spondyloarthropathies

Patients with seronegative spondyloarthropathies (ankylosing spondylitis, psoriatic arthritis, Reiter syndrome, juvenile chronic arthritis) are characterized by negative rheumatoid factor and are often HLA-B27 positive. Any of these spondyloarthropathies can be associated with monarticular disease and a gait disturbance. The spondyloarthropathies frequently involve the sacroiliac joints and spine, as compared to RA.

The involvement of the peripheral joints is frequently asymmetric unlike RA, which is usually symmetric on both sides of the body and in the joints of an affected extremity (Fig. 19-11). Periosteal new bone formation typically occurs in Reiter syndrome and in psoriatic and juvenile arthritis but rarely in RA.[20]

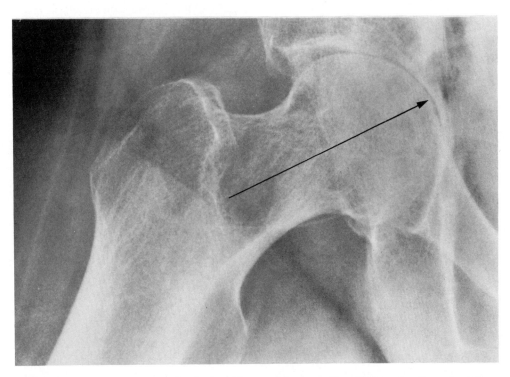

Fig. 19-10. Rheumatoid arthritic hip in a 51-year-old woman. Frog-leg lateral radiograph of the right hip demonstrates that the hip joint is narrowed centrally in the projection of the femoral neck *(arrow)*. There are no osteophytes and no sclerosis. These findings are the opposite of degenerative joint disease.

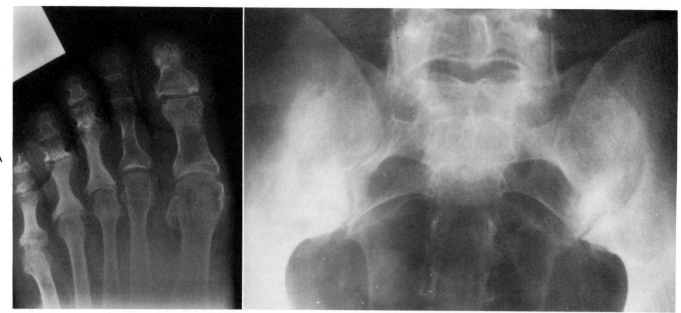

Fig. 19-11. Psoriatic arthritis in a 42-year-old woman. **A,** AP radiograph of the left foot shows asymmetric narrowing of the metatarsophalangeal joints. The second joint is not affected and the first is only mildly affected. Distal joint involvement of the third toe and sclerosis of the third, fourth, and fifth toes (due to periosteal new bone) are characteristic of seronegative spondyloarthropathy. **B,** AP radiograph of the pelvis shows sacroiliitis with marked sclerosis and sacroiliac joint irregularity common to spondyloarthropathies but rare in rheumatoid arthritis. (Reprinted with permission from Demos TC: *Orthopedics* 4:324, 1981.)

Crystalline-induced arthropathies

Patients with acute gait disturbances from crystalline-induced arthropathies are likely to have gout or calcium pyrophosphate dihydrate (CPPD) deposition disease. *Gout* is the term applied to the arthritis resulting from disordered purine metabolism. Gout affects about 3 individuals/1000 population and is two to three times more prevalent than CPPD deposition disease. Idiopathic gout predominantly affects men over age 40 years, whereas CPPD deposition disease occurs in older patients and is more common in women. There may be a family history (6% to 18%) in patients with gout.

CPPD deposition disease, visible as cartilage calcification on radiographs, is often not associated with symptoms. When symptomatic, there is usually monarticular disease (pseudogout). However, CPPD deposition disease is associated with several metabolic disorders, including hyperparathyroidism, hemochromatosis, ochronosis, and Wilson disease.

Gout is arthritis that develops in patients with hyperuricemia. In advanced cases, serum uric acid levels are elevated, monosodium urate monohydrate crystals are deposited in and around joints (tophi), and there may be uric acid nephrolithiasis. Hyperuricemia is defined as a uric acid level greater than 6.8 to 7.0 mg/100 ml (0.4 μmol/L). Hyperuricemia is caused by dietary excess, overproduction of uric acid, or undersecretion of urates. It is not unusual for a patient with gout to have more than one mechanism

causing the elevated serum uric acid level. Supersaturation occurs when the serum uric acid level exceeds 7.0 mg/100 ml, but spontaneous crystal formation usually does not occur at this level unless additional factors come into play. Crystallization (nucleation) is enhanced by cool temperatures, which accounts for the peripheral distribution of gouty arthritis. Nucleation is also aided by the interaction of monosodium urate particles with connective tissue such as cartilage. The monosodium urate crystals may assume the shape of amorphous particles, spherolites, or the more classic needle-shaped crystals. The needle-shaped crystals are negatively birefringent and vary in length from 0.2 to 20 mm, as seen via compensated (red) polarized light microscopy. Failure to identify these crystals in the synovial fluid makes the diagnosis of gout unlikely.

Gouty arthritis typically presents in the first metatarsophalangeal joint (70% of patients). Pain is acute, occurs often at night, and may be precipitated by alcohol, trauma, or another illness. The ankle joint or knee joint may also be the initial site of involvement. The gait is antalgic, and the patient will not bear weight on the extremity. The location of the pain is precise, and there is extreme tenderness of the joint. Swelling and a reddened, shiny skin may simulate a florid cellulitis. In the normal course, pain is maximal within a few hours of onset and then spontaneously resolves in hours to days. The synovial fluid usually contains leukocytes, with a WBC of 10,000 to 70,000. The mucin clot is poor, and the uric

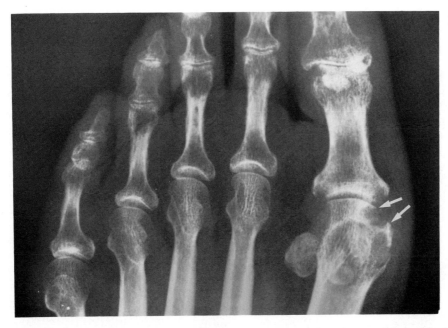

Fig. 19-12. Gout in a 57-year-old man. AP radiograph of the left foot shows erosions of the big toe about the metatarsophalangeal joint. The largest erosion has claw-like overhanging edges *(arrows)* characteristic of gout.

acid and glucose levels are the same as the serum levels of the synovial fluid.

Radiographic abnormalities are seldom found in patients with gout until they have been symptomatic for many years. Joints of the lower extremities are most often affected. The typical radiographic finding is a sharply defined bone erosion near a joint. The erosion is marginal, has a sclerotic rim, and is located beneath the soft tissue mass of a tophus. The erosion is often clasped by bony cortical projections, which have been termed *overhanging edges* and are characteristic of gout (Fig. 19-12). The tophi are sometimes calcified.[22] In contrast to RA, bone density is normal, and the joint spaces are maintained until late in the course of gouty arthritis.

The recommended treatment of acute gouty arthritis is an anti-inflammatory agent. Colchicine has been used most often; however, indomethacin, phenylbutazone, fenoprofen, and naproxen are also effective.

CPPD deposition disease is termed *pseudogout* when it results in acute arthritis (Fig. 19-13). It can also affect multiple small joints, simulating RA, or may cause chronic symptoms in large joints, simulating degenerative arthritis. CPPD deposition disease is classified into three distinct groups: hereditary, idiopathic, and secondary to a metabolic disease. The crystals form at three sites in the joint cartilage: the intra-articular fibrocartilage, the articular hyaline cartilage, and the cartilage where there are tendinous and ligamentous attachments to the bone. The joints most often involved that affect gait include the knee menisci, the ankle, the pubic symphysis, the intervertebral disks, and the hip. *Chondrocalcinosis* is defined as calcification of cartilage. Two other calcium salts in addition to calcium pyrophosphate dihydrate may cause cartilage calcification: hydroxyapatite and, rarely, calcium hydrogen phosphate dihydrate.

Patients with pseudogout are usually elderly women (average age 75 years). There is a 2:1 female-to-male ratio, and affected men tend to be younger (average age of 65 years). This is the reverse of gout.

The acute arthritis of pseudogout affects the knee most often, followed by the ankle, hip, and lumbar vertebrae. The attack is usually confined to one joint, and the onset of pain is not as rapid as seen in gout. The pain tends to peak over 12 to 36 hours, and the intensity of the pain is somewhat less than that experienced in gout. The painful joint appears erythematous, swollen, and warm. The synovial fluid may be puslike in appearance or bloody. There are a large number of leukocytes, and the joint fluid contains calcium pyrophosphate dihydrate crystals, which are short blunt rods or are rhomboidally shaped. Under polarized light microscopy, these crystals show a weakly positive birefringence compared with the strongly negative birefringence of urate crystals. Typical radiographic findings include joint cartilaginous calcifications and varying degrees of joint space destruction.

The most common causes of chondrocalcinosis are hydroxyapatite and CPPD crystals. Calcification caused by CPPD deposition is usually punctate, linear, and delicate and can involve hyaline cartilage, fibrocartilage, and periarticular soft tissue. Hydroxyapatite produces amorphous or coarse calcification in and around joints and bursae. However, cartilage calcification resulting from CPPD dep-

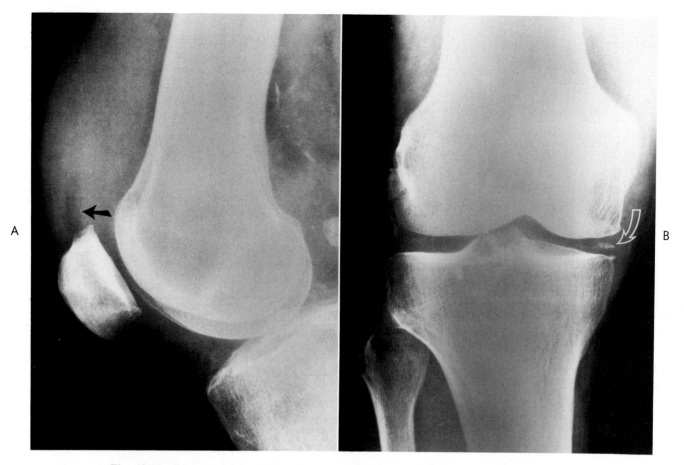

Fig. 19-13. Calcium pyrophosphate dihydrate (CPPD) deposition disease in a 61-year-old man. **A,** Lateral radiograph of the right knee shows a large knee joint effusion distending the suprapatellar extension of the joint and displacing the fat pad *(arrow).* **B,** AP radiograph of the right knee demonstrates chondrocalcinosis with calcification of the medial meniscus *(arrow).*

osition cannot be equated with disease since up to 25% of elderly patients have been found to have chondrocalcinosis. In contrast, CPPD deposition disease can occur in the absence of calcification. It is still possible to suspect the diagnosis when certain patterns of joint space narrowing are encountered. In the knee, isolated patellofemoral narrowing is suspicious for CPPD deposition disease, even if no chondrocalcinosis is present.[23] CPPD deposition disease can lead to marked destruction of a joint similar to a neuropathic joint. This can occur rapidly, especially in the hip.

The treatment for patients with pseudogout includes anti-inflammatory agents, such as indomethacin and phenylbutazone, and many newer nonsteroidal agents. Colchicine tends to have a variable effect but has been used in patients with the chronic form of the disease.

BONE AND JOINT INFECTION
Toxic synovitis

Transient or toxic synovitis is an inflammation of the joint often associated with a recent viral illness and must be differentiated from septic arthritis. The disease is usu-

ally seen in patients between the ages 5 and 10 years. There is a 2:1 male predominance. The hip, knee, or ankle may be involved although gait disturbances are most often caused by hip disease. The child does not appear sick and is usually able to bear weight on the affected extremity. The joint is often held in a position of comfort. There is increased pain with extension or flexion of the joint. Fever occurs in 25% of children, and the ESR is elevated in 50%. The joint aspirate shows only a mild inflammatory reaction, and cultures are negative. The child has spontaneous remission following bed rest. Conservative treatment and close follow-up are necessary because this type of synovitis may be a prelude to Legg-Calvé-Perthes disease (see later discussion).

Acute septic arthritis

Acute septic arthritis is an infection of a joint that can occur in all age groups but is more common in early childhood. The hip and knee are common sites of infection in the infant. Infections of the knee (41%), hip (23%), and ankle (14%) occur most often in later childhood. *Staphyloco-*

cus is the most common organism causing infection, followed by *Pneumococcus*, group A *β-hemolytic Streptococcus*, and *Streptococcus viridans*. *Haemophilus influenzae* infection type B is very common in children under 5 years of age. Gram-negative organisms account for 20% of infections, and a high incidence of *Pseudomonas aeruginosa* infection is found in neonates and drug abuse patients.[24-26]

The joint can become infected from hematogenous spread or direct invasion from surrounding cellulitis or contiguous osteomyelitis. Hematogenous spread occurs most often, and the clinician should determine the primary site of infection. Infants are prone to develop infection. Conditions that increase susceptibility to septic arthritis include the following:

- Following joint instrumentation.
- Chronic arthritis.
- Hemoglobinopathies.
- Immunosuppression.
- Alcoholism.
- Drug abuse.
- Diabetes mellitus.
- Immunodeficiencies.

Infection involves the synovial membrane, which becomes edematous and hyperemic. The synovium produces increased amounts of synovial fluid that distends the joint capsule. Destruction of the joint will result if the increase in intra-articular pressure causes ischemia. Proteolytic enzymes released from neutrophils contribute further to the destruction of cartilage.

Hip joint infection produces hip pain and an antalgic gait. The typical patient usually presents within 3 or 4 days of onset. A child often has a fever (38° to 40° C) and may appear sick when there is an associated abscess or cellulitis. The joint is painful and motion is limited. There is tenderness and warmth over the joint. An infant may only show increased irritability and refuse to walk, crawl, or use the extremity. The painful joint is positioned in a way that maximizes joint volume. The hip is flexed and abducted in external rotation, and the knee is held in slight flexion.

Early diagnosis is crucial in achieving a good outcome. Adults with gout or RA who have septic arthritis may delay seeking treatment because of the mistaken belief that their symptoms represent a flare-up of chronic disease. There may also be a delay when patients are taking glucocorticoids that tend to mask the inflammation.

Joint aspirate in septic arthritis shows a WBC count greater than 100,000, a poor mucin clot, a decreased glucose level, and an elevated protein level. The Gram stain is positive in 75% to 95% of gram-positive infections and 50% of gram-negative infections. Counter-immune electrophoresis (CIE) of the synovial fluid may provide early diagnosis of *Streptococcus* pneumonia or *H. influenzae*.

The patient with gonococcal septic arthritis is likely to be a young adult who presents during or after dissemination of gonococcal disease. Migratory tenosynovitis, arthralgia, vesiculopustular skin lesions, and minimal joint effusion are early findings. The knee, shoulder, wrist, and

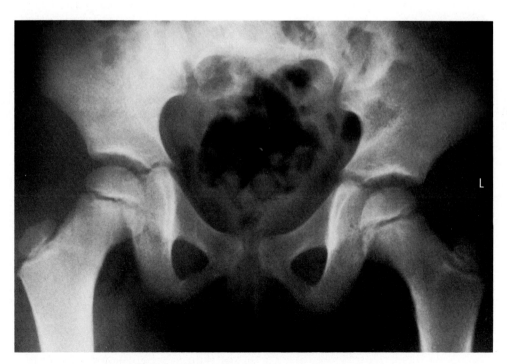

Fig. 19-14. Toxic synovitis in a 5-year-old girl. AP radiograph of the pelvis shows widening of the left hip joint due to joint effusion. The medial aspect of the joint is wider than the opposite side. This widening of the joint space is not specific and could also be due to septic arthritis or early Legg-Calvé-Perthes disease.

interphalangeal joints of the hand are most often involved.

Septic arthritis of the hip in children may be visible on radiographs if the joint effusion displaces the femoral head so that the joint space is widened. Widening can be subtle so that comparison with the normal hip is important (Fig. 19-14). In children, joint effusion associated with toxic synovitis, Legg-Calvé-Perthes disease, and juvenile arthritis will cause the same finding.[27] Ultrasonography can be used to confirm effusion and then to guide aspiration when a septic joint is suspected.[28]

Pyogenic arthritis in adults does not cause bone changes for about 1 week so that aspiration is crucial. Cartilage destruction occurs quickly.

Chronic infection due to fungi and tuberculosis are characterized by osteoporosis, erosion of the non-weight-bearing portions of the bones, and late joint space narrowing.[29]

Lyme arthritis most often presents in the knee with acute symptoms. Radiographs show effusion and erosions.

Treatment consists of parenteral antibiotics, joint drainage, and articular rest. The choice of antibiotic is guided by the patient's age, Gram stain results, and ultimately the culture results.

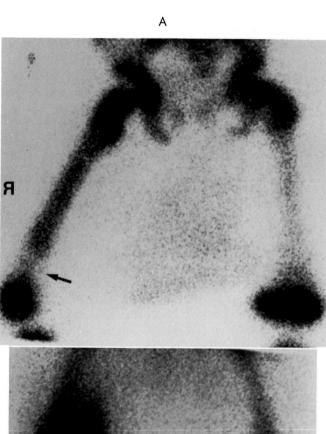

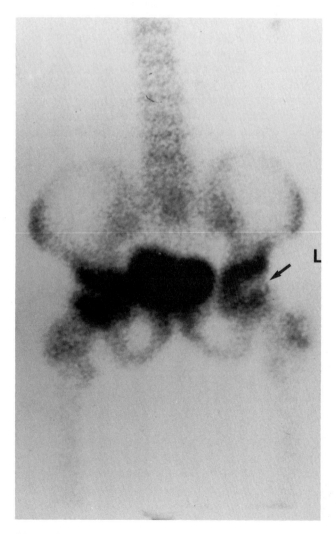

Fig. 19-15. Osteomyelitis in an 11-year-old girl. This delayed image from a three-phase bone scan shows decreased activity in the left femoral head *(arrow)* due to vascular compression. Avascular necrosis could cause a similar appearance.

Fig. 19-16. Osteomyelitis in 2-year-old boy. **A,** Tc 99m–methylene diphosphonate (MDP) bone scan shows increased uptake in the right femur, but there is focal decreased uptake distally due to compromised circulation in that area *(arrow).* **B,** Gallium 67 scan shows intense uptake in the distal right femur *(arrow).*

Osteomyelitis

Osteomyelitis can present as an acute gait disturbance; however, this is usually a late sign. In the early stages the patient may have anorexia, malaise, low-grade fever, and perhaps slight irritability with movement of the involved limb. Later, localized swelling, erythema, tenderness, and limitation of movement of the extremity occur. Osteomyelitis, like septic arthritis, is usually the result of hematogenous spread and is more common in children. The peak age of involvement is 2 to 5 years, and there is a 2:1 male predominance. The WBC may be normal or elevated, and the ESR is generally elevated. In children, the condition has a predilection for the long bones of the lower extremities. It may be difficult to distinguish osteomyelitis from septic arthritis if there is little localized swelling or if the metaphyseal lesion lies within the joint capsule. In osteomyelitis, a sympathetic joint effusion must be distinguished from extension of the infection through the epiphyseal plate into the joint with contamination of the synovial space. The diagnosis can be made by direct needle aspiration of the lesion or by blood cultures.

Bone changes in osteomyelitis are not visible on radiographs for about 10 days. Bone scans (Figs. 19-1, 19-15, and 19-16) and MRI (Fig. 19-17) are highly sensitive and

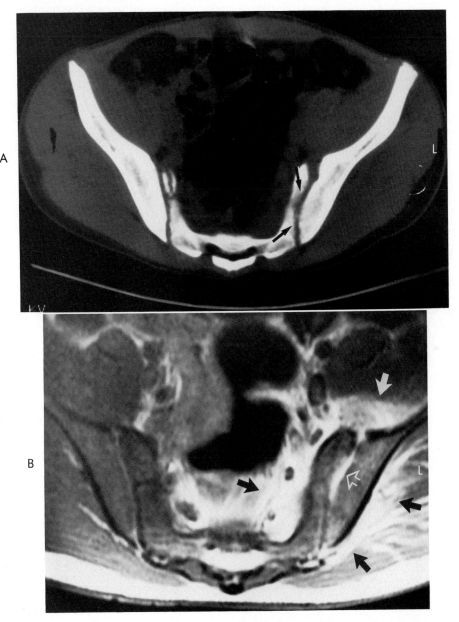

Fig. 19-17. Sacroiliitis. **A,** CT scan shows a widened left sacroiliac joint with poorly defined cortical margins *(arrows).* Radiographs were normal. **B,** T$_1$-weighted image MRI image after intravenous administration of gadolinium shows high signal fluid in the left sacroiliac joint *(open arrow)* and edema of surrounding soft tissue *(arrows).*

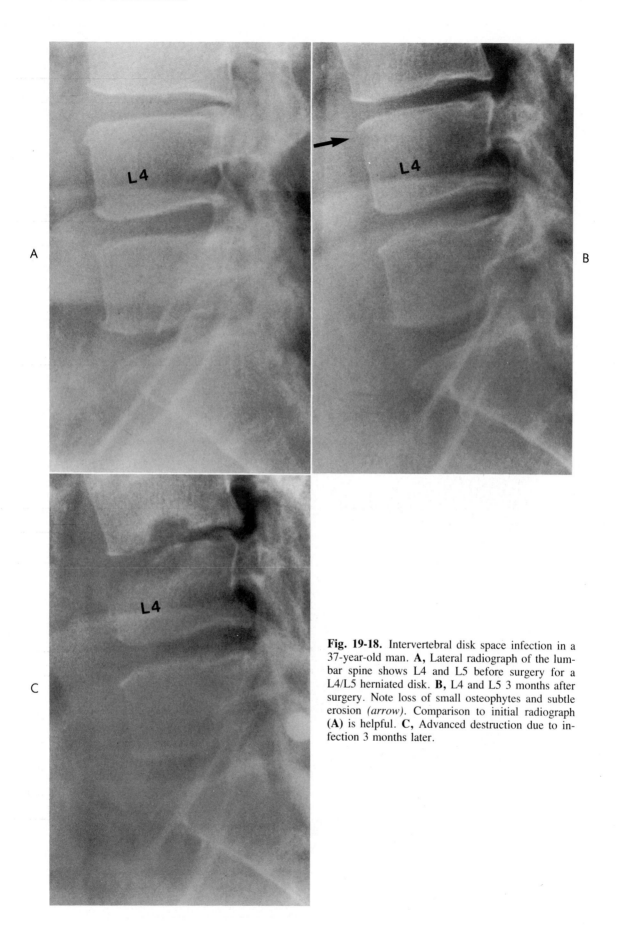

Fig. 19-18. Intervertebral disk space infection in a 37-year-old man. **A,** Lateral radiograph of the lumbar spine shows L4 and L5 before surgery for a L4/L5 herniated disk. **B,** L4 and L5 3 months after surgery. Note loss of small osteophytes and subtle erosion *(arrow)*. Comparison to initial radiograph **(A)** is helpful. **C,** Advanced destruction due to infection 3 months later.

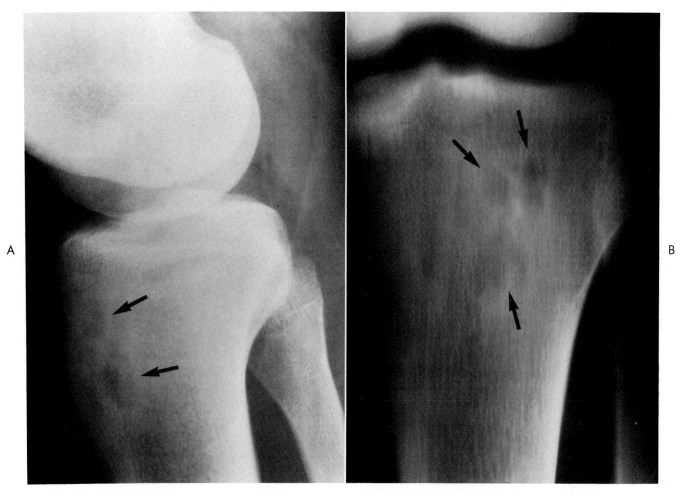

Fig. 19-19. Subacute osteomyelitis (Brodie abscess) in a 27-year-old man. **A,** Close-up of the lateral radiograph of the left knee shows subtle lucencies *(arrows)* of the proximal tibia. **B,** Plain AP conventional tomogram of the proximal tibia shows a cluster of lucencies *(arrows)* with minimal surrounding sclerosis. (Reprinted with permission from Demos TC: *Orthopedics* 2:619, 1979.)

can demonstrate bone abnormalities within 24 hours.[30] Early radiographic findings include bone destruction and periosteal new bone formation[31] (Fig. 19-18). If the patient presents late in the course of the infection, the radiographic appearance can simulate a malignant bone neoplasm.

Subacute osteomyelitis (Brodie abscess) can present as a joint or gait problem involving the hip or knee. There is rarely any periosteal new bone. One or more well-defined lytic lesions are usually present, with surrounding sclerosis varying from minimal to marked[32] (Fig. 19-19). Osteoid osteoma is the primary differential diagnosis. A long, serpiginous lucency is characteristic of subacute osteomyelitis. A gallium 67 scan can be used to differentiate these two processes.

Treatment consists of parenteral antibiotics and rest; in the case of abscess formation, surgical drainage is advocated.

TRAUMA
Stress fracture and stress reaction

A stress fracture can be described as a mechanical disturbance of trabeculae that occurs when normal bone is subjected to repeated episodes of minor trauma. In a child these injuries are usually the result of minor trauma associated with daily activities. The adult is more likely to develop a stress fracture as the result of activities that exceed the usual daily activities. Stress fractures that occur in normal bone are termed *fatigue stress fractures,* whereas those occurring in abnormal bone are termed *insufficiency stress fractures.*

Stress fractures of the tibia, fibula, femur, and metatarsals are quite common and may be associated with injuries to muscles, ligaments, tendons, cartilage, or the joint bursae. A child usually presents with pain and an antalgic limp of gradual onset, but presentation may be sudden. The pain becomes worse after activity or late in the day

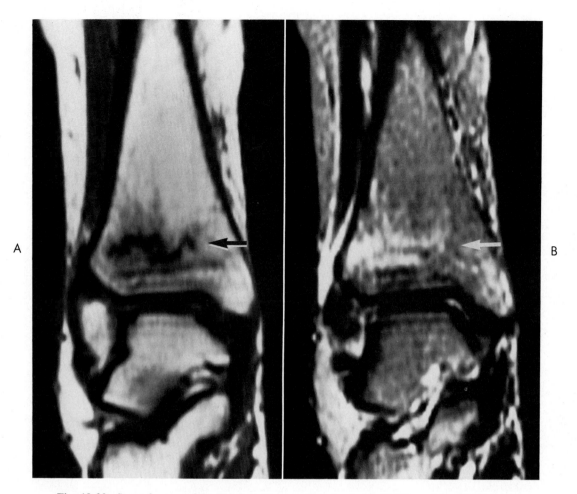

Fig. 19-20. Stress fracture of the tibia in a 52-year-old male. **A,** Sagittal T_1-weighted MRI image shows serpiginous low-signal stress fracture *(arrow)* with surrounding low-signal edema. **B,** Sagittal T_2-weighted MRI image shows high-signal edema at the same site *(arrow)*. (Reprinted with permission from Sacks RM, Salomon CG, and Demos TC: *Orthopedics* 13:1408, 1991.)

and is improved by rest. A history of specific activities, especially sports related, should be sought.

An older child is more likely to suffer from a stress fracture than a younger child because with age the cortical bone becomes less elastic and the periosteum more adherent. Therefore, in the very young child, there are few greenstick and torus fractures and almost no stress fractures. The most common locations of stress fractures in children are the calcaneus, neck or proximal shaft of the femur, proximal and distal tibia, and the distal metatarsals. The site of fractures in adults depends on the activity. Stress fractures of the metatarsal bones (march fractures) in adults are related to walking or running. Stress fractures of the ankle and feet are common in basketball players, whereas knee injuries typically occur in football players and skiers.

Joints affected by stress fractures continue to have full range of motion, with varying degrees of tenderness at the site of the fracture. There is usually little swelling, erythema, or increase in warmth.

Radiographic findings due to stress injuries are delayed and do not become visible for 1 to 3 weeks following the onset of symptoms. Both radionuclide bone scans and MRI, however, can demonstrate the lesion within days[33] (Fig. 19-20). In cortical bone, radiographic signs include periosteal new bone formation, focal cortical thickening, and a lucent fracture line (Fig. 19-21). This is the most common appearance in the shafts of long bones. In cancellous bone, a localized, often linear area of sclerosis is produced by trabecular collapse and endosteal callus. This pattern is common in the calcaneus (Fig. 19-22), pubic symphysis (Fig. 19-23), and the ends of long bones[34] (Fig. 19-24). Stress fractures of the tarsonavicular are especially difficult to identify on standard radiographs. Prolonged symptoms or a positive bone scan should lead to a special navicular radiographic view or a CT scan.[35]

The treatment of patients with stress fractures is reduction of weight bearing. Most patients have spontaneous resolution of their symptoms. If the activity continues, however, a complete fracture may result. Close follow-up

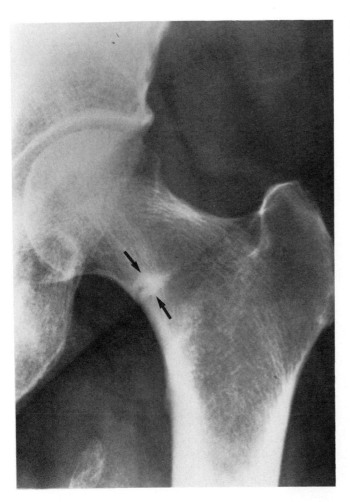

Fig. 19-21. Stress fracture of the femoral neck in a 59-year-old woman. AP radiograph of the left hip shows a lucency through the medial cortex of the femoral neck with surrounding sclerosis *(arrows)*. (Reprinted with permission from Demos TC: *Bone radiology case studies*, New Jersey, 1982, Slack Inc.)

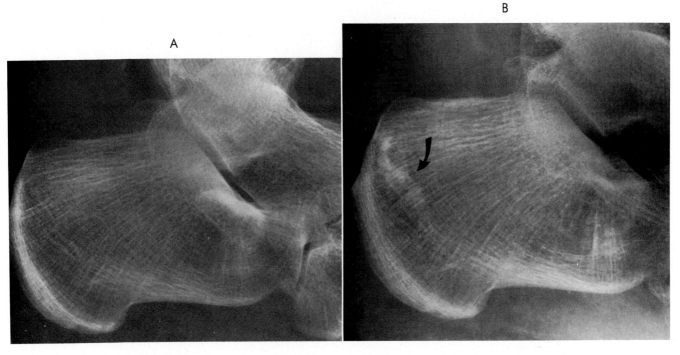

Fig. 19-22. Stress fracture of the left calcaneus in a 61-year-old woman. **A,** Lateral radiograph of the left calcaneus is normal except for osteoporosis. **B,** Sclerotic stress fracture *(arrow)* 2 months later.

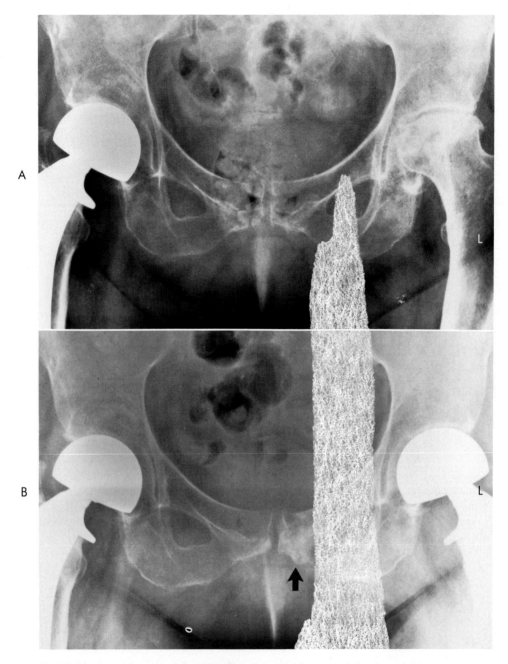

Fig. 19-23. Stress fracture of the pubis in a 61-year-old woman following total hip replacement. **A,** AP radiograph of the pelvis shows generalized osteoporosis, avascular necrosis of the left hip, and a right hip prosthesis. **B,** Six months after a left hip prosthesis, there is sclerosis of the left side of the pubis *(arrow)*.

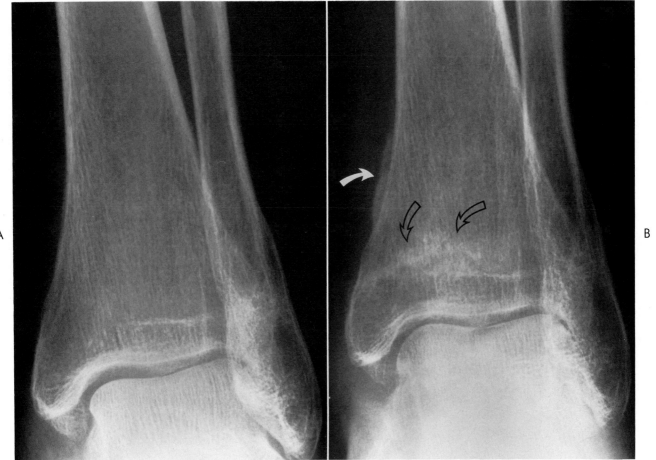

Fig. 19-24. Stress fracture of the tibia in a 61-year-old woman. **A,** AP radiograph of the left ankle shows a normal tibia except for osteoporosis. **B,** Sclerotic stress fracture *(open arrows).* Note
focus of periosteal new bone formation *(white arrows).*

is especially advised in children since avascular necrosis can complicate stress injuries of the hip and feet.

Nonaccidental trauma

Nonaccidental trauma (NAT) should be a consideration in any child under the age of 5 years who presents with a gait disturbance. This is especially true when the history concerning the event is clearly implausible, inconsistent, or there is significant delay in seeking help.

Although the skeletal and soft tissue lesions in NAT may take many forms, any fractures of the ribs, sternum, lateral clavicle, skull, and vertebrae are unusual and should arouse suspicion. Some types of fractures are characteristic of NAT. Metaphyseal corner fractures (small metaphyseal bone fragment) of the long bones occur when the child is held by the trunk or extremities and shaken violently, resulting in rotatory or shearing forces on the long bones. These metaphyseal fractures are common in the distal femur and distal tibia. An isolated spiral fracture of a long bone, especially the femur, should be considered suggestive of NAT when not accompanied by a history of significant trauma, such as falling from a great height or a pedestrian-automobile accident. The mechanism of injury for a spiral fracture of the femur is a rotatory force applied to the leg, at the level of the calf or knee. The ligamentous structures of the knee and hip generally provide good protection of these areas, and the major force is transmitted to the midshaft of the femur. Most fractures occur on the left side because of the right-handed dominance of most persons suspected of NAT. Falls from a bed or sofa seldom produce these types of fractures.

The characteristic metaphyseal corner fracture is a transverse fracture through the metaphysis near the epiphyseal plate. On radiographs this appears as a small metaphyseal bone fragment (corner fracture), a metaphyseal corner lucency, or a curved rim of displaced bone

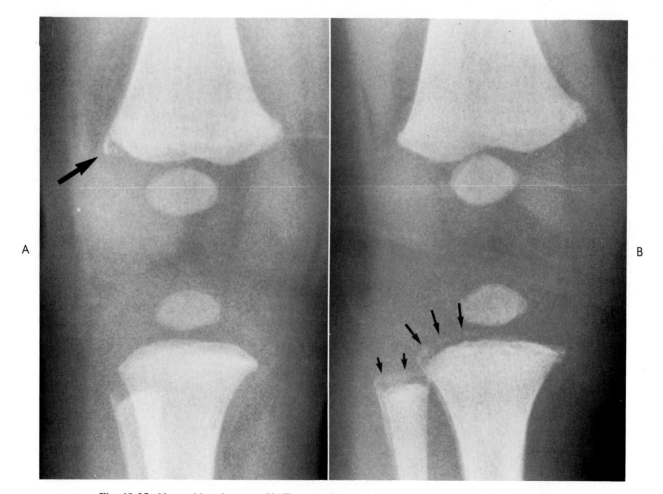

Fig. 19-25. Nonaccidental trauma (NAT) corner fracture and "bucket-handle" fracture. **A,** AP radiograph of the right knee demonstrates a small bone fragment *(arrow)* adjacent to the femoral metaphysis, which is highly suspicious for NAT. **B,** "Bucket-handle" fractures *(arrows)* have the same significance as a corner fracture. The appearance depends on the projection of the bone.

("bucket-handle" fracture). The appearance depends on the projection of the transverse fracture. (Fig. 19-25). All have the same significance. The corner lucency and corner fracture are often subtle and require high-quality radiographs for detection. A "babygram" is not sufficient to diagnose subtle fractures.[36]

NAT resulting in vertebral trauma rarely is the cause of gait disturbance. In these cases the injury occurs when the child is picked up and forced violently into a hard object such as a table edge or slammed downward onto a chair or countertop.

If a child has multiple fractures in varying phases of healing, NAT is a strong possibility. Such multiple fractures are often visible on radiographs. Radionuclide bone scans also have been used to screen for multiple injuries, including subtler and older injuries.[37]

Fractures suggestive of NAT are listed in the box opposite.

Legg-Calvé-Perthes disease

In 1910 Legg in the United States, Calvé in France, and Perthes in Germany described a debilitating disease of the hip. Legg-Calvé-Perthes disease (LCPD) is an ischemic disease of uncertain etiology occurring in children from 3 to 12 years of age (see Chapter 8). There is a 5:1 predominance in boys, and a poor prognosis when LCPD occurs in late childhood. Bilateral disease occurs in 20% of patients. The disease occurs with an increased frequency in ethnic groups from central Europe, Japan, and those of Eskimo origin.[38-40] Infants of low birth weight or abnormal presentation have a high incidence of LCPD. The bone age of children with LCPD demonstrates a delayed maturation of 1 to 3 years when compared with age-matched controls.

Possible causes for LCPD include trauma to the retinacular vessels, vascular occlusion from increased intracapsular pressure, transient synovitis, venous obstruction of the intraepiphyseal vessels, hyperviscosity, and congenital or developmental abnormalities. If one or more of these events occur, the resulting ischemia can cause a loss of enchondral ossification at the physeal plate. Revascularization occurs from the periphery, and new bone is deposited on old avascular bone. The avascular bone is gradually resorbed, causing a difference in the densities of the new vs. the old bone. Subchondral fractures are common during this process of new bone growth. If no subchondral fracture occurs, the patient is usually asymptomatic. When the subchondral fracture occurs, the collapse of bone damages the ingrowing capillaries, causing more ischemia and thus delaying the healing process and making the bone more susceptible to deformity during the remodelling process. Progressive deformity causes a malformed femoral capitus with a short femoral neck. The trochanter is not affected, which causes a change in the normal position of the hip abductors, resulting in a Trendelenburg gait and sign.

The acute presentation of LCPD generally is one of pain

Fractures suggestive of nonaccidental trauma (NAT)

Highly suggestive

Corner fractures
   Distal femur
   Distal humerus
   Distal tibia
   Radius
   Ulna
Isolated fractures
   Scapula
   Sternum
   Ribs
   Vertebrae

Suggestive but not specific

Spiral fractures
   Femur
   Humerus
   Tibia
Separation fractures
   Distal humeral epiphysis
   Distal femoral epiphysis
Metatarsal or metacarpal fractures
Skull fractures
Distal clavicle (acromium) fractures

---

referred to the groin, anterior thigh, or knee. Inflammation in the joint causes an antalgic limp, and there is limited hip motion, especially abduction and internal rotation. Patients present with complaints of dull pain over a period of weeks to months. The pain increases with activity.

The prognosis for LCPD depends on the age of the patient at onset, length of time before discovery, hip mobility remaining, the amount of remodelling and deformity that has occurred during healing, and the onset of osteoarthritis during adulthood.

Radiographs initially show lateral displacement of the femoral head, as indicated by slight widening of the joint space. This is nonspecific and similar in appearance to common transient synovitis. The femoral epiphysis may be smaller because of lack of growth. A curved subcortical fracture of the epiphysis is a relatively early radiographic sign but may only be visible on a frog-leg lateral view. This sign also occurs in adults with avascular necrosis (Fig. 19-26). Later, sclerosis and flattening of the femoral head occur, along with fragmentation (Fig. 19-27). Still later, metaphyseal lucencies represent foci of cartilage.

Radionuclide bone scans and MRI are the most sensitive means of diagnosing LCPD and avascular necrosis in the adult and allow diagnosis much earlier than radiographs[10,41,42] (Figs. 19-28 and 19-29). Even when LCPD is bilateral, the radiographic abnormalities are seldom symmetric. When there is symmetric bilateral fragmenta-

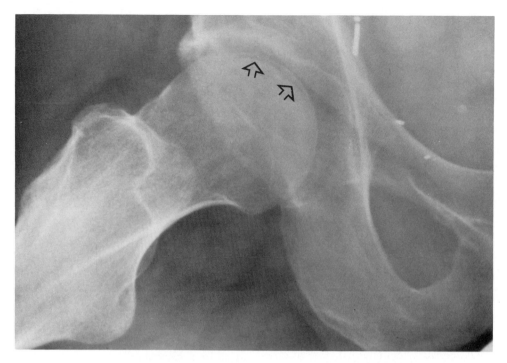

Fig. 19-26. Avascular necrosis of the hip in an adult. Frog-leg lateral radiograph of the right hip demonstrates a thin subcortical lucency *(open arrows)* in the head of the femur. This lucency is an early radiographic sign of avascular necrosis but occurs late in the evolution of the disease.

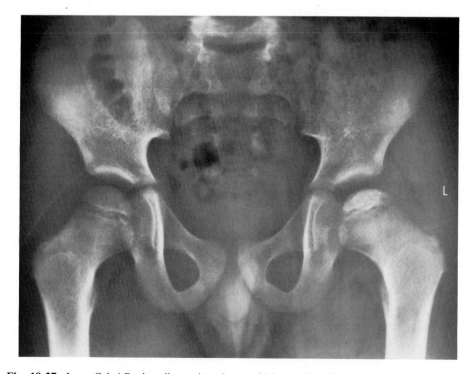

Fig. 19-27. Legg-Calvé-Perthes disease in a 6-year-old boy. AP radiograph of the pelvis demonstrates that the left capital femoral epiphysis is small, sclerotic, flattened, and irregular.

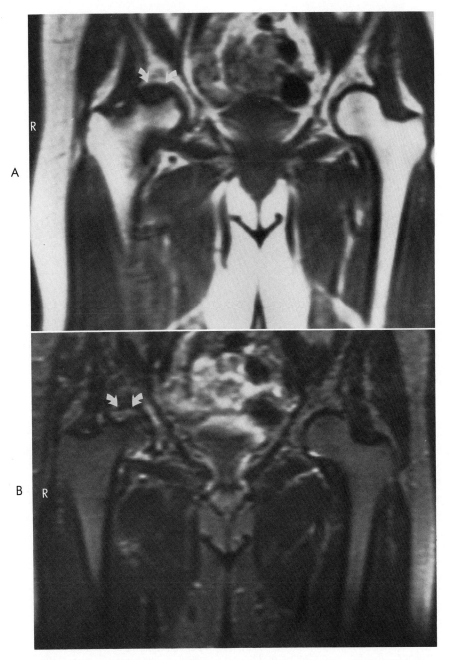

Fig. 19-28. Avascular necrosis in a 74-year-old man. **A,** T_1-weighted MRI image shows a low-signal lesion at the apex of the right femoral head *(arrows)* with a lower signal rim. **B,** T_1-weighted MRI image shows the lesion is now high signal but the low-signal rim is unchanged *(arrows)*. Radiographs were normal.

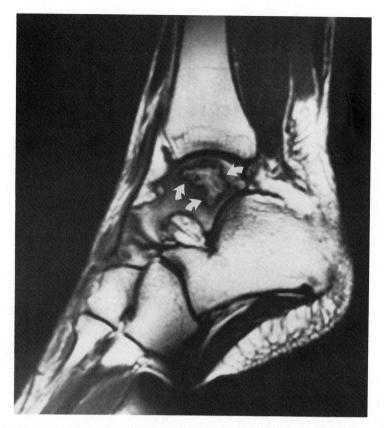

Fig. 19-29. Avascular necrosis of the right talus in a 39-year-old woman. T_1-weighted MRI image shows decreased signal of the talus *(arrows)* with a large irregular subarticular area of higher signal bounded by a rim of no signal, typical of avascular necrosis. Radiographs and conventional tomograms showed only a faint increase in the density of the talus.

tion, other diseases should be considered, including sickle cell disease, Gaucher disease, consequences of steroid therapy, hypothyroidism, and epiphyseal dysplasia.

Treatment goals are to reduce inflammation and hip irritability, restore or maintain maximal hip mobility, and minimize deformity. A regimen of bed rest, reduction of weight-bearing stress, physical rehabilitation for joint mobility, and surgical intervention to correct the deformity and the resulting severe osteoarthritis is suggested.

Slipped capital femoral epiphysis

Slipped capital femoral epiphysis (SCFE) affects predominantly the adolescent male with 5:2 ratio of male to female (see Chapter 8). The males range in age between 13 to 16 years, with a peak age of 13.5 years, whereas the females range in age between 11 to 14 years, with a peak age of 11.5 years.

The hallmark of SCFE is the progressive displacement of the femoral head relative to the femoral neck.[43] It is thought that the initial event may be secondary to minor trauma. There is an increased frequency of SCFE in patients with endocrinopathies. However, the role of some genetic abnormalities and endocrinopathies remains elusive although the common pathway appears to be a loosen-

Disorders associated with slipped capital femoral epiphysis	
Endocrine	*Iatrogenic*
Hypothyroidism	Radiation therapy
Hyperparathyroidism	Chemotherapy
Panhypopituitarism	Growth hormone administration
Pituitary tumor	
Acromegaly	*Metabolic*
Cryptorchidism	Riedel disease
	Renal osteodystrophy
Genetic	Rickets
Klinefelter syndrome	
Down syndrome	*Other*
Turner syndrome	Coxa vara
Marfan disease	Intracranial tumor
Froelich disease	Ovarian dysgenesis

ing or increased ability for migration of the femoral head at the epiphysis. The box above lists various disorders associated with SCFE.

The typical patient presents with dull pain, referred usually to the groin, thigh, or knee. The gait is antalgic and worsens with activity. SCFE is considered to be acute when the slippage is less than 3 weeks old and chronic when it is more than 3 weeks. There is also a small group of patients with acute slippage superimposed on chronic disease. The degree of slippage varies directly with the length of time symptoms have been present. Displacement is described as mild if one third of the surface area of contact between the head and neck has been traversed, moderate when one third to one half of the surface area is involved, and severe when greater than one half of the sur-

face area is involved. The migration of the head distorts the joint capsule and begins to restrict motion so that there is a decrease in the ability to internally rotate and abduct the hip. The patient with chronic slippage may have a Trendelenburg-like gait secondary to a shortened extremity and change in the structural integrity of the hip musculature, especially the major hip adductor, the gluteus medius muscle. Early detection limits deformity and disability. SCFE is bilateral in 25% of patients, but only 40% of these patients have symptoms in both hips at presentation.

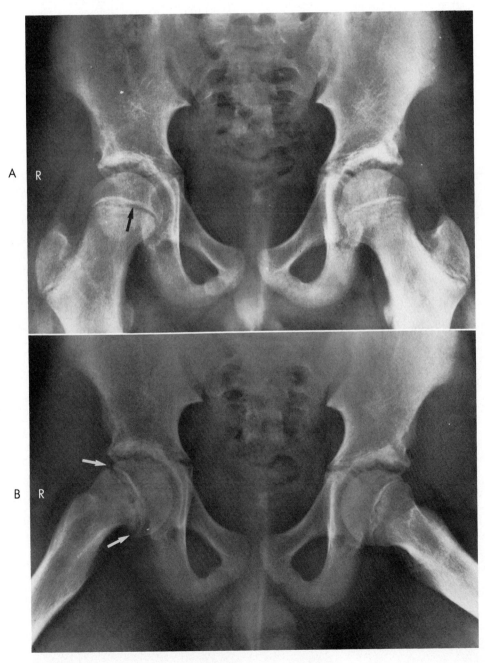

Fig. 19-30. Slipped capital femoral epiphysis in a 14-year-old boy. **A,** AP radiograph of the pelvis shows a slightly widened physis of the right hip *(arrow)* compared to the left hip. No slip is visible. **B,** The frog-leg lateral radiograph shows a slight posterior slip of the right capital femoral epiphysis *(arrows)*, better appreciated when compared to the opposite side.

The first radiographic sign of SCFE is increased lucency or widening of the physis. At this stage, the *preslip stage,* the epiphysis is normally aligned with the femoral neck. When slippage of the capital femoral epiphysis has occurred, it is primarily posterior so that early minimal displacement is best or only seen on a frog-leg lateral radiograph of the hip (Fig. 19-30). When slippage is chronic, the femoral neck becomes curved and there is thickening of the posteromedial cortex.[44]

Avascular necrosis complicates SCFE in about 10% of patients, usually those with moderate-to-severe slippage. Cartilage necrosis and atrophy of cartilage (chondrolysis) leads to degenerative changes in about 5% of patients.

The goal of treatment is to halt the progression of the disease and to re-establish normal joint morphology. Surgical intervention is the treatment of choice. Surgical approaches include epiphysiodesis, fixation, osteotomy, arthrodesis, and total joint replacement. Arthrodesis and

Table 19-2. Tumors associated with gait disturbances

Site	Diagnosis	Age (years)
Femur	Osteochondroma	5-25
Distal femur	Osteosarcoma	10-25
	Chondroblastoma	10-28
	Fibrosis dysplasia	5-20
	Nonossifying fibroma	5-25
	Unicameral bone cyst	5-20
	Aneurysmal bone cyst	5-25
Proximal femur	Chondrosarcoma	25-65
Tibia	Ostechondroma	5-25
Distal tibia	Nonossifying fibroma	5-25
Proximal tibia	Osteosarcoma	10-25
	Chondroblastoma	10-20
	Aneurysmal bone cyst	10-25
Pelvis	Myeloma	50-80
Spine	Myeloma	50-80

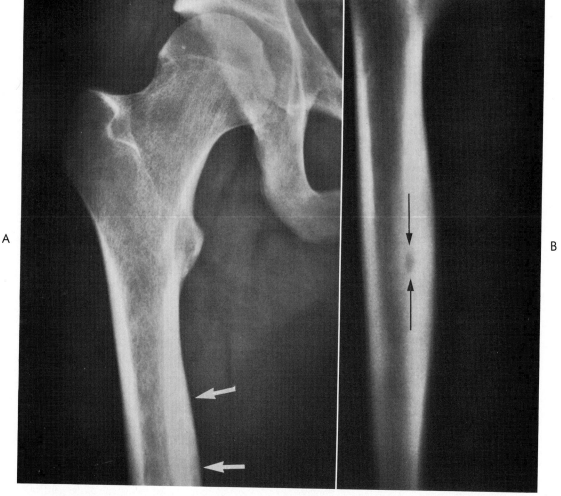

Fig. 19-31. Osteoid osteoma of the femur. **A,** AP radiograph of the femur shows marked thickening of the medial cortex *(arrows).* **B,** Conventional tomogram shows a small lucent nidus *(arrows)* that was obscured by dense cortical bone on the plain radiograph.

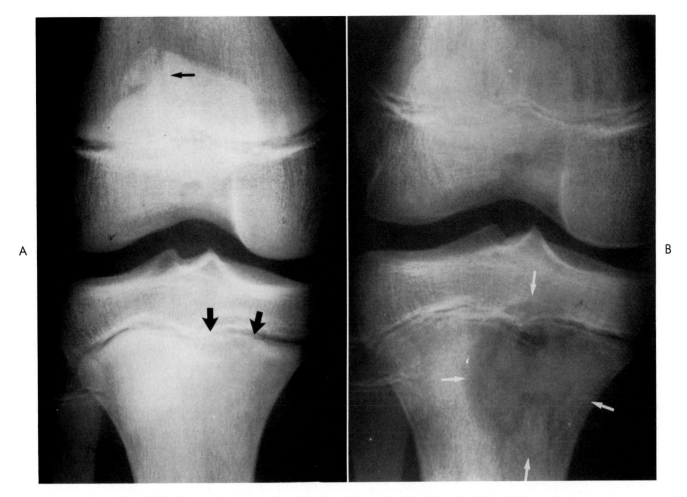

Fig. 19-32. Osteogenic sarcoma in an 11-year-old boy. **A,** AP radiograph of the right knee shows a very subtle difference in the medial and lateral aspects of the tibial metaphysis. The cortex next to the physis is less dense medially *(between vertical arrows)*. Incidentally, there is a bipartite patella *(horizontal arrow)*. **B,** Follow-up AP radiograph 3 weeks later shows obvious destruction of the medial side of the tibial metaphysis *(arrows)*. (Reprinted with permission from Ludkowski P, Demos TC: Orthopedics 4:1036, 1981.)

joint replacement are not optimal because arthrodesis leads to significant loss of joint mobility in this young population, and joint replacement carries the feature of repeated future replacements or structural failure in this physically active age group. However, the use of bed rest, hip spica cast application, and crutch walking have not prevented the sequelae of progression of the disease, avascular necrosis, and chrondrolysis.

NEOPLASTIC DISEASE

Altered gait as a presentation of neoplastic disease is usually a late manifestation but can be the initial sign. Skeletal lesions causing early gait disturbance include tumors of cartilage and bone that have a predilection for the distal metaphyses of the long bones. Bone tumors in the adult population are more often metastatic, and metastases should be considered in patients with breast, prostate, lung, kidney, or gastrointestinal malignancies who have

musculoskeletal complaints. Occasionally the initial presentation of a primary malignancy may be a pathologic fracture.

Neoplasms in the long bones of children or adolescents are closely related to the patient's age and to the location of the neoplasm.[45] Table 19-2 list the tumors that are likely to manifest as gait disturbances.

A neoplasm, malignant or benign, may present on a radiograph taken because of the patient's complaint of pain (Figs. 19-31 and 19-32). Such neoplasms can range from flagrant to subtle lesions, and the radiographic findings may include bone destruction, bone production, periosteal new bone formation, and soft tissue masses.

SUMMARY

A patient with an isolated gait disturbance can have a myriad of diseases. The key to identifying the cause starts with the patient history and physical examination. The physical examination must include a careful and complete evaluation of the gait, posture, and range of motion of the affected limb. The age, history of trauma, and acuity of onset are extremely helpful in refining the investigative process. Plain radiographs may demonstrate pathology or may be normal. If the physical examination is suggestive of an active process and the plain radiographs are not informative, a return visit and re-evaluation of the patient are recommended. Follow-up radiographs, a CT scan, radionuclide bone scan, or MRI should be obtained according to the results of this clinical evaluation.

REFERENCES

1. Tachojian MO: *Pediatric orthopedics,* Philadelphia, 1972, WB Saunders.
2. Hensinger RN: Limp, common orthopedic problems, *Pediatr Clin North Am* 33(6):1355, 1986.
3. Phillips WA: The child with a limp, *Orthop Clin North Am* 18(4):489, 1987.
4. Yablon IG: Limp in childhood, *J Fam Prac* 2(4):291, 1975.
5. Volpe RG: Alteration in gait in neuromuscular disease, *Clin Pediatr Med Surg* 5(3):627, 1988.
6. Sartoris DJ, Resnick D: Plain film radiography: routine and specialized techniques and projections. In Resnick D, Niwayama G, eds: *Diagnosis of bone and joint disorders,* ed 2, Philadelphia, 1988, WB Saunders.
7. Scheible W: Diagnostic ultrasound. In Resnick D, Niwayama G, eds: *Diagnosis of bone and joint disorders,* ed 2, Philadelphia, 1988, WB Saunders.
8. Marchal GJ, Van Holsbeeck MR, Roes M, et al: Transient synovitis of the hip in children: role of ultrasonography, *Radiology* 162:825, 1987.
9. Alazaraki N: Radionuclide techniques, In Resnick D, Niwayama G, eds: *Diagnosis of bone and joint disorders,* ed 2, Philadelphia, 1988, WB Saunders.
10. Murphy WA, Totty WG, Destouet JR et al: Musculoskeletal system. In Lee JKT, Sagel SS, and Stanley RJ, eds: *Computed body tomography with MRI correlation,* New York, 1988, Raven Press.
11. Hensinger RN: Congenital dislocation of the hip, *Orthop Clin North Am* 18(4):597, 1987.
12. Swischuk LE: *Imaging of the newborn, infant and young child,* ed 3, Baltimore, 1989, Williams & Wilkins.
13. Conway JJ, Cowell, HR: Tarsal coalition: clinical significance and roentgenographic demonstration, *Radiology* 92:799, 1969.
14. Sarno RC, Carter BL, and Bankoff MS: Computed tomography in tarsal coalition, *J Comput Assist Tomogr* 8:1155, 1984.
15. Scherr DD: Toeing in and toeing out in children, *Missouri Med,* 73:25, 1976.
16. Staheli LT: Rotational problems of the lower extremities, *Orthop Clin North Am* 18(4):503, 1987.
17. Ozonoff MB: *Pediatric orthopedic radiology,* Philadelphia, 1979, WB Saunders.
18. Dieppe PA, Bacon PA, Bamji AN, et al: *Atlas of clinical rheumatology,* Philadelphia, 1986, Lea & Febiger.
19. Brower AC: Arthritis in black and white, Philadelphia, 1988, WB Saunders.
20. Weissman BN: Spondyloarthropathies, *Radiol Clin North Am* 25:1235, 1987.
21. *Harrison's principles of internal medicine,* ed 12, New York, 1991, McGraw-Hill.
22. Ediken J: Radiologic approach to arthritis, *Semin Roentgenol* 17:8, 1982.
23. Resnick D, Niwayama G: Calcium pyrophosphate dihydrate (CPPD) crystal deposition disease. In Resnick D, Niwayama G: *Diagnosis of bone and joint disorters,* ed 2, Philadelphia, 1988, WB Saunders.
24. Klein RS: Joint infection, with consideration of underlying disease and sources of bacteremia in hematogenous infection, *Clin Geriatr Med* 4(2):375, 1988.
25. Shaw BA, Kasser JR: Acute septic arthritis in infancy and childhood, *Clin Orthop Related Res* 257:212, 1990.
26. Green NE, Edwards K: Bone and joint infections in children, *Orthop Clin North Am* 18(4):555, 1987.
27. Kallio P, Ryoppy S, Jappinen S et al: Ultrasonography in hip disease in children, *Acta Orthop Scand* 56:367, 1985.
28. Novick GS: Sonography in pediatric hip disorders, *Radiol Clin North Am* 26:29, 1988.
29. Edeiken J, Dalinka M, and Karasick D: Edeiken's Roentgen diagnosis of bone disease, Baltimore, 1990, Williams & Wilkens.
30. Gupta NC, Prezio JA: Radionuclide imaging in osteomyelitis, *Semin Nucl Med* 18:287, 1988.
31. David R, Barron BJ, and Madewell JE: Osteomyelitis, acute and chronic, *Radiol Clin North Am* 25:1171, 1987.
32. Miller WB Jr, Murphy WA, and Gilula LA: Brodie abscess: reappraisal, *Radiology* 132:15, 1979.
33. Mink JR, Deutsch AL: Occult cartilage and bone injuries of the knee: detection classification and assessment with MR imaging, *Radiology* 170:823, 1989.
34. Wilson ES Jr, Katz FN: Stress fractures: an analysis of 250 consecutive cases, *Radiology* 92:481, 1969.
35. Pavlov H, Torg JR, and Freiberger RH: Tarsal navicular stress fractures: radiographic evaluation, *Radiology* 148:641, 1983.
36. Kleinman PK: Diagnostic imaging in infant abuse, *AJR* 155:703, 1990.
37. Sty JR, Starshak RJ: Role of bone scintigraphy in the evaluation of the suspected abused child, *Radiology* 146:369, 1983.
38. Thompson GH, Salter RB: Legg-Calvé-Perthes disease, *Orthop Clin North Am* 18(4):617, 1987.
39. Barker DJP, Hal AJ: The epidemiology of perthes disease, *Clin Orthop Related Res* 1986, 209, pp 89-94.
40. Cotler JM: Office management in Legg-Calvé-Perthes syndrome, *Orthop Clin North Am* 13(3):619, 1982.
41. Danigelis JA, Fisher RL, Ozonoff MB et al: ^{99m}Tc-polyphosphate bone imaging in Legg-Perthes disease, *Radiology* 115:407, 1975.
42. Mitchell DG, Kressel HT: MR imaging of early avascular necrosis, *Radiology* 169:281, 1988.
43. Busch MT, Morrissy RT: Slipped capital femoral epiphysis, *Orthop Clin North Am* 18(4):637, 1987.
44. Schoenecker PL: Slipped capital femoral epiphysis, *Orthop Rev* 14:289, 1985.
45. Schubiner JM, Simon MA: Primary bone tumors in children, *Orthop Clin North Am* 18(4):577, 1987.

Hemiplegia and Paraplegia

Mary L. Dunne
Michael P. Earnest
David L. Symonds

The evaluation of a patient with focal weakness challenges the entire system of emergency care, requiring rapid coordination of multidisciplinary attention. In initiating care and directing evaluation, the emergency physician must synthesize the guiding tenets of emergency medicine and neurologic diagnosis and find the "life threat" based on the principles of neuroanatomic localization. This chapter will focus on acute patterns of presentation caused by structural nervous system lesions, on the appropriate radiographic evaluation, and on characteristic radiographic findings.

CLINICAL EVALUATION

The physician confronted with a patient with focal weakness has a critical responsibility: to understand the pathologic process as completely as possible in order to reverse or minimize its effects. Failure to recognize treatable conditions may result in permanent neurologic impairment or death.

It is important to identify patients whose history or physical examination reveals "red flags." These data suggest processes that may require urgent intervention (see the box above).

As in all emergency care, patient history, physical examination, stabilization, and laboratory evaluation should

---

Clinical "red flags" in patients with focal weakness

History

Very rapid onset
Trauma
Headache or spine pain
Recent infection (especially ENT)
Known cancer
Immunosuppression (steroids, chemotherapy, AIDS)
Coagulopathy (especially anticoagulant therapy)
Drug abuse
Alcoholism

Physical examination

Evidence of trauma
Fever
Suppurative focus
Ataxia in absence of intoxication
Hypertension
Bradycardia
Depression of consciousness

---

proceed concomitantly. Appropriate laboratory studies focus on identifying conditions that may contribute to pathology or complicate evaluation or treatment. Patients with acute focal weakness should have complete blood and platelet counts, ESR, blood chemistry analysis (to evaluate renal, hepatic, and cardiac status), and a coagulation profile. Hypoglycemia, which can cause focal neurologic deficit, should be measured by quick bedside testing. Selected patients may require blood cultures, arterial blood gases, sickle cell preparation, or a drug screen. An electrocardiogram and chest radiograph should be assessed.

Early consultation with radiologic, neurologic, and neurosurgical colleagues is essential. Direct and timely discussion of clinical information with consultants allows optimal use of available technology, helps identify patients who may require invasive procedures or surgical intervention, and facilitates an appropriate diagnostic sequence.

None of the preceding procedures need impede the patient's progress to definitive evaluation in the radiology department. When patients leave the emergency department they should be attended by personnel able to recognize and initiate intervention should precipitous deterioration (seizures, dysrhythmias, apnea, brain herniation, or cardiac arrest) occur.

FOCUSED NEUROLOGIC EXAMINATION

As always, the physician must first attend to the ABCs of emergency care: airway, breathing, circulation, and appropriate resuscitation. *D* in this alphabet represents "disability." This paradigm next directs attention to level of consciousness, signs of increased intracranial pressure, and maintenance of spinal immobilization if appropriate. On secondary assessment, attention can be directed to the complaint or finding of focal weakness. Since altered consciousness (see Chapter 15), head trauma (Chapter 3), and spinal trauma (Chapter 9) are considered elsewhere, this chapter will focus on patterns of motor weakness independent of those contexts.

Weakness is used by patients to describe a variety of subjective complaints. The clinician must elicit and elucidate symptoms that vary in their diagnostic importance and prognostic significance, including fatigue, lassitude, faintness, vertigo, and loss of muscular strength. Patients may sometimes use *numbness* to describe motor weakness. The patient may *not* complain of findings that are striking to the examiner, which underscores the importance of an objective, consistently practiced neurologic assessment.

Motor function can be compromised at any level in the motor pathway, from the cerebral cortex to the biochemical milieu of the muscle cell. *Paralysis, palsy,* and *plegia* have different linguistic derivations but are used interchangeably for loss of motor function; *paresis* denotes a lesser degree of impairment. In terms of emergency evaluation, there is no difference in the implications of the descriptors or the physical findings they represent.

The emergency neurologic examination must be appropriate to the setting and the complaint. This initial physical examination directs further diagnostic evaluation and documents a baseline by which future observations are compared.

Beyond assessing level of consciousness and mental status (accomplished informally by interaction with the patient), the focused neurologic examination has five components: eyes (pupils, EOM, corneal reflexes, fundi); face (symmetry); limbs (strength, DTRs, Babinski reflex); cerebellar function (finger to nose, heel to shin, gait); and sensory function. The sensory examination (the most difficult to perform, reproduce, and interpret) is best directed by patient complaint and by any abnormalities found in the rest of the examination. At a minimum, posterior column

Table 20-1. Some common patterns of focal neurologic signs and lesion localization

Distribution of weakness	Usual localization
Hemiparesis	
With facial weakness, hemisensory loss, aphasia, or hemianopia	Cerebral hemisphere
Without other findings	Lacunar infarction deep in cerebral hemisphere or pons
With contralateral cranial nerve findings	Brain stem
With contralateral trunk and limb sensory loss	Cervical spinal cord
Quadriparesis (without eye or bulbar signs)	Cervical spinal cord or area affected by diffuse neuromuscular disease
Paraparesis	Thoracic or lower cord or cauda equina
Monoparesis (most muscles of one limb)	Brachial or lumbar plexus (rule out small cerebral cortex lesion)
Isolated muscles of one limb	Peripheral nerve or spinal root lesion
Bilateral distal arm and leg weakness with numbness	Peripheral polyneuropathy
Bilateral proximal limb weakness without numbness	Muscle or neuromuscular junction
Acute ophthalmoparesis or bulbar weakness with variable extremity weakness	Guillain-Barré, botulism, myasthenia gravis, tick paralysis, diphtheria, organophosphate toxicity

Modified from Earnest ME: Principles of early diagnosis and management. In Earnest ME, ed: *Neurologic emergencies,* New York, 1983, Churchill-Livingstone.

(position, vibration) and spinothalamic (pain) function should be tested distally in each extremity. The sensory examination must be pursued in detail if a spinal cord or peripheral nerve lesion is suspected.

LOCALIZATION

Once the existence of a neurologic problem is established, the physical findings are analyzed to localize the causative lesion in the nervous system. While the emergency physician need not accomplish this precisely, a general location must be postulated in order to guide further diagnostic evaluation (Table 20-1).

In addition to defining weakness in its gross anatomic distribution, differentiating between upper and lower motor neuron characteristics can be essential to localization.

The term *upper motor neuron (UMN)* encompasses all the pathways by which the cerebral cortex influences the cranial nerve nuclei or spinal motor neurons. The corticospinal, or pyramidal, tract descends from the cerebral cortex, decussates in the lower medulla, and continues caudad in the lateral funiculus of the spinal cord to synapse di-

Table 20-2. Upper vs. lower motor neuron lesion findings

Findings	UMNs	LMNs
Tone	Hyperactive	Flaccid
DTRs	Increased	Decreased/absent
Babinski reflex	Present	Absent
Fasiculations	Absent	May be present
Atrophy (if present)	Mild (disuse)	Pronounced (denervation)

rectly or via interneurons with the anterior horn cells (or cranial nerve nuclei). Thus the UMNs begin in the cerebral cortex, end in the spinal cord, and can be interrupted at any level: cortex, white matter, internal capsule, brain stem, or spinal cord.

The term *lower motor neuron (LMN)* encompasses the anterior horn cell (or cranial nerve nucleus), its axon, and its motor end plates in the innervated muscle fibers. The motor nerve fibers of the spinal ventral roots intermingle as the roots join to form plexuses and peripheral nerves. These efferent motor axons combine with afferent sensory axons in the plexuses and peripheral nerves, thus combining motor and sensory functions.

The distribution of weakness from an UMN lesion will vary with location, but certain features are characteristic. Muscles are affected in groups, rather than individually. Antigravity muscles are affected more than others. Muscle tone is increased and tendon reflexes below the level of the lesion become hyperactive. In an acute spinal cord lesion, however, reflexes below the lesion may be temporarily abolished, a condition known as "spinal shock." The Babinski reflex (upgoing toe) is a sign of an UMN lesion. Mild atrophy, from disuse of paralyzed muscles, may be seen with chronic UMN lesions.

In LMN lesions, all voluntary and reflex movements are abolished, muscle tone is reduced, DTRs are reduced or abolished, and the denervated muscle undergoes profound atrophy, losing 20% to 30% of its bulk within 3 months[1] (Table 20-2).

ACUTE HEMIPLEGIA
Radiographic evaluation

Skull radiography. In the absence of trauma, plain radiographs of the skull have no place in the evaluation of patients with acute hemiplegia (or sudden onset of paralysis in the upper and lower extremities on one side of the body). While plain radiographs may be abnormal in rare instances (e.g., shift of calcified pineal gland), they have no bearing on management and only delay definitive evaluation.

For reference, a skull series involves a radiation dose of about 1 rad.[2]

Computed tomography. Computed tomography (CT scan) is currently the most widely available imaging mo-

dality for the definitive neuroradiologic evaluation. It is extremely sensitive in detecting pathology that distorts normal anatomy (hemorrhage, neoplasm, abscess, hydrocephalus); somewhat less sensitive for the detection of brain infarction, arteriovenous malformation (AVM), and aneurysm (depending on size and location); and still less sensitive in detecting white matter disease and leptomeningeal processes. The CT scan may be relatively nonspecific: infection, infarction, and neoplasm can be difficult to distinguish on the scan alone.

Injection of intravenous contrast material serves to heighten differences in tissue density and improve detectability of lesions. Many lesions will "enhance" or demonstrate increased density after intravenous contrast material administration, especially those that are hypervascular (tumor, AVM) or that alter the blood-brain barrier with leakage of contrast material into the abnormal tissue (infarction, abscess, many tumors) (see Chapter 17 and the Appendix).

The CT scan is rapid, requiring approximately 10 minutes for an uninterrupted series of sections for brain imaging. Monitoring and life-support equipment do not interfere with the scan.

The radiation dose varies from 2 to 5 rads depending on technical factors and the number of sections obtained.[2] With a head CT scan the gonadal dose is insignificant.[3]

Disadvantages. Given the relative lack of specificity of the CT scan, additional modalities (MRI, angiography) may be required to further characterize a lesion. The CT scan has contrast resolution limitations, and brain lesions smaller than 5 mm may be missed. The scan is also degraded by bone artifact, and lesions close to dense skull (posterior fossa, base of the brain, temporal lobe) may be obscured.

Despite these factors, the CT scan remains the modality of choice for most emergency neurologic imaging of the central nervous system because of its wide availability, rapid accessibility, and short scanning time.

Magnetic resonance imaging. Magnetic resonance imaging (MRI) uses the magnetic characteristics of tissue protons to create image slices. It involves no ionizing radiation and has no known biologic hazard. While the influence of strong magnetic fields on development has not been determined, no fetal effect has been found after MRI.[4]

Since most brain pathology alters tissue water content such a change is discernable by MRI. In patients with neurologic signs, MRI identifies pathology in 30% more cases than a CT scan.[5] MRI depicts soft tissue anatomy and demonstrates white matter disease far better than a CT scan. Bone exerts little or no signal and has no disturbing influence on images. MRI can be electronically selected in any plane, as compared to the axial images of the CT scan. Edema and abnormal vascularity are readily detectable by MRI without the contrast agents necessary in a CT scan. Intravenous injection of gadolinium, a paramagnetic agent that enhances the process of proton relaxation, per-

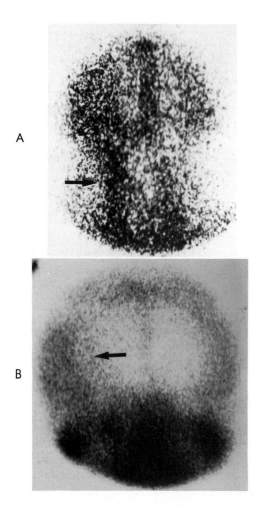

Fig. 20-1. Radionuclide brain scan in herpes encephalitis. **A,** Anterior flow image shows increased activity in the right neck vessels *(arrow).* **B,** Static image demonstrates increased uptake in the lateral and inferior right cerebral hemisphere *(arrow).*

mits even sharper delineation of these lesions. Such enhancement makes it possible to visualize even small lesions and to differentiate between a lesion and its surrounding edema.

Disadvantages. On the negative side, the use of MRI in emergency patients is presently limited. Ferromagnetic objects (such as life-support equipment, cardiac pacemakers, aneurysm clips) cannot be placed in the scanner area. Patients with cochlear implants or ocular metallic foreign bodies should not undergo MRI. A high degree of patient cooperation is required, given the greater vulnerability of MRI to motion artifact and the longer imaging time needed compared to the CT scan. Once the imaging sequence is started, manipulation of the patient is not possible.[6] Also, where MRI is available, the scanner site (which requires magnetic shielding and is often a late addition to the hospital) is apt to be remote from the emergency department.

Given the superior imaging capability and lack of patient hazard, MRI will undoubtedly play an increasingly larger role in emergency diagnosis as the technical limitations are overcome.

Radionuclide brain scan. Radionuclide brain scan has largely been replaced by the CT scan and MRI. While not an emergency imaging technique, it may be useful in patient evaluation in some circumstances, particularly when possibility of a brain lesion is great, the CT scan is negative, and MRI is not available. Such may be the case in herpes encephalitis, metastatic disease, and superficial brain infarction.[2] Radionuclide brain scan can also be used to evaluate cerebral perfusion, brain death, and blood pool lesions such as AVM and aneurysm.

The study has two phases. The *dynamic* phase of rapid sequence images, performed just after radionuclide injection, evaluates cerebral perfusion. The *static* phase is assessed 1 to 3 hours after injection to evaluate the blood-brain barrier (Fig. 20-1).

Ultrasonography. Direct methods of noninvasive carotid artery imaging include real-time B-mode ultrasonographic imaging, Doppler flow mapping, and color flow scanning. These modalities, respectively, evaluate the vessel wall, the vessel lumen, and the presence and direction of blood flow. Duplex ultrasonography or Doppler duplex combines real-time B-mode imaging and Doppler instrumentation with the two crystals in a single transducer.

Real-time B-mode imaging. Ultrasonography evaluates the vessel wall for the presence and character of arteriosclerotic plaque. Plaque with few and similar internal echoes is deemed homogenous; plaque with internal echo signals of varying amplitudes is considered heterogeneous. Heterogeneity denotes ulceration and intraplaque hemorrhage, which has been implicated as a source of cerebral embolism. Ultrasonography appears to be superior to angiography in characterizing these lesions.[7,8]

Doppler ultrasonography. Doppler evaluation detects the increased frequency (representing increased flow velocity) and spectral broadening (representing the mixed velocities of turbulent flow) associated with vascular stenosis (Fig. 20-2). Quantification of the frequency analysis allows estimation of the severity of vascular disease.[9] Doppler imaging reliably characterizes stenosis with lesions that narrow the vessel lumen by more than 50%.[7,8]

Color flow imaging. Color flow imaging is based on pulsed Doppler ultrasonography with color-coded Doppler information superimposed on the real-time image. In essence, flowing blood becomes its own contrast medium. The conventional red and blue colors represent blood flow toward or away from the transducer. Color flow imaging is valuable in detecting channels of flow in areas of tight stenosis and improves the ultrasonographic distinction between high-grade stenosis and occlusion.

Application of Doppler duplex to the vertebrobasilar system is limited. Ultrasonography can aid in the diagnosis of the subclavian steal syndrome, demonstrating reversal of flow in the vertebral artery (the collateral pathway circumventing the subclavian stenosis).

Angiography. Since the advent of the CT scan, MRI, and advanced ultrasonographic techniques, cerebral an-

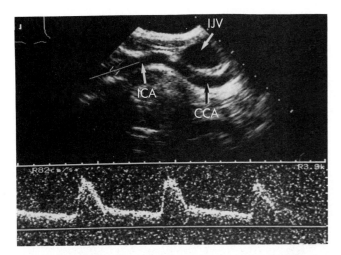

Fig. 20-2. Carotid Doppler duplex. Sagittal ultrasonographic image of the right side of the neck shows common carotid artery *(CCA)*, internal carotid artery *(ICA)*, and internal jugular vein *(IJV)*. Cursor *(line)* in the internal carotid artery identifies location of flow velocity *(displayed at bottom)* measurement.

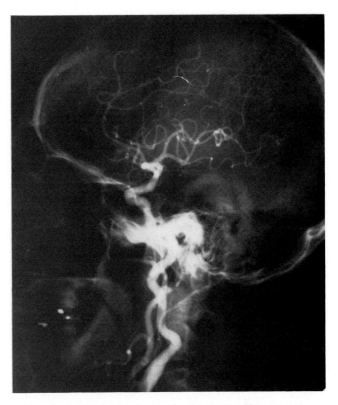

Fig. 20-3. Normal common carotid angiogram, lateral view.

giography is reserved to add specificity to noninvasive diagnosis, to evaluate vascular lesions beyond the spatial resolution of the CT scan and MRI, to evaluate vascular flow, and to evaluate anatomy pre-operatively (Fig. 20-3) (see Chapters 3 and 15).

The procedure consists of fluoroscopic placement of an angiographic catheter and injection of water-soluble contrast material and requires special expertise in both performance and interpretation. The study carries risk even in the most expert hands. Post-angiographic complication rates range from 1% to 12%[10,11] in elective series and include minor puncture site complications, contrast reactions, and (rarely) irreversible stroke and death (1/1000).[12] The radiation dose is significant, involving an average of 30 rads to the target area.[13]

Digital subtraction angiography. In digital subtraction angiography (DSA), the pre-injection "scout" image is electronically subtracted from all subsequent images, which display only the contrast medium in the blood vessels; the rapidly generated computer-intensified and amplified image appears near real-time on video display monitors (Fig. 20-4). With DSA, exact catheter placement becomes less critical, the volume of contrast material may be decreased by 60% to 75%, and the procedure is less time-consuming. Intravenous DSA has been replaced by small caliber catheterization of the brachial or femoral arteries.

However, the final DSA image is of lower quality than conventional angiography. The techniques are often integrated during a single examination to maximize both patient safety and image quality.

Positron emission tomography. Positron emission tomography (PET) involves the injection or inhalation of positron-emitting radionuclides (2-F^{18}fluro-2-deoxy-D-glucose [FDG] or N^{13}-ammonia) for a CT scan. Axial images are generated that reflect regional brain biochemical activity. In stroke, PET demonstrates abnormalities earlier than the CT scan and has been used to distinguish viable from nonviable brain tissue.[14]

The cost of PET instrumentation and the cyclotron required to produce the isotopes limits PET imaging to major medical centers.

Single photon emission computed tomography. Single photon emission computed tomography (SPECT) can be performed using conventional radioisotopes with conventional nuclear medicine cameras that have been modified to rotate 360 degrees around the patient. The images (axial sections similar to those of the CT scan) can demonstrate perfusion abnormalities before the CT scan evidence of infarction (Fig. 20-5). In addition, SPECT may demonstrate perfusion abnormalities in patients with transient ischemic attacks when CT scans are normal. In stroke, the size of the perfusion deficit has been shown to have a predictive value for the degree of neurologic recovery.[15]

SPECT is much less costly and complex than PET. While not an emergency imaging technique, it is being applied in the emergency clinical setting with increasing frequency.

Structural causes of hemiplegia

Stroke. Cerebrovascular disease remains a significant cause of morbidity and mortality. Overall, it is by far the commonest cause of acute hemiplegia.

A

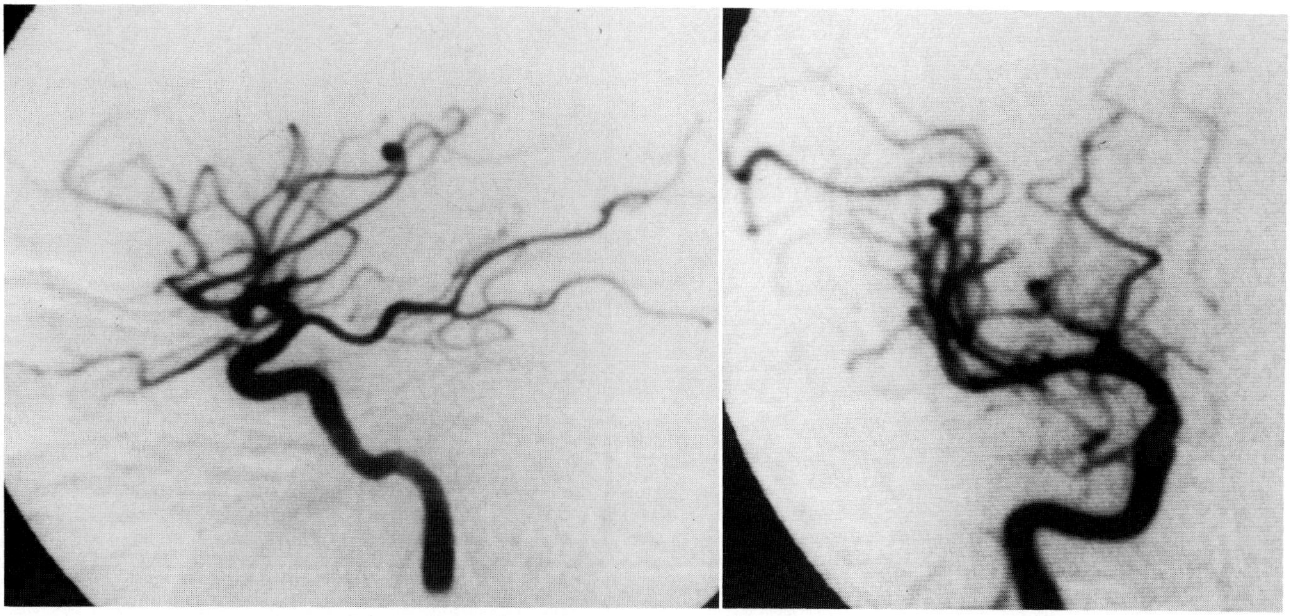

B

Fig. 20-4. Normal intra-arterial digital subtraction cerebral angiogram. **A,** Lateral view. **B,** Anteroposterior view.

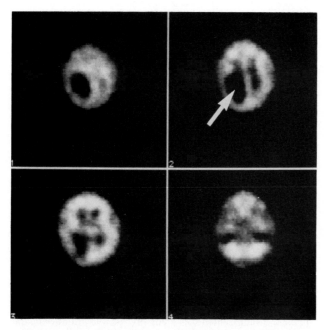

Fig. 20-5. Brain SPECT. Axial brain perfusion images (HM-PAO) demonstrate enlargement of the right lateral ventricle *(arrow)* in a patient with a seizure disorder. (Courtesy Dawn Bedrosian, MD, University Hospital, Denver, Colorado.)

After examining the acutely hemiplegic patient, the clinician will have formed an etiologic postulate based on the patient's demographic, historic, and physical findings. The diagnostic sequence, ideally determined with radiographic and neurologic consultants, generally proceeds as described in the following discussion.

The CT scan demonstrates or excludes parenchymal and large subarachnoid hemorrhage (SAH) and nonstroke mass lesions (the latter may require contrast material for clarification). However, since cerebral infarction is the most common cause of stroke and may not be visualized for hours to days, it will still need to be excluded, as well as encephalitis, meningitis, and subarachnoid hemorrhage (Fig. 20-6).

If meningitis, encephalitis, or subarachnoid hemorrhage are the considered diagnoses, a lumbar puncture should be performed. If acute carotid artery pathology is considered, Doppler duplex and color flow studies can identify patients who are candidates for angiography. If the CT scan is nondiagnostic and the lumbar puncture is negative or not indicated, further evaluation is individualized based on the clinical setting and diagnostic resources.

Ischemic cerebral infarction. Brain infarction commonly develops by two pathophysiologically distinct mechanisms. Blood flow may be blocked by a thrombus, generally from arteriosclerotic narrowing or by an embolus from a more proximal arterial or cardiac source. Less common causes of infarction include profound or prolonged hypotension, blood coagulation disorders, vasculitis, venous thrombosis, and carotid artery dissection.

Cerebral infarction usually occurs in the distribution of a single major vessel; most involve the middle cerebral artery (the main intracranial branch of the internal carotid artery) and affect the lateral aspect of the cerebral hemisphere.

CT scan in cerebral infarction. The CT scan may detect cerebral infarction as early as 3 to 6 hours after onset

ACUTE HEMIPLEGIA: DIAGNOSTIC SEQUENCE

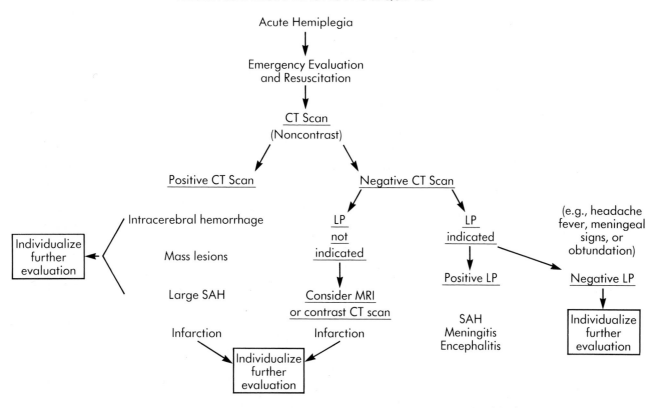

Fig. 20-6. Algorithm for the diagnostic sequence of imaging for acute hemiplegia.

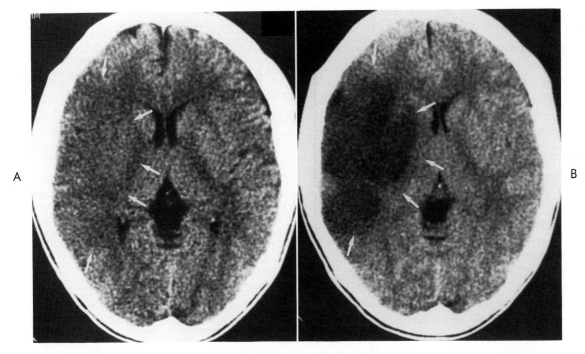

Fig. 20-7. CT scan of an acute cerebral infarction. **A,** Nonenhanced scan 5 hours after the onset of symptoms shows a subtle decrease in the density of gray matter in the right middle cerebral artery territory *(arrows)*. **B,** After 48 hours the infarction has a mass effect and is well defined *(arrows)*.

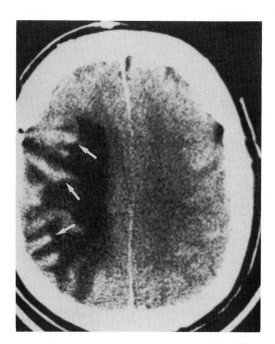

Fig. 20-8. Nonenhanced CT scan of hemorrhagic infarction reveals areas of gyral hemorrhage *(arrows)* in a subacute right middle cerebral artery infarction.

of symptoms. More commonly, an ill-defined low-density area evolves between 1 and 3 days after the insult. Cerebral edema may be seen within hours of infarction, and a large infarction may demonstrate a mass effect. Five percent to 10% of completed infarctions are isodense on a nonenhanced CT scan; contrast enhancement of the infarction can be seen as early as 1 day (Fig. 20-7) but may not be seen for 5 to 7 days after the event.[16-18]

Cerebral infarction is complicated by hemorrhage into the infarction zone in 18% to 23% of cases; such hemorrhagic infarctions are usually the result of embolism but may follow cortical vein or venous sinus thrombosis.[19] Hemorrhagic infarction appears as a high-density wedge-shaped area with ill-defined margins, usually involving the cortex with extension into the white matter (Fig. 20-8).

MRI in cerebral infarction. Although the CT scan has been the "gold standard" for emergency evaluation of suspected cerebral infarction, a significant number of infarctions (50%) are not visible in the first 24 hours and some are not visible for several days.[20] MRI may be positive 2 to 4 hours after the ictus.[3,21] During the acute phase of infarction, ischemia causes cytotoxic and early vasogenic edema, resulting in increased water content in affected brain tissue; those areas yield a higher intensity signal on the T_2-weighted MRI image. In addition, the superior contrast resolution of MRI allows identification of smaller areas of infarction than are visible on the CT scan.[21] Therefore MRI is far superior for imaging the posterior fossa, where bone artifact degrades CT scan images (Fig. 20-9).

Posterior fossa infarction. While posterior fossa infarction is uncommon, it carries a risk of precipitous deterioration. Cerebellar infarction may develop significant

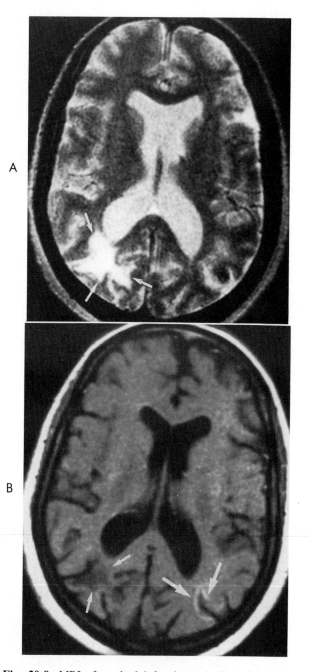

Fig. 20-9. MRI of cerebral infarctions. **A,** T_2-weighted image shows an increased signal *(arrows)* in the gray and white matter from old infarction. **B,** T_1-weighted image after intravenous administration of gadolinium demonstrates a low-intensity old infarction *(small arrows)* on the right and a gyral enhancement in the subacute infarction on the left *(large arrows).*

edema and mass effect, with acute hydrocephalus and brain stem compression (Fig. 20-10). Any patient with demonstrated cerebellar infarction, or with stroke and cerebellar signs, must be closely observed. Deterioration should prompt repeat scanning and preparation to manage brain stem herniation. Neurosurgical decompression of the posterior fossa and excision of the infarcted cerebellar tissue may be necessary.[22]

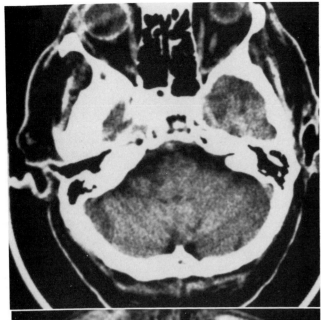

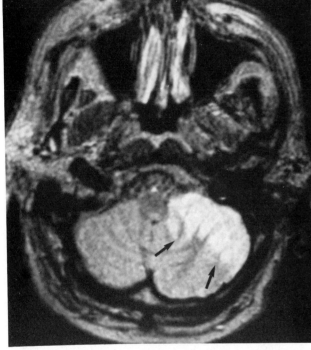

Fig. 20-10. Cerebellar infarction. **A,** Early nonenhanced CT scan does not demonstrate an infarction. **B,** T₂-weighted MRI image 3 days later shows an infarction *(arrows)* involving the anteroinferior left cerebellar hemisphere. (Courtesy David Rubenstein, MD, University Hospital, Denver, Colorado.)

A dangerous cause of brain stem and cerebellar infarction is basilar artery thrombosis. Any patient with suspected posterior fossa ischemia should be closely followed for increasing neurologic signs. If they occur, urgent angiography and anticoagulation must be considered.

Lacunar infarction. As opposed to hemispheric infarction resulting from occlusion in the larger branches of the

Table 20-3. Lacunar syndromes

Syndrome	Lesion location
Pure motor stroke (66%) Hemiplegia *without* aphasia, sensory, or visual field deficits	Internal capsule or pons
Dysarthria (20%) Dysarthria, central facial weakness, clumsiness of fine hand movement, ataxia, dysmetria	Contralateral pons
Pure sensory stroke (10%) Hemisensory numbness/tingling without motor signs or symptoms	Thalamus
Ataxic hemiparesis (4%) Prominent limb clumsiness, plus weakness that affects lower limb more than upper	Corona radiata

carotid or vertebrobasilar systems, lacunar infarctions are small (0.2 to 2.0 cm) lesions deep within the brain caused by thrombosis of small penetrating arteries. Lacunar infarctions are seen in patients with chronic hypertension; they comprise approximately 10% of recognized strokes. "Lacunes" (holes or lakes) are characterized as such by their small size and typical location (putamen, pons, thalamus, caudate nucleus, internal capsule). While some lesions may cause variable or no symptoms, four common clinical syndromes are recognized: pure motor stroke, dysarthrias, pure sensory stroke, and ataxic hemiparesis (Table 20-3).

Patients who manifest these patterns may be clinically recognized as having a lacunar stroke. CT scan will detect 50% to 75% of these infarctions [23] (Fig. 20-11, *A*). Those likely to be missed are less than 5 mm in diameter or located at the level of the pons, where bone artifact compromises visualization of small nonhemorrhagic lesions. MRI, with superior spatial resolution and lack of bone artifacts, more reliably demonstrates lacunar lesions (Fig. 20-11, *B*).

Emergency angiography in ischemic stroke. While the role of angiography in acute ischemic cerebrovascular disease remains controversial, angiography should be considered in certain clinical situations:

- A young patient with apparent stroke, negative CT scan, and rapid neurologic deterioration, especially if signs and symptoms suggest carotid distribution. In such cases, severe carotid stenosis, carotid intraluminal dissection, or aortic dissection should be actively sought; angiography is the definitive test.
- Acute carotid occlusion. This should be considered in the setting of stroke following anterior neck trauma,

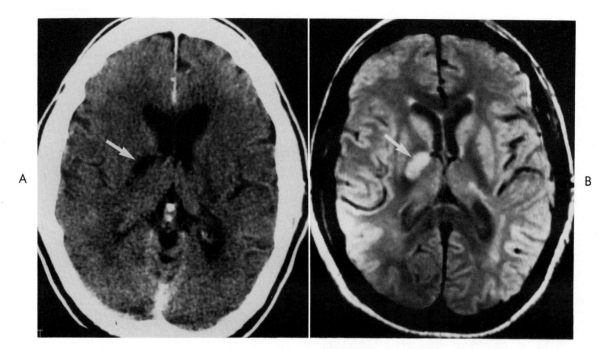

Fig. 20-11. Lacunar infarction. **A,** Nonenhanced CT scan shows a low-density infarction *(arrow)* involving the posterior limb of the right internal capsule. **B,** Infarction is of high intensity *(arrow)* on T$_2$-weighted MRI image.

Anterior and posterior circulation ischemic symptoms

Anterior (carotid)

Hemiparesis
Hemisensory loss
Aphasia
Monocular blindness

Posterior (vertebral-basilar)

Ataxia
Vertigo
Dysarthria
Diplopia
Facial paresthesias
Bilateral limb sensory or motor symptoms
Loss of consciousness
Drop attacks

---

neck surgery, or carotid angiography, or in an acute stroke patient who has anterior neck pain or tenderness. Emergency removal of the carotid thrombus within a few hours of occlusion may reverse the stroke.[24,25]

A young patient with suspected embolic stroke but no clear cardiac source of embolism. Angiography may be required to confirm the mechanism of stroke before anticoagulation.

Transient ischemic attack. Transient ischemic attack (TIA) describes an episode of acute neurologic deficit caused by inadequate blood flow that resolves completely in less than 24 hours. Most TIAs resolve within minutes or hours. While a TIA may reflect involvement of any cerebrovascular territory, symptoms may be usefully divided into two syndromes: anterior, or carotid, and posterior, or vertebrobasilar. The patient's signs and symptoms can often be attributed to one particular vascular territory (see the box opposite).

The two types of TIAs have different implications for management. Anterior circulation TIAs may represent surgically correctable internal carotid artery atherosclerotic disease. Posterior TIAs are associated with the less accessible vertebral and basilar arteries; attempts at surgical intervention have had unacceptable morbidity and mortality.

Although TIA syndromes may resolve within minutes or hours, the emergency physician must initially assume that the patient's symptoms are permanent and may worsen. Symptoms of cerebrovascular ischemia, whether transient or not, mandate urgent evaluation by a CT scan or MRI. Patients with TIAs may demonstrate CT scan abnormalities in 20% of cases.[26,27] MRI has been found to be abnormal in 80% of cases, resulting in the subclassification known as "completed infarctions with transient symptoms."[28,29]

Doppler duplex and color flow studies are used to screen patients for carotid artery lesions amenable to surgical intervention and to identify patients who are candidates for angiography. All patients with TIAs must be evaluated

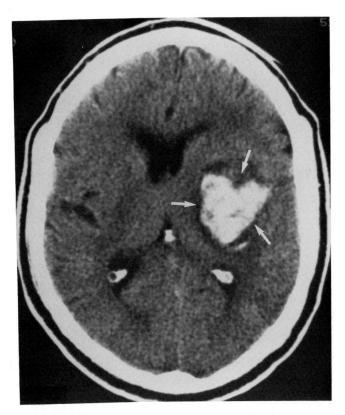

Fig. 20-12. Nonenhanced CT scan of brain hemorrhage demonstrates a large left basal ganglia hematoma *(arrows)* in a patient with hypertension.

for conditions that predispose to cerebrovascular disease (hypertension, cardiac dysrhythmia or valvular disease, diabetes, hyperlipidemia, estrogen use, street drug use, coagulation disorders, syphilis, vasculitis).

Intracerebral (parenchymal) hemorrhage. Nontraumatic intracranial hemorrhage has two distinct mechanisms. Subarachnoid hemorrhage results from the rupture of a vascular lesion on the surface of the brain (see Chapter 17). Intracerebral hemorrhage results from the rupture of a blood vessel deep within the brain substance, common in patients with chronic hypertension (Fig. 20-12). In contrast to patients with ischemic infarction, those with intracerebral hemorrhage are more likely to present with headache and a depressed level of consciousness in addition to sensorimotor deficit. Intracerebral hemorrhage may require expeditious neurosurgical intervention.

Primary intracerebral hemorrhage (ICH) causes approximately 10% of all strokes; 80% of ICHs originate in the cerebral hemispheres (putamen, thalamus, deep white matter), 20% in the brain stem and cerebellum.[30] The most common etiology is chronic hypertension; other contributing mechanisms include arteriolar spasm (the postulated mechanism in pre-eclamptic ICH), localized vasculitis (periarteritis nodosa, viral and rickettsial diseases), blood dyscrasias (anticoagulant therapy, leukemia, polycythemia, sickle cell disease, thrombotic thrombocytopenic purpura,

hemophilia), neoplasms (with erosion of normal vessels or rupture of abnormal tumor vessels), dural sinus thrombosis, and drug abuse.[31]

In most cases, hemorrhage originates from deep penetrating arteries damaged by chronic hypertension with lipohyalinosis, fibrinoid necrosis, and microaneurysm formation. Intimal rupture may lead to a cascade effect, with stretching and rupture of neighboring vessels. The resultant clot may cause mass effect with displacement of adjacent normal tissues, or it may rupture into the ventricular or subarachnoid space.

Cerebellar hemorrhage. Cerebellar hemorrhage is a neurosurgical emergency as the expanding posterior fossa mass leads to brain stem compression and death (Fig. 20-13). Before widespread availability of the CT scan, the mortality of cerebellar hemorrhage was estimated at 65% to 80%.[32] Early diagnosis and prompt intervention can result in complete recovery.

The distinctive presentation of abrupt occipital headache, vertigo, vomiting, and ataxia must be recognized and evaluated with utmost urgency. Often the patient has severe hypertension, few cranial nerve signs, no limb weakness, and severe gait ataxia. Progression of the hemorrhage and mass effect results in tonsillar herniation into the foramen magnum and brain stem compression and upward herniation through the incisura with midbrain compression.

Consultants must be alerted to the suspected diagnosis at the earliest moment so that a CT scan of the posterior fossa may be obtained, and any indicated neurosurgical intervention can proceed with haste.

The traditional view that cerebellar hemorrhage must be treated by excision of the clot has recently been challenged.[19,33,34] In the absence of brain stem compression or hydrocephalus, selected patients may do well with conservative management.

CT scan in intracerebral hemorrhage. The CT scan of ICH is easily identified as a sharply delineated homogenous area of increased density that displaces normal anatomic structures (Figs. 20-12 and 20-13). There may be a surrounding ring of decreased density representing edema. The radiodensity of the clot begins to decrease after several days; it disappears after several weeks, leaving an area of decreased density.

MRI in intracerebral hemorrhage. The MRI characteristics of hemorrhage are complex, involving the temporal evolution of signal changes (Fig. 20-14). While MRI has greater sensitivity to hemorrhage, can better image the posterior fossa, and is more likely to demonstrate underlying pathology (tumor, aneurysm, vascular malformation) than the CT scan, a lesion cannot be characterized as hemorrhagic within the first 1 to 6 hours.[20] As such, CT scan is the preferred early imaging modality.

Angiography in intracerebral hemorrhage. If patient history, physical examination, and hematoma location are typical of hypertensive ICH, no further urgent diagnostic

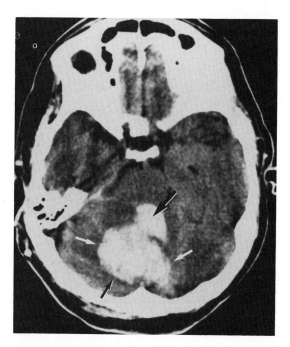

Fig. 20-13. Nonenhanced CT scan of cerebellar hemorrhage shows a large cerebellar hematoma *(small arrows)* with extension into the fourth ventricle *(large arrow).*

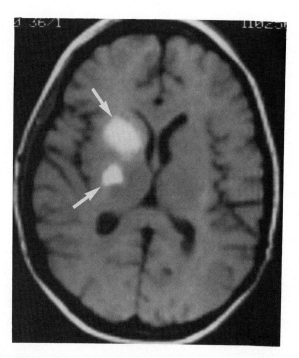

Fig. 20-14. MRI of brain hemorrhage in a young woman with lupus vasculitis. Right basal ganglia hemorrhage *(arrows)* appears of high intensity on the T_1-weighted nonenhanced image.

evaluation may be necessary. However, if the clinical setting or lesion location are not typical of ICH, the etiology is less clear. Angiography may be considered to evaluate the patient for arteriovenous malformation, aneurysm, and tumor as causes of hemorrhage [19,23] (see Chapter 17).

Surgery in intracerebral hemorrhage. Surgery must be considered for certain groups of patients with intracerebral hemorrhage: (1) those with cerebellar hemorrhage and (2) those with large superficially located (frontal, temporal, occipital lobe) hematomas who are either unresponsive to medical treatment or who are critical or acutely deteriorating.

Cerebral venous thrombosis. Cerebral venous thrombosis may complicate suppurative processes or result from a hypercoaguable state (dehydration; sickle cell disease, polycythemia, leukemia; post-operative or hyperestrogenic conditions).

Among healthy young women, venous thrombosis is associated with either the puerperium, the first trimester of pregnancy, or oral contraceptives. It most commonly occurs 1 to 4 weeks postpartum,[1] usually after a normal labor and delivery.[31] While older literature ascribed most strokes during pregnancy to venous thrombosis, arterial occlusion is the more likely cause.[35] While CT scan demonstrates direct signs of cerebral venous thrombosis in 33% of cases, MRI may prove more sensitive.[35]

Stroke in children and young adults. Young adults and children with stroke have a much broader spectrum of etiologies than the arteriosclerosis, hypertension, and diabetes that underly most brain infarctions in older patients. Treatable conditions and predisposing factors must be ac-

tively sought in all aspects of evaluation: history, physical examination, laboratory testing, and radiographic evaluation.

Stroke in children. The incidence of stroke in childhood is approximately 2/100,000 population/year or about half the childhood rate of primary intracranial neoplasms.[36,37] Childhood stroke syndromes may be classified according to the age at onset and the presence or absence of underlying systemic disease. Childhood stroke is not amenable to rigid classification, as the cause of stroke (e.g., sickle cell disease) may cause hemorrhage in one child and thrombosis in another.[38]

Neonatal stroke may occur in the setting of sepsis, acidosis, respiratory distress syndrome, disseminated intravascular coagulation, or congenital heart disease. Stroke at this age may be manifested by hypotonia, bradycardia, apnea, hypotension, or cyanosis. Focal neurologic symptoms are uncommon.[39]

With congenital heart disease, a right-to-left shunt allows venous emboli to reach the cerebral arterial circulation. In lesions that cause chronic cyanosis, polycythemia and hyperviscosity may lead to arterial and venous thrombosis.

A hypercoaguable state can result from a number of other causes, including dehydration, nephrotic syndrome, acute leukemia, thrombotic thrombocytopenic purpura, and, in adolescents, oral contraceptive use and pregnancy. Homocystinuria, a metabolic disorder with the clinical features of marfanoid body habitus and ocular lens dislocation, may be associated with thromboembolic stroke.

Stroke occurs in 5% of patients with sickle cell disease;

children are more likely to have infarction, adults more likely to have intracerebral hemorrhage.[39] Careful management with hypertransfusion appears to decrease the incidence of recurrent stroke.[40]

Purulent venous thrombosis may occur as a complication of ear, nose, sinus, scalp, or facial infection. Stroke may occur as a complication of meningitis, especially if diagnosis is delayed or treatment is incomplete.[39]

Systemic lupus erythematosis (SLE), the only collagen vascular disease in children that affects the central nervous system with any frequency, causes clinically apparent strokes in 3% of patients.[39,40]

Arteriovenous malformation (AVM) is the most common cause of subarachnoid hemorrhage in children,[41] and intracranial hemorrhage is the most common childhood presentation of AVM.[39] Conditions associated with cerebral aneurysm include coarctation of the aorta and polycystic kidney disease (see Chapter 17).

"Acute hemiplegia of childhood" describes the sudden onset of hemiparesis in a previously well child that is not associated with intracerebral hemorrhage or clinically apparent predisposing conditions[42]; such cases comprised 19% of a 10-year Mayo Clinic review of childhood stroke.[37] The number of patients in this category decreases as diagnostic technology and pathophysiologic understanding evolve. Angiography is abnormal in 80% of such cases, with a number of clinicopathologic groups recognized.[43] Among these is Moya-Moya syndrome, which is associated with vascular occlusions at the base of the brain and basal ganglia telangiectasia that has a pathognomonic "puff of smoke" appearance on cerebral arteriography.

Stroke in young adults. The incidence of stroke in patients under 35 years of age is estimated to be 3/100,000 population/year. Using the same parameters, this rate rises to 20 in the 35- to 44-year-old age group, and 63 in the 45- to 54-year-old age group,[39] and doubles in each decade of life thereafter.[44] Between the ages of 15 and 45, initial strokes affect males and females with equal frequency.[44]

The etiology of cerebral infarction in young adults is different from the elderly population and is less often atherosclerotic and more often treatable. Cerebral embolism of cardiac source is the most common cause[45] (Table 20-4).

Brain tumor. Primary brain tumors represent nearly 10% of all neoplasms; they are the most common solid tumor of childhood.[46] While brain tumors are an uncommon cause of acute focal neurologic deficit, hemorrhage into the tumor or acute hydrocephalus may occur abruptly.

Despite the greater sensitivity of MRI in detecting soft tissue lesions, the widely available CT scan is more often used for emergency screening. Small lesions, with diameter equal to or less than the CT section, may not be accurately depicted; similarly, small lesions in areas of bone artifact may be obscured. While a CT scan (and MRI) may not characterize the nature of a mass, integration of the CT scan findings with clinical data has been reported to have a

Table 20-4. Causes of brain infarction in young adults

Causes	Aggregate (%)	Range (%)
Atherosclerosis	20	7-48
Embolism (recognized source)	20	11-31
Nonatherosclerotic arteriopathy	10	0-10
Coagulopathy/systemic	10	2-16
Peripartum	5	2-5
Uncertain cause*	35	27-47

Modified from Hart RG, Miller VT: By permission of the American Heart Association. *Stroke* 14:110, 1983.
*24 of 58 females in this group used oral contraceptives.

predictive accuracy of tumor identification in the range of 85% to 90%.[47,48] Contrast enhancement improves the detection and localization of tumors; the degree and pattern of enhancement may elucidate the tumor type.[47]

While space does not permit a review of the radiographic characteristics of individual tumor types, complications common to all tumors will be considered briefly.

Cerebral edema. Edema is a common sequelae of many brain processes and may add significant volume to the lesion. A variety of pathophysiologic mechanisms produce different forms of edema, including vasogenic (tumor, abscess, hemorrhage, infarction, contusion), interstitial (acute obstruction of CSF flow), and cytotoxic (hypoxia or ischemia).[49]

Intracranial tumors produce vasogenic edema from breakdown of the blood-brain barrier. While the degree of tumor edema varies widely, it is greatest with metastatic carcinoma. Edema (which on a CT scan is of low density compared with normal brain tissue) accumulates mainly in the white matter, with compression and thinning of overlying cortical gray matter.

Interstitial edema from ventricular obstruction appears on the CT scan as a periventricular low density (Fig. 20-15), and on a T_2-weighted MRI as a periventricular high intensity. This edema results from the seepage of CSF across microscopic rents in the ependymal lining of the ventricles.

Tumor hemorrhage. Hemorrhage, overall an infrequent complication of intracranial neoplasm, is more common in particular tumors, including metastases (melanoma, choriocarcinoma, bronchogenic carcinoma, hypernephroma), and primary CNS neuroblastoma, lymphoma, and medulloblastoma.[48] Bleeding may occur within the necrotic tumor center or peripherally around the tumor. The hemorrhage may obscure the tumor itself on the CT scan; an enhanced scan may demonstrate enhancement of tumor tissue at the margin of the hematoma (Fig. 20-16).

Brain metastases. Intracranial metastases occur in 10% of neoplasms; metastases represent 30% of brain tumors.[32,47]

Intracranial metastases have three patterns of spread: to

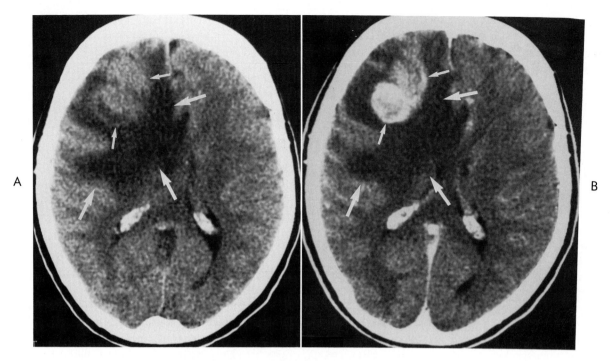

Fig. 20-15. Metastatic sarcoma. Nonenhanced **(A)** and enhanced **(B)** CT scans reveal a large metastatic lesion *(small arrows)* with marked surrounding edema *(large arrows)*.

the brain itself, to the skull and dura, and to the meninges. The most frequent sources of brain metastases are hematogenously spread carcinomas of lung, breast, kidney, and gastrointestinal tract, and malignant melanoma.[32] Certain tumors are particularly likely to spread to the brain: 75% of melanomas, 57% of testicular tumors, and 35% of bronchogenic carcinomas (Fig. 20-17).[51] Patients with systemic cancers that metastasize to the brain often have lung lesions; either their primary tumor is in the lung, or they also have lung metastases (gastrointestinal, breast, or ovarian tumors).[30] A chest CT scan may demonstrate lesions not apparent on the plain chest radiograph.

A cerebral metastasis, a solitary lesion in 47% of cases,[51] usually occurs at the junction of the cortex and white matter.[46,52] Small tumors appear on the CT scan as rounded homogenous high-density or isodense nodules[48]; contrast may be necessary for visualization. Metastatic lesions may cause extensive vasogenic edema. Some small and most large metastases have central necrosis; such lesions appear as ring-like masses with a central lucency and a high-density or isodense rim.[52] Hemorrhage within a lesion causes a high-density appearance.

Skull and dural metastases, common with breast and prostate cancers, are believed to spread via the vertebral venous plexus, which extends from the pelvis to the dural venous sinuses and bypasses the systemic circulation.[1] Metastases to the skull convexity may compress the brain in a manner similar to subdural hematoma. Skull base me-

tastases may involve the cranial nerve roots.[53] A CT scan identification of bony skull metastases is facilitated by using wide window and high-center settings (Fig. 20-18). (see p. 566 for discussion of window width and window level).

Diffuse metastatic involvement of the meninges may be seen with breast and lung carcinoma and lymphoma.[54]

Space-occupying infections

Brain abscess. Brain abscess, the most frequent focal brain infection, is usually a complication of a suppurative focus elsewhere in the body. The clinical presentation of brain abscess is not stereotypic. Fever is not common; symptoms are more suggestive of mass effect than infection, including (in order of frequency) headache, confusion, seizures, and focal deficits.[55]

Approximately 40% of brain abscesses can be traced to otorhinologic infections.[1] In such cases infection may reach the brain by two routes: direct extension from the middle ear or nasal sinuses via osteomyelitis and suppuration or via spread along the venous sinuses into subcortical white matter.[46]

One third of brain abscesses are metastatic, resulting from hematogenous spread of infection from a remote site. Most such abscesses result from a pulmonary focus (bronchiectasis, lung abscess, empyema, bronchopleural fistula). Other sources include skin, dental, and pelvic infections and cardiac pathology (endocarditis, congenital

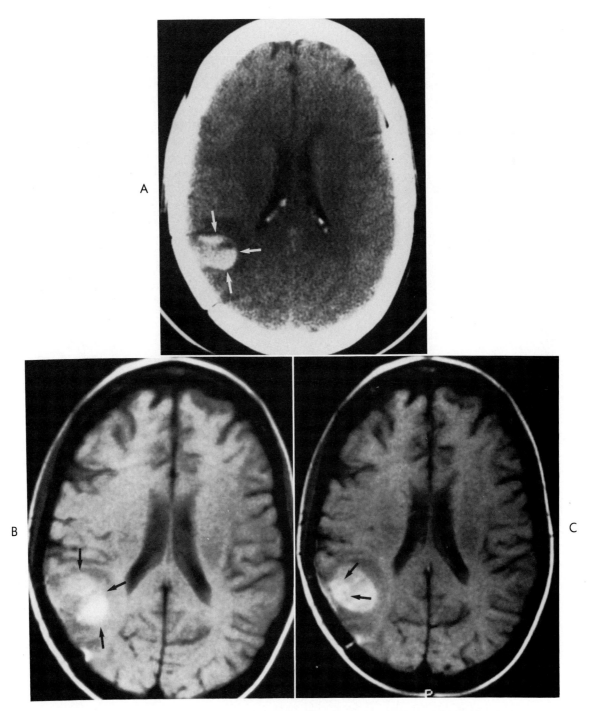

Fig. 20-16. Tumor with hemorrhage. **A,** Nonenhanced CT scan shows a right parietal hematoma *(arrows)*. Enhanced CT scan *(not shown)* did not demonstrate enhancement of the lesion. **B,** Hemorrhage appears of high intensity on nonenhanced T_1-weighted MRI image *(arrows)*. **C,** T_1-weighted MRI image after intravenous administration of gadolinium shows a nodular enhancement *(arrows)* within the hematoma, suspicious for neoplasm. Metastatic melanoma was found at surgery.

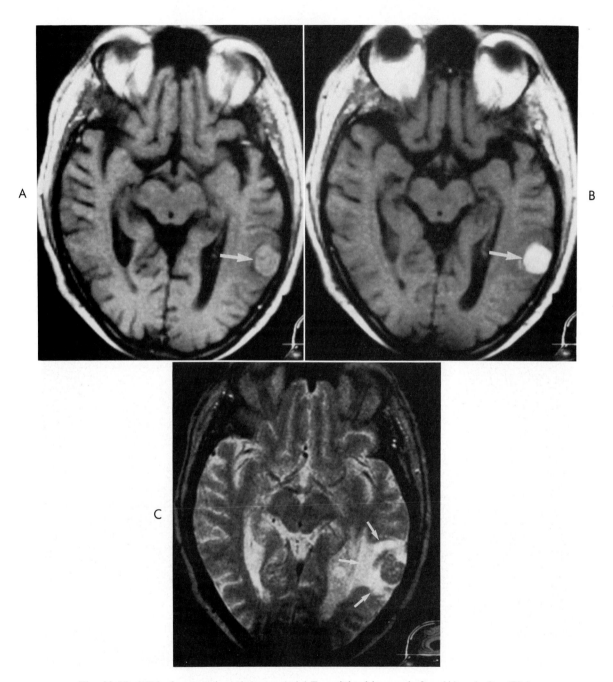

Fig. 20-17. MRI of metastatic melanoma. Axial T$_1$-weighted images before **(A)** and after **(B)** intravenous administration of gadolinium show an enhancing nodule in the gray matter *(arrow)*. T$_2$-weighted image **(C)** demonstrates moderate surrounding edema *(arrows)*.

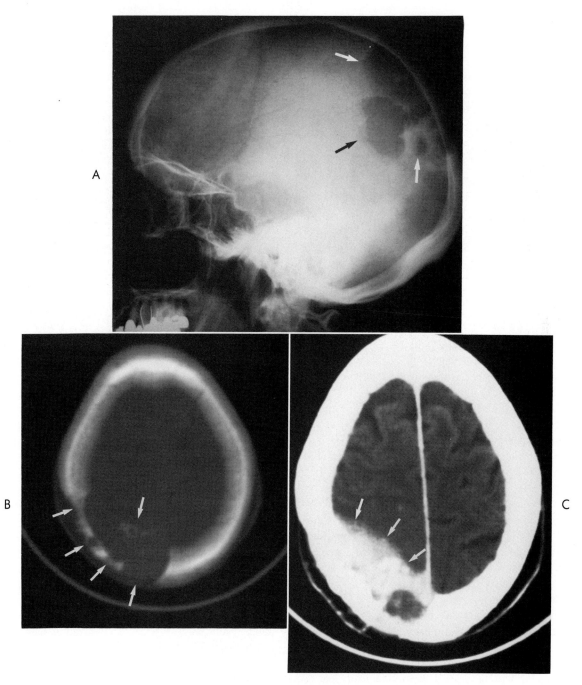

Fig. 20-18. Skull metastasis. **A,** Skull radiograph demonstrates a large lytic lesion from renal cell carcinoma *(arrows)*. **B,** CT bone window setting confirms a lytic expansile lesion *(arrows)*. **C,** CT brain window setting reveals an enhancing epidural tumor *(arrows)*.

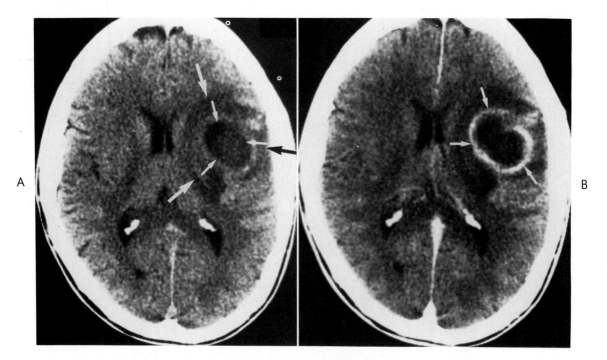

Fig. 20-19. CT scan of a bacterial abscess. **A,** Nonenhanced scan shows a low-density mass *(small arrows)* with surrounding edema *(large arrows)*. **B,** Enhanced scan demonstrates a ring-enhancing lesion *(arrows)* consistent with abscess.

anomalies with right-to-left shunt). Metastatic abscesses usually occur in the distal territory of the middle cerebral artery and are frequently multiple.[1]

In 20% of cases no septic source is found.[17] Brain abscess rarely occurs with bacterial meningitis.[1]

The microbial etiology is mixed, includes anaerobes, and varies with the source of the infection. Enteric flora are associated with otogenic infections, streptococci with a pulmonary source, staphylococci with trauma or surgery. *Actinomyces, Nocardia, Toxoplasma,* and *Candida* abscesses occur in immunosuppressed patients; toxoplasmosis is especially common in patients with AIDS (see Chapter 26). Tuberculosis and syphilis can produce localized brain infections (tuberculomas and gummas); these generally develop insidiously.

Brain abscess often follows a biphasic course. Initially, bacterial invasion causes a focal cerebritis, with poorly circumscribed inflammation. Within days, the intensity of the inflammatory reaction subsides and the infection becomes more localized, with central necrosis, suppuration, and peripheral granulation. The abscess capsule or wall may be identified within 2 weeks of the onset of infection.[1]

CT scan in brain abscess. The CT scan features of brain abscess vary with the stage of evolution of the process. Cerebritis is manifested as an ill-defined area of low density and mass effect. With progression, patchy contrast enhancement may be seen, reflecting blood-brain barrier disintegration.[56] As the abscess cavity and capsule evolve, the CT scan demonstrates a central, round, low-density area (cavity), a ring of higher density (capsule), and a surrounding low-density zone (edema)[46] (Fig. 20-19). Rarely, gas may be visualized within the abscess cavity.[46] An enhanced CT scan shows ring-like enhancement of the capsule. Brain tumors, infarctions, or resolving hematomas may present a similar picture. A radionuclide brain scan may show abnormalities in the cerebritis stage before any specific changes are seen on the CT scan.

MRI in brain abscess. MRI is more sensitive than the CT scan in demonstrating early cerebritis, which is seen as white matter of high intensity on T_2-weighted images. Once developed, central necrosis is of low intensity on T_1- and of high intensity on T_2 spin-echo sequences, as is the peripheral edema. The abscess capsule has a characteristic low intensity on T_2 spin-echo images[3] (Fig. 20-20).

The superior sensitivity of MRI for detection of early cerebritis may be of minimal practical significance, as patients rarely present (or are recognized as having an intracranial process) at this stage.[57]

Treatment. Treatment at the cerebritis stage includes appropriate antibiotics and therapy for cerebral edema. Lumbar puncture is not indicated and may be hazardous because of the risk of herniation.

For encapsulated abscesses, surgical intervention is recommended for culture and drainage; total excision may be attempted if the abscess is superficial and well encapsulated. If deep, multicentric, or near critical areas (motor cortex or speech centers), aspiration and antibiotic injection may be the only surgical treatment possible.

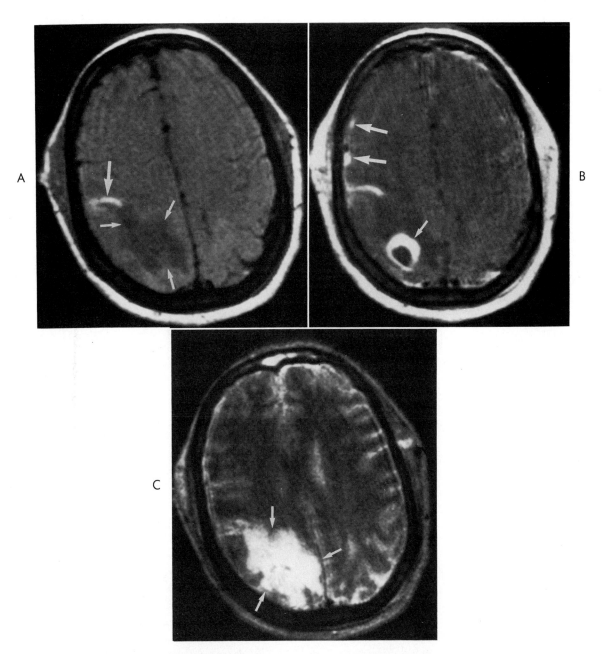

Fig. 20-20. MRI of brain abscess. **A,** Axial nonenhanced T_1-weighted image shows low-intensity white matter edema *(small arrows)* and a small high-intensity hemorrhage *(large arrow)*. **B,** T_1-weighted image after intravenous administration of gadolinium reveals a ring-enhancing lesion *(small arrow)* consistent with an abscess. Also note prominent meningeal enhancement *(large arrows)* due to meningitis. **C,** T_2-weighted image demonstrates high-intensity white matter edema *(arrows)* to better advantage.

Subdural empyema. Subdural empyema (SDE) is a suppurative process located between the inner surface of the dura and the outer surface of the arachnoid. The infection usually extends from the frontal or ethmoid sinuses; less commonly, it originates in the middle ear or mastoid air cells; in rare instances it is metastatic from a pulmonary source. SDE may complicate a penetrating skull wound or craniotomy. The subdural pus depresses the underlying cerebral hemisphere, similar to a subdural hematoma.

The clinical course of SDE after otorhinologic infection is often fulminant, with fever and obtundation progressing to seizures, focal deficit, and coma. Post-operative and post-traumatic SDE may be indolent, with symptoms of slowly progressive mass effect rather than infection.

CT scan in subdural empyema. On the CT scan, SDE may be seen as a low-density crescent-shaped area adjacent to the inner table of the skull; the empyema may be isodense to brain tissue. Enhanced CT scan may demonstrate a thin enhancing rim at the inner margin of the empyema (Fig. 20-21). When present, subjacent cortical cerebritis or infarction may show enhancement, differentiating the process from subacute or chronic subdural hematoma.

MRI in subdural empyema. SDE is more easily visualized and characterized on MRI as the purulent fluid has excellent contrast to adjacent bone and brain. The multiplanar capability of MRI is of advantage as coronal images best demonstrate collections overlying the convexity of the brain. Coronal sections may also demonstrate contiguity of the empyema with the ethmoid or mastoid air cells (Fig. 20-22).

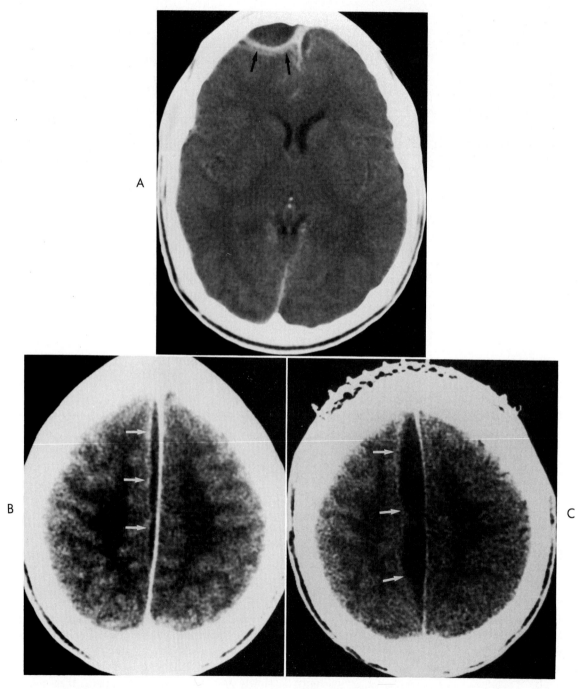

Fig. 20-21. CT scans of epidural abscess and subdural empyema. **A,** Enhanced scan reveals a biconvex low-density extracerebral collection with rim enhancement *(arrows)*. Epidural abscess and frontal osteomyelitis were found at surgery. **B,** Pre-operative enhanced scan of the same patient shows a small interhemispheric subdural fluid collection *(arrows)*. **C,** Ten days after surgery, the interhemispheric fluid collection has increased in size *(arrows)*. Repeat surgery confirmed a subdural empyema.

Treatment. Subdural empyema is a neurosurgical emergency because of its rapidly progressive course. Treatment involves surgical decompression and appropriate antibiotics. The rapid and accurate diagnosis possible since the advent of the CT scan has reduced the mortality for acute SDE from 50% to 10%.[3]

Epidural empyema. Epidural empyema (EDE), a complication of otitis media, mastoiditis, or skull osteo-

myelitis, is a collection of pus between the calvarium and the dura. It is usually manifest by a local inflammatory process with fever and tenderness; it rarely causes focal neurologic signs and symptoms.

CT scan in epidural empyema. The CT scan demonstrates a low-density or isodense lentiform extracerebral collection; an enhanced CT scan demonstrates a well-demarcated rim representing inflamed dura. The character-

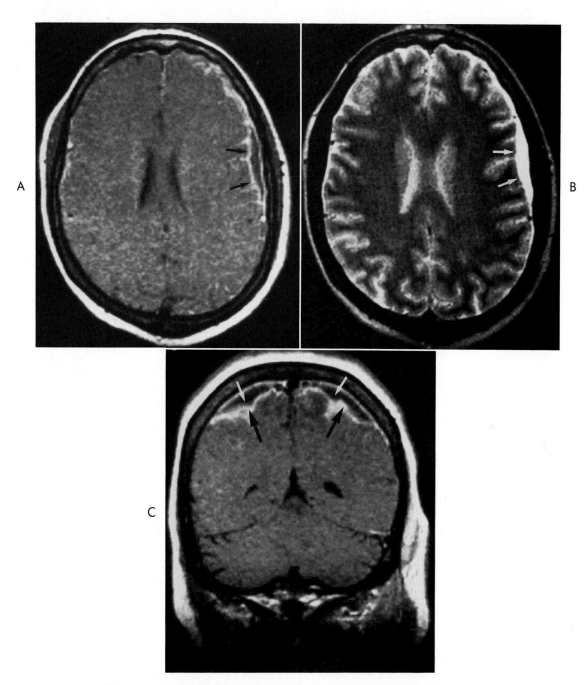

Fig. 20-22. MRI of subdural empyema. **A,** Axial T_1-weighted image after intravenous administration of gadolinium demonstrates a low-intensity subdural fluid collection *(arrows)* in a patient with sinusitis. **B,** Collection is of high intensity on T_2-weighted image *(arrows)*. **C,** Coronal T_1-weighted image after intravenous administration of gadolinium shows bilateral low-intensity subdural fluid collections at the vertex *(white arrows)* with prominent meningeal enhancement *(dark arrows)*. Subdural empyemas were drained surgically. (Courtesy John C Stears, MD, University Hospital, Denver, Colorado.)

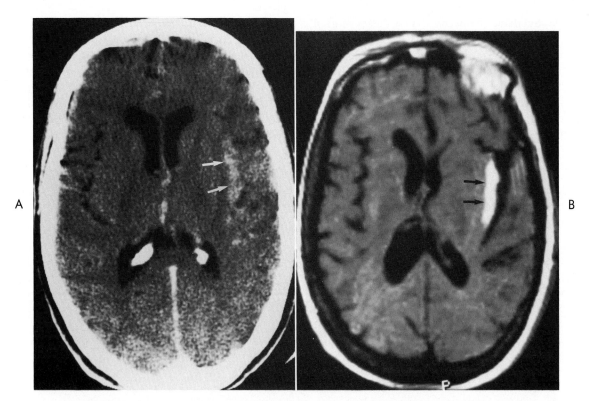

Fig. 20-23. Herpes encephalitis. **A,** Enhanced CT scan reveals enhancement of the left insular cortex *(arrows).* **B,** T₁-weighted MRI image after intravenous administration of gadolinium shows the insular enhancement more clearly *(arrows).* Diagnosis was confirmed by brain biopsy. There is also a high-intensity signal of fat within the superior aspect of the left orbit.

istic shape and displacement of the dura and falx from the calvarium localizes the collection as epidural.

MRI in epidural empyema. Epidural empyema (EDE) is more easily visualized on MRI for the same reasons mentioned with SDE. EDEs are bordered medially by the displaced dura, which is seen as a low-intensity rim.

Treatment. Treatment of epidural empyema consists of appropriate intravenous antibiotics. Skull osteomyelitis may require debridement of diseased bone.

Encephalitis. Herpes simplex virus (HSV) causes the most common yet serious form of encephalitis; the 2000 cases/a year in the United States have a 30% to 70% mortality rate, and the majority of survivors have serious neurologic sequelae.[1] HSV 1 is the usual cause of adult encephalitis; HSV 2 encephalitis is seen in neonates and is related to maternal genital herpetic infection.

While most patients present with fever, headache, mental status changes, and seizures, the propensity of the disease to involve the inferomedial aspects of the frontal and temporal lobes may be manifested in symptoms such as anosmia, olfactory or gustatory hallucinations, bizarre behavior, aphasia, and hemiparesis. Swelling and herniation of the temporal lobes may occur, leading to respiratory arrest.

CT scan in encephalitis. The CT scan is relatively insensitive to the early changes of viral encephalitis, but scattered low-density lesions and blurring of the gray and white matter junction may be seen. With progression of the disease, mass effect and edema predominate. Hetereogeneous contrast enhancement may be seen (Fig. 20-23, *A*).

MRI in encephalitis. MRI detects changes typical of HSV encephalitis earlier than the CT scan[57] and can often more fully delineate the extent of the disease. Initial findings include regions of high-signal intensity on T₂-weighted MRI images; these areas coalesce and a mass effect predominates. Petechial hemorrhage, a common pathologic feature of HSV encephalitis, may be seen as punctate high-intensity areas on T₁-weighted and T₂-weighted images[57] (Fig. 20-23, *B*).

Radionuclide brain scan in encephalitis. Radionuclide brain scan may be positive earlier than CT scan in HSV encephalitis, and electroencephalographic changes (diffuse abnormality with focal epileptiform discharges from one or both temporal lobes) are suggestive but not diagnostic.

Treatment. Prognosis depends largely on early diagnosis (which may require brain biopsy) and early institution of antiviral therapy. Recognition of the characteristic clinical and radiographic signs of HSV encephalitis is crucial, as prompt treatment with acyclovir can improve the outcome of this devastating disease.

Other brain infections. Progressive multifocal leukoencephalopathy and toxoplasmosis are discussed in Chapter 26 on AIDS. While intracerebral manifestations of tropical or parasitic diseases (cysticercosis, malaria, trichinosis, paragonimiasis) may cause mass lesions, seizures or mental status changes are the more characteristic neurologic manifestations.

Nonstructural causes of hemiplegia

Hemiplegia can only be attributed to a nonstructural etiology based on the exclusion of intracranial mass lesion by definitive radiographic evaluation.

Meningitis. Hemiplegia in the context of fever, headache, and meningeal signs mandates the exclusion of a mass lesion, particularly brain abscess, by a CT scan (see Chapter 17).

Demyelinating disease. Multiple sclerosis (MS) may rarely cause acute signs of cerebral origin, including hemiparesis. Establishing a diagnosis of MS is a complex challenge that extends beyond emergency evaluation.

CT scan in multiple sclerosis. The reported incidence of CT scan abnormalities in MS ranges from 33% to 85%.[58] The most common abnormality is focal decreased attenuation in periventricular white matter, representing the characteristic focal areas of demyelination. These "plaques," which are usually multiple and range in size from 5 mm to over 70 mm, may show contrast enhancement during episodes of acute demyelination. Patients with a long history of the disease may be found to have cerebral atrophy, manifested as ventricular and sulcal dilatation.

MRI in multiple sclerosis. MRI demonstrates the plaques in 76% to 100% of patients with definite multiple sclerosis[19] (Fig. 20-24). A gadolinium-enhanced MRI image may differentiate acute from chronic lesions.[3]

Other demyelinating diseases. Foci of high intensity similar to MS plaques may be seen in vasculitis following radiation therapy, in elderly patients with and without dementia, and in children with rare leukodystrophies.[3]

Hemiplegic migraine. Complicated migraine may be impossible to distinguish from cerebrovascular disease. The syndrome of hemiplegic migraine may be associated with a previous history or family history of unilateral motor and sensory symptoms as part of a migraine attack in a relatively young patient.[59,60] The hemiplegia may last hours or even days and may outlast the headache.[61]

Hemiplegia attributed to complicated migraine must be a diagnosis of exclusion in all but the exceptional patient. A negative diagnostic evaluation and a full return to normal functioning corroborate the diagnosis.

ACUTE PARAPLEGIA AND QUADRIPLEGIA

Patients with spinal cord disorders may complain of pain, weakness, paresthesias, and autonomic disturbances, the character and location of which vary with the etiology. Neurologic examination characterizes a spinal cord lesion in its transverse and rostral-caudal involvement; such localization is essential to focus neuroradiographic evaluation.

The classic spinal cord lesion produces LMN signs at

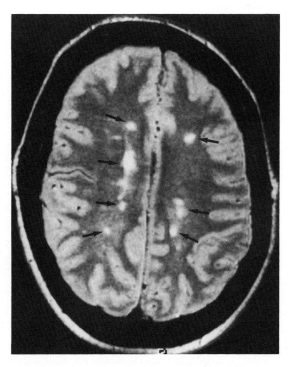

Fig. 20-24. MRI of multiple sclerosis. Axial T_2-weighted image demonstrates multiple white matter high intensities *(arrows)*, representing stages of demyelination.

the level of the lesion, UMN signs below that level, and a sharp sensory "level" at the corresponding dermatome (often two to three segments below the actual cord level).

While location of pain may direct localization to the appropriate cord level, pain may be radicular or referred. Vertebral palpation or percussion may elicit point tenderness over the site of compressive lesions.

Radiographic evaluation

Clinical suspicion of a compressive spinal cord lesion should prompt urgent neurosurgical and neuroradiologic consultation so that evaluation and appropriate intervention may proceed in an optimally coordinated and efficient manner. No procedure should delay definitive diagnosis (myelography or MRI) but should proceed concomitantly with appropriate laboratory evaluation and specialty consultation.

Plain film radiography. Plain radiographs of the spine are immediately available, noninvasive, and may be diagnostically helpful. Plain radiographs are useful to evaluate vertebral alignment, spinal canal size, bony abnormalities, and the status of paravertebral soft tissues. The spinal contents are not visualized on plain radiographs, except when altered by calcified tumors (e.g., meningiomas) or fat-containing lesions.

Conventional tomography. Conventional tomography involves complementary motion of the film and the x-ray tube, blurring all structures except those in the focal plane. While the CT scan and MRI are far superior for detecting

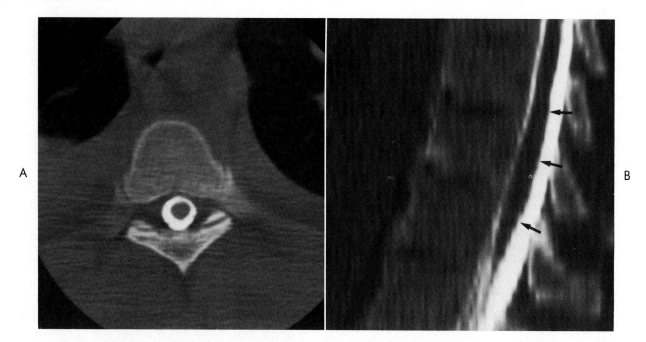

Fig. 20-25. Sagittal reformation. **A,** Axial CT scan with intrathecal contrast material. **B,** Corresponding midline sagittal reformation shows a normal lower thoracic spinal cord and conus medullaris *(arrows)*.

and characterizing lesions, conventional tomography remains useful in certain circumstances, such as assessment of the lateral masses and apophyseal joints following trauma (see Chapter 9).

Myelography. Myelography examines the subarachnoid space via intrathecal injection of contrast material. Air was the earliest contrast material used, followed by a variety of oil-based substances (iodophendylate or Pantopaque), which required removal at the end of the procedure and sometimes produced arachnoiditis. Water-soluble contrast agents (e.g., metrizamide) have been widely used since the 1970s. They may be instilled with a smaller needle (reducing the incidence of post-procedure headache), are resorbed from the central nervous system and excreted by the kidneys, are miscible with CSF (allowing circumferential thecal sac opacification), and may be used with the CT scan (unlike iodophendylate, which produces CT scan artifact). Complications of metrizamide use include headache, nausea, and vomiting; CNS irritation with transient mental status changes; and, rarely, seizures.[69] The newest generation of non-ionic contrast agents, including iohexol and iopamidol, are less toxic to neural tissue.

Diagnostic possibilities prompting myelographic evaluation will influence technique. Lumbar puncture is usually performed at L3/L4 or L2/L3; the amount of contrast material instilled varies with the cord level to be studied.[62] If there is suspicion of complete spinal block, only a small initial volume is used. If there is no obstruction, the usual contrast volume is then injected. If complete block is demonstrated, the upper level of the lesion is usually defined by a post-myelography CT scan; this delayed CT scan (af-

ter 2 to 3 hours) may help delineate the upper extent of the lesion. If necessary, contrast material may be injected via C1/C2 puncture.

The hazards of lumbar puncture are increased in the setting of complete spinal block. The procedure may increase the pressure gradient across the obstruction and precipitate or exacerbate cord compression; removal of CSF may cause herniation of the cord into a decompressed region. Any decision about lumbar puncture in such instances should be made with neurologic or neurosurgical consultants so that the procedure can be performed at the time of myelography, if indicated. An ill-timed lumbar puncture performed before myelography may complicate the second procedure in both performance and interpretation. An "epidural pocket" created by CSF leakage may subsequently obscure, or itself appear to be, a spinal lesion.[63]

Myelography demonstrates lesions that encroach on the subarachnoid space. Extradural lesions, compressing the space from the outside, and intradural extramedullary lesions (between the dura and the spinal cord) are well seen. Intramedullary (within the cord) lesions are less easily seen but may appear as cord widening.

The radiation dose in myelography varies with the level of the spine examined and the amount of fluoroscopy time needed for the study. On average, a patient may require 5 to 10 minutes of fluoroscopy (at 2 to 3 rads/minute) and five to ten spot radiographs (at 0.5 rad/exposure).

Computed tomography. Current CT scanners provide detailed images of the vertebrae, intravertebral disks, and intraspinal and paravertebral soft tissues. The CT scan is most efficiently used to examine short spinal segments identified as areas of concern by clinical examination or plain radiographs. Newer CT scanners are able to generate digital radiographs that serve as scout views for localization of detailed axial sections.

Some lesions are optimally examined in the axial plane of the CT scan; others are better viewed in the sagittal plane. Sagittal CT scan images may be reconstructed by electronically stacking and reslicing the axial images. These images produced by reconstruction remain inferior to direct MRI images in the desired plane (Fig. 20-25).

Visualization of the spinal canal contents on nonen-hanced CT scans varies with location. Visualization of the cord depends on the size of the spinal canal and the volume and contents of the surrounding subarachnoid space, which provides density contrast to the cord proper. The upper cervical (C1/C3) and lower lumbar (L4/L5) areas are best visualized due to their relatively large subarachnoid space and the prominence of epidural veins and fat.

Intrathecal contrast may be used with the CT scan employing a technique similar to that described under myelography (Fig. 20-26). Intravenous contrast material may be of assistance in the evaluation of lesions with abnormal

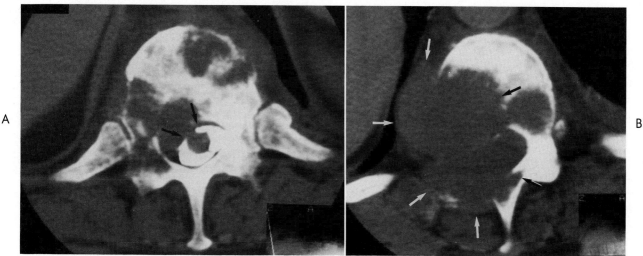

Fig. 20-26. CT myelogram. **A,** CT scan with intrathecal contrast material administration demonstrates a moderate deformity of the dural sac *(arrows)* due to epidural metastases from prostatic carcinoma. **B,** At a slightly higher level, the tumor *(arrows)* completely obliterates the subarachnoid space.

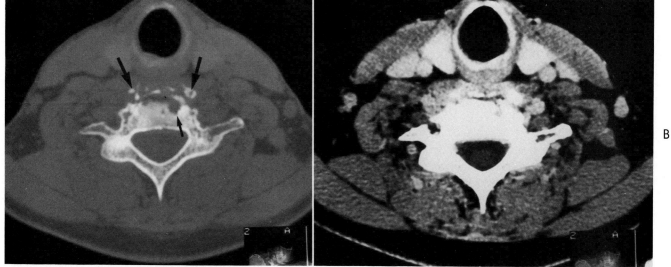

Fig. 20-27. CT scan of the cervical spine at soft tissue and bone window settings. Patient has osteomyelitis and diskitis of C6/C7. **A,** Bone window setting shows bone destruction *(small arrow)* and proliferation *(large arrows)*. **B,** Soft tissue window setting shows the paraspinous tissues to better advantage with no evidence of the epidural abscess (same patient as Fig. 20-33).

vascularity, such as vascular malformations or certain tumors.

The CT scan demonstrates small variations in x-ray attenuation. The examiner can adjust the image appearance by varying the brightness and contrast. The image brightness ("window level") selects the mid-gray value of the image. The image contrast ("window width") selects the range of densities around the chosen mid-gray value, displaying them from black (low attenuation) to white (high attenuation). These two controls are adjusted to visualize an entire density range; different tissues are best visualized by particular window settings. With a spinal CT scan, images are photographed using two different window settings: *soft tissue window* and *bone window* (Fig. 20-27).

Magnetic resonance imaging. Magnetic resonance imaging (MRI) allows direct visualization of the spinal cord. As the spinal cord and CSF have different MRI signal characteristics, they are well visualized and readily differentiated. MRI demonstrates blockage of the subarachnoid space without intrathecal contrast material; compression of the cord may be directly visualized. The use of intravenous paramagnetic contrast material may aid in diagnosis of intramedullary and intradural extramedullary lesions (Fig. 20-28).

No developmental or teratogenic effects have been associated with MRI. When maternal indications mandate diagnostic spinal imaging, MRI may be preferred to the known radiation and contrast risks of the CT scan.[64]

While MRI has become the "gold standard" of spinal cord imaging, its restricted availability and accessibility limits its value in the emergency setting. The same disadvantages previously discussed with MRI brain imaging apply to MRI use in patients with spinal disease. However, despite the longer imaging time, a single MRI scan may be more efficient and require less total time than a CT scan before and after intrathecal contrast administration.

Angiography. Spinal angiography is used to demonstrate vascular abnormalities or vascular tumors within the spinal canal. The technique involves selective catheterization of the spinal arterial supply at multiple levels, with contrast injection and cineangiography at each level. As spinal arteries are small, the risk of toxic or ischemic complications is significantly higher than that associated with cerebral angiography.[65] The advent of digital subtraction imaging has decreased procedure time as well as the volume and concentration of contrast material required.

Spinal angiography is used in the diagnosis and treatment of spinal AVMs, vascular tumors (such as hemangioblastoma), and vascular neoplasms of the spinal column. Endovascular embolization of such lesions may be used pre-operatively to reduce intraoperative bleeding or may be an effective curative or palliative nonsurgical treatment in some cases.[66]

Acute spinal cord compression syndromes

Clinical examination and plain radiographs can localize spinal pathology in the longitudinal axis of the cord (the

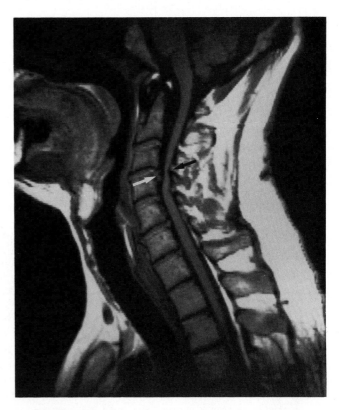

Fig. 20-28. MRI of the cervical spine. Sagittal T_1-weighted scan reveals marked cord flattening at C3/C4 from disk herniation anteriorly and prominent ligamentum flavum posteriorly *(arrows)*.

spinal level), and clinical examination defines its transverse involvement at that level. Further radiographic studies reveal a lesion as extra-axial or extrinsic (outside the cord itself) or intra-axial or intrinsic (within the cord). Spinal tissues may be further subdivided into three compartments. *Extradural* or *epidural* refers to the space between the bony wall of the spinal canal and the dural sac. The intradural extramedullary space is bounded peripherally by the dura and centrally by the spinal cord. The intradural intramedullary space is the spinal cord proper. Such characterization assists in differential diagnosis.

Myelography characterizes a spinal lesion with respect to its anatomic location and the presence and degree of block to CSF flow (Fig. 20-29).

Extradural compartment. The extradural (epidural) space contains fat, nerve roots, blood vessels, and ligaments. The size of the space varies with the region: it is smallest in the cervical area, narrow in the thoracic, and largest at the lumbar level.

Metastatic epidural tumor. Metastatic epidural neoplasm is among the most common causes of acute spinal cord compression; acute myelopathy may be the first manifestation of tumor. Metastatic epidural compression occurs most commonly from epidural extension of bone marrow metastases; other mechanisms include hematogenous spread to the epidural or paravertebral venous plexus and

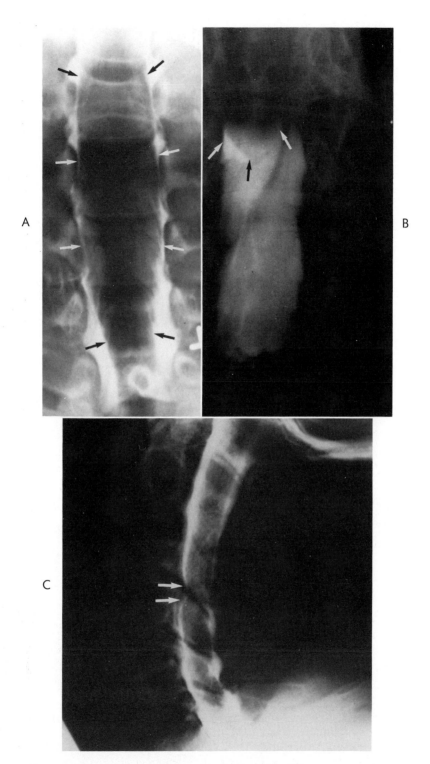

Fig. 20-29. Myelograms of intramedullary, intradural extramedullary, and extradural lesions. **A,** Myelogram with water-soluble contrast material demonstrates a marked enlargement of the cervical cord *(arrows)* due to an astrocytoma. **B,** Pantopaque myelogram shows an intradural extramedullary lesion *(arrows).* Pathologic diagnosis was schwannoma. **C,** Extradural lesion (disk protrusion) causes mild cord indentation *(arrows).* (**B,** Courtesy Delmar Knudson, MD, Denver General Hospital, Denver, Colorado.)

direct extension from metastatic masses or node involvement in the mediastinum or retroperitoneum.

Spinal bone marrow is active even in the elderly; its vascularity renders it a focus for hematogenously disseminated metastases. The expanding metastatic mass encroaches on the epidural space, leading to pressure on the nerve roots or cord. Metastatic epidural cord compression occurs most commonly in the thoracic spine (68%) and less often in the lumbar (17%) and cervical (15%) areas.[67] While any tumor that spreads to bone can cause cord compression, breast, lung, prostate, lymphoma, and myeloma are most frequently seen.[59]

Plain film radiography in epidural metastasis. The initial study of choice for evaluation of metastatic disease is

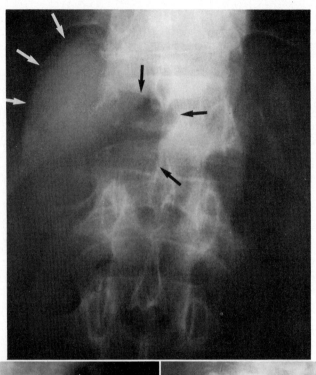

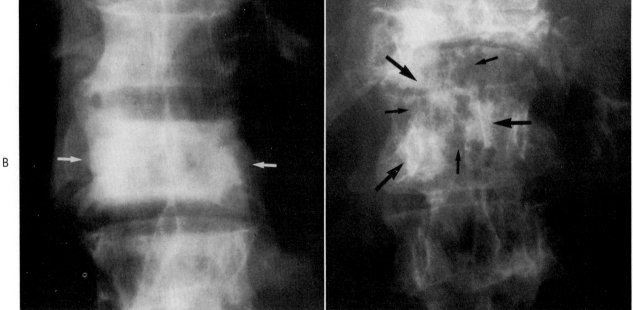

Fig. 20-30. Radiographs of spinal metastases. **A,** Large lytic metastases from a renal cell carcinoma have destroyed the right side of the T12 vertebral body *(arrows).* Also note the paraspinal tumor *(large arrows).* **B,** Blastic metastases *(arrows)* from prostatic carcinoma involve the entire vertebral body ("ivory vertebra"). **C,** Diffuse bony metastases from breast carcinoma show areas of lytic *(small arrows)* and blastic *(large arrows)* involvement.

plain film radiography (Fig. 20-30). Once metastatic compressive symptoms develop, 90% of patients have positive plain radiographs.[68] Spinal metastases may produce a destructive osteolytic process (seen as radiolucency), a sclerotic or osteoblastic reaction of new bone formation (seen as radiodensity), or a mixed process. Osteolytic lesions tend to cause symptoms early, with pain from microfractures within the vertebrae. Osteoblastic lesions may be asymptomatic for some time. Lytic lesions are commonly caused by metastatic lesions from lung, breast, kidney, GI tract, and melanoma; sclerotic lesions are seen with prostate and breast carcinoma, lymphomas, and leukemias.[69] Metastatic disease follows the distribution of red bone marrow, with involvement of the vertebral body, pedicle, and neural arches in descending order of frequency.[50] Vertebral metastases may be multiple and scattered; common findings include loss of vertebral height, destruction of vertebral body cortical edges, and alteration of pedicle appearance on the AP radiograph. Metastases do not ordinarily involve the intervertebral disk, an important distinction from infectious processes.

Radionuclide bone scan. Radionuclide bone scan may be sensitive for detection of osseous pathology but is nonspecific and is not superior to plain radiographs in predicting epidural involvement.[70] The nonspecific information gained during the lengthy acquisition time only delays urgent diagnosis and possible treatment of epidural pathology.

CT scan in epidural metastasis. The CT scan is more sensitive than plain radiographs for detection of osseous spinal metastases and can demonstrate encroachment of the tumor into the epidural space and paravertebral soft tissues (Fig. 20-31). Intrathecal contrast is necessary to demonstrate cord compression. The extradural compression of the subarachnoid space produces a displacement of the contrast column away from the encroaching mass. The extent of the block must be defined so that treatment (emergency radiation therapy or surgery) can be planned.

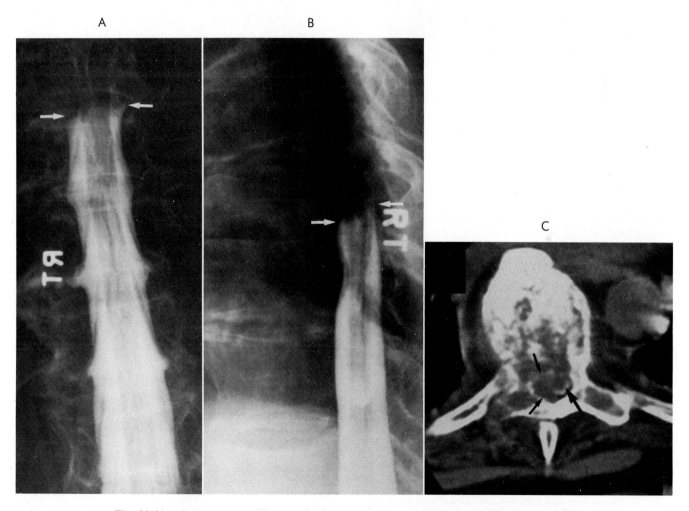

Fig. 20-31. Myelogram and CT scan of epidural metastases. Anteroposterior **(A)** and lateral **(B)** radiographs demonstrate a complete myelographic block *(arrows)* in the mid-thoracic region due to epidural tumor and pathologic fracture. **C,** CT scan after myelography shows the epidural tumor *(small arrows)* and nearly complete obliteration of contrast material surrounding the spinal cord *(large arrow)*. Note permeative destruction of the vertebral body from tumor.

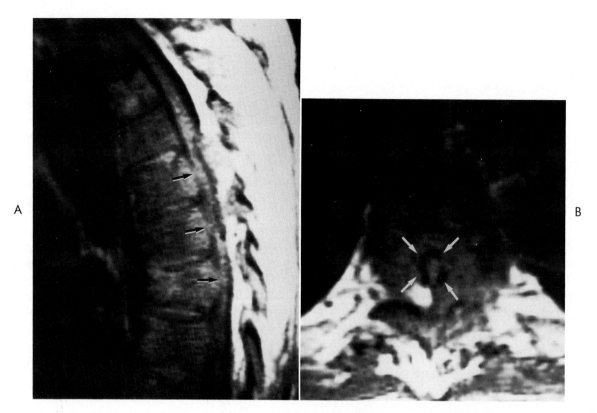

Fig. 20-32. MRI of epidural metastases. Sagittal **(A)** and axial **(B)** T$_1$-weighted MRI images show circumferential cord compression by epidural metastases from a prostatic carcinoma *(arrows)*.

MRI in epidural metastases. MRI is the most sensitive imaging procedure for detecting early metastatic disease of the spine (Fig. 20-32). The entire spinal column can be quickly surveyed in sagittal images, and thin section axial images can be obtained to assess the extent of disease. Tumor replacement of bone marrow (with resultant decreased signal intensity on T$_1$-weighted images), paravertebral involvement, spinal canal compromise, and spinal cord compression can be identified. Use of MRI avoids the lumbar puncture necessary for myelography and intrathecal contrast–enhanced CT scan and, thus, does not have the risks associated with either the invasive procedure or the contrast administration.

While MRI may be the only modality needed to evaluate metastatic spinal disease, there have been cases of myelography-documented epidural compression that have not been apparent on MRI.[65] When a clinically suspected lesion is not detected on MRI, repeat scan after administration of intravenous paramagnetic contrast material may improve detection, or conventional myelography or CT myelography can be performed.

Treatment. Therapy may involve surgical decompression or emergency radiation therapy depending on the lesion, previous radiation therapy, and the patient's status. High-dose steroid therapy (dexamethasone, 100 mg intravenous bolus) may help reduce cord compression and injury before either surgery or radiation therapy. Therapeutic

success is directly related to the patient's neurologic status at the time of diagnosis, making early recognition of great urgency.

Primary extradural tumor. Primary extradural tumors are relatively uncommon. Neurofibromas and meningiomas are the most common (although they more frequently occur intradurally), followed by sarcomas, vascular tumors, chordomas, and epidermoid tumors.[1] Meningiomas and neurofibromas usually occur in the thoracic region, lipomas in the thoracolumbar, and chordomas in the sacral area.[71]

Spinal epidural abscess. Spinal epidural abscess is an uncommon but reversible cause of spinal cord syndrome. It may arise hematogenously or via extension from adjacent vertebral osteomyelitis. Chronic illness, diabetes, immunosuppressive therapy, and intravenous drug abuse are contributing factors. Skin, dental, urinary, and pulmonary infections are common antecedents. Many hematogenous abscesses are associated with recent mild nonpenetrating back injuries; others occur as complications of surgery or lumbar puncture.

Presentation can be characterized as acute or chronic, depending on etiology and clinical evolution. In acute cases, patients appear septic and have fever and leukocytosis; in chronic cases, patients may be afebrile and appear generally well. Sequential clinical stages identified include: (1) localized spinal pain and tenderness, (2) radiat-

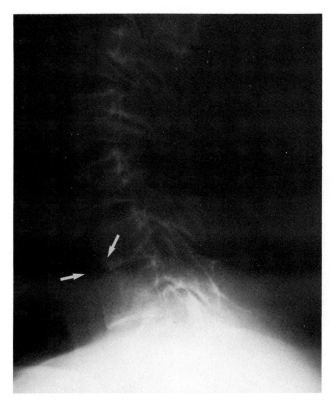

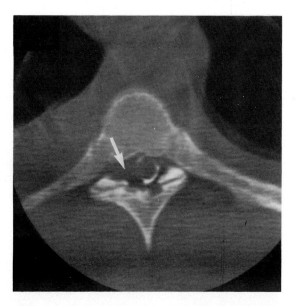

Fig. 20-34. CT scan with intrathecal contrast material administration demonstrates cord compression by an epidural abscess *(arrow).*

Fig. 20-33. Vertebral osteomyelitis. Lateral cervical spine radiograph shows narrowing of the C6/C7 disk space and destruction *(arrows)* of the anteroinferior C6 vertebral body in a patient with osteomyelitis and diskitis (see also Fig. 20-27).

ing pain, (3) limb paresis, and, finally, (4) paralysis and loss of sphincter control.[72] The acute case typically evolves over a period of 7 days; the chronic case may develop over weeks to months.[73] In either case, once weakness develops, paralysis may be complete within hours. As neurologic involvement may appear out of proportion to radiographically apparent manifestations, it has been postulated that neurologic sequelae are in part due to epidural vascular thrombosis and spinal cord infarction.

Most spinal epidural abscesses involve the dorsal epidural space in the thoracic region. In acute hematogenous cases, suppuration extends axially over an average of four spinal segments; chronic cases may have even greater extension.[1] *Staphylococcus aureus* is the most common infecting organism; less often streptococci and gram-negative bacteria are cultured.[74] A wide variety of microorganisms can invade the vertebral column and epidural space, particularly in immunocompromised patients. These include the tubercle bacillus, *Actinomyces, Nocardia, Cryptococcus,* and a variety of other fungi. Parasitic spinal epidural abscesses may be seen in patients from geographic areas where infestations are common.

Plain radiographs in spinal epidural abscess. Plain radiographs, often normal with acute hematogenous infection, may reveal osteomyelitis, although radiographic findings lag behind pathologic changes, signs, and symptoms by

2 to 8 weeks.[75] Early manifestations include loss of trabeculation and erosion of the vertebral body subchondral plate, narrowing of the intervertebral disk space, and involvement of the adjacent vertebral body (Fig. 20-33). Vertebral collapse may follow. Later, anterior osteogenesis occurs, with development of a bridge between the involved vertebral bodies and obliteration of the interspace. Soft tissue densities may be seen if paravertebral abscesses are present.

CT scan in spinal epidural abscess. The CT scan shows indistinctness of epidural soft tissue, replacement of epidural fat with higher density tissue, and narrowing of the subarachnoid space. Intrathecal contrast helps visualize the cord and thecal sac and defines any block (Fig. 20-34). The CT scan can also serve as a guide for needle aspiration and culture. If osteomyelitis is present, the CT scan demonstrates findings much earlier than plain radiographs, with lytic fragmentation of involved vertebrae and irregularity of vertebral end plates.[73] If there is no associated bony infection, the CT scan appearance may be difficult to distinguish from that of neoplasm.[15]

MRI in spinal epidural abscess. The role of MRI in the diagnosis of epidural abscess is less clear. As the signal intensity of epidural inflammatory collections may be similar to adjacent CSF, epidural abscess may be difficult to appreciate unless there is a definite soft tissue component or cord compression[76] (Fig. 20-35). MRI may be helpful in detecting associated diskitis or osteomyelitis.

Treatment. Treatment has traditionally involved urgent surgical decompression. In recent years, some authors have advocated nonsurgical therapy in selected patients: those with minimal or no loss of spinal cord function (in whom any deterioration prompts surgical decompression)

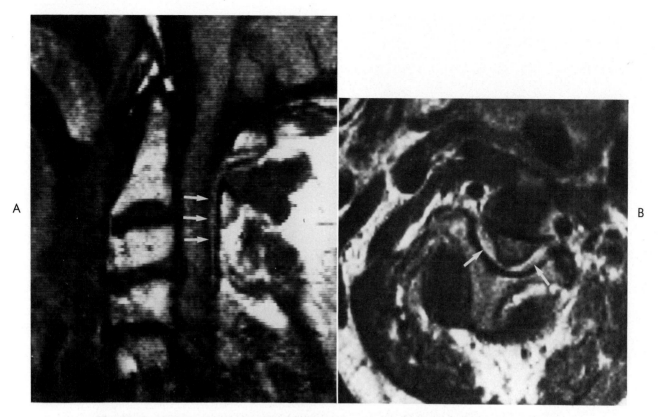

Fig. 20-35. MRI of epidural abscess. **A,** Sagittal T_1-weighted image reveals increased dorsal epidural soft tissue at C2 and C3 *(arrows).* **B,** Abscess shows increased signal on T_2-weighted image *(arrows).* (Courtesy Michael Mestek, MD, Denver General Hospital, Denver, Colorado.)

and patients with severe concomitant medical problems who are poor surgical risks.[77]

Spinal epidural hematoma. Spinal epidural hematoma, while rare, is an important cause of acute spinal cord compression. Bleeding may result from primary or medication-related coagulation defects, trauma, or from rupture of a vascular malformation. Many cases are spontaneous and idiopathic.[78,79] Patients experience abrupt and progressive localized back pain; signs and symptoms of cord compression may rapidly follow.

Radiographic findings in spinal epidural hematoma. Plain radiographs are normal in most cases. On a CT scan, the hematoma, spreading through the epidural space, is seen as a spindle- or crescent-shaped area of high density. This may be difficult to distinguish from other epidural processes, as the high density of the hematoma (80 Hounsfield units) is not easily recognized with the wide windows used for spinal imaging.[15] Myelography demonstrates an epidural mass with partial or complete block but is not specific for the nature of the lesion (Fig. 20-36). MRI demonstrates the spinal epidural hematoma mass within hours of onset; the hematoma is isointense to the cord on T_1-weighted images and may have heterogeneous signal intensity on T_2-weighted images.[78]

Treatment. Treatment consists of surgical decompression of the hematoma and evaluation of any identified un-

derlying condition. Surgery may be contraindicated in some instances of coagulopathy.

Central disk herniation. On occasion a ruptured intravertebral disk may produce acute myelopathy. Midline disk herniation may compress the spinal cord, especially in the thoracic region or in patients with narrow spinal canals. Immediate laminectomy is indicated (see Chapter 18).

Spinal stenosis/spondylosis. See Chapter 18 for discussion.

Intradural extramedullary compartment. Primary tumors of the spinal canal arise most commonly in the intradural extramedullary space; neurofibromas and meningiomas are the most common.[15]

Neurofibromas occur most frequently in middle age and are slightly more common in females. With neurofibromatosis, multiple lesions are the rule. Neurofibromas may be "dumbbell" in shape, extending through the vertebral foramen to form intra- and extra-spinal masses connected by an isthmus of tumor. Plain radiographs may show erosion of the spinal canal, intervertebral foramina, or associated ribs. On a nonenhanced CT scan the tumor may be seen as a slightly high-density mass relative to the spinal cord, or the spinal cord and tumor may be isodense and difficult to visualize if the subarachnoid space is obliterated.[80] An enhanced CT scan delineates the cord margins and usually

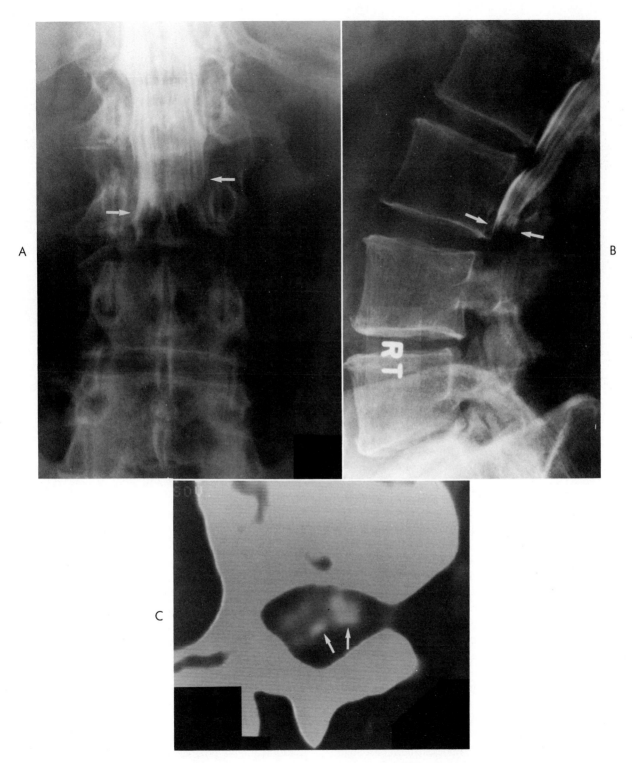

Fig. 20-36. Spinal epidural hematoma. Anteroposterior **(A)** and lateral **(B)** myelogram radiographs of the lumbar region demonstrate a block due to an epidural hematoma *(arrows)* at L2/L3 (site of a recent diagnostic lumbar puncture). **C,** Post-myelogram CT scan demonstrates compression of the dural sac by a dorsal epidural mass *(arrows)*. (Courtesy Delmar Knudson, MD, Denver General Hospital, Denver, Colorado.)

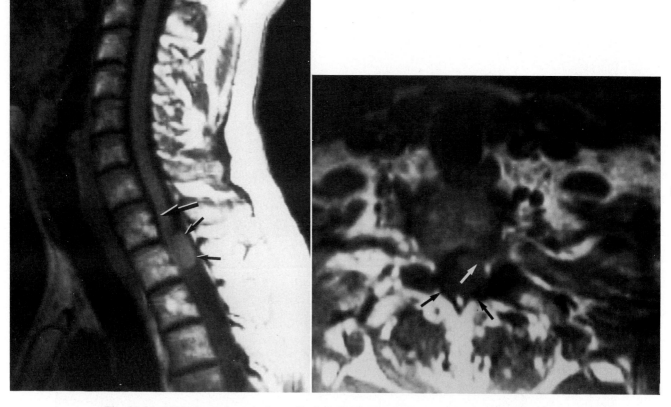

Fig. 20-37. MRI of spinal meningioma. Sagittal (**A**) and axial (**B**) T_1-weighted MRI images show an intradural extramedullary lesion *(small arrows)* compressing and displacing the spinal cord *(large arrows)* anteriorly.

shows enhancement of the tumor. A high-resolution CT scan may demonstrate both the mass and cord displacement as will CT myelography and MRI. Intradural extramedullary location is inferred from displacement and compression of the spinal cord and widening of the subarachnoid space above and below the tumor.

Meningiomas, most often seen in elderly females, are usually midthoracic. They may be calcified, sometimes to the extent of being demonstrable on plain radiographs. On a CT scan meningiomas are high density relative to the spinal cord and may enhance after contrast material administration. Calcification may interfere with delineation on post-myelography CT scan, as both the subarachnoid space and the mass are of high density.[65] On MRI, meningiomas are isointense to the spinal cord but are easily seen because of excellent contrast to CSF; calcifications are seen as foci of low intensity[65] (Fig. 20-37).

Less common masses include lipomas, dermoids, and inflammatory lesions. "Drop metastases" occur from spinal seeding of more rostrally located CNS tumors, such as medulloblastomas and ependymomas; intradural metastases of extraneural tumors occur rarely but may be seen with melanoma and bronchogenic carcinoma.[15] "Carcinomatous meningitis" or "meningeal carcinomatosis" (diffuse metastatic involvement of the meninges and spinal roots)

may be seen with breast and lung carcinoma and lymphoma.[54]

Intramedullary compartment. The spinal cord begins at the medulla oblongata and ends in the conus medullaris at the level of L1/L2 in the adult and L3 in the newborn. On a CT scan, the cord is of higher density than the surrounding CSF, but it may be difficult to visualize when the surrounding subarachnoid space is small (as in the normal thoracic cord or when pathologic processes expand the cord or narrow the subarachnoid space). Intrathecal contrast material helps delineate pathologic alteration of spinal cord margins.

MRI makes possible direct demonstration of intramedullary lesions. Abnormal intensity of cord tissue and cord expansion can be visualized; solid and cystic lesions may be differentiated.

Syringomyelia and hydromyelia. Syringomyelia and hydromyelia are progressive lesions of the spinal cord consisting of variably extensive cavitation ("syrinx," tube) within the central cord. Hydromyelia refers to a cyst lined with ependymal cells derived from enlargement of the central canal of the cord; it is associated with congenital malformations, such as Arnold-Chiari and Dandy-Walker syndromes. Syringomyelia refers to a cyst lined with glial cells, resulting from cavitation of the cord. It may be idio-

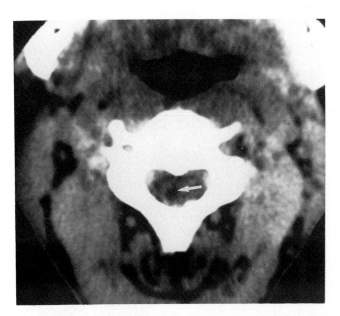

Fig. 20-38. Nonenhanced CT scan of hydrosyringomyelia shows syrinx *(arrow)* to the right of the midline in the upper cervical cord.

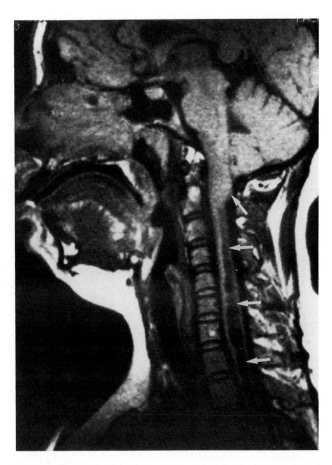

Fig. 20-39. MRI of hydrosyringomyelia. Sagittal T_1-weighted image reveals a low-intensity syrinx *(small arrows)* in a patient with Chiari I malformation. Note the low-lying cerebellar tonsils *(large arrows)*.

pathic or result from trauma, tumor, hemorrhage (hematomyelia), infarction, arachnoiditis, or radiation myelitis. Idiopathic syringomyelia begins in the cervical cord and may extend downward or upward into the medulla (syringobulbia).

Signs and symptoms vary with the level and horizontal involvement of the cord. The clinical syndrome (syringomyelic syndrome or brachial amyotrophy) is characterized by segmental weakness and atrophy of hand and arm muscles with loss of tendon reflexes and segmental sensory loss of the dissociated type (loss of pain and temperature sense, preservation of touch) in a "cape-like" distribution (neck, shoulders, arms). Pain in the areas of sensory impairment is a complaint in one third to one half of patients.[23]

Radiographic findings. The term *hydrosyringomyelia (HSM)* is used radiographically as no modality differentiates between the two conditions.

In cases of congenital malformation, plain radiographs may show associated abnormalities, such as an enlarged foramen magnum, enlarged spinal canal, and basilar invagination.

The CT scan shows cord cysts as low-density regions; cord diameter may be unchanged, increased, or decreased (Fig. 20-38). Intrathecal contrast material reaches the cavity by direct diffusion or via the fourth ventricle; delayed imaging may demonstrate opacification of the cyst.

MRI is ideal for detecting HSM, as sagittal imaging characterizes the lesion in its rostral-caudal extent and surveys the cord for associated pathology (Fig. 20-39).

Treatment. Treatment of progressively symptomatic HSM is surgical decompression.

Intramedullary compartment. Ependymoma is the most common intramedullary neoplasm, usually affecting the conus medullaris and filum terminale. Astrocytomas are next in frequency. Much less common are hemangioblastomas, metastatic foci, and lymphoma.[80]

Common CT scan findings are a decrease in cord density and localized increase in cord diameter; intrathecal contrast material improves visualization of cord distortion.

MRI directly demonstrates cord expansion and abnormal intensity (usually increased) of lesions. Sagittal imaging is especially valuable, as 15% of intramedullary neoplasms have tumor-associated cysts extending in one or both directions[81] (Fig. 20-40).

Spinal cord arteriovenous malformation. Spinal cord arteriovenous malformation (CAVM) occurs more frequently in males (73%)[59]; the mean age of presentation is in the mid-twenties.[82] The malformation may be located within the cord or on its surface and is supplied by the anterior and posterior spinal arteries. Hemorrhage into the cord and subarachnoid space is the most common presentation, followed by presentation of acute nerve root syndrome with root or back pain and weakness; impotence and bladder and bowel dysfunction are often associated.[59,66]

Radiographic findings. Plain radiographs may indicate

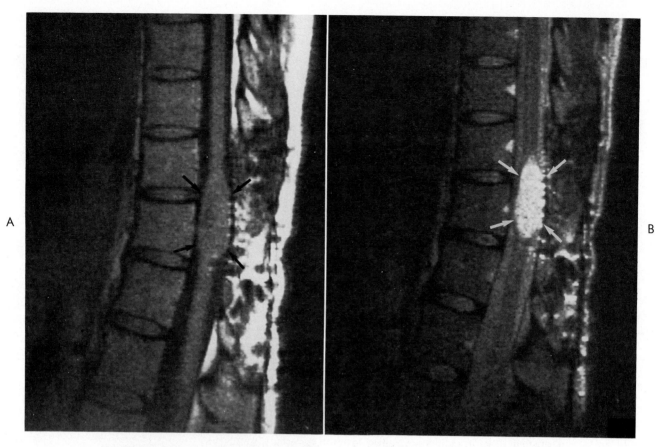

Fig. 20-40. MRI of intramedullary tumor. Sagittal T_1-weighted (**A**) and T_2-weighted (**B**) images demonstrate an astrocytoma of the thoracic cord *(arrows)*. The lesion is isointense on the T_1-weighted image and of high intensity on the T_2-weighted image.

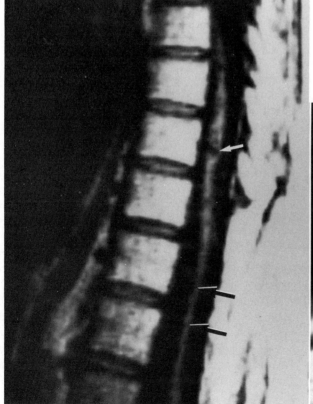

Fig. 20-41. MRI of a spinal cord arteriovenous malformation (CAVM). **A,** Sagittal T_1-weighted image shows an enlarged vessel *(small arrow)* within the thoracic spinal cord with an atrophic cord located distally *(large arrows)*. **B,** Axial T_2-weighted image confirms the intramedullary location of the abnormal vessel *(arrow)*.

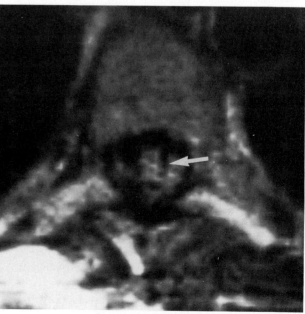

an expanding intraspinal process, with spinal canal widening or erosion of a pedicle or posterior vertebral body.

The CT scan best visualizes these CAVMs with dynamic scanning (scans obtained in rapid sequence), which may demonstrate abrupt and brief enhancement of the abnormal vessels. The cord size may be normal, increased (if hematoma is present), or decreased (if atrophy has supervened).[83] Myelography may clearly demonstrate the CAVM (67%), may demonstrate partial or total block without characterizing the lesion (13%), or may fail to demonstrate small lesions (7%).[59]

While experience is limited, MRI may be useful in characterizing the extent and location of these CAVMs (Fig. 20-41). It may prove to be the study of choice for noninvasive post-treatment imaging.

Angiographic evaluation is crucial, both for pre-operative anatomic localization and characterization and for possible embolic therapy.

Non-mass causes of spinal cord syndrome. There are several causes of spinal cord syndrome.

Anterior spinal artery syndrome. Because the posterior spinal arteries have a richer anastomotic blood supply, hypoperfusion more frequently occurs in the territory of the anterior spinal artery, which supplies the anterior two thirds of the cord. In anterior spinal artery syndrome, infarction involves the spinothalamic tracts (pain and temperature) without affecting the posterior columns (vibration and position sense). Acute back pain is followed by weakness and dissociated anesthesia below the lesion with paralysis of sphincter function. Causes include thrombotic or embolic occlusion, aortic aneurysm, aortic angiography or surgery, arteritis, profound hypotension, and "the bends."

Evaluation includes the exclusion of a spinal mass; treatment is directed toward the underlying condition.

Radiation myelopathy. Radiation myelopathy occurs as a complication of radiation therapy. It may be seen in patients whose "port" encompasses the spinal cord (e.g., thoracic cord segments in lung cancer or Hodgkin's disease). The spinal cord tolerates 4000 to 5000 rads in conventional fractions; the risk is dose related and is significant beyond this level.[75]

The onset of symptoms is insidious and progressive, with painless paresthesias and weakness. Diagnosis depends on the exclusion of a compressive lesion, particularly metastases.

SUMMARY

Patients commonly present to the emergency department with the acute onset of hemiplegia and paraplegia. In some of these patients, these devastating symptoms may be reversible, depending on the etiology. The etiologies are diverse and require individual therapeutic management. Unless the etiology is determined and the therapy is instituted expeditiously, these patients' symptoms may become irreversible. It is for this reason that there should be

a systematic clinical approach to accurate and timely diagnosis, based on history, physical examination, and the radiographic role of the appropriate imaging modality.

REFERENCES

1. Adams RA, Victor M: *Principles of neurology,* ed 4, New York, 1989, McGraw-Hill.
2. Mestek M: Effective use of radiologic tests in neurologic emergencies. In Earnest MP, ed: *Neurologic emergencies,* New York, 1983, Churchill-Livingstone.
3. Deck MD, Weingarten K: Computed tomography and magnetic resonance imaging of the central nervous system. In Youmans JR, ed: *Neurological surgery,* ed 3, Philadelphia, 1990, WB Saunders.
4. Lowe TW, Weinreb J, Santos-Ramos R et al: Magnetic resonance imaging in human pregnancy, *Obstet Gynecol* 66:629, 1985.
5. Brant-Zawadski M, Norman D, Newton TH, et al: Magnetic resonance of the brain: the optimal screening technique, *Radiology* 152:71, 1984.
6. Dillon WP: Magnetic resonance imaging of the head and neck. In Goldberg HI, Higgins CB, Ring EJ, eds: *Contemporary imaging: magnetic resonance imaging, computed tomography, and interventional radiology,* St Louis, 1985, CV Mosby.
7. Grant EG, Wong W, Tessler F et al: Cerebrovascular ultrasound imaging, *Radiol Clin North Am* 26(5):1111, 1988.
8. McGahan JP, Lindfors KK, and Caroll BA: Diagnostic ultrasound in neurological surgery. In Youmans JR, ed: *Neurological surgery,* ed 3, Philadelphia, 1990, WB Saunders.
9. Persson AV, Powis Rl: Recent advances in imaging and evaluation of blood flow using ultrasound, *Radiol Clin North Am* 70:6, 1241, 1986.
10. Anderson DC, Fischer GG: Impact of digital subtraction angiography on carotid evaluation, *Stroke* 16:23, 1985.
11. Pollak EW: Noninvasive cerebrovascular imaging: a prerequisite for angiography? *Am J Surg* 144:203, 1982.
12. Mani RL, Eisenberg RC, McDonald EJ et al: Complications of cerebral arteriography: analysis of 5000 procedures. I. Criteria and indications, *Am J Roentgenol* 131:861, 1978.
13. Brahme FJ: Neuroradiology. In Weiderholt W, ed: *Neurology for non-neurologists,* New York, 1988, Grune & Stratton.
14. Maurer AH: Nuclear medicine: SPECT comparisons to PET, *Radiol Clin North Am* 26(5):1059, 1988.
15. Mark LP, Haughton VM: CT scanning of the spine. In Haaga JR, Alfidi RJ, eds: *Computed tomography of the whole body,* vol I, St Louis, 1988, CV Mosby.
16. Davis IC, Ackerman RH, Kistler JP et al: CT of cerebral infarction: hemorrhagic contrast enhancement and time of appearance, *Comput Tomogr* 1:70, 1977.
17. Modic M: Cerebrovascular disease of the brain. In Haaga JR, Alfidi RJ, eds: *Computed tomography of the whole body,* vol I, St Louis, 1988, CV Mosby.
18. Pullicino P, Kendall BE: Contrast enhancement in ischemic lesions, *Neuroradiology* 19:235, 1980.
19. WHO Task Force on Stroke and Other Cerebrovascular Diseases: Stroke 1989. Recommendations on stroke prevention, diagnosis, and therapy, *Stroke* 20(10):1407, 1989.
20. Dunkley BC, Brant-Zawadski M: MRI evaluation of the stroke patient, *Hosp Physician* March, 33, 1990.
21. Ramadan NM, Deveshwar R, and Levine SR: Magnetic resonance and clinical cerebrovascular disease, *Stroke* 20(9):1279, 1989.
22. Earnest MP: Emergency diagnosis and management of brain infarctions and hemorrhages. In Earnest MP, ed: *Neurologic emergencies,* New York, 1983, Churchill-Livingstone.
23. Kappelle LJ, Ramos LM, and van Gijn J: The role of computed tomography in patients with lacunar stroke in the carotid territory, *Neuroradiology* 31:316, 1989.
24. Goldstone J, Moore WS: Emergency carotid artery surgery in neurologically unstable patients, *Arch Surg* 111:1284, 1976.

25. Najafi H, Jaird H, Dye WS et al: Emergency carotid thromboendart-erectomy: surgical indications and results, *Arch Surg* 103:610, 1971.

26. Kinkel PR, Kinkel WR, and Jacobs L: NMR imaging in patients with stroke, *Semin Neurol* 6:43, 1986.

27. Salgado ED, Weinstein M, Gurlan AJ et al: Proton MR imaging in ischemic cerebrovascular disease, *Ann Neurol* 20:502, 1986.

28. Bogousslavsky J, Regli F: Cerebral infarction with transient signs (CITS): Do TIAs correspond to small deep infarcts in internal carotid artery occlusion? *Stroke* 15:536, 1984.

29. Waxman SO, Toole JF: Temporal profile resembling TIA in the setting of cerebral infarction, *Stroke* 14:433, 1983.

30. Caplan LR, Kelly JJ: *Consultation in neurology,* Toronto, 1988, BC Decker.

31. Donaldson JV: Neurologic complications. In Burrow GN, Ferris TF: *Medical complications during pregnancy,* Philadelphia, 1988, WB Saunders.

32. Meschan I, Osborne AG: Roentgen signs of disease entities of the brain and leptomeneges by computed tomography. In Meshcan I, ed: *Roentgen signs in diagnostic imaging,* ed 2, vol III, Philadelphia, 1985, WB Saunders.

33. Scheinberg P: Controversies in the management of cerebral vascular disease, *Neurology* 38:1609, 1988.

34. Shenken HA, Zavala M: Cerebellar strokes: mortality, surgical indications, and results of ventricular drainage, *Lancet* 2:429, 1982.

35. Srinwaran K: Cerebral venous and arterial thrombosis in pregnancy and the puerperium: a study of 135 patients, *Angiology* 34:731, 1983.

36. Dunn DW, Epstein LG: *Decision making in child neurology,* Toronto, 1987, BC Decker.

37. Schoenberg BS, Mellinger JF, and Schoenberg DG: Cerebrovascular disease in infants and children: a study of incidence, clinical features, and survival, *Neurology* 28:763, 1978.

38. Gold AP: Stroke in children. In Rowland LP, ed: *Merritt's textbook of neurology,* Philadelphia, 1989, Lea & Febiger.

39. Golden GS: Stroke syndromes in childhood, *Neurol Clin North Am* 3(1):59, 1985.

40. Russell MO, Goldberg HJ, Hodson A et al: Effects of transfusion on arteriographic abnormalities and on recurrence of stroke in sickle cell disease, *Blood* 63:162, 1984.

41. Moyes P: Intracranial and intraspinal vascular anomalies in children, *J Neurosurg* 31:271, 1969.

42. Gold AP, Carter S: Acute hemiplegia of infancy and childhood, *Pediatr Clin North Am* 23(3):413, 1976.

43. Golden GS: Strokes in children and adolescents, *Stroke* 9(2):169, 1978.

44. Burns RA: Stroke in young adults. In Rowland LP, ed: *Merritt's textbook of neurology,* Philadelphia, 1989, Lea & Febiger.

45. Grindal AB, Cohen RJ, and Saul SF: Cerebral infarction in young adults, *Stroke* 9(1):39, 1978.

46. Wilson CB: Current concepts in cancer: brain tumors, *New Engl J Med* 300(26):1469, 1979.

47. Baker HL, Houser OW, and Campbell JK: National Cancer Institute Study: evaluation of computed tomography in the diagnosis of intracranial neoplasm, I. Overall results, *Radiology* 136:91, 1980.

48. Kieffer SA: Intracranial neoplasms. In Haaga JR, Alfidi RJ, eds: *Computed tomography of the whole body,* vol I, St Louis, 1988, CV Mosby.

49. Klatzo I: Neuropathologic aspects of brain edema, *J Neuropathol Exp Neurol* 26:1, 1967.

50. Zimmerman RA, Bilaniuk LT: Computed tomography of acute intratumoral hemorrhage, *Radiology* 135:355, 1980.

51. Posner J, Chernick NL: Intracranial metastasis from systemic cancer, *Adv Neurol* 19:575, 1978.

52. Potts DG, Abbott GF, and vonSneidern JV: National Cancer Institute Study: evaluation of computed tomography in the diagnosis of intracranial neoplasms, III. Metastatic tumors, *Radiology* 136:657, 1980.

53. Greenberg HS, Deck MD, Vikram B et al: Metastases to the base of the skull: clinical findings in 43 patients. *Neurology* 31:530, 1981.

54. Adams RA, Hochberg FH: Neoplastic disease of the brain. In Braunwald E, Isselbacher KJ, Petersdorf RG et al, eds: *Harrison's textbook of internal medicine,* ed 11, New York, 1987, McGraw-Hill.

55. Henry GL, Little N: *Neurologic emergencies,* New York, 1985, McGraw-Hill.

56. New PF, Davis KR: The role of CT scanning in the diagnosis of infections of the central nervous system. In Remington J, Swartz M, eds: *Current clinical topics in infectious diseases,* New York, 1980, McGraw-Hill.

57. Sze F, Zimmerman RD: The magnetic resonance imaging of infections and inflammatory disease, *Radiol Clin North Am* 26:839, 1988.

58. Lane B: Leukoencephalopathies and demyelinating disease. In Haaga JR, Alfidi RJ, eds: *Computed tomography of the whole body,* vol I, St Louis, 1988, CV Mosby.

59. Glista GG, Mellinger JF, and Rooke ED: Familial hemiplegic migraine, *Mayo Clin Proc* 50:307, 1975.

60. Prensky AL: Migraine and migraine variants in pediatric patients, *Pediatr Clin North Am* 23(3):461, 1976.

61. Welch KM: Evaluation and management of severe headache. In Earnest MP, ed: *Neurologic emergencies,* New York, 1983, Churchill-Livingstone.

62. Khan A, Marc JA, Chen M et al: Total myelography with metrizamide through the lumbar route, *AJNR* 2:85, 1981.

63. Earnest MP: Safe and effective use of lumbar puncture. In Earnest MP, ed: *Neurologic emergencies,* New York, 1983, Churchill-Livingstone.

64. Pavlicek W: Safety considerations. In Stark DD, Bradley WG, eds: *Magnetic resonance imaging,* St Louis, 1988, CV Mosby.

65. Zimmerman RD, Weingarten K, Johnson CE et al: Neuroradiology of the spine. In Youmans JR, ed: *Neurological surgery,* ed 3, Philadelphia, 1990, WB Saunders.

66. Choi S, Bernstein A: Surgical neuroangiography of the spine and spinal cord: imaging in neuroradiology, Part II, *Radiol Clin North Am* 26(5), 1988.

67. Cairncross JG, Posner JB: Neurologic complications of systemic cancer. In Yarbro JW, Bornstein RD, eds: *Oncologic emergencies,* New York, 1981, Grune & Stratton.

68. Greenberg HS, Kim JH, and Posner JB: Epidural spinal cord compression from metastatic tumor: results with a new treatment protocol, *Ann Neurol* 8:361, 1980.

69. Meschan I: Radiology of the spine. In Meschan I, ed: *Roentgen signs in diagnostic imaging,* ed 2, vol III, Philadelphia, 1985, WB Saunders.

70. Rodichok LO, Ruckdeschel JL, Harper GR et al: Early detection and treatment of spinal epidural metastases: the role of myelography, *Ann Neurol* 20:696, 1986.

71. Pryse-Phillips W, Murray TS: *Essential neurology,* ed 3, 1986, Medical Examination.

72. Hulme A, Dott NM: Spinal epidural abscess, *Br Med J* 1:64, 1958.

73. Carey ME: Infections of the spine and spinal cord. In Youmans JR, ed: *Neurological surgery,* ed 3, Philadelphia, 1990, WB Saunders.

74. Kaufman DM, Kaplan JG, and Litman N: Infectious agents in spinal epidural abscesses, *Neurology* 30:844, 1980.

75. Schold SC: Diagnosis and treatment of spinal cord compression and acute myelopathy. In Earnest MP, ed: *Neurologic emergencies,* New York, 1983, Churchill-Livingstone.

76. Masaryk TJ, Modic MT: Lumbar spine. In Stark DD, Bradley WG, eds: *Magnetic resonance imaging,* St Louis, 1988, CV Mosby.

77. Leys D, Lesoin F, Viaud C et al: Decreased mortality from acute bacterial spinal epidural abscess using computed tomography and nonsurgical treatment in selected patients, *Ann Neurol* 17:350, 1985.

78. Avrahami E, Tadmor R, Ram Z et al: MR demonstration of spontaneous acute epidural hematoma of the thoracic spine, *Neuroradiology* 31:89, 1989.

79. Baker AS, Ojemann RG, Swartz MN et al: Spinal epidural abscess, *N Engl J Med* 293:463, 1975.

80. Mandybur TI: Intracranial hemorrhage caused by metastatic tumors, *Neurology* 27:650, 1977.

81. New PF, Shoukimas GM: Thoracic spine and spinal cord. In Stark DD, Bradley WG, eds: *Magnetic resonance imaging,* St Louis, 1988, CV Mosby.

82. Rosenblum B, Oldfield EH, Deppman SL et al: Spinal arteriovenous malformations: a comparison of dural arteriovenous malformations and intradural AVMs in 81 patients, *J Neurosurg* 67:795, 1987.

83. DiChiro G, Doppman JL, and Wener L: Computed tomography of spinal cord arteriovenous malformations, *Radiology* 123:351, 1977.

Additional readings

Arta JF: Multiple sclerosis and cranial lesions, *Arch Neurol* 37:738, 1980.

Calandre L, Gomnara S, Bermejo F et al: Clinical-CT correlation in TIA, RIND, and strokes with minimum residuum, *Stroke* 15:663, 1984.

Dublin A, Djindjian M: Angiography of the spine and spinal cord. In Youmans JR, ed: *Neurological surgery,* ed 3, Philadelphia, 1990, WB Saunders.

Murphy FK, Mackowiak P, and Lieby J: Management of infections afflicting the nervous system. In Rosenberg RN, ed: *The treatment of neurologic disease,* New York, 1979, Spectrum.

Stone DB, Bonfiglio M: Pyogenic vertebral osteomyelitis: diagnostic pitfall for the internist, *Arch Intern Med* 112:491, 1963.

Uhlenbrock D, Seidel D, Gehlen W et al: Magnetic resonance imaging in multiple sclerosis: comparison with clinical, CSF, and visual evoked potential findings, *AJNR* 9:59, 1988.

Zee C, Han J, and Segall H: Infectious processes of the brain. In Haaga JR, Alfidi RJ, eds: *Computed tomography of the whole body,* vol I, St Louis, 1988, CV Mosby.

Zee C, Han J: Neuroradiology. In Hennings RJ, Jackson DC, eds: *Handbook of critical care neurology and neurosurgery,* New York, 1985, Praeger.

Zimmerman RA, Bilaniuk LT: Imaging of tumors of the spinal canal and cord: imaging in neuroradiology, II, *Radiol Clin North Am* 26(5):965, 1988.

C H A P T E R *21*

Vaginal Bleeding and Pelvic Pain

Jean Abbott
David Thickman

Genitourinary complaints in the female are frequently seen in the emergency department. Pelvic pain and vaginal bleeding are the most common presenting gynecologic complaints. Determination of the existence of a pregnancy is a critical first step in the evaluation of a woman of childbearing age, although pregnant women can have nonpregnancy-related causes of pelvic pain or bleeding. The surgical emergencies of ectopic pregnancy, appendicitis (see Chapter 13), and ovarian torsion must always be considered. Additionally, the complications of intrauterine pregnancy or of pelvic infection are important differential diagnoses. Emergency imaging studies of the female pelvis are valuable in identifying these conditions. There are other, nonemergency conditions for which imaging studies can be scheduled, such as the evaluation of an asymptomatic palpable pelvic mass. Ultrasonography, in particular, plays an important role in the evaluation of female patients presenting to the emergency department with pelvic complaints.

ANATOMIC AND PHYSIOLOGIC CONSIDERATIONS IN PELVIC IMAGING

The female pelvis can be divided into two parts. The *true pelvis* has a basin-shaped contour and is bounded by the pubic symphysis and pubic rami anteriorly, the sacrum and coccyx posteriorly, and the perineal musculature inferiorly. The *false pelvis* is superior to the true pelvis and is bounded by the abdominal wall anteriorly, the iliac bones laterally, and the sacral promontory posteriorly. In the evaluation of the pelvis, determination of uterine size, shape, and contents, as well as identification of the ovaries and posterior cul-de-sac, are essential.

Uterine shape varies with distention of the adjacent bladder and rectum, as well as with cyclic changes in the menstrual cycle. The axis of the nonpregnant uterus is usually anterior to the vaginal axis (anteverted) and anterior to the cervical axis (anteflexed). Retroflexion is a normal variation seen in about 25% of women.[1] Endometrial thickness varies depending on the patient's age and the degree of ovarian (hormonal) stimulation of the endometrium. The thickness fluctuates from 1 to 6 mm during the menstrual cycle and is thinnest following menstruation. The normal prepubertal uterus is relatively small, being 3 cm in length and 1 cm in width and depth. During the reproductive years the uterus enlarges, with maximal normal dimensions of 7 cm × 4 cm × 5 cm. Further enlargement typically occurs with pregnancy and leiomyoma formation. Postmenopausally, the uterine size normally decreases to a maximum of 7 cm in length and 1 to 2 cm in transverse dimensions[2] (Fig. 21-1).

The ovaries are elliptically shaped and have a variable axis and location. In the nulliparous woman, they are located in the ovarian fossa on the posterolateral wall of the true pelvis and immediately adjacent to the ureter, obturator nerve, and internal iliac vessels. In the parous woman, location is extremely variable. Because ovarian shape may vary, size is best measured by total volume (length × width × height divided by 2). Whereas the average ovar-

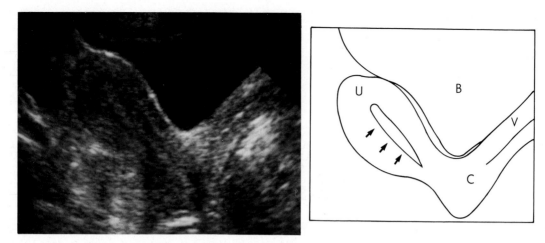

Fig. 21-1. Longitudinal ultrasonogram of the normal female pelvis. Normal echogenic stripe of the endometrial canal *(arrows)* is seen in the middle of the smoothly contoured uterus *(U)*. *B*, Urinary bladder; *C*, cervix; *V*, vagina.

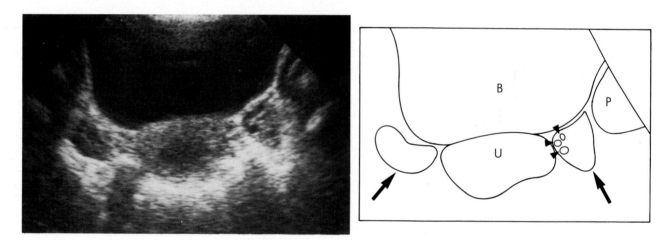

Fig. 21-2. Transverse ultrasonogram of the normal female pelvis. The ovaries *(arrows)* are seen on either side of the uterus *(U)*. Normal follicles *(arrowheads)* are present in the left ovary. *B*, Urinary bladder; *P*, ileopsoas muscle; *U*, uterus.

ian volume during reproductive years is about 6 ml, normal maximal volume may be as much as 14 ml (Fig. 21-2). The premenarchal female and postmenopausal woman both have much smaller ovaries, with maximum volumes of approximately 1 ml and 2.5 ml, respectively.[2] Ultrasonographically, the ovaries are homogeneous structures with an echotexture similar to or slightly less than that of the myometrium. They frequently contain echogenic or anechoic follicles.

The physiology of the ovaries is important in understanding imaging variations. Cystic follicles that measure up to 3 cm occur during the first half of the menstrual cycle (the proliferative phase) in ovulating women. When they are greater than 2.5 cm, they are considered follicular "cysts."[2] During the second half of the menstrual cycle (the secretory phase), the corpus luteum, a physiologic ovarian cyst, is formed at the site of ovulation. This cyst may become as large as 10 cm in diameter and is often

visible by ultrasonography[1] (Fig. 21-3). Corpus luteum cysts rarely last more than 6 weeks and do not occur in the absence of ovulation. They produce the classic ultrasonographic appearance of a cyst: an anechoic mass (no internal echoes), smooth walls, a well-defined posterior wall, and posterior acoustic enhancement. Simple cysts may undergo hemorrhage or rupture. Ultrasonographically, hemorrhagic cysts are complex masses containing internal echoes. Ruptured cysts may no longer be palpable[3] or visible ultrasonographically; the only clue that the cyst existed may be fluid in the cul-de-sac.[1]

The normal fallopian tubes are about 10 to 14 cm in length and cannot usually be visualized by transabdominal sonography. However, they may be seen if enlarged as a result of inflammation (hydrosalpinx), if there is an ectopic pregnancy, or if they are surrounded by fluid. The fallopian tubes can be seen during transvaginal ultrasonography.[4]

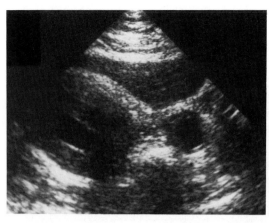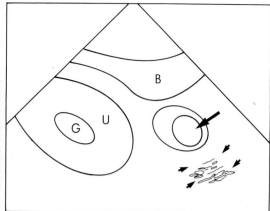

Fig. 21-3. Transverse ultrasonogram of the female pelvis with an early pregnancy. Corpus luteum cyst *(arrow)* is present in the left ovary. There is posterior acoustic enhancement *(small arrows)*. *B,* Urinary bladder; *U,* uterus; *G,* gestational sac.

The posterior cul-de-sac is a space formed by the peritoneal reflection posterior to the uterus and anterior to the rectosigmoid colon. It normally contains a small amount of peritoneal fluid because it is the most dependent portion of the peritoneal cavity in the supine position. Fluid in the cul-de-sac is visible in several pathologic conditions, but it is occasionally a normal finding, most often occurring within 5 days preceding menstruation[5] (Fig. 21-4).

IMAGING OF THE FEMALE PELVIS

The role of plain radiography of the pelvis is limited but valuable in some circumstances. It is an excellent method of assessing the skeletal portions of the pelvis. In addition to bony elements, plain radiography provides a preliminary survey of some of the soft tissues. For example, the urinary bladder is identified by its surrounding fat, and the borders of the pelvic musculature are similarly identified. Furthermore, an abnormal pattern of intraluminal bowel gas or any extraluminal gas can be a sign of significant disease. Additionally, calcifications or other abnormal shadows and foreign bodies can yield significant diagnoses. Intravenous, gastrointestinal, or genitourinary contrast material can selectively enhance the usefulness of pelvic radiographs.

Although plain radiography provides a survey of the pelvis and can provide useful information in some situations, ultrasonography has become the mainstay for imaging evaluation of the pelvis, especially in the female. Ultrasonography provides for a detailed examination of the urinary bladder, uterus, adnexa, cul-de-sac, and major pelvic vasculature. In some circumstances, bowel lesions can be seen, although bowel gas generally hinders ultrasonographic study of the gastrointestinal tract.

Two approaches to imaging the pelvis have been used. *Transabdominal sonography* (TAS) images the pelvic organs from the anterior abdominal wall through the distended urinary bladder, which displaces the gas-containing

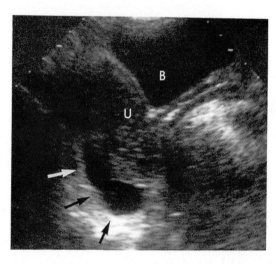

Fig. 21-4. Longitudinal ultrasonogram of the female pelvis. Peritoneal fluid *(arrows)* in the cul-de-sac is seen as a crescentic anechoic collection posterior to the uterus *(U)*. *B,* urinary bladder.

bowel out of the true pelvis, thereby providing a ultrasonographic window for viewing pelvic organs. Newer *endovaginal sonography* (EVS) has been used to visualize organs of the true pelvis using a transducer placed in the vagina. This shortens the distance between the uterus and adnexa and the transducer, thus permitting use of a higher-frequency transducer, which produces sharper images (Fig. 21-5). This procedure is well tolerated by patients, who generally prefer this method of examination to the bladder fullness required for TAS. Although EVS can easily and accurately answer questions in the emergency evaluation of patients, it does not provide complete information if the gravid uterus, enlarged ovaries, or pelvic masses extend above the true pelvis. In such cases, TAS should be performed as well.

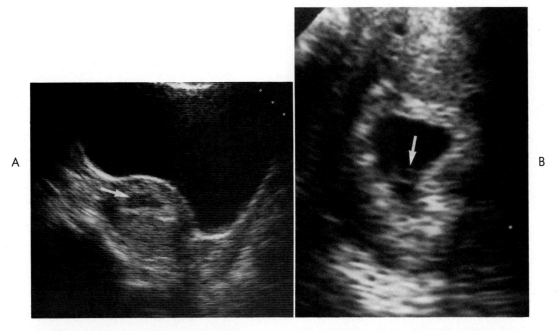

Fig. 21-5. A, Transabdominal ultrasonogram shows a well-defined gestational sac within the uterus (*arrow*), but no parts are identified. **B,** Endovaginal ultrasonogram shows a well-defined sac, which contains a yolk sac *(arrow).*

IMAGING DURING PREGNANCY

Ultrasonography has no known adverse effects on the fetus during pregnancy and is more accurate than a menstrual history for dating the pregnancy. It has been used routinely in the first and second trimesters. Additionally, it produces beneficial emotional effects, such as the relief of anxiety in patients with threatened miscarriage or high-risk pregnancy, as well as the promotion of early maternal bonding and maternal behavior modification (e.g., smoking cessation).[6]

First trimester

During pregnancy, uterine enlargement occurs in a predictable manner. The first change is hypertrophy of the endometrial lining. Because the ultrasonographic appearance of the endometrium varies in thickness throughout the menstrual cycle, a thick endometrium is not a reliable indicator of early intrauterine pregnancy (IUP). The appearance of a gestational sac may be mimicked by the decidual reaction occurring with extrauterine pregnancy (a "pseudogestational" sac). The differentiation between these entities cannot be made reliably by ultrasonography.[7]

There are several early ultrasonographic signs of intrauterine gestation. The *intradecidual sign,* a focal thickening or sac embedded within the endometrium causing enlargement on one side of the endometrial cavity, is a very early, subtle sign of IUP.[8] The *double-decidual sac sign* (DDSS) has a positive predictive value for IUP of about 95%.[9] This finding is believed to result from the *decidua parietalis,* which is separated by fluid in the endometrial cavity from the *decidua capsularis* surrounding the gestational

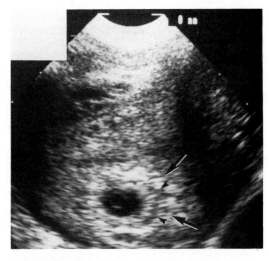

Fig. 21-6. Transverse view of the uterus shows a well-formed intrauterine gestational sac containing a yolk sac. Thin crescentic rim of decreased echoes *(arrowheads)* is fluid between the decidua parietalis and the decidua capsularis. The adjacent echogenic rim *(arrows)* completes the double-decidual sac sign.

sac (Fig. 21-6). The double-decidual sac sign can usually be identified by 42 days after the last menstrual period by TAS. A more reliable sign is identification of the *yolk sac* within the gestational sac, which, if identified, is a 100% confirmation of an IUP[9] (see Fig. 21-5). Another reliable but infrequently identified sign of IUP is the *double-bleb sign,* the ultrasonographic visualization of the amniotic sac and yolk sac sandwiching the embryo of a 5½ -week pregnancy.[10]

Table 21-1. Relationship of gestational age, hCG levels, and transvaginal ultrasonographic findings

		β-hCG (mIU/ml)	
Ultrasound findings	Days from last menstrual period	First international reference preparation	Second international standard
Sac	34.8 ± 2.2	1309 ± 155	914 ± 106
Fetal pole	40.3 ± 3.4*	5113 ± 298*	3783 ± 683
Fetal heart motion	46.9 ± 6.0*	17,208 ± 3772*	13,178 ± 3898*

*$P < 0.05$ when compared with the sac.

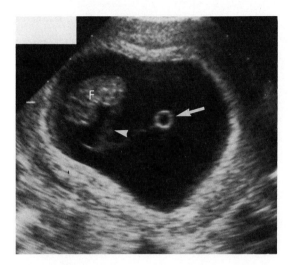

Fig. 21-7. Ultrasonogram of an early pregnancy. The fetus *(F)* is seen within the amniotic sac. Crown-rump length is 22 mm (9 weeks). Secondary yolk sac *(arrow)* and umbilical cord *(arrowhead)* are noted.

Ultrasonographic findings in the pregnant patient with a possible ectopic pregnancy

Indicative of IUP
  Double-ring sign
  Double gestational sac
  Intrauterine fetal pole
  Intrauterine fetal heart activity
Diagnostic of an ectopic gestation
  Ectopic fetal heart activity or fetal pole outside uterus
Suggestive of an ectopic gestation
  Cul-de-sac fluid without IUP
  Adnexal mass (any type) without IUP
Indeterminate
  No intrauterine findings
  Single gestational sac
  Multiple intrauterine echoes

The most reliable sign of IUP is ultrasonographic identification of the embryo, which can be identified and measured by 6½ weeks of gestation (Fig. 21-7). Fetal heart activity can be seen within the embryo or even before the embryo is distinctly identified.[8] Only identification of the embryo or fetus itself can be used reliably to differentiate an IUP from a ectopic pregnancy (see the box above). It must always be remembered that an IUP can coexist with an ectopic pregnancy (incidence 1:7000 to 1:30,000), although on a practical basis, identification of an IUP is sufficient to exclude ectopic pregnancy for the purposes of patient management.[8]

Quantitative human chorionic gonadotropin (hCG) levels correlate well with gestational age and ultrasonographic landmarks in the first trimester (Table 21-1). The "discriminatory zone" is the quantitative hCG level at which a normal IUP can reliably be seen on ultrasonography. This concept is extremely helpful in the emergency department if a quantitative hCG level can be obtained quickly, or if the stable pregnant patient can be referred for ultrasonography and gynecologic follow-up within 24 hours. However, caution must be taken in the interpretation of current publications relating gestational sac size to hCG levels because different hCG units are used by different investigators (9.3 mIU/ml International Reference Preparation [IRP] = 5.0 mIU/ml Second International Standard = 1 ng).[11] In addition, the threshold for identification of the early normal IUP depends on the equipment used as well as the skill of the operator. In general, gestational landmarks are seen with EVS about a week before they can be seen with TAS. Table 21-1 indicates the current hCG levels at which first-trimester landmarks of pregnancy can be visualized ultrasonographically with TAS and EVS. With EVS, a gestational sac should be seen with a hCG of 3600 mIU/ml (IRP), and with TVS, a gestational sac of 4 mm may been seen quite often, corresponding to an hCG of 1025 mIU/ml (IRP).[12,13] Because the mean sac diameter increases at about 1 mm/day during the first few weeks of gestation, ultrasonographic studies that fail to identify a gestational sac should be repeated 7 to 14 days later to allow time for growth to occur.[14]

During the first trimester, the corpus luteum is usually visible until 7 to 8 weeks, with involution occurring as the placenta takes over the hormonal sustenance of the early pregnancy. The corpus luteum in pregnancy normally reaches 3 cm in size; it is considered cystic if it is larger, but it may reach 10 cm in diameter in some normal pregnancies[2] (see Fig. 21-3). The corpus luteum may also be seen in association with ectopic gestations.

Second and third trimesters

Ultrasonographic examinations are mainly requested by the emergency physician after the first trimester to identify fetal heart activity when Doppler-imaged heart tones cannot be detected and to evaluate the placenta for position and possible separation (abruptio placentae). Fetal heart activity that is absent on ultrasonographic examination or is outside of the range of normal rates (120 to 160 beats/min) requires urgent obstetric referral for fetal monitoring and assessment of fetal well-being.

After 12 weeks of gestation, the placenta is ultrasonographically visible as an intermediate, echogenic, soft tissue structure adjacent to the uterine wall. In the first trimester, the placenta frequently appears to cover the endometrium completely and may be difficult to differentiate from decidua. At 20 weeks of gestation, the placenta covers one fourth of the endometrial surface, and may be low lying or encroach on the cervix, suggesting some degree of placenta previa. At term, more than 90% of all placentas identified as overlapping the cervix in the second trimester have "migrated" from the cervix. Two factors are involved: (1) whereas true placental movement does not occur, a change in relative position of the placenta occurs with elongation of the lower uterine segment; and (2) a full maternal bladder can compress the lower uterine segment and create the false impression of placenta previa on ultrasonographic study.[14]

CLINICAL PRESENTATIONS
Vaginal bleeding

Patients with vaginal bleeding can accurately be separated into those who are pregnant and those who are not because of the advent of sensitive qualitative hCG tests. Human chorionic gonadotropin is secreted from the inception of blastocyst implantation, about 3 to 4 days before a missed menstrual period. A threshhold of 10 to 50 mIU/ml (IRP) is common for qualitative pregnancy tests, is achieved within 2 to 3 days of implantation, and almost always yields positive results even in abnormal pregnancies.[15] Ultrasonography is most frequently used in the emergency setting in the evaluation of the patient who is bleeding in early pregnancy, both to determine viability and to locate the pregnancy. In the nonpregnant patient, a tissue diagnosis is often important to establish the cause of bleeding. Imaging is usually less urgent, although it may be part of the workup of the patient with persistent abnormal or increased bleeding.

Vaginal bleeding in the pregnant patient. The differential of vaginal bleeding in the first trimester of pregnancy includes several important entities. Although pain-

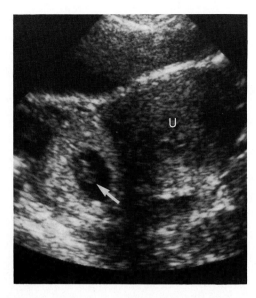

Fig. 21-8. Transverse ultrasonogram of the pelvis shows a well-formed gestational sac outside of the uterus *(U)* containing a fetal pole *(arrow)*.

less bleeding or spotting may be associated with a normal pregnancy, it can also portend a threatened miscarriage, molar pregnancy, or ectopic pregnancy. In the patient with pain and vaginal bleeding, the differential diagnosis includes ectopic pregnancy, normal IUP, IUP with rupture of a corpus luteum cyst, ovarian torsion, and the various stages of threatened or inevitable miscarriage. In the second and third trimester, abruptio placentae is a major concern, particularly when bleeding is painful. Suspicion of placenta previa is also an indication for ultrasonography.

Threatened miscarriage. With accurate, early pregnancy tests, it has become apparent that large numbers of pregnancies end in miscarriage. Recent reports indicate a risk of miscarriage of 25% to 33% in pregnant women.[16] Although ultrasonography is not mandatory in the emergent evaluation of the patient with a threatened miscarriage, several goals are accomplished by scheduling early imaging for the patient. Because ectopic pregnancy presents with painless vaginal bleeding in a small number of cases, the identification of the pregnancy as intrauterine is extremely useful. In addition, determination of the status of an IUP may facilitate early termination of a nonviable gestation. Recently, it has been suggested that ultrasonographic studies at 7½ weeks or later can define pregnancy status into three groups: a fetus with heart activity (normal pregnancy), a fetus with crown-rump length greater than 15 mm but without cardiac activity (fetal death), and a sac without fetus (anembryonic gestation).[17] Molar pregnancies can also be identified by ultrasonography. In the woman with an anembryonic gestation, a dilatation and curettage can be performed early, with tissue review to ensure that the pregnancy was indeed intrauterine.

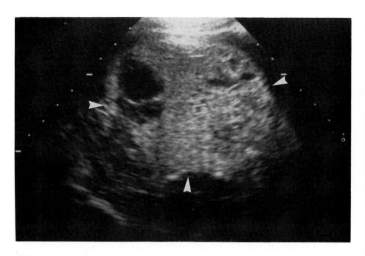

Fig. 21-9. Transverse ultrasonogram of a molar pregnancy. Uterus *(arrowheads)* is enlarged and contains echogenic tissue with multiple cystic spaces of varying sizes.

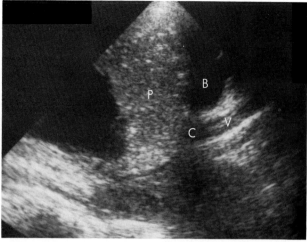

Fig. 21-10. Longitudinal ultrasonogram of placenta previa. The placenta *(P)* covers the cervix *(C)*. *B*, Urinary bladder; *V*, vagina.

Evidence of a viable fetus with heart activity is an encouraging prognostic sign in threatened abortion. Although the risk of fetal loss for patients with vaginal bleeding in the first trimester of an IUP is 50% or greater, the risk with demonstrated fetal heart activity is only about 5%.[18] Although determination of fetal viability is not emergent, the value of giving appropriate advice and counsel to women with threatened miscarriage cannot be underestimated.

Ectopic pregnancy. It is important to exclude ectopic pregnancy (Fig. 21-8) in patients with vaginal bleeding in the first trimester. Because the landmarks of early pregnancy are better seen with EVS than with TAS, it is recommended that the patient either have EVS or, if TAS is "indeterminate," receive further evaluation by EVS if the possibility of an ectopic pregnancy is high.

In the patient whose last menstrual period occurred more than 56 days earlier or whose quantitative hCG level is greater than 6000 mIU/ml (IRP), a normal viable IUP should reliably be seen with TAS.[19] If the uterus is empty or the gestational age is earlier, EVS should be performed. With the endovaginal approach, the intrauterine gestation may be seen as early as a 1000 mIU/ml (IRP) hCG level by an experienced ultrasonographer with good technical equipment.[20] With EVS, both IUPs and actual ectopic gestations can be seen more frequently, and the number of patients with indeterminant results is minimized. In a recent prospective study of patients with possible ectopic pregnancy, 38 of 145 could be diagnosed by TAS and another 98 of 145 could be diagnosed with EVS performed the same day, with only 1 false-positive diagnosis of ectopic pregnancy.[21] Currently, the threshold for accurate identification of IUP depends on the skill of the ultrasonographer and radiologist. Emergency department physicians must be familiar with the accuracy of early IUP identification in their institution.

Molar pregnancy. Molar pregnancy (Fig. 21-9) may cause first- and second-trimester vaginal bleeding. The classic molar pregnancy appearance on ultrasonographic examination is that of a "snow storm," a relatively homogeneous intrauterine echogenic mass containing small cystic spaces, representing overgrowth of placental tissue without fetal development. In a partial molar pregnancy, a fetus may be present, and ultrasonographic diagnosis of the molar nature of the pregnancy rests on the exuberance of placental tissue surrounding the pregnancy.

Vaginal bleeding in the second and third trimesters. Placenta previa typically presents as painless bleeding in the second or third trimester, accounting for about 10% of bleeding during the latter half of gestation. The incidence of placenta previa at term is about 0.5%. As described previously, placenta previa occurs more often in the second trimester and can readily be identified by ultrasonography[13] (Fig. 21-10).

Abruptio placentae accounts for about 15% to 20% of patients with bleeding in the second and third trimesters. It is a cause of considerable fetal mortality because separation of more than 25% of the placenta results in fetal oxygen compromise and potential hypovolemia. At times, ultrasonographic findings are subtle, particularly with acute hemorrhage, and it may be difficult to differentiate normal placenta from clot. Retroplacental thickening and subtle echotexture differences should be sought in the appropriate clinical setting (Fig. 21-11). Marginal placental separations and small amounts of bleeding are often not detected, and the diagnosis must be suspected clinically in the woman with vaginal bleeding and any uterine irritability or evidence of fetal distress by monitoring. When abruptio placentae is identified ultrasonographically, it may be useful in predicting outcome. Retroplacental hemorrhages and large amounts of bleeding (>60 ml) are associated with

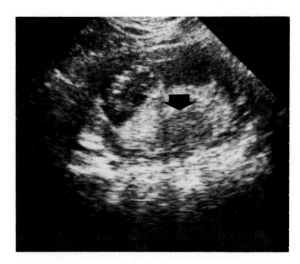

Fig. 21-11. Abruptio placentae with retroplacental thickening (*arrow*) and subtle echotexture differences.

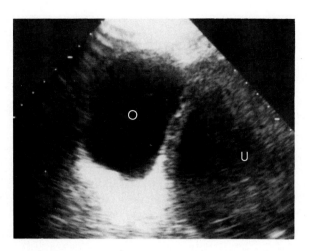

Fig. 21-12. Transverse view of the pelvis in a pregnant patient. Large cystic structure *(O)* to the right of the uterus *(U)* is an ovarian torsion. The patient had an underlying dermoid of the ovary.

75% fetal mortality.[22] Subchorionic bleeding and bleeding of less than 60 ml have a more favorable outcome.[23]

Vaginal bleeding in the nonpregnant patient. In the nonpregnant patient, vaginal bleeding has a differential diagnosis that includes several systemic conditions, including coagulopathy, endocrine abnormalities, and liver disease. Organic or structural causes of vaginal bleeding in the nonpregnant patient include ovarian cyst, carcinoma (particularly over age 30 years) and leiomyoma, which occur in approximately 40% of women over age 35 years.[24] Although imaging studies may be helpful in making these diagnoses, they rarely need to be performed in the emergency department.

Pelvic pain

In the woman who presents with pelvic pain, the differential diagnosis between pain in pregnancy and pain in the nonpregnant patient is important.

Pelvic pain in the pregnant patient. Ectopic pregnancy is discussed under the section on vaginal bleeding in pregnancy. Other causes of pain in the first trimester include stretching of the parovarian structures, torsion of the ovary (see later discussion), and most often, corpus luteum cyst rupture. The corpus luteum sustains the pregnancy during the first 6 to 8 weeks, is normally cystic, and may reach 10 cm in diameter. Clinically, rupture of the corpus luteum cyst is often difficult to distinguish from the presentation of ectopic pregnancy; both cause sudden lower peritoneal irritation and pain in early pregnancy (see Fig. 21-3). A corpus luteum cyst may be seen both with an ectopic pregnancy and an IUP. Ultrasonographically, the typical corpus luteum cyst is a sharply demarcated anechoic structure with posterior acoustic enhancement. However, with rupture or hemorrhage, the ultrasonographic appearance may become complex or solid and may mimic other adnexal pathologic states, including ec-

topic pregnancy.

Pain in the second half of pregnancy may be associated with ovarian torsion, abruptio placentae, or nongynecologic emergencies, such as pyelonephritis, renal calculi, appendicitis, diverticulitis, and spontaneous hepatic or splenic rupture that may be subcapsular. These conditions are discussed in other chapters, but they present a diagnostic imaging dilemma because the patient should not be exposed to excessive ionizing radiation during pregnancy. In these circumstances, ultrasonography can be quite helpful in the evaluation.

Pelvic pain in the nonpregnant patient. The differential diagnosis of pelvic pain in the nonpregnant patient consists of appendicitis (see Chapter 13), ovarian disease (including ruptured cyst, distention of a large cyst, or adnexal torsion), and pelvic inflammatory disease. Other diagnoses that may require consideration in the patient with pelvic pain include endometriosis, degeneration of fibroids, hematomas within the pelvis, and incarcerated hernias.

Adnexal torsion. Ovarian or fallopian tube torsion is a difficult clinical and radiographic diagnosis. Clinical suspicion is based on severe, unilateral pain, often associated with nausea, vomiting, and other symptoms of ischemia, but with scant or absent peritoneal signs. Adnexal tenderness and fullness may be present. It is believed that enlargement or imbalance causing an increased polarity of the ovary or adnexa is required for torsion; therefore the enlarged ovary with a cyst or mass is most susceptible (Fig. 21-12). Torsion can occur premenarchally, postmenopausally, or after hysterectomy. About 20% of torsions occur during pregnancy.[25]

Because it is rare for a normal-sized ovary to twist, identification of normal ovarian size and texture by ultrasonography may be helpful in excluding torsion. Doppler ultrasonography has not been proved to reliably measure

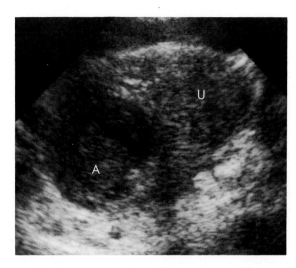

Fig. 21-13. Transverse ultrasonogram of tubo-ovarian abscess. Large, complex, slightly hypoechoic mass representing the abscess *(A)* is seen to the right of the uterus *(U)*.

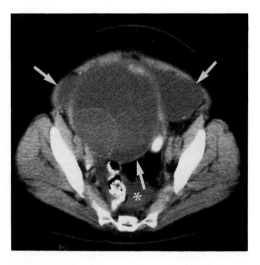

Fig. 12-14. Pelvic CT scan of a 68-year-old female patient shows a large, multi-septale cystic mass *(arrows)* consistent with a serous cystadenoma of the ovary. Note free posterior peritoneal fluid *(asterisk)*.

altered blood flow in ovarian torsion, although engorged vessels can occasionally be seen. The use of ultrasonography is mainly to identify a large ovary with enlarged follicles or an enlarged cystic, complex adnexal mass and to exclude other diseases within the pelvis. No imaging studies should delay laparoscopy or surgical exploration if the suspicion of torsion is high.

Pelvic inflammatory disease. Pelvic inflammatory disease (PID) is another difficult clinical diagnosis. Clinical accuracy in recognizing PID is only 66%. The sequelae of chronic pain, infertility, and ectopic pregnancy occur at least as frequently with clinically mild disease as with severe disease.[26] Ultrasonography is rarely of assistance in the simple, uncomplicated case of PID. However, when a mass is palpated or suspected, ultrasonography may be of use in identifying a large tubo-ovarian abscess (TOA) (Fig. 21-13). Differentiation of an inflammatory mass (phlegmon) from an actual abscess is often problematic. If an abscess is seen, ultrasonography is often used to follow the size of the abscess and to determine whether it is resolving with conservative management or if surgical intervention is required.[27]

Palpable pelvic masses. Further indication for ultrasonography is an asymptomatic mass palpated on pelvic examination. This rarely requires emergency imaging, however, and a routine outpatient workup can be pursued. Determination of the cystic or solid nature of the mass and its size may be extremely helpful in guiding the differential diagnosis and approach to the patient. CT scans may be a useful adjunctive measure (Fig. 21-14). In the postmenopausal woman, any palpable adnexa should be imaged.[2] In addition, the enlarged uterus in the woman in later reproductive years may require imaging to identify fibroids and other masses.

SUMMARY

Although plain radiography has limited usefulness in the evaluation of the patient with pelvic complaint, ultrasonography has become an invaluable adjunct to the physical examination in both the pregnant and the nonpregnant female. In the patient with pelvic pain in pregnancy, the use of ultrasonography is urgent. In the nonpregnant patient, ultrasonography may be useful in identifying the patient at risk for ovarian torsion, appendicitis, or complicated PID. For the patient with an asymptomatic or symptomatic palpable mass within the pelvis, ultrasonography is likewise a useful modality. As a valuable tool in management of the obstetric patient, ultrasonographic studies may be emergently obtained when critical for patient care and may be scheduled from the emergency department for routine evaluation of pregnant patients.

REFERENCES

1. Droegemueller W, Herbst AL, Mishell DR et al: *Comprehensive gynecology,* St Louis, 1987, Mosby–Year Book.
2. Neiman HL, Mendelson EB: Ultrasound evaluation of the ovary. In Callen PW, ed: *Ultrasonography in obstetrics and gynecology,* Philadelphia, 1988, WB Saunders.
3. Hibbard LT: Corpus luteum surgery, *Am J Obstet Gynecol* 135:666, 1979.
4. Levi CS, Lyons EA, Lindsay DJ et al: Normal anatomy of the female pelvis. In Callen PW, ed: *Ultrasonography in obstetrics and gynecology,* Philadelphia, 1988, WB Saunders.
5. Davis JA, Gosink BB: Fluid in the female pelvis: cyclic patterns, *J Ultrasound Med* 5:75, 1986.
6. Waldenstrom U, Nilsson S, Fall O et al: Effects of routine one-stage ultrasound screening in pregnancy: a randomized controlled trial, *Lancet,* September 1988, p 585.
7. Marks WM, Filly RA, Callen RW et al: The decidual cast of ectopic pregnancy: a confusing ultrasonographic appearance, *Radiology* 133:451, 1979.
8. Yeh H-C, Goodman JD, Carr L et al: Intradecidual sign: a US criterion of early intrauterine pregnancy, *Radiology* 161:463, 1986.

9. Nyberg DA, Mack LA, Harvey D et al: Value of the yolk sac in evaluating early pregnancies, *J Ultrasound Med* 7:129, 1988.
10. Yeh H-C, Rabinowitz JG: Amniotic sac development: ultrasound features of early pregnancy—the double bleb sign, *Radiology* 166:97, 1988.
11. Leach RE, Ory SJ: Modern management of ectopic pregnancy, *J Reprod Med* 34:324, 1989.
12. Nyberg DA, Filly RA, Mahony BS et al: Early gestation: correlation of hCG levels and sonographic identification, *AJR* 144:951, 1985.
13. Goldstein SR, Snyder JR, Watson C et al: Very early pregnancy detection with endovaginal ultrasound, *Obstet Gynecol* 72:200, 1988.
14. Nyberg DA, Callen PW: Ultrasound evaluation of the placenta. In Callen PW, ed: *Ultrasonography in obstetrics and gynecology,* Philadelphia, 1988, WB Saunders.
15. Romero R, Kadar N, Copel JA et al: The effect of different human chorionic gonadotropin assay sensitivity on screening for ectopic pregnancy, *Am J Obstet Gynecol* 153:72, 1985.
16. Wilcox AJ, Weinberg CR, O'Connor JF et al: Incidence of early loss of pregnancy, *N Engl J Med* 319:189, 1988.
17. Pridjian G, Moawad AH: Missed abortion: still appropriate terminology? *Am J Obstet Gynecol* 161:261, 1989.
18. Simpson JL, Mills JL, Holmes LB et al: Low fetal loss rates after ultrasound-proved viability in early pregnancy, *JAMA* 258:2555, 1987.
19. Romero R, Kadar N, Jeanty P et al: Diagnosis of ectopic pregnancy: value of the discriminatory human chorionic gonadotropin zone, *Obstet Gynecol* 65:357, 1985.
20. Bernaschek G, Rudelstarfer R, and Csaicsich P: Vaginal sonography versus serum human chorionic gonadotropin in early detection of pregnancy, *Am J Obstet Gynecol* 158:608, 1988.
21. Timor-Tritsch IE, Yeh MN, Peisner DB et al: The use of transvaginal ultrasonography in the diagnosis of ectopic pregnancy, *Am J Obstet Gynecol* 161:156, 1989.
22. Nyberg DA, Mack LA, Benedetti TJ et al: Placental abruption and placental hemorrhage: correlation of sonographic findings with fetal outcome, *Radiology* 164:357, 1987.
23. Sauerbrei EE, Pham DH: Placental abruption and subchorionic hemorrhage in the first half of pregnancy: US appearance and clinical outcome, *Radiology* 160:109, 1986.
24. Farrell RG: Abnormal vaginal bleeding in ob/gyn emergencies: the first 60 minutes. In Farrell RG, ed: Rockville, Md, 1986, Aspen
25. Hibbard LT: Adnexal torsion, *Am J Obstet Gynecol* 152:456, 1985.
26. Westrom L: Effect of acute pelvic inflammatory disease on fertility, *Am J Obstet Gynecol* 121:707, 1975.
27. Landers DV, Sweet RL: Current trends in the diagnosis and treatment of tuboovarian abscess, *Am J Obstet Gynecol* 151:1098, 1985.

CHAPTER 22

Scrotal Pain and Enlargement

Jean Abbott
David Thickman

Early surgical exploration is mandatory in the male with acute scrotal pain and suspected testicular torsion, but imaging modalities are indicated in the patient with a less acute presentation, pain of unknown cause, painless scrotal swelling, or swelling after direct trauma. Urgent imaging is rarely required for the asymptomatic patient with a nonacute scrotal enlargement or mass, but such imaging may be helpful before surgery.

ANATOMIC AND PHYSIOLOGIC CONSIDERATIONS IN SCROTAL IMAGING

The scrotum contains the testis, epididymis, vas deferens, and vestigial remnants such as the appendix testis; all are surrounded by the visceral tunica vaginalis. The interior of the scrotal pouch is lined with tunica vaginalis that is embryonically continuous with the parietal peritoneum. The dartos is a smooth muscle within the scrotal sac. The cremaster muscle, within which the testis is suspended, surrounds the scrotal contents. The spermatic cord traverses the inguinal canal and contains the ductus deferens and the blood vessels, nerves, and lymphatics that supply the testis (Fig. 22-1). The blood supply to the scrotal contents is both through arteries within the spermatic cord (which supply the testis and epididymis) and through the internal and external pudendal arteries outside the spermatic cord (which supply the scrotum and penis).[1,2]

The normal testis is vertical. The visceral tunica vaginalis attaches posteriorly to the scrotal sac and prevents rotation of the testis within the scrotum. If the testis is inade-

quately fixed to the scrotal sac, rotation within the tunica vaginalis can occur, resulting in torsion of the testis. Likewise, remnants of the müllerian duct system may undergo torsion and become ischemic (particularly in children). The most common of these remnants, the testicular appendix, is superior and anterior to the testis.

The testis has two functions: spermatogenesis (exocrine function) and hormonal secretion (endocrine function). Ischemia of only 1 to 3 hours results in a decrease in spermatogenesis, although the functional significance of this is unclear. Irreversible changes occur after 6 to 8 hours of ischemia, but the dysfunction depends on the degree of rotation and periods of spontaneous detorsion. Long-term sequelae of ischemia on ipsilateral and contralateral testicular function are currently unclear.[3,4]

IMAGING THE SCROTAL CONTENTS

Imaging studies should never delay surgical exploration for a presumed testicular torsion because rapid detorsion is crucial to the preservation of testicular function.[3,5] In the patient with an unclear diagnosis, however, three techniques for scrotal imaging may be useful to the emergency physician: radionuclide scan, ultrasonography, and Doppler imaging.

The radionuclide scan uses the intravenous radioisotope technetium 99m to identify areas of the scrotum with normal blood flow. This scan takes less than 30 minutes when proper equipment and personnel are available. Two phases of imaging are used: the angiographic, or flow, phase shows arterial flow to the scrotum; the delayed phase shows the isotope taken up in normal tissue (Fig. 22-2). The venous circulation may also be seen in the delayed phase.[1]

The radionuclide scan is useful in detecting occult ischemia of the testis, avascular areas such as hydroceles, or areas of increased flow caused by inflammation or tumor. In the neonate, testicular size precludes adequate imaging.[6] Because inflammation may occur in conjunction with isch-

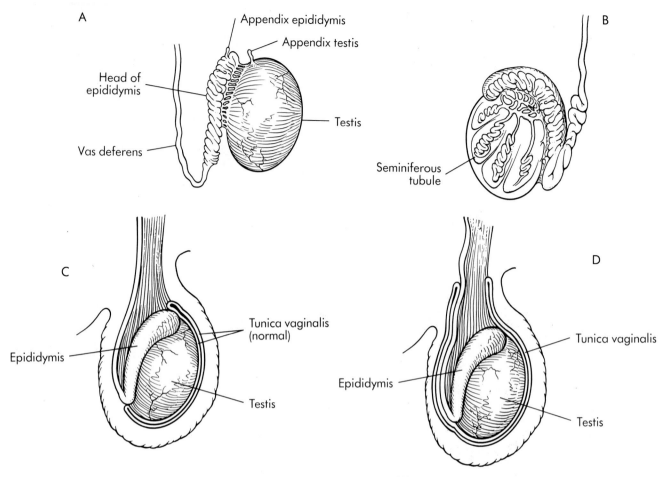

Fig. 22-1. The scrotum and its contents in the adult male. **A,** Schematic demonstrates the normal structures of the testis. **B,** Cross-sectional schematic demonstrates seminiferous tubules and epididymis. Schematics representing the normal (**C**) and abnormal (**D**) relationship between tunica vaginalis and the scrotal walls.

emia (e.g., with testicular torsion of more than 24 hours), false-positive and false-negative scan results may occur in the presence of testicular ischemia. For the same reason, masses, tumors, and abscesses frequently cannot be differentiated from one another by this scan. Therefore surgical exploration is required for definitive diagnosis of abnormalities detected by the CT scan. The major emergency department need for the radionuclide scan is to confirm the presence of blood flow in the patient with a clinical diagnosis of epididymitis or other nonsurgical presentation when the diagnosis is uncertain.[3]

Ultrasonography of the scrotum requires special ultrasonographic equipment that allows for good resolution of near fields. An acoustic window may be obtained by imaging through the opposite testis or by using various water baths. Ultrasonography can differentiate tissues of different acoustic properties within the scrotum, separating bowel gas, hydrocele fluid, abscesses, and hematomas from normal testicular tissue. The normal testis is homogeneous and of moderate echogenicity. The epididymis is similar in echotexture to the testis. The tunica vaginalis is a hypoechoic rim around the testis.

Ultrasonography is most useful in differentiating testicular from extratesticular masses and in detecting inhomogeneity within testicular tissue, which is virtually always abnormal but nonspecific.[7] When the scrotum is enlarged, ultrasonography can differentiate a simple or uncomplicated hydrocele or bowel herniation from a hematoma or infectious process. A hydrocele is an anechoic fluid collection outside the testes. With bowel herniation, an echogenic complex mass containing gas or showing peristalsis is seen. Hematomas and infections typically appear as complex masses and cannot be reliably differentiated from one another by ultrasonography. With ultrasonography, the testis can also be evaluated for intrinsic abnormality.[8] In acute scrotal trauma, ultrasonography may be useful in differentiating testicular disruption from scrotal hematomas with an intact testicle. It may also be useful in the patient with acute scrotal pain when a normal radionuclide scan has excluded torsion.[9]

Doppler imaging is a bedside technique for demonstrating blood flow to the testis and for monitoring return of

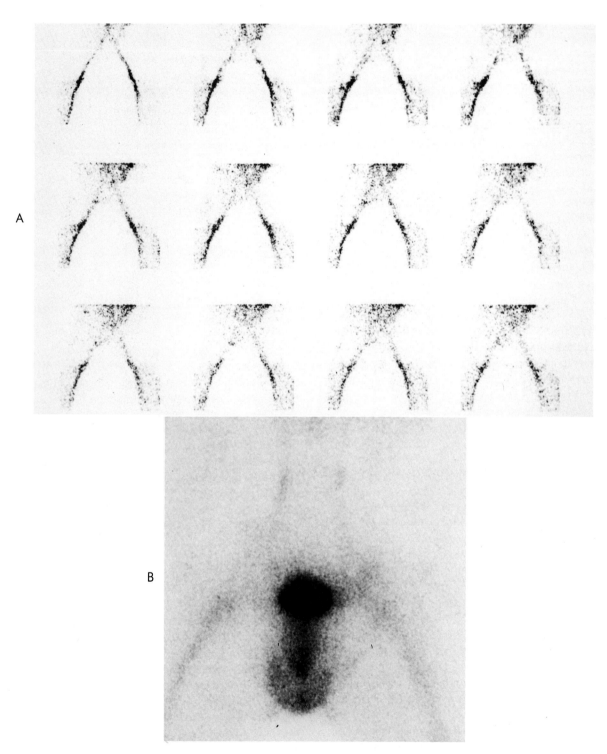

Fig. 22-2. Technetium 99m scan of scrotum. **A,** Normal vascular (early) phase. **B,** Normal static (delayed) phase.

blood flow after emergency department detorsion attempts in treating testicular torsion. Although useful in early ischemia, the accuracy of Doppler imaging diminishes as soon as reactive scrotal inflammation occurs with torsion. The technique is considered unreliable in most clinical situations.[10]

CLINICAL PRESENTATIONS
Scrotal pain

Acute unilateral scrotal pain is a common male genitourinary presentation in the emergency department. The differential diagnosis includes testicular torsion, torsion of scrotal appendages, epididymitis, tumor, scrotal trauma with scrotal hemorrhage or testicular rupture, and acute hernia, hydrocele, or varicocele. Critical is the accurate differentiation of surgical disease (testicular torsion or rupture) from disease that can be treated medically (e.g., epididymitis). Clinical differentiation of testicular torsion from epididymitis (the usual dilemma) is difficult. Although epididymitis is rare before puberty and torsion is uncommon after the first 2 decades of life, overlap in history, age, symptoms, and clinical signs is sufficiently great that the physician cannot rely on these alone to exclude surgical disease.[11,12] If the patient lacks clear signs of infection and testicular torsion is thought to be present, surgical exploration is the procedure of choice because each imaging modality has pitfalls and all delay the reversal of ischemia. Even if symptoms are present for more than 12 hours, surgery is still indicated to determine if the ischemia was subtotal, to confirm the diagnosis, and to perform preventative orchioplexy of the opposite testicle.[13]

Testicular torsion. The radionuclide scan is the imaging modality of choice if the diagnosis of torsion is unclear and the clinical presentation does not warrant immediate surgical exploration. Classic radionuclide scan findings include decreased blood flow in spermatic cord vessels and in the testis, with normal blood flow to scrotal skin (Fig. 22-3). Occasionally, it is useful to quantify blood flow so that subtle ischemia may be recognized.[13] Because blood flow may also be provided by arteries not within the spermatic cord, findings after 6 to 12 hours of ischemia are more variable, and a cold spot with a rim of increased flow (the "halo" sign) may be seen with late or missed torsion.[3] Overall, the accuracy of the radionuclide scan in the diagnosis of torsion is high: sensitivity in several study series ranges between 89% and 95%.[1,12] Accuracy is decreased in children under 10 years of age in whom the risk of torsion is also highest. In this age group, surgical exploration should be the procedure of choice.[1] False-positive scan findings demonstrating decreased uptake in the area of the testis can occasionally be seen with an overlying hernia or hydrocele if imaging is done in only one plane.[14] False-negative scan findings can occur with torsion of over 24 hours' duration, with partial ischemia, or with spontaneous detorsion. In any of these clinical settings, cautious inter-

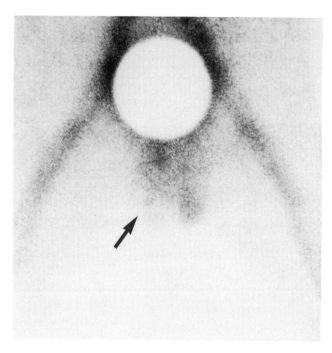

Fig. 22-3. Technetium 99m scan (static phase) of testicular torsion with decreased activity on the right (*arrow*).

pretation of imaging is necessary, and surgical exploration may be required to resolve the problem.[6]

Ultrasonography is not useful in the diagnosis of torsion because a completely normal testicular image may be present with acute ischemia. Although hyperechogenicity may be seen, it is a late finding.[6] Testicular torsion occasionally occurs after groin trauma.[2] Although ultrasonography is the imaging modality of choice in trauma, the radionuclide scan should be used to exclude torsion if no evidence of testicular rupture or fluid collection is seen in the post-traumatic patient with a painful swollen testicle (see later discussion).

Torsion of the appendix testis. In children, torsion of the vestigial appendix testis occurs almost as frequently as torsion of the testis itself.[11] If the clinical presentation is early, the findings of ischemic pain and point tenderness (the "blue dot" sign with transillumination) at the superior pole of the testis and a normal nontender testis may avoid unnecessary surgery. The radionuclide scan can confirm normal testicular blood flow, particularly in older children. When the patient presents with prolonged ischemia, symptoms and clinical findings are less localized and exploration may be required to avoid any further delay in the diagnosis of testicular ischemia.[2]

Epididymitis. Epididymitis can often be diagnosed clinically when the patient has a gradual onset of pain, focal tenderness over the epididymis, pyuria, and urethral discharge.[15] In cases in which the clinical picture is not so clear, both the radionuclide scan and ultrasonography can be useful in establishing the diagnosis and excluding surgical disease. The radionuclide scan demonstrates increased radioisotope uptake through the spermatic vessels as well as superiorly and laterally to the testis (Fig. 22-4). Occasionally, some increased uptake within the testis occurs if an element of orchitis is present. The radionuclide scan is particularly useful in patients over the age of 24 years (in whom the diagnosis of torsion is rare but possible) and should be performed if clear evidence of genitourinary infection is not present. Likewise, the radionuclide scan can define the degree of inflammation and identify potential complications.[1]

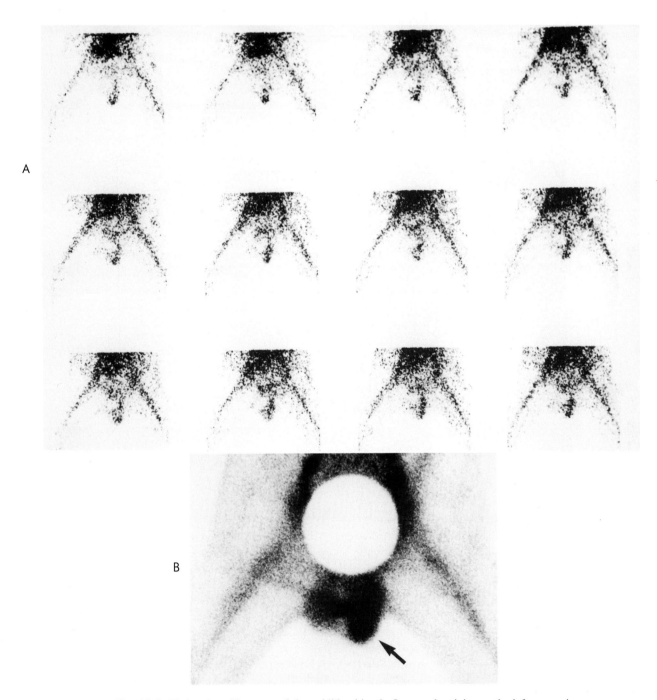

Fig. 22-4. Technetium 99m scan of the epididymitis. **A,** Increased activity on the left occurs in the vascular phase, indicating increased flow on the side with epididymitis. **B,** In the late phase, increased activity on the left reflects the inflammatory response in the inflamed epididymis (*arrow*).

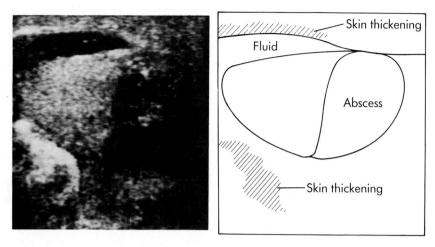

Fig. 22-5. Longitudinal ultrasonogram demonstrates an intratesticular abscess with skin thickening posteriorly and anteriorly.

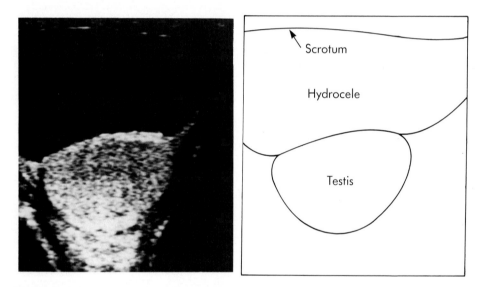

Fig. 22-6. Transverse ultrasonogram with anterior anechoic fluid collection from a hydrocele. The homogeneous testis is posterior to the fluid collection.

Ultrasonography also can be used to confirm inflammation of the epididymis, which appears enlarged with diffuse or focal increased echogenicity. The testis should appear homogeneous, although severe disease may be accompanied by orchitis and inhomogeneity within the testis itself. Caution should be exercised in attributing testicular abnormalities to inflammation alone (as opposed to tumor or abscess) when using either imaging modality, unless the clinical setting is clearly one of epididymo-orchitis. Follow-up imaging must be obtained to demonstrate resolution of testicular abnormalities.[6] Infectious complications such as abscess or necrosis within the testis can be identified by ultrasonography (Fig. 22-5). Intratesticular abscesses usually require immediate exploration and drainage to prevent extension of the infection.[1,16]

Scrotal enlargement

Enlargement of the scrotum, with or without pain, may be caused by several diseases that can be recognized by radiographic imaging. The evaluation of an enlarged scrotum, however, is generally not an emergent diagnostic dilemma. Ultrasonography is particularly useful in recognizing fluid collections and intratesticular and extratesticular masses and for demonstrating testicular location when scrotal enlargement precludes accurate palpation of the testis.

Hydrocele. A hydrocele may represent a spontaneous fluid collection within the tunica vaginalis, or it may occur as a result of epididymitis, torsion, or even tumor.[17] Ultrasonography may be useful to define the hydrocele if the testis cannot be palpated (Fig. 22-6).

Varicocele. Acute scrotal enlargement, particularly on

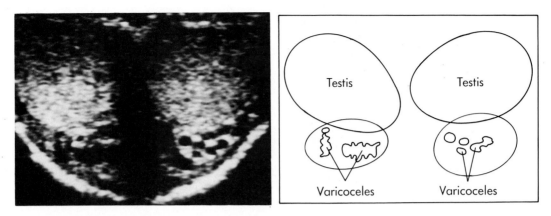

Fig. 22-7. Varicoceles. Transverse ultrasonogram of both testes demonstrating 2 to 4 mm serpiginous hypoechoic varicoceles in both epididymi.

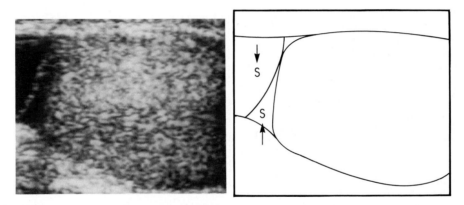

Fig. 22-8. Spermatocele*(s)* *(arrows)*. Longitudinal ultrasonogram of a cystic structure in the head of the epididymis.

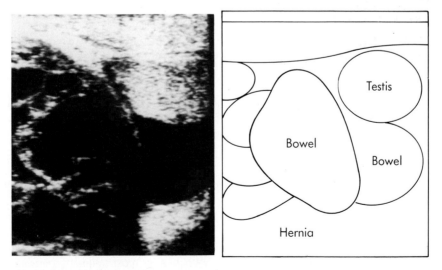

Fig. 22-9. Scrotal hernia. Longitudinal ultrasonogram with bowel seen posteriorly and superiorly to the testis.

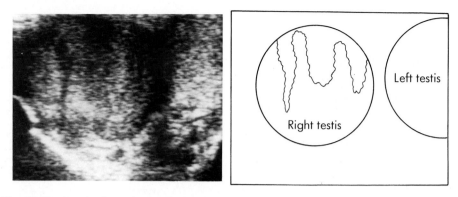

Fig. 22-10. Anaplastic seminoma. In the transverse ultrasonogram of both testes, diffuse inhomogeneity with hypoechoic areas is seen within the right testis, representing anaplastic seminoma. The left testis is normally homogeneous.

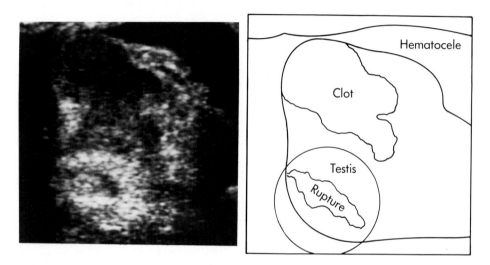

Fig. 22-11. Hematocele. Transverse ultrasonogram demonstrates hypoechoic hematocele within the scrotal sac, as well as a testicular disruption caused by traumatic rupture.

the left side, may result from incompetence of the spermatic veins and resultant varicocele, which is palpated as a soft, beady enlargement of the spermatic cord. Although rarely emergent, ultrasonography is probably most useful as a noninvasive imaging modality when the clinical diagnosis is in doubt, since venous reflux can be demonstrated with position changes and a valsalva maneuver (Fig. 22-7).

Spermatocele. Likewise, a cystic collection of sperm may be seen in the head of the epididymis by ultrasonography, but rarely does this cause symptoms (Fig. 22-8).

Hernia. Ultrasonography in the case of hernia will demonstrate a complex echogenic mass containing air and showing peristalsis (Fig. 22-9).

Testicular tumors. Malignant and benign tumors of the testes may be identified by either a radionuclide scan or ultrasonography, but no characteristic pattern of abnormality exists. Masses may have increased or decreased density and flow and may demonstrate a combination of findings. Although ultrasonography can be helpful in dif-

ferentiating intratesticular from extratesticular masses, exploration is required to define the type of tumor and its malignant potential (Fig. 22-10).

Acute post-traumatic scrotal swelling and pain

In the patient with blunt injury to the groin, the differential diagnosis includes several entities, and the need for surgical intervention must be ascertained. Ultrasonography can accurately diagnose testicular fracture that requires immediate surgical repair (Fig. 22-11). The diagnoses of scrotal hematoma (within the skin), hematocele (acute blood collection within the scrotal sac but with an intact testis), and urinary extravasation from urethral rupture (which presents with an "onion-peel" collection of scrotal fluid) can also be made by ultrasonography.[8] When acute post-traumatic pain and swelling (see Chapter 7) occur in the absence of any findings on ultrasonographic examination, a radionuclide scan is indicated to exclude the rarer traumatic complication of testicular torsion.[2]

SUMMARY

Scrotal imaging is unnecessary in the young patient with acute scrotal pain presumed to be caused by torsion. Rather immediate surgical exploration is required without delay. In the patient with testicular pain of longer duration in whom the diagnosis of epididymitis is more likely, the radionuclide scan can accurately differentiate inflammatory changes of epididymitis from ischemia. Ultrasonography is useful to define scrotal enlargement from masses or fluid collections and to demonstrate testicular integrity following direct trauma.

REFERENCES

1. Eshghi M, Silver L, and Smith AD: Technetium 99m scan in acute scrotal lesions, *Urology* 30:586, 1987.
2. Kursh ED: Traumatic torsion of the testicle, *Urology* 17:441, 1981.
3. Thomas WEG, Williamson RCN: Diagnosis and outcome of testicular torsion, *Br J Surg* 70:213, 1983.
4. Nagler HM, Deitch AD, and White R: Testicular torsion: temporal considerations, *Fertil Steril* 42:257, 1984.
5. Cass AS, Cass BP, and Veeraraghavan K: Immediate exploration of the unilateral acute scrotum in young male subjects, *J Urol* 124:829, 1980.
6. Lightner DJ, Grand F, and Lange PH: Noninvasive scrotal imaging techniques. In McCullough DL, ed: *Difficult diagnoses in urology,* New York, 1988, Churchill Livingstone.
7. Rifkin MD, Kurtz AB, Pasto ME et al: Diagnostic capabilities of high-resolution scrotal ultrasonography: prospective evaluation, *J Ultrasound Med* 4:13, 1985.
8. Hricak H, Jeffrey RB: Sonography of acute scrotal abnormalities, *Radiol Clin North Am* 21:595, 1983.
9. Bird K, Rosenfield AT, and Taylor KJW: Ultrasonography in testicular torsion, *Radiology* 147:527, 1983.
10. Bickerstaff KI, Sethia K, and Murie JA: Doppler ultrasonography in the diagnoses of acute scrotal pain, *Br J Surg* 75:238, 1988.
11. Melekos MD, Asbach HW, and Markou SA: Etiology of acute scrotum in 100 boys with regard to age distribution, *J Urol* 139:1023, 1988.
12. Levy OM, Gittelman MC, Strashun AM et al: Diagnosis of acute testicular torsion using radionuclide scanning, *J Urol* 129:975, 1983.
13. Nakielny RA, Thomas WEG, Jackson P et al: Radionuclide evaluation of acute scrotal disease, *Clin Radiol* 35:125, 1984.
14. Krubsach AJ, Akhtar R: Caudal view: aid in testicular scanning, *Clin Nucl Med* 12:614, 1987.
15. Williams RCN: Death in the scrotum: testicular torsion, *N Engl J Med* 296:6, 1977.
16. Vordermark JS, Buck AS, Brown SR et al: The testicular scan: use in diagnosis and management of acute epididymitis, *JAMA* 245:2512, 1981.
17. Dunn EK, Macchia RJ, and Soloman NA: Scintigraphic pattern in missed testicular torsion, *Radiology* 139:175, 1981.

CHAPTER 23

Nontraumatic Hematuria

Suzanne Z. Barkin
Ellen Taliafero

Hematuria is always a significant finding although the degree of hematuria does not necessarily reflect the severity or significance of the underlying condition. Frequently a harbinger of serious urinary tract disease, hematuria may be present grossly or microscopically. It may occur as an isolated finding or in association with systemic signs and symptoms such as fever or pain. Following trauma, hematuria indicates renal injury although the injury is rarely clinically significant (see Chapter 7). The finding of two or more red blood cells (RBCs) in a centrifuged urine specimen or five or more RBCs in a noncentrifuged specimen is defined as hematuria.[1,2] Individuals without hematuria may have up to 8000 RBCs/mm^3 of glomerular origin when measured by light microscopy. Renal origin for hematuria is usually associated with the presence of concomitant casts and significant proteinuria; erythrocytes are usually dysmorphic.[3]

INCIDENCE AND IDENTIFICATION

The incidence of patients presenting with hematuria in the emergency department is unknown. In a population-based study, 2.3% of patients with confirmed asymptomatic microscopic hematuria had significant disease.[4] A comparable study at the Mayo Clinic reported an incidence of 0.5% to 1.8%.[5] Reports in the pediatric literature have revealed an incidence of 4.1% of microscopic hematuria

on at least one occasion in the 8- to 15-year age group.

Microscopic hematuria may be identified by one of two methods: a dipstick test or a microscopic examination of the urinary sediment. The dipstick test results are positive if there is lysis of RBCs, detecting hemoglobin at a minimal concentration of 0.003 mg/L, corresponding to 10,000 RBCs/mm^3 or 1 or 2 RBCs/high-power field (HPF). It is reported that 24% of negative dipstick readings, 82% of trace readings, and 100% of positive dipstick readings have 10 RBCs/mm^3 or greater.[6] Microscopic examination of a centrifuged specimen will also reveal RBCs. Dysmorphic RBCs are most often found with glomerular disease, whereas a more normal uniform shape and size are associated with disorders of a nonglomerular origin. One study suggested that, if there are less than 14% dysmorphic cells, extrarenal disease should be suspected. If there are more than 14% dysmorphic cells, intrarenal disease is common.

Gross hematuria is suggested by the color of the urine. In alkaline urine, gross hematuria is accompanied by a red tint; in acid urine, gross hematuria may appear smoky or brown. A smoky appearance requires 2 to 3 million RBCs/mm^3.[7-9]

ETIOLOGIC CONSIDERATIONS

Nontraumatic hematuria typically accompanies serious urologic disease. The degree of hematuria does not reflect the significance of the underlying condition. Initial hematuria not persisting throughout urination reflects urethral bleeding caused by calculi, neoplasm, or infection. Hematuria occurring near the end of voiding usually results from involvement of the bladder neck, prostate, or posterior urethra. Hematuria throughout voiding represents disorders of the bladder neck, ureters, or kidneys. After infection, benign prostatic hypertrophy, and renal calculi, neoplasm is the most likely cause of hematuria. The frequency of specific causes of hematuria varies widely[10] (Table 23-1). Hematuria may occur in patients with bleeding disorders

Table 23-1. Causes of hematuria

Underlying conditions	Frequency (%)
Infection	0-24
Nephrolithiasis	4-25
Prostatic hypertrophy	0-23
Urethritis	1-24
Neoplasm	2-18
Glomerulonephritis	0-10
Trauma	5-10

or those who are taking anticoagulation medications. These patients must be fully investigated; in one series of 16 patients, 13 had urologic disease.[11]

Upper urinary tract disease

Upper tract disease, accounting for about 40% of cases of hematuria, may be glomerular or nonglomerular in origin (see the box opposite).

Glomerular hematuria from the kidneys may be a manifestation of a variety of abnormalities of an infectious, autoimmune, or familial nature. Glomerulonephritis, either primary or secondary to a systemic disease, is common and is often accompanied by proteinuria and RBC casts. Exercise may also induce hematuria, particularly in endurance runners. It usually persists up to 24 to 48 hours after exercise.

Nonglomerular hematuria is associated with tubulointerstitial, renovascular, or systemic disease. Arteriovenous fistulas, renal artery embolism and thrombosis, and renal vein thrombosis may be causal factors. Concomitant medication may also produce drug-induced hematuria. Familial bleeding problems, anticoagulants, sickle cell anemia, polycystic kidney disease, or diabetes are other possible causes. Finally, hematuria may be secondary to renal cell carcinoma, particularly in older patients.

Renal colic with gross hematuria is associated with disease in the kidney or ureter. If a wormlike clot is passed, the lesion is frequently a neoplasm in the kidney or renal pelvis.

Lower urinary tract disease

Approximately 60% of hematuria is caused by lower urinary tract disease (see the box opposite). Bladder neoplasms (squamous and transitional cell carcinomas), infection (cystitis), varices, diverticula, foreign body presence, and calculi may be causes. Benign prostatic hyperplasia (BPH) is the most common cause of gross hematuria in men 60 years of age and older; prostatitis and neoplasm must also be considered. Ureteral disease may include calculi, papillomas, or congenital defects, with the latter frequently contributing to the formation of calculi.

Hematuria in the catheterized patient represents a special problem because catheterization itself may cause he-

---

Hematuria: differential considerations

Upper urinary tract disease

KIDNEY
Infection: pyelonephritis, cystitis
Inflammation and autoimmune disorders: acute and chronic glomerulonephritis, Goodpasture syndrome, Wegener granulomatosis, lupus erythematosus, Henoch-Schönlein purpura, nephrotic syndrome, blood transfusion reaction
Trauma and exercise
Metabolic disorders: calculi (uric acid, calcium phosphate, cystine); diabetes
Congenital disorders: polycystic kidney, medullary sponge kidney, hydronephrosis, hemangioma and arteriovenous malformation, hereditary nephritis and hematuria, bleeding diathesis, sickle cell anemia
Vascular disorders: renal vein or artery thrombosis or embolism, embolic glomerulonephritis, subacute bacterial endocarditis
Neoplasms: papillomas, hypernephromas, Wilm's tumor, oncocytoma
Intoxication: sulfa drugs, mercury and other heavy metal poisoning, aspirin, methicillin

URETER
Trauma
Metabolic disorders: calculi
Congenital disorders: bands, aberrant vessels

Lower urinary tract disease

BLADDER
Infection: cystitis
Inflammation: Hunner ulcer
Trauma: foreign body presence, rupture, instrumentation
Metabolic disorders: calculi
Neoplasms: papilloma, transitional cell carcinoma, squamous cell carcinoma
Congenital disorders: bleeding diathesis

PROSTATE
Infection: prostatitis
Inflammation: benign prostatic hypertrophy (BPH)
Neoplasms: carcinoma

URETHRA
Infection: *Neisseria gonorrhoeae, Chlamydia trachomatis,* and others
Trauma: manipulation, foreign body presence
Metabolic disorders: calculi
Congenital disorders: stricture
Neoplasms

maturia in 17% of patients. However, such hematuria is usually microscopic, with under 3 RBCs/HPF.[12]

Pseudohematuria

Pseudohematuria results when the urine is red but both the microscopic and the dipstick examination findings are negative. The causes include:

- Anthocyanins in beets and berries.
- Phenolphthalein in alkaline urine.
- Pyridium.
- Heavy concentration of urates.
- Porphyria.
- Vegetable dyes used for food coloring.

Red or brown urine without RBCs may also result from free hemoglobin and myoglobin.

NORMAL RADIOGRAPHIC ANATOMY

Retroperitoneally, the anterior and posterior renal fasciae define the normal perirenal space (see Chapter 7). The fasciae form a cone-shaped space, extending inferomedially toward the lower lumbar vertebrae and psoas muscles. Radiographic visualization of the renal silhouette is permitted by the radiolucency of the perinephric fat within the fasciae. The outer one third of the renal substance is cortex (nephrons), which has terminal branches of collecting tubules extending from the medulla into it at regular intervals.

The inner two thirds of the renal substance is medulla composed of collecting tubules, proximal and distal convoluted tubules, loops of Henle, and connective tissue. The arterial blood supply to the medulla is primarily from the vasa recta. The medulla receives less than 20% of the total renal blood flow, with about 80% perfusing the cortex through the interlobular arteries. The medullary pyramids culminate in papillae, which are surrounded by a part of the collecting system called calyces and which ultimately drain urine into the renal pelvis. The right kidney usually lies slightly inferior to the left, with the renal shadow in adults normally measuring between 12 to 14 cm in length and the two kidneys varying by 1.5 to 2 cm. However, measurements depend on patient size and state of hydration and can be quite variable. Kidneys are anatomically directed inferolaterally.

The ureters pass from the renal pelvis and across the upper portion of the psoas muscles to the sacral promontory and insert into the bladder wall.

INDICATIONS, LIMITATIONS, AND SEQUENCE OF RADIOGRAPHIC EVALUATION

Radiographic evaluation should focus on defining the anatomic and functional nature of lesions causing hematuria. The diagnostic evaluation of symptomatic patients with microhematuria is controversial. An aggressive evaluation may be especially important in patients over 40 years of age. Microscopic hematuria in patients over 40 years of age is frequently a sign of major urinary tract le-

sions, which are detected in 20% of individuals, of which 10% are malignant.[4,13,14]

A supine abdominal radiograph provides only presumptive evidence of a calculus. Radiographic densities may be noted. Phleboliths, or spheric masses with hollow (lucent) centers in the pelvic veins, may be seen frequently. Calcified mesenteric lymph nodes may be noted. Radio-opaque calculi are those composed of calcium oxalate, cystine, calcium phosphate, or magnesium-ammonium phosphate. Uric acid stones, blood clots, and sloughed papillae may be seen as negative shadows on the intravenous pyelogram (IVP). Most renal stones (90%) are radio-opaque.

The standard radiographic, diagnostic step in the evaluation of the patient with hematuria and normal creatinine remains the intravenous pyelogram (IVP) or excretory urogram with nephrotomography. The IVP is helpful in that it provides excellent visualization of the urinary tract. Tumors, calculi, and urinary tract obstruction, as well as congenital or anatomic abnormalities, may be defined.[15] An IVP establishes the diagnosis of calculous disease in 96% of cases and can delineate the severity of obstruction[16] (Fig. 23-1).

An IVP is the primary diagnostic test in the evaluation of renal colic. Following injection of a contrast material a 30-second nephrogram is taken, followed by urograms at 5 or 10 minutes. A delay in the appearance of contrast material (nephrographic phase) on the nephrogram may be noted. An IVP can evaluate the delay in filling, the location of the obstruction, and the degree of hydronephrosis. The degree of dilatation of the ureter above the calculus should be noted. Helpful findings and specifics to look for include:

- Increased and prolonged nephrographic phase.
- Delay in appearance time of contrast material in the calyces.
- Dilatation of the collecting system and ureter down to the level of the calculus.

This may progress to incorporate a persistent and intense nephrographic phase with delay in calyceal appearance (Fig. 23-2).

The IVP may be curative because the hyperosmolar load of contrast material given may assist the passage of calculi. However, cessation of pain may also signify the onset of complete obstruction (Fig. 23-3).

Following trauma (see Chapter 7), an IVP may be indicated in selected cases. Patients with gross hematuria or microscopic hematuria accompanied by shock after blunt trauma require evaluation, as do those with penetrating trauma when there is suspicion of renal involvement. Although, historically, microscopic hematuria following blunt trauma without shock has occurred, data suggest that an IVP may not be justified because of the low incidence of injuries requiring surgical intervention (i.e., IVP demonstrates either contusion or normal kidneys). Many authors suggest that, if there are less than 50 RBCs/HPF, the initial urinalysis should be repeated in several hours in the

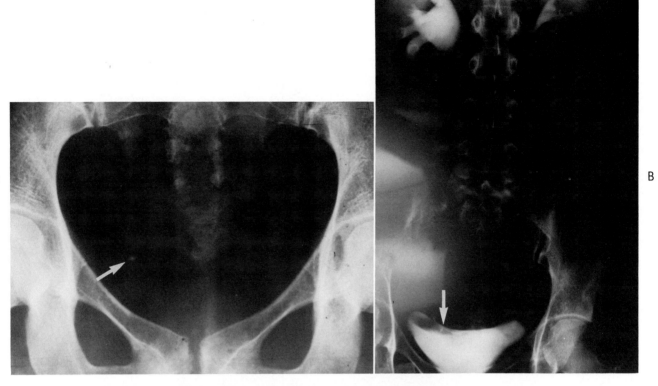

Fig. 23-1. A, Preliminary film of an intravenous pyelogram (IVP) demonstrates a right ureteric calculus *(arrow)* at the ureterovesical junction. B, Same patient 2 hours after injection of intravenous contrast material. Urogram shows a partial obstruction of the right upper urinary tract and edema of the ureter at the level of the calculus *(arrow)*.

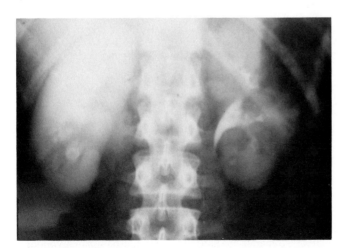

Fig. 23-2. Right ureterovesical calculus causing increased and prolonged nephrographic phase. This urogram, taken 60 minutes after injection of intravenous contrast material, demonstrates a delayed initial visualization of the calyceal system on the right.

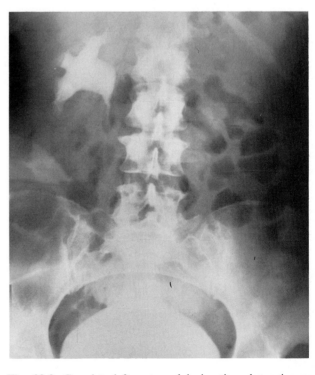

Fig. 23-3. Complete left ureteropelvic junction obstruction on the left, demonstrated on IVP.

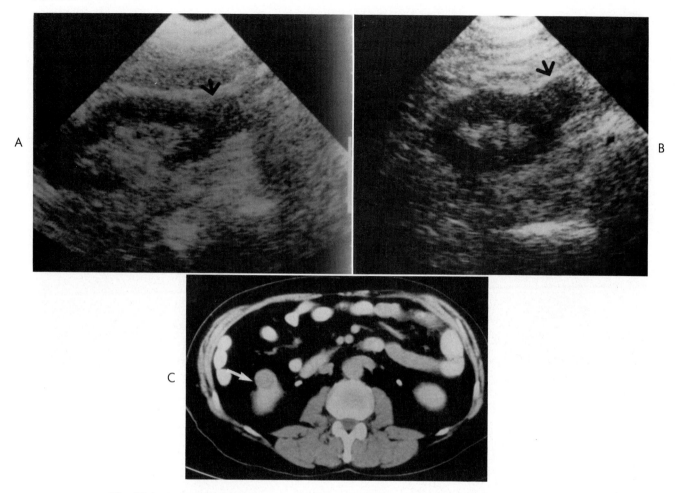

Fig. 23-4. A, Longitudinal ultrasonogram of the right kidney shows a 2.5 cm, solid, slightly hyperechoic mass *(arrow)* within the inframedial aspect of the lower pole. **B,** Transverse ultrasonogram of the right kidney of same patient shows a slightly hyperechoic mass *(arrow)*. **C,** CT scan of the same patient demonstrates a solid lesion *(arrow)* anterior to the inferior pole of the right kidney. The lesion is of very low density, with minimal wall thickening. No change in the lesion was seen with intravenous contrast material administration. Nephrectomy was performed. Pathologic diagnosis was oncocytoma (benign renal neoplasm).

Table 23-2. Protocol for monitoring hematuria

	Perform IVP	Observe and monitor urinalysis
Gross hematuria (≥50 RBCs/HPF)	Yes	No
Microscopic hematuria (<50 RBCs/HPF) and significant physical findings*	Yes	No
Microscopic hematuria and no significant physical findings	No	Yes

*Significant physical findings include hypotension, flank pain, tenderness, or ecchymosis.[17-19]

stable patient and that an IVP should be performed only if there is persistent hematuria. A suggested protocol for monitoring hematuria following blunt trauma is given in Table 23-2.

Ultrasonography can detect renal and prostatic masses and is useful in distinguishing between solid and cystic renal masses (Fig. 23-4, *A* and *B*). Ultrasonography is an excellent screening modality and can be used for many glomerular conditions. In addition, it provides additional information about the relation to surrounding tissues and the patency of the vena cava. Ultrasonography lacks sensitivity with respect to lesions of the anterior bladder wall, and renal calculi may not be identified.[20]

The CT scan and, recently, magnetic resonance imaging (MRI) can provide excellent resolution of renal masses (Fig. 23-4, *C*). Both these modalities are effective in the

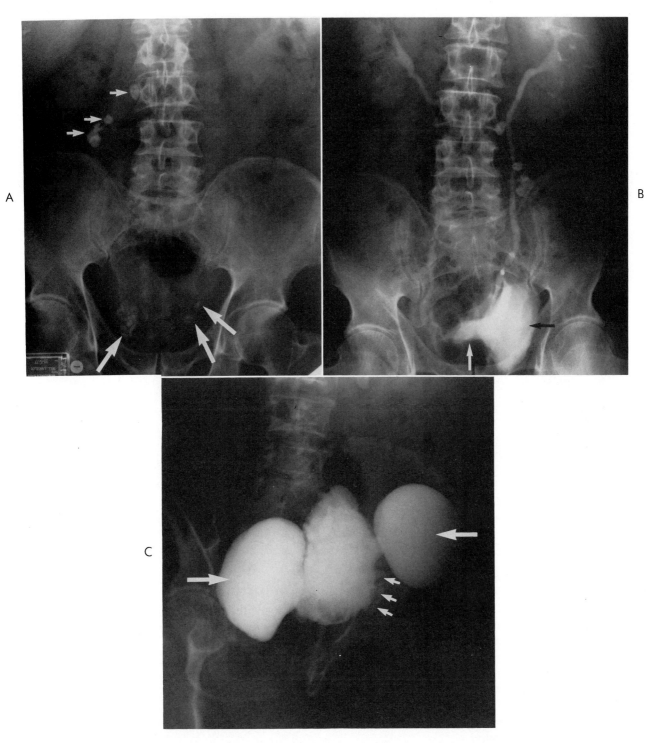

Fig. 23-5. Bladder diverticula. **A,** Preliminary film demonstrates multiple pelvic calcifications suggestive of bladder calculi or ureteral calculi (*large arrows*) as well as calcified lymph nodes (*small arrows*) within the right midabdomen. **B,** Prone view of intravenous pyelogram (IVP) demonstrates nonobstructed ureters, an uplifted and incompletely filled bladder (*vertical arrow*), and a large right bladder diverticulum (*horizontal arrow*) containing multiple calculi. **C,** Voiding cystogram confirms the presence of both right and left bladder diverticula (*large arrows*) containing multiple calculi. Note multiple small bladder diverticula (*small arrows*).

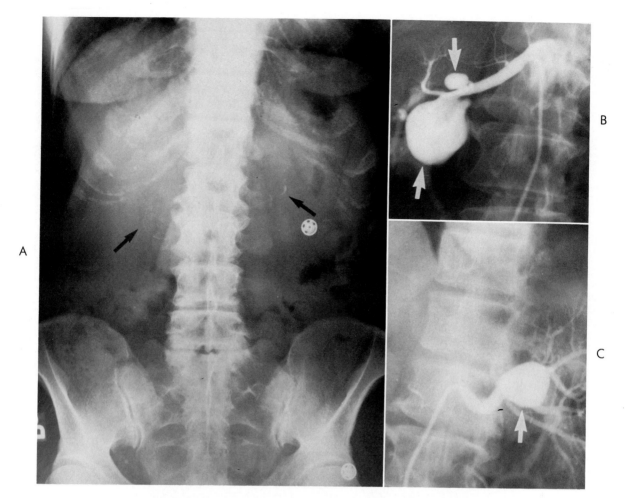

Fig. 23-6. A, Angiograms of a renal artery aneurysm. Preliminary film demonstrates bilateral curvilinear radio-opacities (*arrows*) suggestive of vascular calcifications. Selective right (**B**) and left (**C**) renal angiograms confirm the presence of bilateral renal artery aneurysms (*arrows*).

investigation of the perirenal areas as well as pelvic pathologic states.[21]

The voiding cystourethrogram (VCUG) provides anatomic information about the bladder and urethra, helping to determine if there are masses, lacerations or perforations, diverticula, or functional abnormalities (Fig. 23-5). Reflux, presenting as recurrent urinary tract infections and (less commonly) hydronephrosis, can be determined. Usually a VCUG is not performed in the emergency department unless trauma is suspected.

Angiographic studies are often required in the evaluation of patients with abnormal IVPs in whom vascular lesions are suspected (Fig. 23-6). As discussed in Chapter 7, such studies are indicated in the evaluation of the patient with an acutely injured kidney when there is persistent and significant hematuria, decreased or absent opacification of the kidney on the IVP, and evidence of retroperitoneal hemorrhage. The CT scan may be substituted because it provides anatomic definition of the kidneys, ureters (with contrast material), and retroperitoneal space.

SUMMARY

Microscopic hematuria noted on a nontraumatic basis requires evaluation. A systemic approach is warranted.

REFERENCES

1. Thompson C: Hematuria: a clinical approach, *Am Fam Physician* 33:194, 1986.
2. Blau EB: Hematuria in children: is it cause for alarm? *Postgrad Med* 79:65, 1986.
3. Schaeffer AJ, Del Greco F: Other renal diseases of urologic significance. In Walsh PC, Gittes RF, Permutter AD et al: *Campbell's urology,* Philadelphia, 1986, WB Saunders.
4. Mohr DN, Offord KP, Owen RA et al: Asymptomatic microhematuria and urological disease, *JAMA* 256:224, 1986.
5. Woolhandler S, Pels RJ, Bor DH et al: Dipstick urinalysis screening of asymptomatic adults for urinary tract disorders, *JAMA* 262:1215, 1989.
6. Arm JP, Peile EB, Rainford DJ et al: Significance of dipstick haematuria. I. Correlation with microscopy of the urine. *Br J Urol* 58:211, 1986.
7. Fairley KF, Birch DF: Hematuria: a simple method for identifying glomerular bleeding, *Kidney Int* 21:105, 1982.
8. Pillsworth TJ, Haver VM, Abrass CK et al: Differentiation of renal

from non-renal hematuria by microscopic examination of erythrocytes in urine, *Clin Chem* 33:1791, 1987.

9. Kincaid-Smith P: The investigation of patients with haematuria, *Ann Acad Med (Sing)* 16:232, 1987

10. Bauer DC: Evaluation of hematuria in adults, *West J Med* 152:305, 1990.

11. Ramayya GR, Hemingway D, and Desmond AD: Hematuria in patients with bleeding disorders, *Postgrad Med* 61:969, 1985.

12. Hockberger RS, Schwartz B, and Connor J: Hematuria induced by urethral catheterization, *Ann Emerg Med* 16:550, 1987.

13. Ritchie AD, Bevan EA, and Collier BJ: Importance of occult haematuria found at screening, *Br Med J* 292:681, 1986.

14. Kassirer JP: The wild goose chase and the elephant's relevance, *JAMA* 256:256, 1986.

15. Jones MW, Cox R, Davies KI et al: The value of the pre-clinic intravenous urogram in the earlier diagnosis of the cause of haematuria, *Br J Urol* 62:11, 1988.

16. Corriet D, Thompson IM: The value of retrograde pyelography for fractionally visualized upper tracts on excretory urography in the evaluation of hematuria, *J Urol* 138:554, 1987.

17. Heinz S: Hematuria after blunt trauma. In Barkin RM: *The emergently ill child,* Rockville, Md, 1987, Aspen Publishers.

18. Halsell RD, Vines FS, Shatney CH et al: The reliability of excretory urography as a screening examination for blunt trauma, *Ann Emerg Med* 16:1236, 1987.

19. Lieu TA, Fleisher GR, Mahboubi S et al: Hematuria and clinical findings as indications for intravenous pyelography in pediatric blunt renal trauma, *Pediatrics* 82:216, 1988.

20. Jequier S, Cramer B, and Petitjeanroget T: Ultrasongraphic screening of childhood hematuria, *J Can Assoc Radiol* 38:170, 1987.

21. Tackett RE, Gaum LD: Urological emergencies. In Stine RJ, Marcus RH, eds: *A practical approach to emergency medicine*, Boston, 1987, Little, Brown.

CHAPTER *24*

Foreign Body

Peter T. Pons
Marsha J. Heinig

Radiographic studies obtained on the patient who presents with a complaint of a possible foreign body should be performed in an orderly, thoughtful way, tailored to the nature of the foreign object in question and its suspected location. Diagnostic imaging serves as a valuable adjunct to determine the presence and location of such foreign objects.

GENERAL PRINCIPLES

Great emphasis should be placed on the diagnosis and subsequent removal of foreign bodies. Occasionally, the foreign body can pose either an immediate or potential life threat to the patient. For instance, a foreign body in the trachea is an *immediate* life threat, whereas an object lodged in the esophagus (which may lead to perforation and mediastinitis) or a swallowed drug-filled balloon or condom (which may lead to toxic complications) represents a *potential* life threat.

In most cases, however, although the object itself is not a life threat, there are numerous reasons for confirming its presence and removing it. When located in the lumen of a hollow viscus or organ (i.e., bronchus, esophagus, bowel, or urethra), it may cause obstruction or problems related to obstruction, such as atelectasis. The object may become lodged, exert pressure on adjacent tissues, and produce necrosis and possible perforation, or it may serve as a nidus

for an infection that does not respond to treatment until the object has been removed.

In general, radiographic studies are indicated when (1) the presence of a foreign body cannot be determined by physical examination, (2) assistance is needed to identify its location, or (3) additional information is needed to ascertain involvement of or injury to underlying structures.

The radiographic technique or modality used to confirm the presence of a foreign body (plain radiograph, contrast study, xeroradiography, ultrasonography, or computed tomography) will be determined by the nature of the foreign material and the suspected location. Plain radiography is usually tried first if the object is thought to be radio-opaque. If the object is embedded in soft tissue, soft tissue technique (low KVP) is used to highlight the material. Examples of radio-opaque objects include metal, rocks or gravel, glass,[1,2] bone fragments, and other hard, dense materials. Contrast studies are generally reserved for radiolucent objects in the esophagus. Xeroradiography and ultrasonography are rarely indicated. A CT scan is indicated when specific definition of the relationship of the foreign body to anatomic structures is required (e.g., relation of a foreign object in the orbit to the globe). Organic material is notoriously difficult to visualize radiographically because it has a density similar to human tissue. If the radiographic appearance or density of a foreign object is uncertain and a piece of the material is available for examination, it may be tested by placing it on the patient, marking its location, and obtaining radiographs to ascertain whether or not it can be visualized by plain film radiography.

FOREIGN BODY IN SOFT TISSUES

In the evaluation of any emergency patient with an open wound, the mechanism of injury should be ascertained to determine if a foreign object could be embedded in the wound. Often patients will raise this possibility themselves or will be aware of the object and indicate its presence. Retained foreign material should also be considered in any patient who has had multiple visits for recurrent soft tissue infections localized to the site of prior trauma.

Clinical findings

In many instances the foreign body is easily and readily diagnosed by simple physical examination. The object may be detected visually or by careful palpation and exploration of the wound. Objects in proximity to tendons, joints, blood vessels, nerves, or ducts should be considered to have possibly caused injury to those structures. Careful distal function evaluation and wound exploration are essential to assess structural integrity.

Special mention must be made of the eye and orbit. Missile-like penetration can occur in individuals engaged in metal grinding, lawn mowing, or other activities, which can propel small objects or fragments of material at high velocity. Physical examination often may appear quite innocuous, suggesting nothing more serious than conjunctival or scleral irritation or corneal abrasion. However, tonometry (revealing ocular pressure that is lower in the injured eye compared with the opposite globe) coupled with patient history, may suggest a ruptured globe, which warrants further investigation.

Diagnostic imaging

Plain film radiography is usually sufficient to confirm the presence of foreign material in soft tissue when the object cannot be ascertained by physical examination alone. Generally, soft tissue technique should be specified when requesting radiographs of the extremities, and three views, anteroposterior (AP), lateral, and oblique provide adequate information about the object and its location (Fig. 24-1). Standard (non–soft tissue technique) radiography is used when evaluating the cranial vault, thorax, or abdomen for foreign body penetration or the bone structures for fracture (e.g., gunshot wound of an extremity) (Figs. 24-2 and 24-3). Tangential or coned-down views with attention to the specific area of interest should be considered if the initial survey is negative and clinical indications of a retained foreign object are strong. Although rarely used, xeroradiography, if available, can provide excellent definition of a foreign object. The CT scan is particularly valuable in localizing objects, with particular attention to the relationship of the object to adjacent anatomic structures and its path of travel (Fig. 24-4). Angiography is indicated when there is significant concern that the proximity of the foreign object to a major vessel has injured that vessel. How-

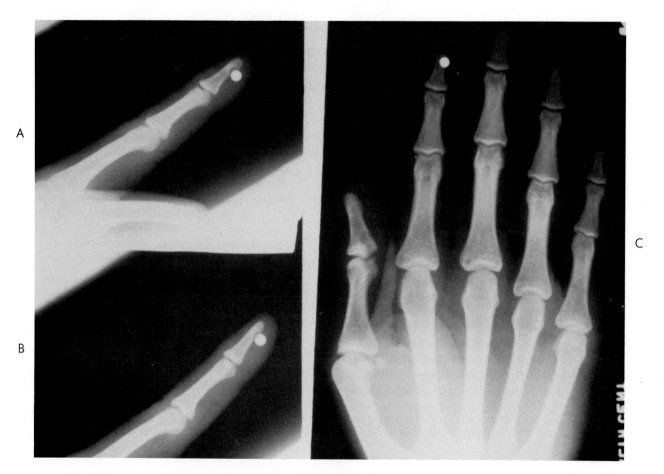

Fig. 24-1. Lateral (**A**), oblique (**B**), and anteroposterior (**C**) radiographs of the index finger following a BB shot wound of the distal phalanx. (From Rosen P, Baker FJ II, Barkin RM, et al.: *Emergency medicine: concepts and clinical practice,* ed 2, St Louis, 1988, CV Mosby.)

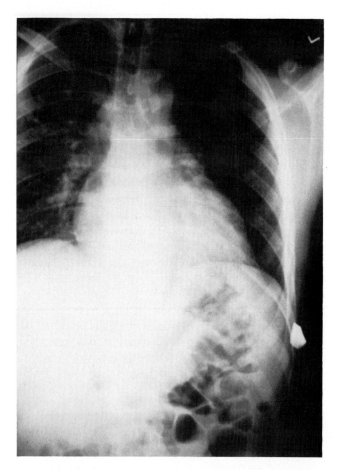

Fig. 24-2. Posteroanterior chest radiograph of a patient following a stab wound of the left chest. Broken knife blade is embedded in soft tissue.

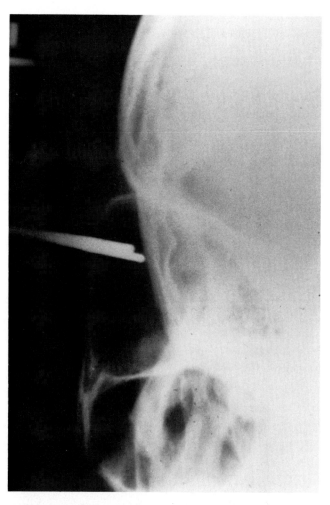

Fig. 24-3. Orbit radiograph of a patient involved in a fight and struck with a metal comb (pick). There are embedded metallic foreign bodies in the orbital wall.

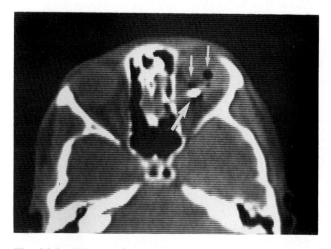

Fig. 24-4. CT scan of the orbit and skull, showing a BB shot *(large arrow)* of the orbit with disruption of the globe and air in the orbit and globe *(small arrows)*.

ever, surgical exploration and repair should not be delayed in favor of angiography when vascular injury is obvious on physical examination.

Treatment

Removal of foreign bodies can frequently be accomplished directly through the original wound. If necessary, the wound opening may be extended to explore the injury adequately, as well as to locate and remove the object. If the foreign body is located some distance from the entry site, it is often preferable to make a separate incision. In all cases a bloodless field is necessary to conduct a thorough exploration and removal.[3] Small foreign bodies located deep within soft tissues, such as a bullet in the gluteal muscles, are often left in place. Removal is undertaken only if the object is likely to cause problems and if the potential benefit of removal outweighs the potential risk and morbidity of the surgical procedure.

When difficulty is encountered locating the object during exploration and removal attempt, fluoroscopy can provide direct visualization. If fluoroscopy is not available, another technique can be used that involves placing different-gauge needles at right angles to each other in the soft tissues in proximity to the foreign body and performing repeat radiographs. The relationship of the needles to the foreign body can aid in localizing the object and guiding the exploration.[2]

Vascular or neurologic injuries warrant immediate referral to a surgeon.

FOREIGN BODY IN THE GASTROINTESTINAL TRACT

Foreign objects may be located anywhere along the length of the gastrointestinal (GI) tract. The sites most often involved where foreign objects can lodge and cause symptoms that result in the person seeking medical attention include the hypopharynx, esophagus, and rectum. Typically, objects that become lodged fall into one of two categories: sharp, pointed objects that become impaled or large, blunt objects that lodge at points of anatomic constriction.

Although a sharp object may be impaled at any site in the GI tract, the pharynx, hypopharynx, and esophagus are most often involved. The classic example is a fish bone stuck in the vallecula or pyriform sinus. Blunt objects may become lodged at any point of narrowing that cannot distend to allow passage. In the esophagus, the post-cricoid

area, aortic arch, and esophagogastric junction are common sites for impaction to occur. The ileocecal junction may also prevent passage of large objects. The rectal sphincter can permit retrograde introduction of objects but often prevents expulsion.

Pharynx and esophagus

In most cases the patient is able to provide a useful history.[4] Patients may complain that they can feel the sharp object (most often a fish or poultry bone) sticking in their throat, especially with swallowing, or feel an object stuck in the esophagus, which they are unable to pass any further.[5]

Clinical findings. Patients may state that they are unable to swallow their secretions and are drooling, or they may complain of blood-tinged sputum production. The patient often can accurately localize the foreign body and therefore should be asked to demonstrate where it is felt. Children may have shortness of breath and signs of tracheal obstruction from a large esophageal foreign body compressing the relatively soft cartilage of the trachea. Rarely, patients who did not seek early medical attention may sustain a serious complication secondary to perforation of the esophagus, including mediastinitis, aortic erosion with exsanguinating hemorrhage, pulmonary abscess, or pneumothorax.[4,6-8]

Foreign bodies of the pharynx or hypopharynx are often visualized by careful physical examination using indirect or direct laryngoscopy. Topical anesthesia of the mucosa may be needed to visualize adequately the base of the tongue, epiglottis, vallecula, and pyriform sinuses. Direct laryngoscopy is valuable as the initial step since a visualized foreign body can be removed at the same time. Abra-

Fig. 24-5. Lateral (**A**) and anteroposterior (**B**) radiographs of the cervical spine demonstrate a button located in the pyriform sinus *(arrow)*.

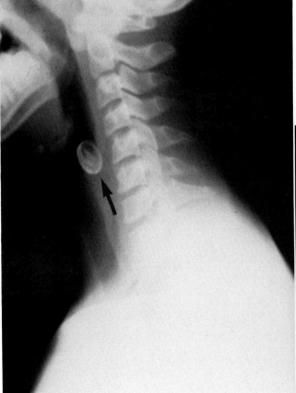

A

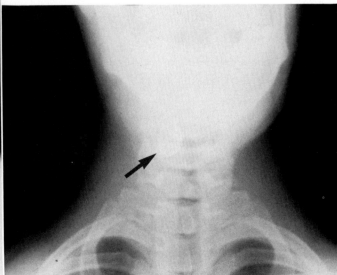

B

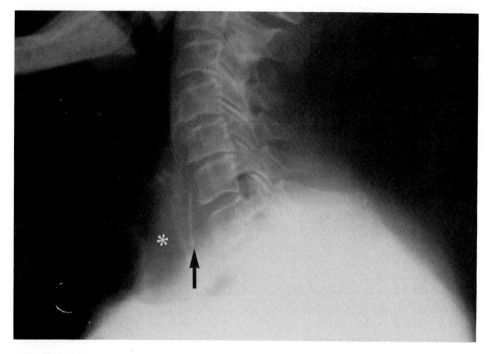

Fig. 24-6. Lateral radiograph of the cervical spine reveals a poultry bone *(black arrow)* lodged in the esophagus (note location posterior to tracheal air column) *(asterisk)*. (From Rosen P, Baker FJ II, Barkin RM et al: *Emergency medicine: concepts and clinical practice,* ed 2, St Louis, 1988, CV Mosby.)

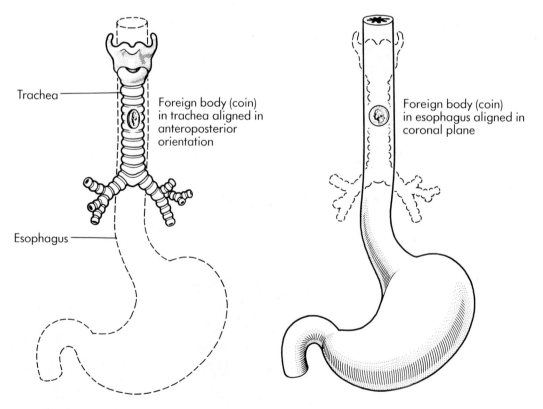

Trachea

Foreign body (coin) in trachea aligned in anteroposterior orientation

Esophagus

Foreign body (coin) in esophagus aligned in coronal plane

Fig. 24-7. Sagittal (on-end) orientation of a tracheal foreign body and coronal (en face) orientation of an esophageal foreign body. (From Rosen P, Baker FJ II, Barkin RM et al: *Emergency medicine: concepts and clinical practice,* ed 2, St Louis, 1988, CV Mosby.)

sions or lacerations caused by the object should also be noted since these may account for the patient's symptoms, even in the absence of the foreign body itself. Finally, careful palpation of the neck to determine the presence of subcutaneous emphysema should be performed in all patients who may have an impaled sharp object or delayed presentation. Such emphysema indicates esophageal or pyriform sinus perforation.

Diagnostic imaging. Radiographic evaluation is the next step when the foreign object cannot be located by physical examination[5] or the object is clearly esophageal in location. Plain film radiography can be used if the foreign body is thought to be radio-opaque. AP and lateral radiographs of the cervical spine (using soft tissue technique) and a standard chest radiograph often reveal the location of the object (Fig. 24-5). The object can further be confirmed as being in the esophagus by noting that the object is posterior to the tracheal air column (Fig. 24-6) and by the tendency for flat objects such as coins to align themselves in the coronal plane of the esophagus (Fig. 24-7). This situation is in contrast to tracheal foreign bodies. Since the trachea has a longer AP diameter than coronal because of the orientation of the incomplete cartiliginous rings, the tracheal foreign body will present sagitally rather than coronally as in the esophagus. Plain radiographs should also be carefully reviewed for air in the soft tissues and mediastinum, suggesting esophageal perforation.

Contrast study of the esophagus is indicated if the object is not visualized by plain film radiography and the patient remains symptomatic. Three types of radio-opaque contrast material are available for evaluation of the gastrointestinal tract: barium, high-osmolality water-soluble contrast (meglumine diatrizoate, gastrograffin), and low-osmolality non-ionic water-soluble contrast (iohexol, iopamidol). Barium is relatively contraindicated if there is a likelihood of perforation, particularly into the mediastinum since it may cause a mediastinitis. High-osmolality water-soluble contrast (gastrograffin) is contraindicated when there is a risk of aspiration (e.g., high obstruction), possible communication to the lungs or bronchial tree, or possible small bowel obstruction.[9,10] In the lungs, gastrograffin can cause chemical pneumonitis, pulmonary edema, and possible death.

For cases of suspected esophageal perforation, initial fluoroscopy with non-ionic contrast (iohexol or iopamidol) is recommended. If initial fluoroscopy is negative for perforation, barium should then be used for better definition of anatomy. The column of contrast material is evaluated for contour, for filling defects representing the foreign body (Fig. 24-8), and for passage into the stomach. If a small, sharp object is suspected, barium-soaked cotton balls may be swallowed by the patient so that the cotton will catch on the small impaled object that could not be seen on the initial contrast study.

Treatment. Foreign bodies located in the pharynx or hypopharynx can usually be removed with a forceps or clamp during direct visualization. Esophageal foreign bodies often pose a greater challenge. Blunt objects lodged in the proximal or midesophagus may be extracted either by esophagoscopy, which may require general anesthesia, or Foley catheter balloon technique.[11] In the latter instance, the patient is placed in a head-down position, a Foley catheter is passed beyond the object, the balloon is inflated using contrast material, and under fluoroscopic monitoring, the catheter is slowly and gently withdrawn, thus pulling the object along with it.[12-14] Precautions to prevent aspiration of the object once it reaches the pharynx should be taken.[15,16]

The choice of esophagoscopy vs. balloon extraction depends on the resources available, physician experience, consultant preference, and the length of time the object has been in place. Objects that have been lodged for more than 24 hours should be removed under direct visualization, thus allowing inspection of the esophageal wall. Unsuccessful balloon extraction warrants esophagoscopy to remove the object. Esophagoscopy is also indicated for

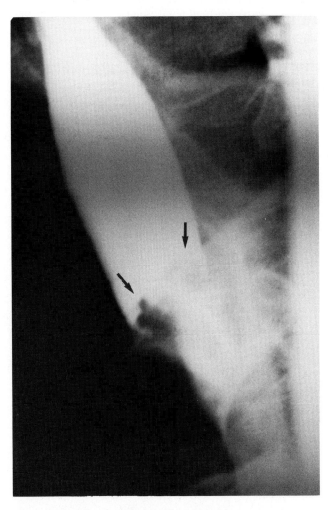

Fig. 24-8. Barium esophagogram demonstrates complete obstruction of the esophagus caused by an impacted meat bolus *(arrows).*

sharp, pointed objects lodged in the esophagus that are not amenable to removal by other techniques.

The patient with distal esophageal food impaction may be treated in several ways. Intravenous administration of glucagon has been described to relieve distal obstruction in numerous case reports.[17-21] Glucagon acts to decrease smooth muscle tone at the lower esophageal sphincter and to allow passage of the bolus. Care should be taken to administer glucagon slowly because, given rapidly, it can cause nausea and vomiting with possible esophageal rupture if the esophagus is obstructed. The administration of gas-forming agents has also been described in the treatment of food impaction. Carbon dioxide, produced by first drinking 15 ml of tartaric acid solution (18.7 g/100 ml) then 15 ml of sodium bicarbonate (10 g/100 ml), pushes the bolus into the stomach.[22] Alternatively, prepackaged gas-forming agents ("fizzies" used in upper GI examinations) along with glucagon may be administered, followed by 250 ml of water.[23] This technique has been reported to be successful in two thirds to three quarters of patients; however, if the impaction is longstanding (greater than 6 hours), it is less likely to succeed.[24] Enzymatic degradation of an impacted food bolus using a papain slurry is no

longer recommended.[19,25] Life-threatening medical problems result if papain should spill into the mediastinum from an unrecognized esophageal perforation.

Disk or button battery ingestion is of special concern because batteries are not sealed biologically and may leak their contents. These batteries may contain mercury, lithium, silver, nickel, zinc, cadmium, or potassium hydroxide in high concentration (40% to 45%).[26-29] Leakage may result in heavy metal poisoning, especially mercury,[29] or liquefaction necrosis from the potassium hydroxide.[30] Any time a disk battery has been ingested, its location should be determined, and, if lodged in the esophagus, it should be removed immediately.[29,31] If the battery is located in the stomach, it can be managed by observation for passage through the bowel. A blood test for heavy metal levels should be obtained if the battery is noted to have come apart on follow-up examination.[31]

Finally, a repeat esophagogram is indicated following removal or passage of an impacted object to confirm esophageal patency and to exclude a stricture. Older patients who may have esophageal motility disorders or obstructive lesions, which are often neoplastic, should be referred for further evaluation.[24]

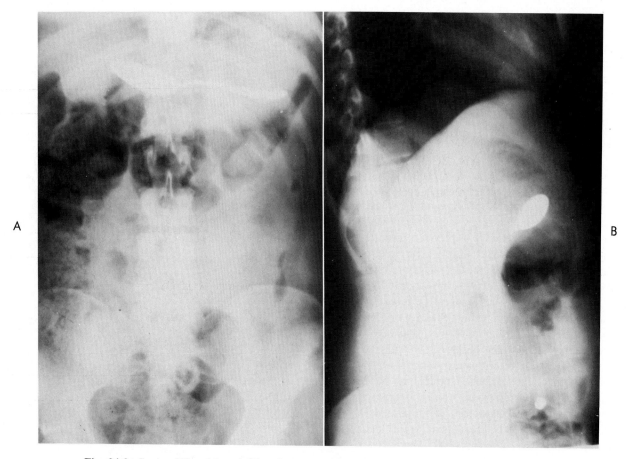

Fig. 24-9. Supine (**A**) and lateral (**B**) radiographs of the abdomen show a spoon swallowed by a psychiatric patient. (From Rosen P, Baker FJ II, Barkin RM et al: *Emergency medicine: concepts and clinical practice,* ed 2, St Louis, 1988, CV Mosby.)

Stomach and bowel

Clinical findings. In most cases the history of foreign body ingestion is available from and provided by the patient. Often, these ingestions occur when individuals, particularly children, hold small objects in their mouths or lips and accidentally swallow them. Occasionally, psychiatric patients swallow a variety of objects, prisoners ingest objects such as silverware or razor blades in an effort to get out of jail, and drug pushers swallow drug-filled balloons or packets to conceal the drugs in transport (i.e., body packing) or to prevent police seizure as evidence.

Diagnostic imaging. Physical examination is generally unremarkable in cases of foreign bodies in the stomach and bowel, and the diagnosis may be confirmed by radiography only if the ingested object is radio-opaque (Fig. 24-9). Usually an abdominal radiograph is sufficient to make the diagnosis (Fig. 24-10).

Treatment. In most cases, if the foreign object has passed through the esophagus and reached the stomach, it

will usually traverse the entire GI tract uneventfully and be expelled within several days. Confirmation of passage of the foreign body can be made by examination of the stools. In most cases the patient can be followed clinically as an outpatient without follow-up radiography; however, if there is concern that the object will not progress through the bowel, repeat studies may be obtained.[32] If a foreign body has not moved on two radiographic examinations taken over 24 hours or the patient shows signs of bowel obstruction or perforation, surgical intervention is indicated.

Patients who have swallowed balloons containing heroin, cocaine, or other illicit drugs should be admitted to the hospital under close observation to detect signs and symptoms of overdose, to initiate emergency treatment in the event of balloon rupture, or to document passage of the ingested drug.[33]

Rectum

Clinical findings. The overwhelming majority of foreign objects lodged in the rectum result from retrograde insertion, often as an accidental result of autoerotic behavior. In many instances the patient is in significant discomfort from the object, and this discomfort is compounded by embarrassment and anxiety.

The general physical examination is usually unremarkable. The foreign object may be palpated during digital rectal examination. Signs of peritoneal irritation suggest perforation of the bowel by the object.

Diagnostic imaging. Diagnostic radiography is indicated if the foreign object cannot be felt on rectal examination or if there is concern about perforation. A plain radiograph of the abdomen will often demonstrate the object (Fig. 24-11). If perforation is suspected, an upright radiograph to detect free air under the diaphragm should be obtained. Additionally, a water-soluble contrast enema may help exclude perforation, following removal of the foreign body.

Treatment. In most cases, extraction of the foreign body can be accomplished by insertion of a proctoscope or vaginal speculum in the rectum to visualize the end of the object and grasp it with forceps. The object is then withdrawn through the scope or speculum or, if it is too large, it is extracted as the scope or speculum is being removed. The colonic mucosa may become adherent to the object and create, in effect, a vacuum that prevents removal. In these situations the "vacuum" can sometimes be broken by passing a Foley catheter beyond the object and insufflating some air.

Rarely, if the foreign body is small, it can be hooked by the examining finger during rectal examination and removed. Surgical intervention is necessary if the object cannot be removed rectally or perforation has occurred.

If the object is successfully extracted transrectally, sigmoidoscopy should be performed to examine the bowel wall and ensure its integrity. Hospital admission is usually not necessary unless laceration or perforation of the bowel wall has occurred.[34]

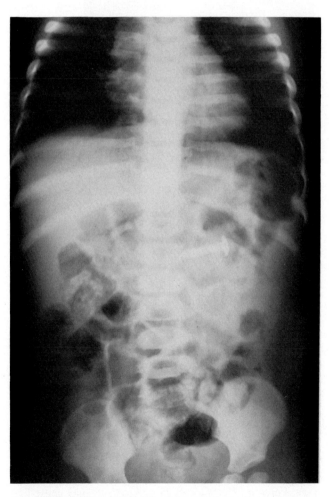

Fig. 24-10. Supine radiograph of the abdomen of a pediatric patient following ingestion of a screw. Patient was observed and passed the object uneventfully. (From Rosen P, Baker FJ II, Barkin RM et al: *Emergency medicine: concepts and clinical practice,* ed 2, St Louis, 1988, CV Mosby.)

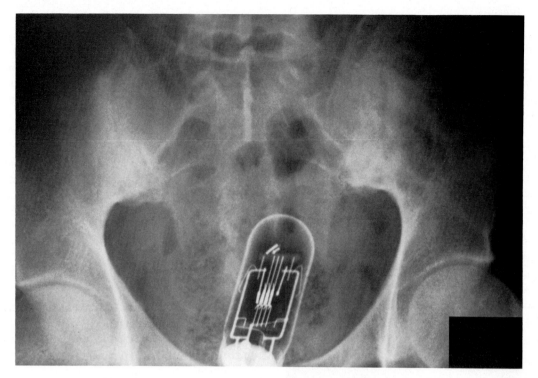

Fig. 24-11. Pelvic radiograph demonstrates a light bulb in the rectum.

FOREIGN BODY IN THE AIRWAY AND RESPIRATORY TRACT

Patients with foreign bodies of the airway and respiratory tract present with a wide variety of symptoms and signs, ranging from none to complete respiratory and cardiac arrest. Each year in the United States, approximately 2000 children die from foreign body airway obstruction.[35] Death also occurs in adults and has been termed the "cafe coronary."

Clinical findings. History of the inhalation or aspiration of a foreign object is usually available from adult patients who do not have complete airway obstruction. Small objects may be aspirated by workers who keep objects such as pins or nails in their mouths.[36] The "cafe coronary" involves aspiration of a bolus of food, often meat, which is larger than the esophagus can accommodate or which has not been chewed sufficiently. This often occurs in patients with alcohol consumption or patients who have upper dentures. These patients may not realize that the food bolus is too large to swallow.[37]

It may be difficult to differentiate the "cafe coronary" from an actual myocardial infarction. The patient with airway obstruction is initially conscious but unable to speak, the patient having a myocardial infarction is conscious and able to speak, and the patient in cardiac arrest is unconscious. The public should be taught the sign for airway obstruction, which is to grasp the trachea between the thumb and first two fingers to indicate an airway problem.

Children also may aspirate food, small toys, or other objects that they have placed in their mouths. This may occur when the child is playing or running and falls, thus aspirating the foreign body. Foods such as hot dogs and nuts are often aspirated and should not be fed to young children (under age 3 years).[35,37-41] Foreign body aspiration should be considered in any child who presents to the emergency department with sudden onset of respiratory distress, whether or not the presence of a foreign body is known.[35] In addition, this diagnosis should be considered in a child who presents with an atypical pneumonia, unilateral wheezing, or recurrent episodes of pneumonia in the same segment of the lung.[42]

The physical findings depend on the location of the object, the degree of obstruction, and the length of time the object is present.[43] Complete airway obstruction follows a progression that begins with the patient being in obvious distress, unable to speak or move any air. This is followed by loss of consciousness, cessation of respiratory effort, but continued cardiac activity with a pulse and blood pressure. If the obstruction is not relieved, complete cardiac arrest ensues.[44]

Small foreign bodies that do not cause tracheal obstruction can present with a variety of findings. The physical examination may be completely unremarkable in many cases. Foreign objects located in a bronchus may cause local irritation and coughing, localized wheezing, or stridor over the involved area. If the object completely obstructs a bronchus, breath sounds will be absent distal to the obstruction. Foreign bodies that act as a one-way valve may

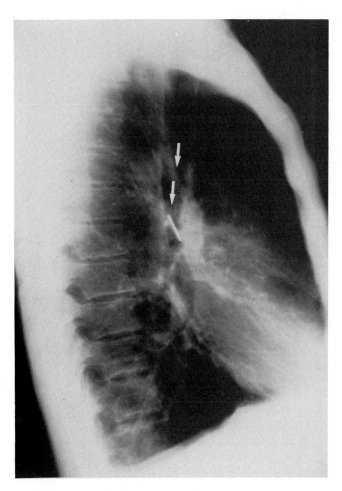

Fig. 24-12. Lateral chest radiograph shows an aspirated coin in the trachea *(white arrows)* at the level of the carina. (From Rosen P, Baker FJ II, Barkin RM et al: *Emergency medicine: concepts and clinical practice,* ed 2, St Louis, 1988, CV Mosby.)

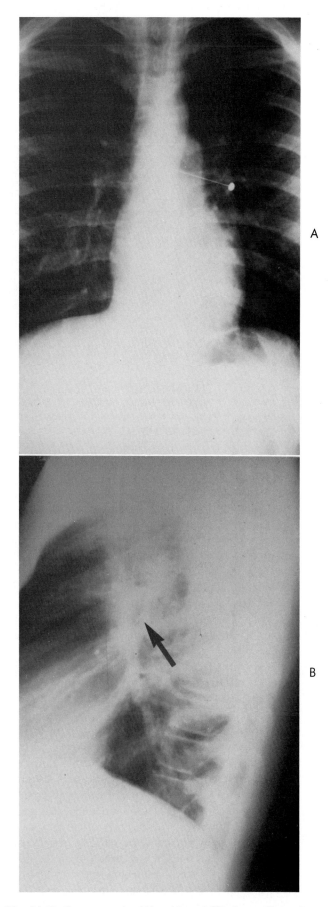

Fig. 24-13. Posteroanterior **(A)** and lateral **(B)** chest radiographs demonstrate an inhaled hat pin *(arrow)* in the left mainstem bronchus.

allow air entry during inspiration but no exit during expiration; thus the involved lung becomes hyperinflated. If the object has been present long enough for the distal lung to become infected, the patient may present with symptoms and signs of pneumonia or bronchitis, including fever, pleuritic chest pain, and cough that may be productive of sputum.

Diagnostic imaging. Standard chest radiography is the primary method of confirming the diagnosis of inhaled foreign object in patients with incomplete or no evidence of obstruction. (Complete obstruction warrants immediate, aggressive intervention and not radiographic confirmation.) Occasionally the foreign body can be visualized within the tracheal or bronchial air column on both the posteroanterior and the lateral radiographs, thus documenting aspiration (Figs. 24-12 and 24-13). If a foreign body is suspected but not visualized on the chest radiograph, inspiratory and expiratory film studies may provide additional information suggesting that an object is, in fact, present. If

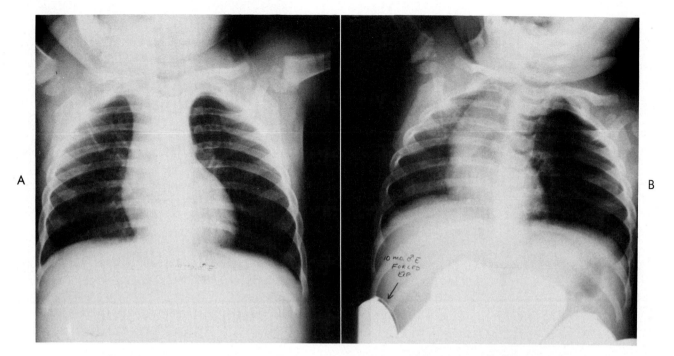

Fig. 24-14. A, "Normal inspiratory" chest film in a child with a left mainstem bronchus foreign body. **B,** "Forced expiratory" film shows a hyperinflated lung on the left with shift of the mediastinum to the uninvolved right side. (From Rosen P, Baker FJ II, Barkin RM et al: *Emergency medicine: concepts and clinical practice,* ed 2, St Louis, 1988, CV Mosby.)

the foreign body is acting as a one-way valve, the involved lung will appear hyperinflated on both films, and the heart and mediastinum will appear to shift to the uninvolved side on the expiratory film. If the object has caused obstruction, the segment of lung distal to the site will subsequently become atelectatic, the diaphragm will appear elevated, and the mediastinum will shift toward the involved side on both films because of loss of volume.[39] Forced expiratory films are indicated in young children suspected of foreign body aspiration. In general, there will be air trapping on the involved side, resulting in shift of the mediastinum away from the involved side (Fig. 24-14).

Treatment. Treatment of complete airway obstruction caused by a foreign body must be accomplished as rapidly as possible, and patient survival often depends on the action of witnesses, bystanders, or first responders. It is exceedingly rare for the emergency physician to affect the outcome in any way unless on the scene.

In adults and older children, the abdominal thrust is the first procedure to be attempted to relieve the obstruction. A brief thrust is applied to the epigastrium to produce a sudden increase in intrathoracic and intratracheal pressure and force the object out of the trachea into the pharynx, where it may be expelled or retrieved. This maneuver may be repeated several times if not successful on the first attempt. Digital removal of a foreign object may also be attempted by sweeping the pharynx. Great care must be exercised to prevent further impaction of an object located at the tip of the sweeping finger. If a laryngoscope and

Magill forceps are available, as well as personnel trained in their use, direct visualization with attempted removal of the object may be performed. The patient must be carefully observed subsequent to a Heimlich maneuver to ensure that no internal injuries were caused by the maneuver.

The optimal method of management of the young, choking child remains controversial. Data are limited regarding the initial intervention that should be attempted. Chest thrusts, abdominal thrusts, and back blows each have proponents. The American Academy of Pediatrics, the American Heart Association, and the National Academy of Science recommend the following: with the patient in a head-down position, four back blows followed by chest thrusts should be attempted, and repeated as necessary until the obstruction is relieved. Skilled personnel may attempt intubation or cricothyrotomy.[45]

If the obstruction cannot be cleared by these methods and the patient has lapsed into unconsciousness, cricothyrotomy can be accomplished by placing one or more large-gauge needles through the cricothyroid membrane.

Trained individuals can perform cricothyrotomy using any tools and material available, such as a knife and any hollow tube or a scalpel and endotracheal tube. In most cases the lodged object will be located at the introitus of the trachea and thus be above a tube inserted via the cricothyroid membrane. Rarely, the object will have passed beyond the cords and be lodged more distally in the trachea. In such a circumstance, attempts should be made to push the object past the carina into a mainstem bronchus, using an endotracheal tube; this allows ventilation of the nonobstructed lung.

In patients with incomplete obstruction or those with no findings, the role of the emergency physician is to diagnose. Removal of the foreign body involves bronchoscopy of the patient under general anesthesia. The patient must be properly positioned to prevent the foreign body from slipping into the uninvolved side, and care must be taken to avoid fragmentation of the object. If the object cannot be grasped by standard bronchoscopy forceps, a Fogarty catheter may be used in the same fashion as the Foley catheter for esophageal foreign body. It is passed beyond the object, the balloon is inflated, and the object is gently pulled out.[46,47]

SUMMARY

The diagnosis and removal of foreign bodies pose unique challenges for the emergency physician. Patients may present with symptoms that range from minimal to life-threatening, and the emergency physician must be prepared to pursue the appropriate sequence of investigations when time permits or to intervene aggressively when it does not.

REFERENCES

1. Whelan GP: The radiopacity of glass in soft tissue, *JACEP* 4:401, 1975.
2. Tandberg D: Glass in the hand and foot, *JAMA* 248:1872, 1982.
3. Marquis GP: Radiolucent foreign bodies of the hand: case report, *J Trauma* 29:403, 1989.
4. Nandi P, Ong GB: Foreign body in the oesophagus: review of 2394 cases, *Br J Surg* 65:5, 1978.
5. Haglund S et al: Radiographic diagnosis of foreign bodies in the oesophagus, *J Laryngol Otol* 92:1117, 1978.
6. Singh B et al: A fatal denture in the oesophagus, *J Laryngol Otol* 92:829, 1978.
7. Okafor BC: Lung abscess secondary to esophageal foreign body, *Ann Otol Rhinol Laryngol* 87:568, 1978.
8. Kawakami M et al: Pyopneumothorax due to perforation of the esophagus with an ingested fish bone, *Sci Rep Res Inst Tohoku Univ* 25:1, 1978.
9. Brick SH, Caroline DF, Leu-Tooff AS et al: Esophageal disruption: evaluation with iohexol esophagography, *Radiology* 169:141, 1988.
10. Bell KE, McKinstry CS, and Mills JOM: Iopamidol in the diagnosis of suspected upper gastro-intestinal perforation, *Clin Radiol* 38:165, 1987.
11. Dunlap L, Oregon E: Removal of an esophageal foreign body using a Foley catheter, *Ann Emerg Med* 10:101, 1981.
12. Bancewics J: Oesophageal bolus extraction by balloon catheter, *Br Med J* 1:1142, 1978.
13. Campbell JB, Davis WS: Catheter technique for extraction of blunt esophageal foreign bodies, *Radiology* 108:438, 1973.
14. Nixon GW: Foley catheter method of esophageal foreign body removal: extension of applications, *AJR* 132:441, 1979.
15. Campbell J, Quattromani F, and Foley L: Foley catheter removal of blunt esophageal foreign bodies: experience with 100 consecutive children, *Pediatr Radiol* 13:116, 1983.
16. Campbell J, Foley C: A safe alternative to endoscopic removal of blunt esophageal foreign bodies, *Arch Otolaryngol* 109:323, 1983.
17. Marks HW, Lousteau RJ: Glucagon and esophageal meat impaction, *Arch Otolaryngol* 105:367, 1979.
18. Ferrucci JT Jr, Long JA Jr: Radiologic treatment of esophageal food impaction using intravenous glucagon, *Radiology* 125:25, 1977.
19. Glauser J et al: Intravenous glucagon in the management of esophageal food obstruction, *JACEP* 8:228, 1979.
20. Handal K, Riordan W, and Siese J: The lower esophagus and glucagon, *Ann Emerg Med* 9:577, 1980.
21. Trenkner S, Maglinte D, Lehman G, et al: Esophageal food impaction treatment with glucagon, *Radiology* 149:401, 1983.
22. Rice B, Spiegel P, and Dombrowski P: Acute esophageal food impaction treated by gas-forming agents, *Radiology* 146:299, 1983.
23. Kaszar-Seibert DJ, Korn WT, Bindman DJ et al: Treatment of acute esophageal food impaction with a combination of glucagon, effervescent agent, and water, *AJR* 154:533, 1990.
24. Zimmers TE, Chan SB, Kouchoukos PL et al: Use of gas-forming agents in esophageal food impactions, *Ann Emerg Med* 17:693, 1988.
25. Giordano A, Adams G, Boies L Jr et al: Current management of esophageal foreign bodies, *Arch Otolaryngol* 107:249, 1981.
26. Litovitz T: Button battery ingestions, *JAMA* 249:2495, 1983.
27. Temple D, McNeese M: Hazards of battery ingestion, *Pediatrics* 71:100, 1983.
28. Votteler T, Nash J, and Rutledge J: The hazard of ingested alkaline disk batteries in children, *JAMA* 249:2504, 1983.
29. Kulig K, Rumack C, Rumack B et al: Disk battery ingestion, *JAMA* 249:2502, 1983.
30. Willis GA, Ho WC: Perforation of Meckel's diverticulum by an alkaline hearing aid battery, *Can Med Assoc J* 126:497, 1982.
31. Rumack B, Rumack C: Disk battery ingestion (editorial), *JAMA* 249:2509, 1983.
32. Selivanov V, Sheldon G, Cello J et al: Management of foreign body ingestion, *Ann Surg* 9:187, 1984.
33. Fainsinger MH: Unusual foreign bodies in bowel, *JAMA* 237:2225, 1977.
34. Barone JE, Yee J, and Nealon TF Jr: Management of foreign bodies and trauma, *Surg Gynecol Obstet* 156:453, 1983.
35. Aytac A et al: Inhalation of foreign bodies in children: report of 500 cases, *J Thorac Cardiovasc Surg* 74:145, 1977.
36. Templer J et al: Foreign bodies of the airways, external ear canal, and upper digestive tracts, *Mo Med* 75:217, 1978.
37. Harris CS, Baker SP, Smith GA et al: Childhood asphyxiation by food, *JAMA* 25:2231, 1984.
38. Bose P, El Mikatti N: Foreign bodies in the respiratory tract, *Ann Roy Coll Surg Engl* 63:129, 1984.
39. Salzberg AM, Krummel T: Respiratory foreign bodies, *Top Emerg Med* 4:8, 1982.
40. Cohen SR, Lewis GB, Jr, Herbert WI et al: Foreign bodies in the airway, *Ann Otolaryngol* 89:437, 1980.
41. Kero P, Puhakka H, Erkinjuntti M et al: Foreign body in the airways of children, *Int J Pediatr Otorhinolaryngol* 6:51, 1983.
42. Banks W, Botsic WP: Elusive unsuspected foreign bodies in the tracheobronchial tree, *Clin Pediatr* 16:31, 1977.
43. Goldsher M et al: Paradoxical presentation in children of foreign bodies in trachea and oesophagus, *Practitioner* 220:631, 1978.
44. Dailey RH: Acute upper airway obstruction, *Med Clin North Am* 1:261, 1983.
45. Abman SH, Fan LL, and Cotton EK: Emergency treatment of foreign-body obstruction of the upper airway in children, *J Emerg Med* 2:7-12, 1984.
46. Sam HS et al: Fogarty catheter extraction of foreign bodies from tracheobronchial trees of small children, *J Thorac Cardiovasc Surg* 77:240, 1979.
47. Kosloske AM: The Fogarty balloon technique for the removal of foreign bodies from the tracheobronchial tree, *Surg Gynecol Obstet* 155:72, 1982.

PART FOUR

Special Considerations

Management of the Emergency Patient in Radiology

James J. Mathews
Harold J. Matthies

The primary goal of this chapter is to provide the emergency physician and radiologist with guidelines to the management of the patient in the radiology department. Acutely injured or ill patients should be carefully monitored when they leave the emergency department, where all treatment and resuscitative modalities are readily available, and are transported to the radiology department, an environment in which all too often there are neither the mechanical devices nor the trained personnel to handle an abrupt deterioration in a patient's condition. The use of sedation to ensure that adequate studies are obtained and the use of prophylaxis to prevent reaction to contrast material in high-risk patients as well as treatment of anaphylactoid reactions to contrast material should also be emphasized.

TRANSPORTING AND MONITORING THE EMERGENCY PATIENT

Unstable patients are the nemesis of obtaining safe and adequate radiographic studies. They often arrive from the emergency department without adequate precautions being taken.[1] The transportation phase may be well covered by experienced personnel, but, during the actual procedure,

the patient may be left for extended periods of time with only a radiology technician in attendance. These personnel often are not equipped nor trained to recognize the early signs of a deteriorating patient nor can they institute therapy to either prevent or reverse the developing problem. In teaching hospitals, the individual assigned to accompany the patient is often the least experienced member of the team, but it must be stressed that the individual observing the patient should be experienced enough to recognize early signs and symptoms of deterioration and to provide at least initial care. Ideally, a resident physician and an experienced registered nurse (RN) should accompany the transport of an unstable patient in the teaching hospital, but the manpower logistics of staffing often prevent such ideal coverage. In the nonteaching hospital, the team might consist of two RNs or an RN and an emergency medical technician (EMT) with good clinical skills. In either case one of the transport team members should remain in close proximity to the patient and provide frequent reassessment. At any sign of deterioration of the patient's condition, backup support should be immediately available. Adequate equipment and supplies should either accompany the patient to the radiology department or should be on site.

Many hospitals have substantially reduced these problems by locating extensive radiology facilities within the geographic confines of the emergency department. Portable radiographic studies are also helpful in reducing transfers, but they must be used judiciously.[2,3] Even when radiology equipment is located in the emergency department, patients may be in the actual radiology department area for extended periods of time and may not be appropriately monitored. An experienced member of the team should be assigned the responsibility for monitoring the patient. In addition, many patients will still require transport for specialized studies, such as a CT scan. In busy facilities that deal with a high level of trauma, consideration should be given to installing a CT scanner within the emergency department. This will markedly reduce the number of unstable patients leaving the emergency department for diagnostic studies. Another suggestion that should be considered is to add a radiologist to the trauma response team to ensure early and efficient planning for obtaining radiographic studies.[4]

To ensure safe transport and monitoring for unstable patients, a plan should be developed beforehand, with clear delineation of the respective responsibilities of each member of the team. Patients who are to receive a specialized radiographic study on their way to an intensive care area or to the surgical suite are a frequent source of nursing disputes over responsibilities. This type of argument is impossible to resolve at the time and should be worked out before the need arises. There should be effective and realistic backup systems built in, so that the patient is not placed at risk because the staff is too small in number to allow someone to monitor the patient while the radiographic studies are being done. Hospital administration cannot ignore this type of "down time" for nursing, and the patient escort must be considered in the overall staffing plans of the units involved. These are not luxury positions but are mandatory for the safe and effective management of patients. Careful facility planning and upgrades can reduce the frequency of this problem substantially, but it will never be completely resolved. These patients also represent a high-risk group for malpractice litigation.

It is a truism of emergency medicine that the patient with the horrible, clear-cut injury gets expeditious and comprehensive care. A patient with a gaping hole in the chest from a shotgun blast moves rapidly through the emergency department to either the operating room or the morgue. However, the patient with blunt trauma who requires extensive workup to determine the extent of internal injuries is much more difficult for both emergency department and radiology personnel to handle. The risk to these patients is that they lull the staff into a false sense of security since they may be stable over a long period of time. As the workup continues to unfold and more and more results are negative, less and less attention is paid to the patient. At some point, a decision may be made to obtain head and abdomen CT scans, transportation is called, and the patient is transported to the radiology department. This practice is often appropriate for diagnosis but is dangerous to patient stability. The patient should be carefully reassessed before going to the radiology department, and this reassessment should be compared to previous results and charted. If there is any question regarding the patient's stability, it is best to err on the side of caution and to assign a member of the team to remain with the patient. One of the most unsettling sounds to an emergency physician is the announcement of a cardiac arrest code in the radiology department shortly after an emergency patient has been sent for radiographic studies. Judicious use of personnel and frequent reassessment of patients may prevent an unexpected and frequently irreversible arrest.

MAINTENANCE OF PROPER VENTILATION

Patients who are intubated with or without assisted ventilation represent a special problem in the radiology department. If the patient is being ventilated, it is mandatory that this procedure be continuous. Medical personnel, nevertheless, must be adequately shielded to prevent x-ray exposure while attending the patient, and, if exposure is repetitive, they should wear radiation detection badges. The practice of personnel stepping outside the room when a radiograph is taken is inappropriate and should be avoided. The advent of portable volume ventilators is changing the way such patients are managed, because these devices are an effective means of ensuring ventilation and thus reducing personnel requirements and risks. Whoever remains with the patient must be familiar enough with these devices to recognize problems and to be able to take over ventilation in the event of equipment malfunction.

Obstruction of the airway and ventilatory failure frequently occur in unstable patients. If there is any doubt regarding the adequacy of the airway or ventilation, the patient should be intubated and the airway secured before transport for radiographic evaluation. Another reason to consider intubation is if heavy sedation will be required to obtain a cooperative patient. Standard radiographic studies and CT scans are impossible to obtain in moving patients, and, if the patient is unable to cooperate, sedation and physical restraints are often necessary to ensure interpretable results.

RESUSCITATION

No matter how carefully patients are evaluated and monitored, it is impossible to completely prevent an unexpected acute change in a patient's status. When this occurs within the confines of the emergency department, full resuscitative efforts can be brought to bear. The situation is much different when deterioration occurs in the radiology department. There is all too often chaos, and, by the time order is established, the chances of a good result are reduced or lost. Simply relying on the response of a code team is not adequate to ensure a safe environment for patients in radiology. Staff radiologists should be capable of initial resuscitation, but it is very important to have someone available with advanced cardiac life support capability. At a minimum, Basic Life Support (BLS) training should be provided for technicians.

INSTITUTING PROTOCOLS FOR HANDLING EMERGENCY PATIENTS

In addition to training and certification, radiology departments should develop a staff nurse position charged with the responsibilities of developing and instituting protocols for treatment of emergencies, for inservice training to technicians, and for monitoring patients. Examples of such protocols are provided in the box on p. 625. These are presented only as guidelines, as specifics will undoubtedly vary from institution to institution. In smaller departments, the protocol development function can be met by

Examples of protocols for use in the radiology department

I. Critical Care Policy for Monitoring Patients in the Radiology Department:
  1. All patients will be monitored in the waiting area by the department nurse.
  2. When any critically ill patient is transferred from a floor, a nurse or physician must accompany the patient.
  3. If the patient coming to the radiology department has special problems that the department needs to be aware of, the floor nurse in charge of the patient will notify the chief technician or the departmental nurse.
  4. Transportation of spinal cord–injured patients on Stryker frames will be done with the patient in the supine position and with the arms securely strapped to the frame.
  5. If a spinal cord–injured patient with tongs in place must be transferred to an x-ray table from the Stryker frame, the neurosurgical or orthopedic resident in charge of the patient must be present during the transfer.
  6. Patients who are critically ill will have their procedures expedited while in the department. *The patient will remain on the x-ray table until completion of the test.*
  7. If the patient is receiving IV fluids or oxygen therapy, the IV infusion and oxygen-tank level will be monitored by the departmental nurse.
  8. With transfer of any patient from an intensive care unit, the chief technician and the departmental nurse will be made aware of the patient's status before transfer. The patient must be accompanied by a housestaff member (not a medical student) and, if necessary, also by a nurse. The physician or nurse will remain with the patient throughout the procedure and will accompany the patient back to the unit.
  9. If the patient is being maintained on a mechanical ventilator, the patient will be accompanied by a respiratory therapist or other experienced personnel to maintain proper ventilation.
  10. During the hours when the departmental nurse is not working, the patient's unit nursing station will be contacted with any special patient problems. With any critically ill patients, if deemed necessary by the chief technician on duty, the patient's unit will have to designate a nurse or house officer to stay with the patient for the duration of the examination.
II. Monitoring Policy for Departmental Drug Reaction Kits:
  1. Each x-ray room that contains a drug reaction kit should be monitored daily by the departmental nurse or chief technician.
  2. A daily record of this monitoring should be kept and be made available in the x-ray room.
  3. In the event that the drug reaction kit is opened or removed from its designated room, it should be restocked and replaced before the next patient is examined in the x-ray room.

an assigned nursing supervisor or by an interested staff radiologist on a part-time basis.

Adequate equipment and supplies need to be immediately available to medical personnel. A full crash cart with an electrocardiographic monitor-defibrillator should be stationed in the radiology area. If this is not economically feasible in small hospitals, a minimum number of basic agents for treatment of anaphylaxis and for ventilatory support should be located within the department for immediate use by radiologic personnel. The necessary equipment and supplies for advanced cardiac life support (ACLS) should be located nearby. In all departments, all personnel should be completely familiar with the protocol for mobilizing the code team and obtaining the necessary equipment.

Implementation of the preceding suggestions should produce several positive results. First, there should be a decreased number of unstable patients sent to the radiology department. Second, when it is necessary for patients to be transported, adequate supervision will be ongoing. Finally, education of radiologic personnel will result in better chances for resuscitation of those patients who deteriorate unexpectedly, whether they arrive from the emergency department or from other areas of the hospital to the radiology department.

SPLINTING

Splinting is a mandatory aspect of management during the initial care and assessment of the acutely injured patient.[5] Effective splinting of an acute fracture minimizes the risk of further injury, reduces bleeding, and decreases the pain associated with the fracture. If severe pain persists after the splint is applied, it is very suggestive of an inadequate splint that needs to be reapplied.

Long bone fractures are a common occurrence in the patient population of both the emergency and radiology departments. It is the role of the emergency physician to apply proper splinting to suspected fractures after initial assessment, to evaluate the neurovascular integrity of the injured extremity, and to rule out an open fracture. If the patient is brought to the facility by paramedics, the injury will often be immobilized and dressed. In general, these injuries should be unwrapped and reassessed, and the splint and dressing then reapplied.

Once the extremity is stabilized and other serious injuries have been ruled out, the patient may be sent for radiographic studies. Because most splinting devices are radiolucent or are constructed in such a way that the radio-opaque parts will not interfere with interpretation, there is no need to remove the splint for preliminary radiographs. In most cases only anteroposterior (AP) and lateral radiographs are required to determine if an obvious fracture exists and to assess the extent of displacement of the fracture. If the initial radiographic findings are negative and there has been appropriate consultation with the emergency physician, the splint may be removed and a full radiographic series obtained. On occasion, a patient may be sent from the emergency department with a fracture that is not splinted. A common setting for this occurrence is that a patient may have sustained a horrendously obvious injury to one area of the body that may obscure other injuries. If the technician suspects a long bone fracture that is not splinted, medical personnel should be notified immediately and the appropriate stabilization obtained.

In conclusion, the radiology technician should not remove splints until initial scout radiographs are obtained and until removal is discussed with the medical team. Any injured extremity should be handled with care until the radiographic results prove to be negative. If the pain from an injury seems to be excessive in contrast to the external appearance, the technician should notify the emergency physician, and the injury should be reassessed. If there is any doubt, splinting should be applied until initial radiographic screening studies are completed. Immobilization and radiographic evaluation of suspected spinal injuries are discussed elsewhere in this text (see Chapter 9). In general, full immobilization should be ensured until the initial screening radiographs are obtained, and the results are determined to be negative. In the cervical spine, all seven vertebrae should be visualized before stabilization is removed. Even then, if there are neurologic complaints consistent with spinal injury or if the patient experiences severe tenderness over the spine, immobilization should be maintained until the patient is fully cleared by an appropriate consultant. Finally, if a patient with suspected spinal injury begins to complain of numbness or tingling during the radiographic study, evaluation should cease immediately and the emergency medical staff should be notified.

SEDATION

Agitated or intoxicated patients are common in the emergency department. Often these patients present with serious injuries that require extensive radiographic assessment. Physical restraints are often used in this circumstance, but, to obtain adequate studies, these patients may also require sedation. This is also a frequent requirement in the pediatric population. Several commonly used agents are discussed in the following paragraphs, and their dosages and how to use them are summarized in Table 25-1.

Many of these agents, especially the narcotics, produce both sedation and analgesia. The practitioner should be familiar with several agents and be prepared to deal with any untoward reactions. In recent years, the use of sedatives and analgesics has generated a great deal of discussion, especially in the pediatric literature. This is a changing field, but, currently, the agents discussed are considered relatively safe and are widely used. With the advent of new agents with rapid onset, shorter duration of action, and more predictable results, the long-established regimen in the pediatric population of Demerol, Phenergan, and Thorazine (DPT) should be reconsidered.[6] In many institutions, use of this combination in the emergency department mandates short-term admission to observe for de-

Table 25-1. Common sedatives used in the emergency department

Agent	Dose	Route
Chloral hydrate	25-50 mg/kg/24 hrs *Total:* 500 mg-1 g	Oral or rectal
Narcotics		
Morphine sulfate	1 mg/kg *Total:* 5 mg (more may be used if needed)	IM or IV
Meperidine (Demerol)	1-2 mg/kg *Total:* 100 mg (*Note:* commonly used with hydroxyzine, 0.5-1 mg/kg, IM only)	IM or IV
Fentanyl (Sublimaze)	2-4 μg/kg given in 50 μg increments in adults and in 25 μg increments in children *Total:* 400 μg in adults (more may be used if needed)	IV only
Benzodiazapines*		
Diazepam (Valium)	2-20 mg depending on age and responses; 10 mg usual, maximum IM	IM or IV
Midazolam (Versed)	0.1-0.3 mg/kg to desired effect	IM or IV

*Note: These agents are most commonly used with narcotics. When administered by IV, the narcotics are given first. Midazolam may be mixed with the narcotic when IM administration is used. Meperidine and midazolam are not recommended for children <3 years of age.

layed effects of these drugs. Often this is the only reason for admission and is another reason why shorter acting agents should be used. Whenever sedatives are used as adjuncts in the assessment of patients in the emergency department, certain risks are incurred. These risks need to be minimized, and the patient should be carefully observed for any evidence of complications of the sedation. Included in these potential problems are respiratory depression, untoward interactions with intoxicants consumed by the patient before arrival, and loss of the ability of the emergency physician to assess changing mental status. Although serial evaluation of mental status remains an important aspect of clinical assessment, its overall importance has been reduced by the widespread availability of the CT scan. Nonetheless, a careful neurologic examination should be documented before the use of sedatives, and, subsequently, the medical and surgical consulting services should be made aware that the use of sedatives is planned.

In intoxicated patients and patients with underlying respiratory disease, the risk of respiratory depression during sedative use is greatly increased. These agents should be used with the greatest caution in this setting, and the patient should be monitored for evidence of respiratory compromise. If there is any question regarding the adequacy of the airway or ventilation, the airway should be secured and the patient mechanically ventilated during the procedure and until the pharmacologic effects have resolved.

If the type of ingested agent is known, any potential interaction can be anticipated and prepared for, and specific drugs may be chosen that do not interact with the ingested agent. Often the intoxicant, or more commonly the combination of drugs ingested before arrival, is unknown so that an unsuspected reaction may occur. Careful monitoring of the patient will prevent this problem from going unrecognized and will allow for early intervention to occur.

Chloral hydrate

Chloral hydrate is an agent with a long history of use and a wealth of clinical experience behind it. It remains an extremely effective sedative and is the agent of choice in the pediatric population for procedures such as a CT scan, MRI, and EEG if the child does not require analgesia. The actual mechanism of action is not fully understood, but the effect is on the central nervous system. When given in therapeutic doses, chloral hydrate is extremely safe.

Its use requires minimal equipment and monitoring. The usual dose of 25 mg/kg to a total of 500 mg is given either by mouth or by rectum. If the hypnotic effect is desired, the dose may be increased to 50 mg/kg up to a 1-g total. Onset of action is within ½ to 1 hour. One drawback is that the duration of action is from 4 to 9 hours, and there is no specific agent to reverse the drug's effects.

Although chloral hydrate is generally a safe drug, potential complications exist. These include coma from overdose, respiratory depression, and delirium if pain is present. Some degree of respiratory depression almost always occurs, but this is usually not a clinically significant problem. Respiratory depression is a much greater risk, however, when other depressants such as ethanol and barbiturates are present, and chloral hydrate should be avoided in these circumstances.

Narcotics

The opiates are among the oldest of therapeutic agents available to the practitioner.[7] A great deal of effort has been expended in developing synthetic agents to enhance the benefits of this class while eliminating the untoward side effects—especially addiction, respiratory depression, and hypotension. Currently, none of these attempts have been completely successful, and these problems remain whenever narcotics are used. Fortunately, there is a specific agent that can reverse the undesirable side effects of narcotics: naloxone.

Morphine sulfate. Morphine sulfate (MS) remains a mainstay of therapy in the emergency department for both its sedative and analgesic effects. In the acute situation, IV use is recommended. Incremental doses are given until the desired effect is observed. Onset of action by this route oc-

curs in minutes, and the effects persist for several hours. Respiratory depression may occur, especially at high doses or if the agent is given too rapidly. The patient must be carefully observed for this problem, and ventilatory support provided or the effects reversed with naloxone. Another common side effect is hypotension, which is generally brief and is readily reversed with fluids. Morphine has wide use, especially during painful orthopedic manipulations and for sedation of agitated patients to obtain studies such as a CT scan. In the agitated patient with suspected intracranial injury, MS is an ideal sedating agent for a CT scan. The usual dose is 0.1 mg/kg to a maximum of 5 mg. If the desired effect is not obtained, an additional dose can be administered, but significant respiratory depression is more likely to occur, especially after the procedure is completed. As with all narcotics, MS affects the perception of pain within the CNS. MS may also be used IM, and this route has advantages in the very young or in other patients in whom IV access is difficult. The same dosage is recommended, and similar precautions and monitoring should be done. When given IM, MS activity in the patient is prolonged for 3 to 4 hours.

Meperidine. Meperidine (Demerol) is a synthetic opioid. It is commonly administered IM, but IV usage is acceptable. Onset is rapid, generally within 10 minutes when given IM, and peaks within 30 to 50 minutes. The duration of action is 2 to 4 hours. This agent is frequently used with hydroxyzine (Vistoril), a tranquilizer unrelated to phenothiazines or benzodiazepines. This combination should be given only by deep IM. Because hydroxyzine potentiates the CNS depressant effects of opiates, it is suggested that the dose of the narcotic should be reduced by 25% to 50%. The usual dose of meperidine is 1 to 2 mg/kg, either IM or IV, to a maximum of 100 mg. If used with hydroxyzine, the dose is reduced to 0.5 mg to 1 mg/kg. Hydroxyzine is given in a dose of 1 mg/kg IM. It has a wide range of safety, and overdosage is rare. While it relieves the nausea of opiates, it does not increase the analgesic effect. Meperidine should not be used in patients with head trauma or other conditions associated with increased intracranial pressure or in patients on MAO inhibitors.[8] Respiratory depression is a common side effect, as it is with all narcotics.

Fentanyl. Of the newer synthetic narcotics, fentanyl (Sublimaze) has had the most widespread usage. Fentanyl has a mode of action in the CNS that is similar to other opiates, but it is extremely potent. It is estimated that this agent is 25 to 100 times more potent than morphine on an equal-dose basis. The effects of fentanyl are reversed by naloxone. Because of this agent's potency and its rapid onset, fentanyl is most often administered intravenously. This may be a drawback in certain situations in which IV access is difficult. The rate of administration is extremely critical because almost all cases of acute respiratory depression occur when the drug is given too rapidly. A suggested rate is 0.5 μg/kg/minute, with a maximum rate of 25 μg/minute. Naloxone should be ready for use. The usual dose in the emergency department is 2 to 4 μg/kg given in 50 μg aliquots in adults and 25 μg aliquots in children. These boluses are given over 1 to 1.5 minutes, and the patient is continually monitored. The usual adult dose is less than 400 μg, but it is common to use more to obtain the desired analgesic effect.

The side effects of fentanyl are similar to other narcotics. Respiratory depression is perhaps a greater risk because of the potency and rapid onset of this agent. Apnea may occur with minimal change in mental status, especially if the rate of administration has been excessive. This can also occur, as in all narcotics, after the painful stimulus is over. This is somewhat less of a risk with fentanyl because of its very short duration of action. Fentanyl appears to have a higher risk of producing thoracic muscle rigidity, the "wooden chest syndrome." This reaction impairs ventilation and is generally seen at high doses, but it can also occur if the rate of infusion is too rapid. This untoward effect is reversible with naloxone. Increased intracranial pressure and hypotension are less of a concern than with other opiates. Moreover, unlike MS, fentanyl does not induce hypotension in the supine patient. A final side effect that is often used as a clinical marker for onset of action is facial pruritus. The cause of this reaction is unknown.

Benzodiazepines

Benzodiazepines are a large class of agents with many shared similarities of action.[9,10] As a group, these agents all have muscle relaxant, anxiolytic, anticonvulsant, and sedative and hypnotic effects. There is significant variation as to the degree of action of a specific benzodiazepine or its given effect. Also these drugs have major differences in dose response that must be remembered when they are used. The most widely used of this class of drugs is diazepam (Valium). Of the newer agents, midazolam (Versed) has undergone a number of clinical trials, especially in the pediatric population.

Diazepam (Valium). Diazepam is an extremely effective and widely used benzodiazepine in the emergency department setting for all cases where this class of drugs is indicated. It can be used by all routes, but in the emergency department it is most commonly given intramuscularly or intravenously. The dosage is from 2 mg to 20 mg (0.1-0.5 mg/kg in the pediatric age group), depending on the patient's size and age and the desired therapeutic effect. In general, 10 mg is the maximum IM dose. Almost all effects of this drug occur within the CNS. At high doses, there is direct neuromuscular blockade. Onset of action occurs within 5 minutes when given intravenously and peaks within 30 minutes. The drug is given at a rate of less than 5 mg/minute and is titrated to effect. Generally this agent is very safe, and true untoward interactions are uncommon. Diazepam is frequently administered intravenously with narcotics, especially for orthopedic manipulations. The narcotic is given first, followed by diazepam. Major effects subside within 2 to 3 hours although blood

levels may rise 6 to 12 hours later as a result of enterohepatic circulation. This agent remains the benzodiazepine of choice for use in adult emergency medicine.

Midazolam (Versed). Midazolam (Versed) is a short-acting benzodiazapine with CNS activity.[11] Used alone, it produces a short period of conscious sedation and amnesia for the event. These properties make it an excellent premedication for surgery. It also has an additive and synergistic effect for narcotics. It does not produce analgesia but reduces the requirements for narcotics by alleviating the anxiety associated with pain. Because of its short duration of action, this agent has been widely recommended for use in the pediatric population.[12-16]

The usual dosage of midazolam is 0.1 to 0.3 mg/kg. This may be given either intravenously or intramuscularly. Onset is within 15 minutes when given intramuscularly and within 3 minutes when administered intravenously. The peak effect occurs at 30 to 60 minutes by either route and dissipates over the next 1 to 2 hours. Frequent checks of the patient's vital signs should be made until the patient is reasonably alert.

Most commonly, this agent is used with narcotics. The combination of midazolam and a narcotic has essentially replaced the old "Demerol, Phenergan, and Thorazine" (DPT) cocktail. The major reasons are improved efficacy, predictability of effects, and a much shorter duration of action, eliminating the need for long-term observation. In general, the narcotic should be given first in usual doses, followed by midazolam. When given intramuscularly, the drugs may be mixed. The combination of meperidine and midazolam is not recommended for children under 3 years of age, and, as stated earlier, fentanyl should be used only intravenously. When used with narcotics, the onset of action of midazolam is more rapid—less than 2 minutes when given intravenously. Peak sedation time is also reduced. This combination is extremely effective, especially for the patient in pain who requires orthopedic manipulation.

The potential complications of midazolam are respiratory depression, hypotension, and hallucinations if pain is present. Whenever it is used with narcotics, the effects of respiratory depression and hypotension must be observed carefully, and the patient's vital signs monitored at frequent intervals.

Currently, a specific antagonist for the benzodiazepines has not been approved for general clinical use, but the drug flumazenil does have satisfactory reversal potential.[17-21] When this agent is released, the combination of narcotics and benzodiazepines will clearly be a safe and effective method of producing sedation, as both classes will be able to be rapidly reversed.

ANAPHYLACTOID REACTIONS

Acute generalized reactions can occur with the use of contrast material in 1% to 2% of all radiographic procedures in unselected patients.[22-24] If a patient has had a pre-

---

Prophylaxis for administration of contrast material

I. Use nonionic (low-osmolarity) contrast material
II. Nonemergent procedure
  A. Pretreat patient as follows:
    1. Prednisone 50 mg po 13 hours before, 7 hours before, and 1 hour before the procedure.
    2. Diphenhydramine 50 mg po 1 hour before the procedure.
    3. Ephedrine 25 mg po 1 hour before the procedure.
      a. Do not use if severe hypertension is present.
  B. Ensure emergency therapy is available.
III. Emergent procedure
  A. Administer hydrocortisone 200 mg IV immediately and repeat q 4 hour until study is completed.
  B. Give diphenhydramine 50 mg IM 1 hour before the study.
  C. Consider also ephedrine 25 mg po 1 hour before the study.
  D. In the hyperacute patient, these agents should be given as long as possible before the procedure.

Treatment of anaphylactoid reactions

Immediate in all patients with hypotension, bronchospasm, or laryngeal edema
1. Administer 0.01 ml/kg up to 0.3 ml of aqueous epinephrine, 1:1000 IM; repeat twice at 15-20 minute intervals if needed.

Other agents and modalities
1. Diphenhydramine, IV or IM, 1.25 mg/kg up to 50 mg; may suffice if uticartia only is present.
2. Hypotension: in addition to epinephrine, volume expansion and corticosteroid should be given (5 mg/kg up to 200 mg of hydrocortisone).
3. Bronchospasm: in addition to epinephrine, aqueous hydrocortisone, as described above, should be given. Aminophylline may be indicated and oxygen should be administered.
4. Laryngeal obstruction: endotracheal intubation or tracheostomy should be performed, and oxygen should be administered.
5. Respiratory arrest: oxygen, intubation, and mechanical ventilation should be performed as needed.
6. Cardiac arrest: CPR and further therapy should be performed as needed.

---

vious reaction to contrast material, the incidence rises to as high as 35%.[25] The reaction can range from mild urticaria to profound hypotension and shock and is nonimmunologically induced. IgE antibodies have not been demonstrated. Pretesting to determine patients at risk has not been successful.[26] The use of nonionic contrast material has helped to reduce the risk of reaction but has not eliminated it. These nonionic agents should be used in patients with a previous history of a reaction, and, in time, they may replace the ionic agents even in unselected patients.

If possible, contrast-enhanced radiographic studies should be avoided in patients with a history of prior reaction, and alternative diagnostic imaging studies should be used. If the study is mandatory, suggested pretreatment regimens are presented in the box opposite. If followed, these regimens, coupled with nonionic agents, have been shown to markedly reduce the incidence of contrast reaction.[27,28]

Treatment of anaphylactoid reactions is the same as for IgE antibody–mediated allergic reactions. The treatment is outlined in the box below. It is essential that, whenever contrast material is used, emergency treatment must be immediately available, and the radiographic personnel performing the procedure must be well versed in the initial care of patients who have a reaction to contrast material. If, in addition to pretreatment, nonionic agents are used, significant reactions to contrast material can be virtually eliminated.[29] Currently, the universal use of nonionic agents has been limited by expense. However, their use is indicated for the high-risk group, and eventually universal use is predicted (see Appendix).

SUMMARY

One of the most discouraging events in the practice of emergency medicine is the patient who abruptly deteriorates or experiences an unanticipated complication in the radiology department. Such an event frequently results in recriminations and feelings of guilt on the part of the personnel involved. Preplanned management of the sick or severely injured patient while in the radiology department will contribute toward eliminating such a tragic occurrence. However, even with the best preparation, unexpected events can occur. The radiology department must have adequate equipment and backup to treat patients, and all radiology department staff must have adequate training to recognize a deteriorating patient early enough so that intervention will be successful. Of utmost importance is the recognition that radiologists are part of the overall healthcare team and must be included in planning the management of the desperately ill or injured emergency patient.

REFERENCES

1. Nesbitt WR: Pitfalls in emergency care, *J Fam Pract* 2(5):333, 1975.
2. Eisenberg RL, Akin JR, and Hedgcock MW: Optimal use of portable and stat examination, *AJR* 134:523, 1980.

3. Gleadhill DN, Thompson JY, and Simms P: Can more efficient use be made of x-ray examinations in the accident and emergency department? *Br Med J* 294:945, 1987.

4. Daffner RH, Diamond DL: Trauma radiology: an integrated approach, *Appl Radiol* 17(1):51, 1988.

5. Shaw DC, Heckman JD: Principles and techniques of splinting musculocutaneous injuries, *Emerg Med Clin North Am* 2(2):391, 1989.

6. Goulding R, Helliwell PJ, and Kim AC: Sedation of children as outpatients for dental operations under general anesthesia, *Br Med J*, p. 855, 1957.

7. Jaffe H, Martin R: Opioid analgesics and antagonists. In Goodman et al, eds: *The pharmacological basis of therapeutics,* ed 7, New York, 1985, MacMillian Publishing.

8. Kaufman JS: Drug interactions involving psychotherapeutic agents. In Simpson S, ed: *Drug treatment of mental disorders,* New York, 1976, Raven Press.

9. Havey SC: Hypnotics and sedatives. In Goodman et al, eds: *The pharmacological basis of therapeutics,* New York, 1985, MacMillian Publishing.

10. Baldessarini RJ: Drugs and the treatment of psychiatric disorders. In Goodman et al, eds: *The pharmacological basis of therapeutics,* New York, 1985, MacMillian Publishing.

11. Dundee JW, Halliday et al: Midazolam: a review of its pharmacological properties and therapeutic use, *Drugs* 28:519, 1984.

12. Rita L et al: Intramuscular midazolam for pediatric preanesthetic sedation: a double-blind controlled study with morphine, *Anesthesiology* 63:528, 1985.

13. Weissman B et al: Midazolam sedation for computed tomography in children: pharmacokinetics and pharmacodynamics, *Ann Neurol* 16(3):410, 1984.

14. Wilton NCT et al: Preanesthetic sedation of preschool children using intranasal midazolam, *Anesthesiology* 59(6):972, 1988.

15. Feld LH et al: Premedication in children: oral versus intramuscular midazolam, *Anesthesiology* 69(3A):745, 1988.

16. Diament MJ, Stanley P: The use of midazolam for sedation of infants and children, *AJR* 150(2):377, 1987.

17. Hennis FJ et al: Antagonism of midazolam sedation by flumazenil: a placebo-controlled study in patients recovering from intravenous anesthesia with high doses of midazolam, *Eur J Anaesth* 5(6):369, 1988.

18. Jensen S et al: Flumazenil used for antagonizing the central effects of midazolam and diazepam in outpatients, *Acta Anaesth Scand* 33(1):26, 1989.

19. Hojer J et al: The effect of flumazenil in the management of self-induced benzodiaxzepine poisoning: a double-blind controlled study, *Acta Med Scand* 224(4):357, 1988.

20. Sullivan GF, Wade DN: Flumazenil in the management of acute drug overdosage with benzodiazepines and other agents, *Clin Pharmacol Ther* 42(3):254, 1987.

21. Roncari B et al: Pharmacokinetics of the new benzodiazephine antagonist in man following intravenous and oral administration, *Br J Clin Pharmacol* 22(4):421, 1986.

22. Davies P, Roberts MB, and Royiance J: Acute reactions to urographic contrast media, *Br Med J* 2:434, 1975.

23. Witten DM, Hirsh FD, and Hartmann GW: Acute reactions to urographic contrast media: incidence, clinical characteristics, and relationship to history of hypersensitivity states, *Am J Roentgenol Radium Ther Nucl Med* 119:832, 1973.

24. Coleman WP, Ochsner SF, and Watson BE: Allergic reactions in 10,000 consecutive intravenous urographies, *South Med J* 57:1401, 1964.

25. Witten DM: Reactions to urographic contrast media, *JAMA* 231:974, 1982.

26. Fischer JW, Doust VL: An evaluation of pretesting in the problem of serious and fatal reactions to excretory urography, *Radiology* 103:497, 1972.

27. Greenberger PA, Patterson R, and Radin RC: Two pretreatment regimens for high-risk patients receiving radiographic contrast media, *J Allergy Clin Immunol* 74(4):540, 1984.

28. Greenberger PA, Patterson R, and Tapio CM: Prophylaxis against repeated radiocontrast media reactions in 857 cases, *Arch Intern Med* 146:2197, 1985.

29. Greenberger PA, Patterson R: Personal communication, October 1989.

Acquired Immune Deficiency Syndrome

Beatrice D. Probst
Kevin J. Kirshenbaum
Robert P. Cavallino

The human immunodeficiency virus (HIV or HIV-1), previously called lymphadenopathy-associated virus (LAV) and human T-cell lymphotrophic virus type III (HTLV-III), causes acquired immune deficiency syndrome (AIDS). Infection with HIV and its major consequence, AIDS, are health problems worldwide, reported in more than 100 countries. An estimated 800,000 to 1,200,000 people in the United States are presently infected with HIV, most of them remaining undiagnosed.

Like other retroviruses, HIV establishes lifelong infection by integrating its genome into the host cell. HIV is cytopathic for selected T4 cells (helper cells). The virus replicates in helper T lymphocytes, monocytes, and macrophages that express the T4 (CD4) receptor due to direct viral infection.

The definition for AIDS was revised in 1987 to identify four stages in the HIV infection/disease process. Group I (the first stage) indicates acute infection with the HIV virus while group II indicates a seropositive but otherwise asymptomatic individual. Group III indicates persistent

Table 26-1. Groups in the United States at risk for HIV infection

Groups	Percentages
Homosexual or bisexual males	65%-75%
IV-drug abusers	15%-17%
Persons with hemophilia	16%
Heterosexual contacts (of high-risk groups)	2%-4%
Unknown or incompletely determined	3%

generalized lymphadenopathy for more than 3 months, and group IV indicates the presence of a secondary infection or malignancy in an HIV-infected individual. Declining CD4 cell counts in seropositive individuals (group II) without evidence of secondary infection or malignancy predict the likelihood of the person developing AIDS within the following 18 months. CD4 cell counts less than 500 are associated with the greatest risk of opportunistic infection and progression to symptomatic HIV infection.[1]

Prospective studies of asymptomatic carriers have indicated that between 15% to 45% will develop AIDS within 7 years of the initial infection. Epidemiologic data indicate that transmission of the virus occurs almost exclusively through contact with blood, semen, and vaginal secretions. The virus is transmitted most effectively by way of a large inoculum of blood.

The number of AIDS cases reported each year continues to increase; however, the rate of increase has steadily declined. Although new infections continue to occur, the rate of new infections among several groups, including homosexual men, appears to have decreased, which may have major implications for the overall incidence of new infection.[1]

The groups of people at recognized risk for HIV infection in the United States has remained stable during the first 8 years of reporting[2] (Table 26-1). However, as the number of new infections continues to increase (an additional 250,000 cases in 1991), the use of the emergency department by patients with AIDS is likely to increase as well. A level-one trauma center/emergency department in an indigent urban area found that 7.8% of their critically ill or injured patients were infected with HIV (an increase of nearly 5% in 1 year).[3]

Patients who come to the emergency department with known HIV infection have recognized complications of HIV within specified organ system categories. The largest category of involvement is pulmonary (31.6%), followed by neuropsychiatric (21%), constitutional (19%), and gastrointestinal (14%).[4] The increased incidence of HIV-infected patients presenting to the emergency department requires that physicians be knowledgeable concerning potential medical complications of the disease, its clinical presentation, and its radiographic correlations.

PULMONARY DISORDERS

Patients presenting to the emergency department with known or suspected AIDS often require evaluation of respiratory symptoms, such as dry cough, dyspnea, shortness of breath, fever, or chest pain. Plain chest radiographs should be obtained initially to rule out life-threatening problems and to direct subsequent investigation. Despite limitations, radiographic interpretation plays an important role in the initial workup and management of a suspected AIDS patient. Although there is considerable overlap in

the radiographic appearance of many of the common AIDS-related pulmonary diseases (see the box below), diagnostic priorities can be established.

Pneumocystis carinii pneumonia

In two thirds of patients, *Pneumocystis carinii* pneumonia (PCP) is the initial AIDS diagnosis. Clinically, the pulmonary symptoms are often preceded by weeks of constitutional symptoms, such as weight loss, night sweats, and diarrhea.[5] Ultimately, the pulmonary symptoms predominant with cough, fever, and shortness of breath. Bilateral, diffuse, or perihilar interstitial infiltrates are a common radiographic presentation in AIDS patients. This is the classic appearance of *Pneumocystis carinii* pneumonia (PCP) seen in up to 86% of AIDS patients with pulmonary involvement[5,6] (Fig. 26-1). Initially, the pattern is granular or reticulogranular, but, with progressive disease, patchy or diffuse alveolar air-space consolidation appears, resembling pulmonary edema. Although the disease is typically described as bilateral, unilateral diffuse or focal infiltrates are still consistent with PCP (Fig. 26-2).

Cavitation and pneumatocele formation are unusual radiographic findings in PCP but have been reported. Cystic parenchymal changes have been documented in up to 7% of patients with PCP. These are of uncertain origin but may predispose the patient to spontaneous pneumothorax[7] (Fig. 26-3). Cavitation is more often seen with infection caused by fungal, mycobacterial, and bacterial pneumonias.

Clinically significant *Pneumocystis carinii* infection may be diagnosed in the absence of infiltrates or other chest radiographic findings in up to 20% of patients with AIDS. Therefore, in the appropriate clinical setting, a normal chest radiograph does not exclude pulmonary infection with *Pneumocystis* organisms.[8-10]

Radiographic signs: differential diagnosis of AIDS-related pulmonary diseases

Diffuse infiltrates
PCP
PCP plus other infections (CMV, MAI, MTB, *Candida* sp., *Toxoplasma* sp., and fungal infections)
PCP plus KS
Idiopathic interstitial fibrosis
TB
KS

Cavitation
Septic emboli (addicts)
PCP

Adenopathy
MTB and MAI
Fungal infection
KS
Lymphoma

Pleural disease
KS
Pyogenic bacterial pneumonia

Focal infiltrates
Pyogenic bacterial pneumonia
PCP
MTB

Nodules
KS
Fungal infection
Septic emboli

Miliary disease
Histoplasmosis sp. infection
Cryptococcis sp. infection
MTB

PCP indicates *Pneumocystis carinii* pneumonia; *CMV*, cytomegalovirus; *MAI*, *Mycobacterium avium intracellulare*; *MTB*, *Mycobacterium tuberculosis* infection; *KS*, Kaposi sarcoma; *TB*, tuberculosis.

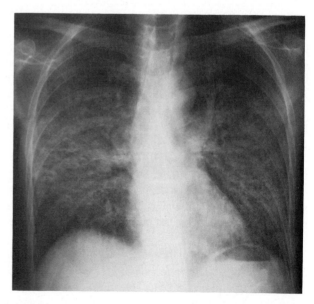

Fig. 26-1. *Pneumocystic carinii* pneumonia (PCP). PA radiograph demonstrates the classic appearance, showing bilateral perihilar and lower lobe interstitial infiltrates.

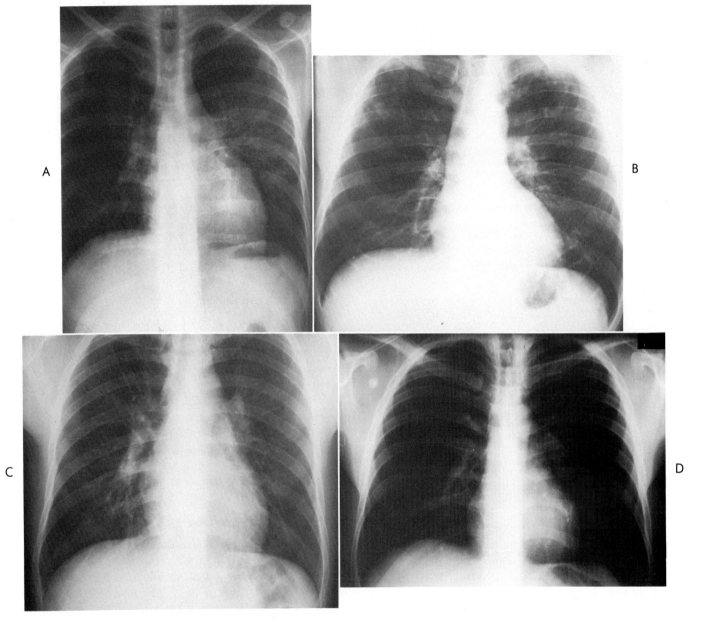

Fig. 26-2. Atypical radiographic presentation of PCP. **A,** Asymmetric disease. PA chest radio-graph shows an asymmetric pulmonary interstitial consolidation, which is most prominent in the left upper lobe. PCP presents with asymmetric disease in 1% to 5% of cases. **B,** Nodular disease. PA chest radiograph shows bilateral apical scattered nodules, which are more suggestive of a my-cobacterial infection. **C,** Hilar adenopathy. PA chest radiograph shows a left hilar adenopathy with no pulmonary infiltrates. Only 2% to 4% of PCP infection presents solely with a hilar or mediastinal adenopathy. **D,** Normal radiographic appearance. PA chest radiograph shows no ra-diographic evidence of disease although a transbronchial biopsy proved PCP.

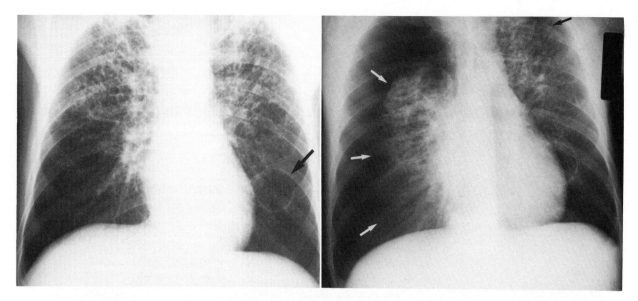

Fig. 26-3. PCP; cavitary disease. **A,** PA chest radiograph shows bilateral interstitial infiltrates, predominantly in the upper lobes, and numerous thin-walled cavities, varying in size with the largest in the left lower lobe *(arrow).* **B,** Spontaneous pneumothorax developed in the same patient. PA chest radiograph shows bilateral pneumothoraces *(arrows)* with a nearly complete collapse of the right lung.

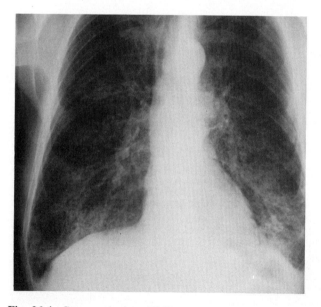

Fig. 26-4. Cytomegalovirus (CMV) pneumonia. PA chest radiograph shows extensive bilateral interstitial infiltrates, which are indistinguishable from PCP. CMV pneumonia is the most common form of CMV infection in AIDS patients.

The diagnosis of PCP is usually made by examination of tissue obtained after performance of bronchoscopy with bronchial lavage and transbronchial biopsy. The treatment regimen usually consists of sulfamethoxazole-trimethoprim administered for a total of 21 days. Should toxic reactions to the drug require discontinuation or should patients fail to improve, the sulfamethoxazole-trimethoprim therapy should be switched to pentamidine-isethionate therapy.[11]

Cytomegalovirus pneumonia

Cytomegalovirus (CMV) pneumonia is the most common form of CMV infection in AIDS patients, but its contribution to morbidity and mortality in these patients has been questioned. Only rarely has it been found to be the sole causative pathogen of respiratory failure. Radiographically, it is indistinguishable from the bilateral interstitial infiltrates associated with PCP[12] (Fig. 26-4). Diagnosis requires histologic demonstration of viral inclusion bodies.[7] Several drugs, including ganciclovir, have been used for treatment, but none has proved effective. The diagnosis of CMV pneumonia is not suggested until other more likely causes have been ruled out.

Mycobacterium organisms

Hilar and mediastinal lymphadenopathy is not a feature of uncomplicated PCP. Their presence should indicate an independent or co-existent pathologic condition such as Kaposi sarcoma, lymphoma, or mycobacterial infection.

Pulmonary tuberculosis is increasingly observed in AIDS patients, afflicting more than 10% of patients with HIV and may appear before the development of any AIDS stigmata.[7] It is more common in the chronically ill, high-risk groups of IV-drug abusers and Haitians rather than in homosexuals or recipients of contaminated blood products. Several features distinguish mycobacterial infections in AIDS patients from such infections in the general population. The chest radiographic pattern is consistent with primary tubercular infection with hilar and mediastinal lymphadenopathy and noncavitating infiltrates distributed equally to upper and lower lung fields (Fig. 26-5, *A*). This pattern exists despite evidence suggesting that reactivation is the mechanism of

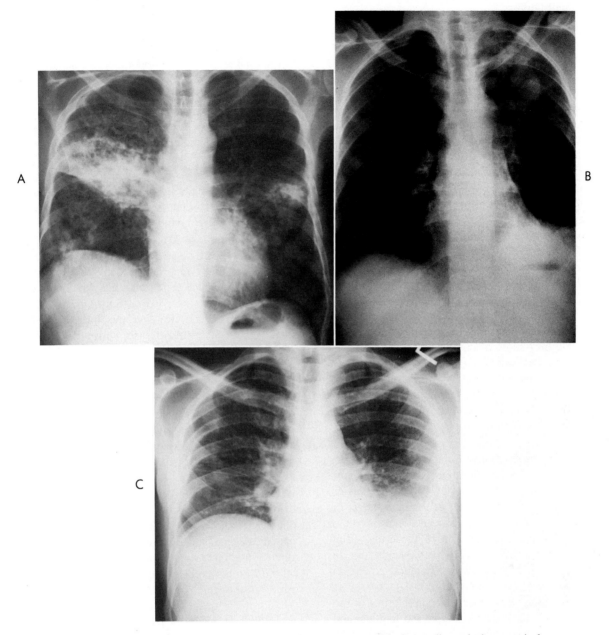

Fig. 26-5. Mycobacterial tuberculosis **A,** Typical appearance. PA chest radiograph shows typical bilateral noncavitary pulmonary infiltrates. **B,** Atypical appearance. PA chest radiograph shows multiple left apical nodules and a left pleural effusion, which is an atypical finding in an AIDS patient. **C,** Atypical appearance. PA chest radiograph shows a left pleural effusion, representing tuberculous pleuritis.

mycobacterial infections.[13] Apical or cavitary diseases have not routinely been observed because these portend a relatively intact immune system (Fig. 26-5, *B* and *C*).

The sputum cultures in these patients are less likely to yield acid-fast organisms. AIDS patients, however, have an increased incidence of extrapulmonary and lymphatic involvement. Treatment with conventional antituberculosis agents has been fairly successful in these patients.

Atypical mycobacteria, including *Mycobacterium avium intracellulare* (MAI), is seen in 10% to 20% of AIDS patients sometime during their lifetime and is usually widely disseminated at the time of diagnosis. Patients usually present with fever, dyspnea, cough, and weight loss, which are symptoms difficult to attribute solely to nontubercular mycobacterial infection. Radiographic correlation is equally nonspecific, with adenopathy; diffuse, patchy, alveolar infiltrates; multiple nodules; and miliary disease all being possible manifestations.[6,14] The diagnosis requires sputum culture or confirmation of disease at an extrapulmonary site. Treatment of MAI complex is unsatisfactory. Again, as with mycobacterial tuberculosis, cavitation has not been observed in AIDS patients with MAI.

Bacterial pneumonia

The reported incidence of bacterial pneumonia varies widely among AIDS patients, from 3% in chart reviews to 35% at autopsy, with the majority of cases caused by *Streptococcus pneumoniae* or *Haemophilus influenzae.* Other bacteria, including *Legionella pneumophilia,* have been demonstrated, alone or in association with other infections, most notably PCP. *Streptococcus pneumoniae* occurs more frequently in AIDS patients than in the general population. This organism is more likely to have multilobar involvement on chest radiographs. The clinical presentation of *S. pneumoniae* in these patients is not significantly different from that in a normal host, with acute onset of fever and a productive cough. The clinical course in AIDS patients, however, is more severe, with a longer time to defervescence and a longer course of antibiotic therapy required.

H. influenzae is very similar to *S. pneumoniae* in its incidence, clinical presentation, and patient response to treatment. Occasionally, *H. influenzae* infection can present radiographically as diffuse interstitial infiltrates indistinguishable from those of PCP.

Patients with HIV who have a diagnosis of bacterial pneumonia are at increased risk for the development of subsequent episodes. The chest radiographic presentation is reported to be different for each episode.

Fungal disease

Cryptococcus neoformans. Compared with the incidence of other opportunistic infections, fungal pneumonia is unusual, occurring in less than 5% of AIDS patients. *Cryptococcus neoformans* is the most common fungal organism isolated and is usually associated with brain or meningeal involvement at the time of diagnosis. Clinically, the patient presents with chest pain, weight loss, fever, dyspnea, and cough that may be productive. The duration of symptoms varies from a few days to several months. Chest radiographic appearance at the time of presentation is variable and includes single and multiple nodules that may progress to confluence or cavitation[12] (Fig 26-6, *A* and *B*). Mediastinal lymphadenopathy and segmental or diffuse interstitial infiltrates have also been found. *Cryptococcus neoformans* can be recovered from bronchial alveolar lavage fluid. Histologic confirmation is possible with transbronchial biopsy or open lung biopsy. Treatment with amphotericin B, alone or in combination with flucytosine, is effective in approximately half of patients.

Histoplasma capsulatum. In AIDS patients, *Histoplasma capsulatum* infection has been reported in both endemic and nonendemic areas, with most cases caused by reactivation of latent infection. Disseminated histoplasmosis is an indicator disease for the diagnosis of AIDS in patients with laboratory evidence of HIV infection and is not necessarily confined to patients from endemic areas.[14] AIDS patients with histoplasmosis present with constitu-

tional symptoms such as weight loss, myalgia, fever, chills, and diarrhea, which have often persisted for months before the diagnosis.[15] Dyspnea and cough can occur. Chest radiographs, when abnormal, reveal diffuse interstitial infiltrates or, less commonly, evidence of miliary disease, nodules, cavitary lesions, or adenopathy. Chest radiographs, however, may also be normal in patients with disseminated histoplasmosis documented by blood or bone marrow cultures. Associated infections with *Pneumocystis carinii* pneumonia, disseminated *Mycobacterium avium intracellulare,* and mucocutaneous herpes simplex virus are common.[12] The majority of the patients respond to treatment with amphotericin B, but, as with *Cryptococcus neoformans,* relapse is common.

Coccidioides immitis. Coccidioidomycosis occurs in up to 27% in AIDS patients living in endemic areas, a number that likely represents reactivation of latent infections. Clinically, the patient presents with chronic wasting illness, fever, and weight loss much like AIDS patients with histoplasmosis. However, respiratory symptoms are more prominent in this disease, with a dry or productive cough, dyspnea, and pleuritic chest pain. Chest radiographs typically reveal diffuse nodular or interstitial infiltrates.[12] Other patterns, such as single nodular lesions, hilar or mediastinal adenopathy, cavitary lesions, and a miliary infiltrate, have also been described. Diagnosis is generally made on biopsy, disclosing thick-walled spherules. The clinical course of coccidioidomycosis in AIDS patients is fulminant, despite treatment with amphotericin B.[15]

Other fungal infections typically associated with immune dysfunction are not commonly seen in AIDS patients. *Aspergillus* species is not thought of as a significant pulmonary pathogen, despite its occurence in a number of studies. It is more likely to be diagnosed in AIDS patients related to other predisposing factors, such as steroid therapy or neutropenia (Fig. 26-6, *C*). *Candidia* organism infection of the trachea, bronchi, or lungs has been designated by the Centers for Disease Control (CDC) as one of the indicator diseases used to establish a diagnosis of AIDS. Despite being the single most common fungal infection seen in AIDS patients, *Candida* species is not a frequent pulmonary pathogen.[15] Little is known about the clinical or radiographic presentation of candidiasis pneumonia in AIDS patients.

Noninfectious illnesses

Kaposi sarcoma. Approximately 25% to 35% of patients with AIDS have Kaposi sarcoma (KS), most commonly in the subgroup of homosexual or bisexual males. Pulmonary KS occurs in approximately 20% of patients with the epidemic form of KS and is usually preceeded by cutaneous or visceral involvement.[12,14,16] Patients with pulmonary KS present with fever, cough, and dyspnea that can be clinically indistinguishable from other pulmonary opportunistic infections in AIDS patients. The radio-

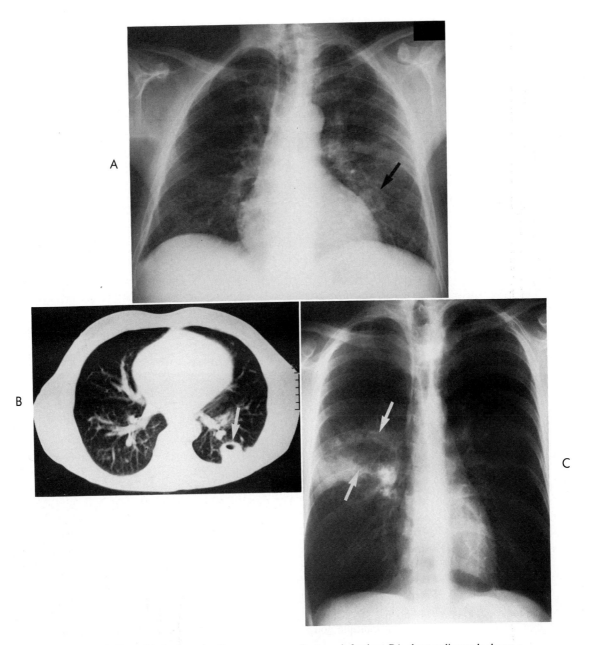

Fig. 26-6. Fungal infection. **A,** *Cryptococcus neoformans* infection. PA chest radiograph shows a large, thick-walled cavity in the left lower lobe *(arrow)*. **B,** CT scan through lower lung fields shows the same thick-walled cavity in the left lower lobe *(arrow)*. **C,** Bronchopulmonary aspergillosis. PA chest radiograph shows a large right middle lobe consolidation with a central cavity *(arrows)*.

graphic findings of KS have not changed significantly from the pre-AIDS era. Pulmonary involvement tends to be focal and randomly scattered throughout the pulmonary parenchyma. Hilar and mediastinal adenopathy, nodular infiltrates, and particularly large pleural effusions should make one suspect a diagnosis of KS (Fig. 26-7, *A*). A nonspecific diffuse interstitial pattern that is indistinguishable from that seen in other pulmonary opportunistic infections has also been reported[17] (Fig. 26-7, *B*).

Premorbid diagnosis by fiberoptic bronchoscopy is difficult but should be pursued to distinguish KS from other opportunistic infections that may be treatable. Otherwise, the diagnosis of pulmonary KS allows for temporary and palliative treatment with combination chemotherapy. Those patients with concurrent opportunistic infections have approximately two and one-half times the mortality of those without opportunistic infections.

AIDS-related lymphoma. Although both Hodgkin and non-Hodgkin lymphoma (NHL) have been reported in AIDS, the NHL occurs more frequently. AIDS-related lymphomas tend to be highly aggressive neoplasms with poorly differentiated histologic subtypes and an overall

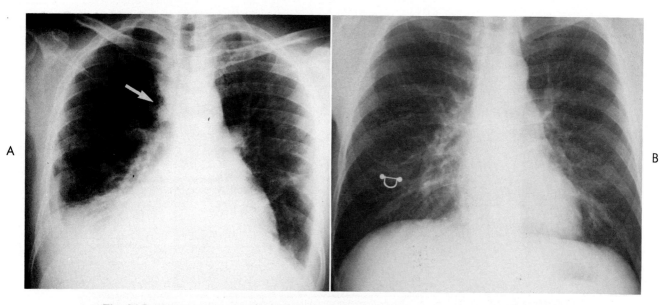

Fig. 26-7. Kaposi sarcoma. **A,** PA chest radiograph shows bilateral interstitial infiltrates, pleural effusions, and a right paratracheal adenopathy *(arrow)*. Findings are suggestive but not diagnostic of Kaposi sarcoma. **B,** PA chest radiograph shows diffuse bilateral interstitial infiltrates with a right hilar adenopathy, indistinguishable from PCP. Frequently, there is concurrent involvement with pulmonary Kaposi sarcoma (5% to 20%). Metallic nipple ring over the right lung field is an incidental finding.

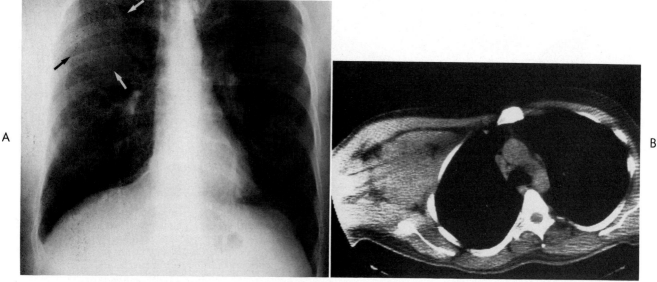

Fig. 26-8. Non-Hodgkin lymphoma of the chest wall. **A,** PA chest radiograph shows a subtle, diffuse, increased density over the right upper chest *(arrows)*. **B,** CT scan shows a large, right axillary soft tissue mass abutting the chest wall.

poor prognosis. NHLs are almost always extranodal and tend to involve multiple organ systems. Thoracic involvement is relatively rare given the frequency of extranodal involvement and can also be difficult to document (Fig. 26-8). Reported radiographic findings include isolated mediastinal and hilar lymphadenopathy, as well parenchymal infiltrates, nodules, and pleural effusions. Biopsy of hilar and mediastinal lymph nodes or pulmonary parenchyma is the only means of diagnosis.[12,14]

Lymphocytic interstitial pneumonia. Lymphocytic interstitial pneumonia (LIP) is a component of lymphoproliferative disorders of the lung and is characterized by diffuse infiltration of the interstitium with a mixture of lymphocytes, histocytes, and plasma cells. LIP associated with AIDS (HIV stages II to IV) occurs predominately in the Haitian population who have positive findings for HIV.[16] The Centers for Disease Control classifies children with serologically positive results for HIV and with lymphocytic interstitial pneumonia as having AIDS.[18] The etiologic factors of LIP are uncertain; possibly, they represent a direct and specific immune response to HIV pulmonary infection.[19]

Clinically and radiographically, LIP may be indistinguishable from other opportunistic infections manifested by fine-to-coarse reticulonodular infiltrates or superimposed, patchy alveoli infiltrates. Diagnosis requires either open lung biopsy or transbronchial biopsy. Clinical response is variable following appropriate immunosuppression.[12]

CENTRAL NERVOUS SYSTEM DISORDERS

The clinical manifestation of AIDS frequently involves central nervous system (CNS) disorders. Neuropsychiatric involvement represents the second largest category of known HIV-infected patients presenting to the emergency department.[3] In 20% of reported cases of patients with AIDS, neurologic illnesses are the presenting manifestations.[20] In autopsy-based studies, 80% of adult patients with AIDS have neuropathologic abnormalities, and at least half of these patients have had a neurologic disease during the course of their illness.[21]

The clinical features alone may not always point to the neurologic abnormality in AIDS patients. Nonfocal symptoms such as altered mental status and confusion may be seen with toxoplasmosis. Alternately, focal motor deficits, seizures, and headaches may be seen in the AIDS dementia complex (ADC). Neuroimaging studies, therefore, are important in making a diagnosis and in guiding therapy. Recent studies have suggested that magnetic resonance imaging (MRI) may be more sensitive than the CT scan in detecting intracranial lesions in patients with AIDS.[14] Common indications for neuroimaging in AIDS patients include decreased mental status, a change in the level of consciousness, headache, seizures, focal motor deficits, and cranial nerve palsies. Neuroradiographic findings generally fall into four categories, with the most common being cerebral atrophy. Other patterns include single or multiple mass lesions, focal or diffuse white matter disease, and leptomeningeal or ependymal disease.

Cerebral atrophy

Subacute encephalitis or AIDS dementia complex (ADC) is the most common cause of chronic neurologic dysfunction in HIV-infected adults. Dementia develops most commonly in patients with other manifestations of HIV infection, but it may also be the initial or predominant feature of the infection. The frequency of ADC is estimated to be 2% to 3% in the otherwise asymptomatic HIV carrier and is said to be as high as 50% in males with lymphadenopathy syndrome.[21] Evidence supports an etiologic role for HIV in this encephalopathy although the exact pathogenic mechanism is unknown. The syndrome consists most commonly of progressive dementia that first appears as a confusional state accompanied by mild fever or mild metabolic derangement. Other reported symptoms are focal motor deficits, seizures, signs of frontal lobe damage, headache, or behavioral changes.[22,23]

In general, radiographic studies of these patients is unrevealing but should be pursued to rule out potentially treatable illnesses or infections. The CT scan frequently shows mild generalized cortical atrophy characterized by enlargement of the sulci and ventricles (Fig. 26-9). Occasionally, low-density lesions in the white matter may be visualized. Both supratentorial and infratentorial atrophy may be present. Patients with atrophy appear to be at greater risk for subsequent development of intracranial mass lesions.[14,24]

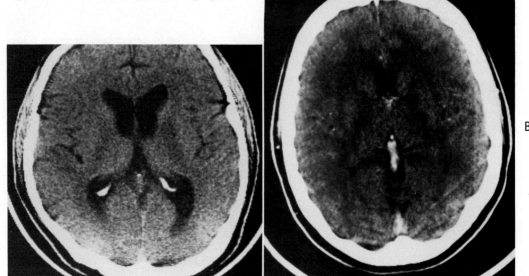

Fig. 26-9. Subacute encephalitis. **A,** Nonenhanced CT scan shows a diffuse central and cerebral cortical atrophy. Findings are indistinguishable from HIV encephalitis. **B,** Normal scan for comparison.

Mass lesions

Toxoplasma gondii. In patients with AIDS, focal space-occupying lesions of the central nervous system (CNS) result most commonly from neoplasms or infection. *Toxoplasma gondii,* an obligate intracellular protozoan, is the most common cause of this, occurring in approximately 10% of all AIDS patients. It appears to be more common in Haitian patients with AIDS than in other groups of AIDS patients, which is consistent with the higher prevalence of toxoplasmosis in the general population of tropical regions.[22] Life-threatening illness results from reactivation of a previously acquired infection. In the brain, this causes a necrotizing encephalitis.

The presentation usually includes focal deficits, often with an altered level of conscienceness. Approximately 15% of patients present with seizures. The focal deficits are often preceded by nonfocal deficits, such as lethargy and confusion, for several days to weeks. Headache and fever are commonly present. Diffuse findings may simulate ADC.[22] The CT scan has proved extremely useful for diagnosing toxoplasmic encephalitis, revealing rounded lesions that are single or multiple and isodense or of low

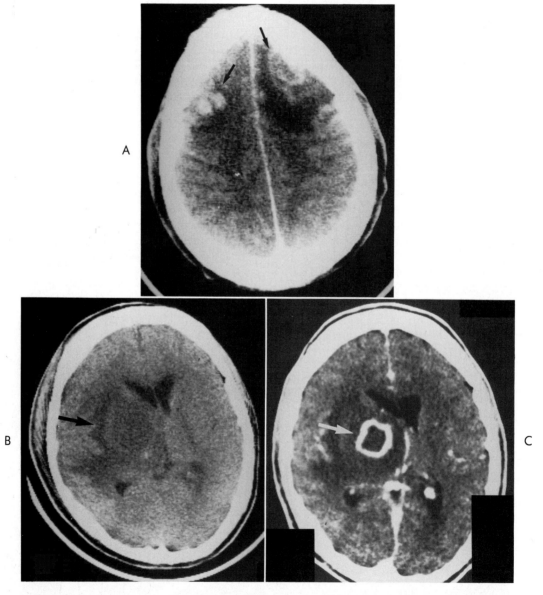

Fig. 26-10. Toxoplasmosis. **A,** Enhanced CT scan shows bilateral frontal lobe masses *(arrows)* with considerable surrounding edema and mass effect. Multiple lesions are most common. **B,** Nonenhanced CT scan shows a single (less common) low-density mass lesion *(arrow)* in the right basal ganglion. **C,** Enhanced CT scan shows an internal capsule, demonstrating typical ring enhancement *(arrow)* with surrounding edema and mass effect.

density (Fig. 26-10, *A*). Single lesions are less common. Surrounding edema is common and usually moderate to marked. When contrast material is given, the lesions enhance in either ring or nodular fashion in over 90% of patients (Fig. 26-10, *B* and *C*). The cerebral cortex and subcortical gray matter are the most common locations of in-fection.[14,22,24] The diagnosis is made clinically, followed by trial treatments with pyrimethamine and sulfadiazine. Response is usually evident after 2 weeks of therapy. Recurrence, however, is common when medication is discontinued. Biopsy is reserved for patients for whom therapy fails or who are clinically atypical for toxoplasmosis.[25,26]

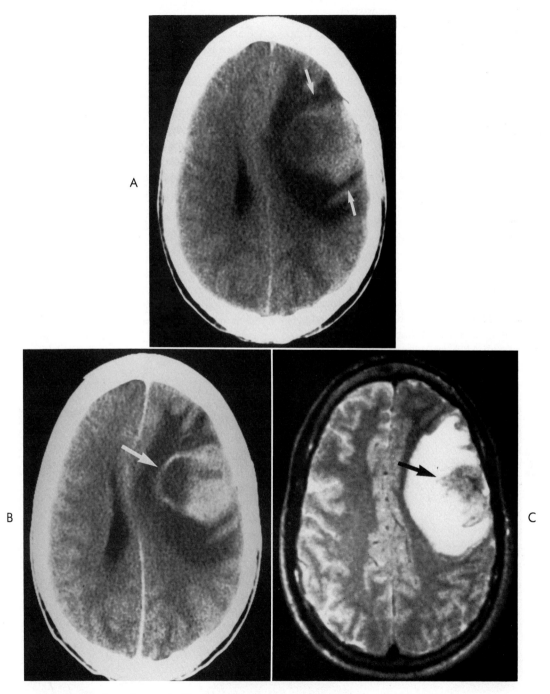

Fig. 26-11. Lymphoma. **A,** Nonenhanced CT scan shows a solitary, slightly high-density mass *(arrows)* in the left frontotemporal lobes. **B,** Enhanced CT scan demonstrates a nodular ring enhancement *(large arrow)* and a central low density, corresponding to central necrosis (rarely seen in non–AIDS patients with CNS lymphoma). **C,** Axial T_2-weighted MRI image shows an isointense mass *(arrow)* with central and surrounding peripheral, high-signal intensity, representing central necrosis and surrounding edema with mass effect, respectively.

Aggressively searching for the diagnosis is crucial because it is the most common treatable form of CNS involvement in AIDS patients.

Lymphoma. After toxoplasmosis, the next most common focal lesion is primary CNS lymphoma, which is found in approximately 6% of all AIDS patients at autopsy.[24] Patients with primary CNS lymphoma usually present with progressive mental deterioration, seizures, gait impairment, or cranial nerve dysfunction. Focal neurologic deficits and headache are less common as compared with toxoplasmosis. Typically, symptoms progress indolently for several weeks before medical attention is sought. Primary CNS lymphoma initially and preferentially involves the brain parenchyma so that cerebral spinal fluid findings do not usually show malignant cells.

The CT scan findings in about half of all AIDS patients are similar to CNS lymphoma in non-AIDS patients, demonstrating a single isodense or high-density lesion that enhances homogeneously with contrast material administration. Another 50% of AIDS patients with primary CNS lymphoma have lesions that show ring enhancement with central low density, correlating with central necrosis and mimicking *Toxoplasma gondii* abscesses (Fig. 26-11). In half of the AIDS patients, the CT scan demonstrates multiple lesions most commonly in the supratentorial gray or white matter (compared with only 14% of non-AIDS–related lymphoma). Prognosis is generally poor despite the high radiosensitivity of these lymphomas. Most patients survive less than 2 months.[14] Intracranial metastatic lesions in patients with AIDS are quite unusual, occurring in

only 2% of NHLs. NHL usually presents as leptomeningeal or ependymal disease rather than as parenchymal masses.[24] Kaposi sarcoma only rarely metastasizes to the brain.

Fungal and mycobacterial tuberculosis. Although unusual, fungal infections and mycobacterial infections may occasionally present as mass lesions in patients with AIDS. Fungal infections are common, occurring in as many as 15% of AIDS patients, but these infections usually present as meningitis rather than as mass lesions.[14] Intracranial tuberculosis has been recently described in 10 patients with AIDS (HIV stages II to IV).[27] The CT scan findings included ring-enhancing lesions (with one proving to be an acute tubercular abscess on biopsy) and low-density nonenhancing cortical areas. Although rare, tuberculoma or tubercular abscess should be considered in a differential diagnosis of intracranial mass lesions, especially in patients with IV-drug abuse or Haitians with AIDS. Although *Cryptococcus* organism infection is the most common CNS fungal infection in AIDS patients, it usually causes a subacute or chronic meningitis. The CT scan may demonstrate cerebral atrophy or hydrocephalus or may be entirely normal. Cryptococcomas are a rare cause of intracranial masses (Fig. 26-12).

Cerebral vascular complications. Cerebral vascular accidents were noted in up to 7% of AIDS patients in one study series and must be included in a differential diagnosis of mass lesions in patients with AIDS.[26] Intracerebral hemorrhage may result from coagulopathies, hemorrhage caused by intracranial neoplasms, or necrotizing angiitis involving intracranial vessels. Bacterial endocarditis may

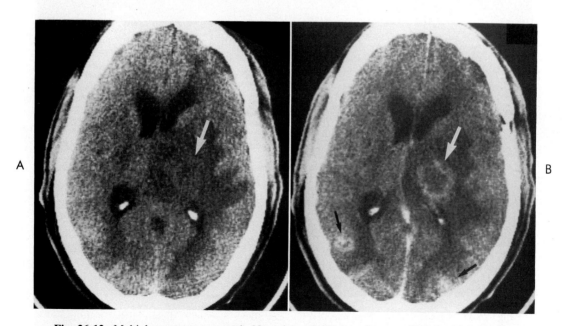

Fig. 26-12. Multiple cryptococcomas. **A,** Nonenhanced CT scan shows an ill-defined low-density mass lesion *(arrow)* in the left thalamic region. **B,** Enhanced CT scan demonstrates a ring enhancement *(arrow)* with extensive surrounding vasogenic edema. In addition, the right parietal and left occipital mass lesions are seen with nodular and solid enhancement demonstrated, respectively *(small arrows).*

cause the development of mycotic aneurysms, which may rupture and cause subarachnoid or intracerebral bleeding. Cerebral infarctions may be secondary to vascular occlusion from disseminated intravascular coagulation (DIC) and emboli related to endocarditis. Meningovascular encephalitis is another cause of cerebral infarctions in AIDS patients. The clinical presentation and imaging characteristics of infarctions and hemorrhage are usually distinguishable from mass lesions.[14]

White matter disease

Viral infections. White matter disease is common in AIDS patients and is usually the result of viral infections, including HIV, CMV, papovavirus, varicella-zoster virus, and herpes simplex virus. In most cases the cause of white matter disease is probably the result of HIV encephalitis although there are no distinguishing features to differentiate this from white matter diseases related to other causes. Pathologically, HIV encephalitis is diagnosed by the presence of multinucleated giant cells found in the white matter of cerebral and cerebellar hemispheres. There are few reports of imaging characteristics of HIV encephalitis. The most common finding is that of cortical atrophy. MRI is much more sensitive to abnormalities of white matter than is the CT scan.[14]

CMV is a common infection of the brain in AIDS patients. It is found on pathologic examinations in 25% of all AIDS patients, but symptomatic disease is uncommon.[14] Patients with symptomatic infections usually have normal

CT scans. This is not surprising because most often the infection is microscopic (glial nodules in gray and white matter) without gross histologic abnormalities.[14,24] Encephalitis produced by other viruses of the herpes group occurs in AIDS patients although their occurrence is overshadowed by ARD and nonviral infections. Herpes simplex encephalitis has been recorded in several patients with AIDS. The typical presentation includes fever and focal neurologic deficits similar to herpes encephalitis in patients without AIDS.[26] The CT scans are nonspecific or normal as compared with immunocompetent individuals in which the CT scans reveal low-density temporal and inferior frontal nonenhancing lesions. MRI subsequently reveals white matter abnormalities. The diagnosis can only be definitely established by temporal lobe biopsy.

Progressive multifocal leukoencephalopathy. Progressive multifocal leukoencephalopathy (PML) effects 2% to 7% of patients with AIDS.[24] Reactivation of papovavirus (usually JC virus) under conditions of immunoincompetence leads to this progressive demyelinating disease. In AIDS patients, it presents as altered mental status or as focal neurologic signs of aphasia, hemiparesis, and ataxia, which progress over weeks until death.[22]

Characteristic CT scan findings are low-density lesions, either single or multiple in the cerebral white matter that do not enhance with administration of contrast material nor exhibit mass effect nor are associated with edema (Fig. 26-13, A). The CT scan findings usually underestimate the degree of neurologic impairment.[14,22] The findings are

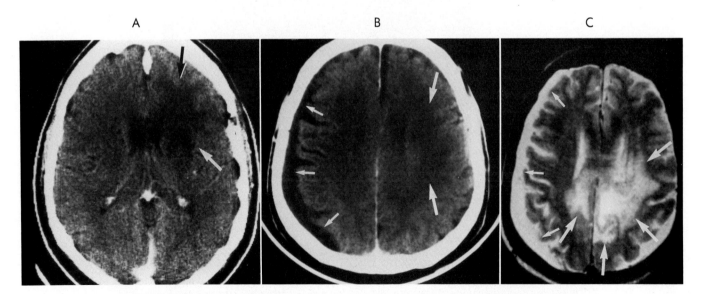

Fig. 26-13. Progressive multifocal leukoencephalopathy. **A,** Enhanced CT scan shows a subtle focal area of decreased density in the left subcortical frontal white matter (most common location) *(arrows)*. Typically, no significant mass effect or enhancement is demonstrated. **B,** Enhanced CT scan shows a vague low density in the left temporo-parietal white matter *(arrows)*. There is no significant mass effect. A right hemisphere subdural hygroma is incidentally noted *(small arrows)*. **C,** T$_2$-weighted MRI image shows a high-signal intensity in the left temporo-parieto-occipital lobes, extending across the midline and involving the corpus callosum *(arrows)*. A right hemisphere subdural hygroma is incidentally noted *(small arrows)*.

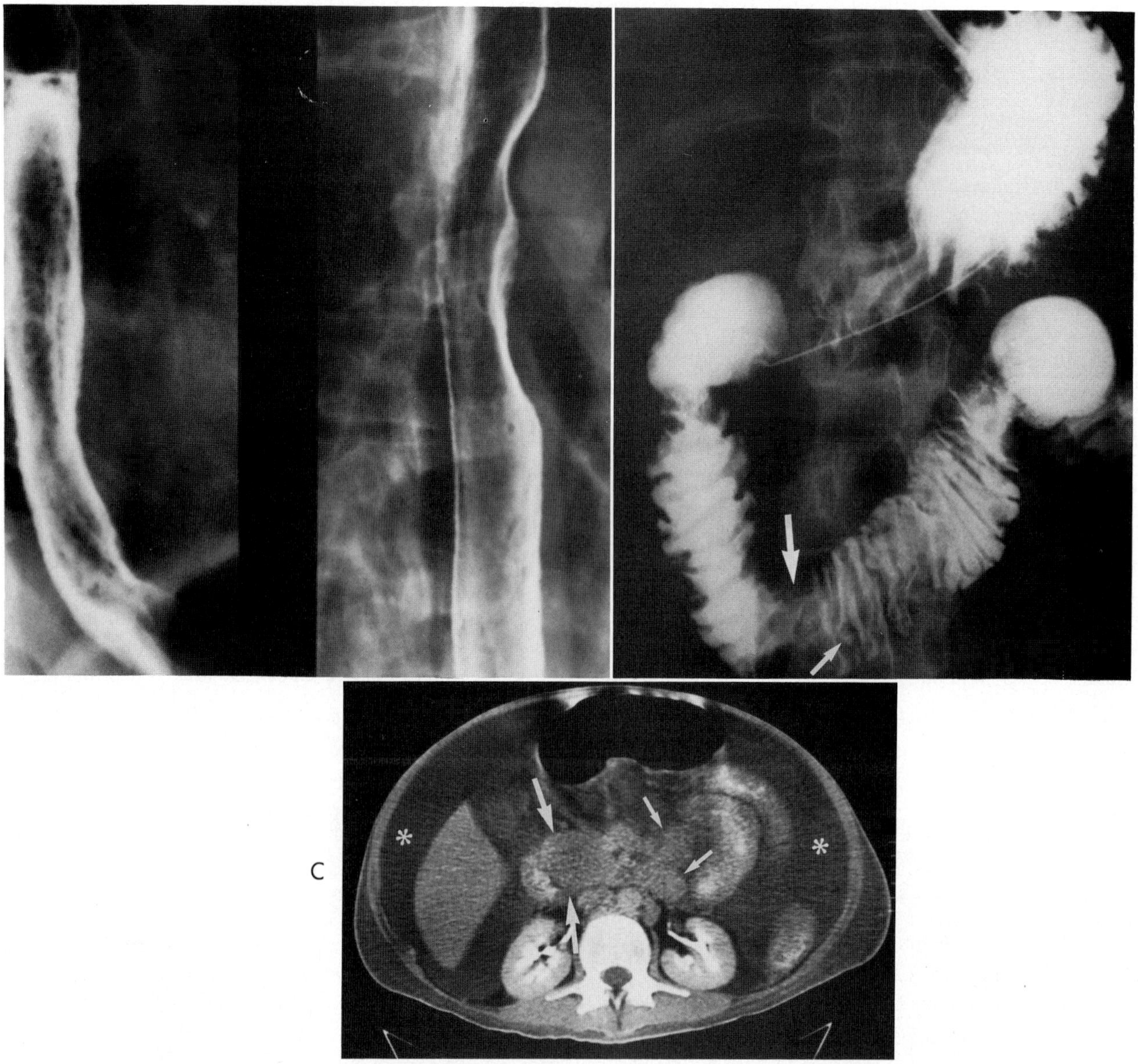

Fig. 26-14. Gastrointestinal manifestations related to AIDS. **A,** Candidiasis esophagitis. Diffuse filling defects caused by mucosal plaques along with extensive ulceration are scattered throughout the esophagus. Candidiasis is the most common AIDS-related gastrointestinal infection and the most common cause of esophagitis in AIDS patients. **B,** Kaposi sarcoma. Early radiograph from a small bowel examination shows discrete submucosal nodules with relative preservation of mucosal folds involving the proximal third portion of the duodenum *(large arrow)*. An ulcerated nodule *(small arrow)* is shown. **C,** Kaposi sarcoma. CT scan of the same patient showing a 2 × 3 cm low-density soft tissue mass *(large arrows)* abutting and involving the proximal third portion of the duodenum. Associated ascites *(asterisks)* and retroperitoneal lymphadenopathy *(small arrows)* are evident.

usually more striking with MRI than with the CT scan (Fig. 26-13, *B* and *C*). The disorder is progressive, with a mean time to death following diagnosis of 18 months. There is no effective treatment.

Leptomeningeal and ependymal disease

Septic meningitis. Although AIDS patients with meningitis may present to the emergency department requiring urgent clinical evaluation, neuroimaging does not contribute significantly to the diagnosis. If neuroimaging is indicated, an enhanced CT scan is superior to MRI in evaluating leptomeningeal or ependymal disease. Meningitis may be caused by HIV, CMV, fungal (especially *Cryptococcus* species), mycobacterial, *Toxoplasma gondii,* or *Treponema pallidum* infections.

Aseptic meningitis. HIV appears to be the most common cause of acute and chronic aseptic meningitis in AIDS patients, with the disorder occurring in up to 13% of patients.[14]

Acute aseptic meningitis may be a manifestation of primary HIV infection, with clinical features of fever, headache, and meningeal signs as well as cranial nerve involvement.[23] CSF monopleocytosis and protein elevation is found. Isolation of HIV from the CSF has been documented in these patients. CT scans and MRI rarely show abnormality of the leptomenigi, but atrophy and white matter changes secondary to HIV infection may occur.

Fungi and mycobacteria. *Cryptococcus neoformans* is the most common fungal infection of the CNS in AIDS patients. Clinically, these patients present with symptoms of meningitis, such as headache, confusion, and meningeal signs. Cryptococcal antigen titers are elevated in the CSF.[14,26] Neuroimaging study findings are usually normal or demonstrate cortical atrophy. Despite treatment with amphotericin B, the prognosis is extremely grave. Mycobacterial infections producing meningitis in AIDS patients are relatively rare.

Lymphoma. In 1% to 2% of AIDS patients, systemic lymphoma may metastasize to the CNS, usually affecting the meninges. Primary CNS lymphoma may also spread along the leptomeningial or ependymal pathways. Enhanced CT scans demonstrate an enhancement of the leptomeninges or ependyma that is nodular or irregular in pattern.[14]

CONSTITUTIONAL DISORDERS

Constitutional symptoms such as fever, weight loss, cachexia, and malaise constitute the third largest category of presentation by HIV-infected patients to the emergency department. Pulmonary or central nervous system diseases are often preceded by constitutional symptoms, and, therefore, a careful history and physical examination is warranted to identify potential diseases in those organ systems. If evidence for disease is found in an organ system, then radiographic evaluation can be directed toward this system. Isolated constitutional symptoms, although of im-

portance, rarely warrant emergency department radiographic evaluation unless one is searching for specific organ system disease. The severity of symptoms will guide subsequent disposition of the patient to either inpatient or outpatient evaluation.

GASTROINTESTINAL DISORDERS

Gastrointestinal complaints are the fourth largest organ system category represented in emergency department patients with HIV infection.[3] Candidiasis, CMV, cryptosporidiosis, histoplasmosis, isosporiasis, salmonellosis, and unusual mycobacteria account for the majority of nonneoplastic diseases (Fig. 26-14, *A*). Many patients may be infected with multiple organisms. Multiple sites are shown to be involved in 64% of patients. Neoplasms (Kaposi sarcoma) and lymphomas are also seen in the gastrointestinal tract of AIDS patients (Fig. 26-14, *B* and *C*). Many of these entities produce radiographic findings that may suggest a specific diagnosis. Rarely, however, is diagnostic radiographic evaluation of gastrointestinal complaints necessary in the emergency department. Radiographic demonstrations of the diagnostic features of gastrointestinal tract abnormalities in AIDS patients is usually reserved for the hospitalized or outpatient setting.

SUMMARY

Emergency department visits by HIV-infected patients are expected to increase in the future. Both the emergency physician and the radiologist are faced with the challenge of recognizing the many clinical manifestations of AIDS with their matching protean radiographic appearances. While any organ system can be affected by the AIDS virus, the central nervous system, pulmonary, and gastrointestinal systems are most often involved. Radiographic demonstration of certain abnormalities is often striking although not often specific.

Early recognition of HIV-related diseases demands a careful history and physical examination by the emergency physician. Subsequent diagnostic radiographic investigation is crucial in identifying the presence of opportunistic infections and neoplasms and in guiding further diagnostic evaluation.

REFERENCES

1. American Medical Association: *HIV early care: AMA physician guidelines,* Chicago, 1991, AMA Health Sciences.
2. American College of Physicians: *Medical knowledge self assessment program VIII: part A—book 5.* Philadelphia, 1988, American College of Physicians.
3. Kelen G et al: Substantial increase in human immunodeficiency virus (HIV-1) infection in critically ill emergency patients: 1986 and 1987 compared. *Ann Emerg Med* 18(4):378, 1989.
4. Kelen G et al: Human immunodeficiency virus infection in emergency department patients: epidemiology, clinical presentations, and risk to heath care workers—the John Hopkins experience, *JAMA* 262(4):516, 1989.
5. Clement, MJ et al: Diagnosis of pulmonary diseases, *Clin Chest Med* 9(3):497, 1988.
6. Golden J et al: The radiology of pulmonary disease: chest radiogra-

phy, computed tomography, and gallium scanning, *Clin Chest Med* 9(3):481, 1988.

7. Federle M: A radiologist looks at AIDS: imaging evaluation based on symptom complexes, *Radiology* 166(2):553, 1988.

8. Cohen B et al: Pulmonary complications of AIDS: radiologic features, *Am J Radiol* 143:115, 1984.

9. Goodman J et al: Pneumocystis with normal chest x-ray film and arterial oxygen tension, *Arch Intern Med* 143:1981, 1983.

10. Israel H et al: Hypoxemia with normal chest roentgenogram due to *Pneumocystis carinii* pneumonia: diagnostic errors due to low suspicion of AIDS, *Chest* 92(5):857, 1987.

11. Kaplan L et al: Treatment of patients with acquired immunodeficiency syndrome and associated manifestations, *JAMA* 257(10):1367, 1987.

12. Naidich D et al: Radiographic manifestations of pulmonary disease in the acquired immunodeficiency syndrome (AIDS), *Semin Roentgenol* 22(1):14, 1987.

13. Pitchenik A et al: The radiographic appearance of tuberculosis in patients with the acquired immune deficiency syndrome (AIDS) and pre-AIDS, *Am Rev Respir Dis* 131:393, 1985.

14. Federle M et al: *Radiology of AIDS,* New York, 1988, Raven Press.

15. Fels A: Bacterial and fungal pneumonias, *Clin Chest Med* 9(3):449, 1988.

16. Longo D et al: Malignancies in the AIDS patient: natural history, treatment strategies, and preliminary results, *Ann NY Acad Sci* 437:420, 1984.

17. Garay S et al: Pulmonary manifestations of Kaposi's sarcoma, *Chest* 91(1):39, 1987.

18. Oldham S et al: HIV-associated lymphocytic interstitial pneumonia: radiologic manifestations and pathologic correlation, *Radiology* 170(1):83, 1989.

19. Centers for Disease Control: Revision of the case definition of acquired immunodeficiency syndrome for national reporting—United States, *Ann Intern Med* 103:402, 1985.

20. Berger J et al: Neurologic disease as the presenting manifestation of acquired immunodeficiency syndrome, *South Med J* 80(6):683, 1987.

21. Dalakas M et al: AIDS and the nervous system, *JAMA* 261(16):2396, 1989.

22. Levy R et al: Neurological manifestations of the acquired immunodeficiency syndrome (AIDS): experience at UCSF and review of the literature, *J Neurosurg* 62:475, 1985.

23. Gabuzda D et al: Neurologic manifestations of infection with human immunodeficiency virus, *Ann Intern Med* 107:383, 1987.

24. Jeffrey B et al: Radiologic imaging of AIDS, *Curr Probl Diagn Radiol* 17:3, 1988.

25. Luft B et al: Toxoplasmic encephalitis, *J Infect Dis* 157(1):1, 1988.

26. McArthur J: Neurologic manifestations of AIDS, *Medicine* 66(6):407, 1987.

27. Bishburg E et al: Central nervous system tuberculosis with the acquired immunodeficiency syndrome and its related complex, *Ann Intern Med* 105:210, 1986.

APPENDIX

A P P E N D I X

Principles of Modalities

Constance S. Greene
Steven M. Montner

OVERVIEW OF PRINCIPLES OF MODALITIES
Conventional radiography

Conventional radiography uses ionizing radiation or x-rays, which are produced by bombardment of a target element by a stream of electrons in a vacuum tube. An object between the x-ray source and the receptor produces an image by attenuating the x-ray beam, analogous to a shadow. Attenuation in this case is reduction in the intensity of the x-ray beam as it traverses matter by either the absorption or the deflection of photons from the beam.

The image is created on photographic film, which is inherently sensitive to photons in the x-ray range, darkening with increasing exposure. The sensitivity is enhanced by placing the film between two screens that emit light in response to x-ray bombardment, thus reducing the intensity of the x-ray beam necessary to create an image. The combination of film and screen is optimized for the type of radiographic work desired, such as chest vs. extremity radio-

graphs. In fluoroscopy, the image is received on an image intensifier that is linked to a television monitor for viewing or to a VCR for recording.

Computed tomography

Computed tomography (CT scan) also uses ionizing radiation to produce an image. In this case an x-ray tube creates the beam but electronic radiation detectors receive the image. In most conventional (third generation) scanners, the x-ray tube and opposing array of detectors rotate around the patient. Average time required to obtain each image ranges from 3 to 5 seconds. Computer reconstruction produces an image that may be displayed on a television monitor, recorded on film, or stored on magnetic disk, tape, or optical disk.

Images are displayed as cross-sectional views, taken in an approximately horizontal plane. More limited images may also be electronically reconstructed in the sagittal and coronal planes. Recently images have been displayed three-dimensionally. The window level (brightness) or window width (contrast) are adjustable depending on the area of the body under consideration. Furthermore, administration of intravenous iodine can be used to enhance vascular or highly vascularized structures, allowing better differentiation from surrounding tissue.

Diagnostic ultrasonography

Ultrasonography uses no ionizing radiation and so is well suited for the evaluation of pregnant patients. It depends on the interaction of high frequency sound waves with tissue. These interactions consist of transmission, reflection, refraction, diffraction, scatter, and absorption. A piezoelectric material such as quartz or lithium sulfate generates a sound wave when an electric current is applied. This same crystalline material is capable of detecting a sound wave; in this case the crystal itself generates an electric current. When the sound wave traverses a material such as soft-tissue, some of the sound is reflected back to the transmitter. The time delay between transmitted and received signal is proportional to the depth of the reflecting surface of the material being studied. The ratio of the intensity between received and transmitted signal characterizes the tissue under consideration. A computer in the ultrasound equipment is able to reconstruct an image of the object, based on its interactions with the sound beam.

Ultrasonography is very useful in studying certain abdominal and pelvic structures. However, since air does not adequately transmit sound, overlying bowel gas can completely obscure regions of potential pathology. Furthermore, the thoroughness of the examination is highly dependent on the operator and is best left in experienced hands.

Magnetic resonance imaging

Magnetic resonance imaging (MRI) uses no ionizing radiation. Instead it depends on the behavior of the atomic nuclei of the tissue under study when exposed to a radiofrequency (RF) while in a magnetic field. This behavior depends on the physical and chemical environment within the tissue as well as external factors that are part of the measurement process. To simplify, the nuclei are subject to a brief radio signal while in a magnetic field, causing them to radiate a signal themselves. By applying a magnetic field with a spatial variation, or gradient, along three axes, a selective imaging plane may be obtained. A computer reconstructed image is obtained from the data, which may be displayed on a television monitor, printed on film, or stored on magnetic disk, tape, or optical disk.

Images are displayed as cross-sectional views *without* the restriction to a horizontal plane as with the CT scan in the coronal, sagittal, and axial planes. MRI provides excellent contrast in soft tissues and is exceptionally useful for studying the central nervous system. However, while very sensitive to differences in tissue type, it can be nonspecific in characterizing an abnormality.

Nuclear medicine

Radionuclide studies consist of administering small doses of short-lived radioactive compounds, radioisotopes, to the patient. These may be administered intravenously, inhaled, or instilled through a catheter. Radionuclides emit gamma-rays, and the most common elements in use are technetium, xenon, thallium, gallium, and iodine. The radioactive elements are generally tagged to a larger molecule or compound that may have an affinity for a particular type of tissue. For example, in lung perfusion studies, the technetium is attached to a micro albumin aggregate (MAA) of very small particle size. These temporarily lodge in pulmonary capillaries, allowing an image of the pulmonary perfusion to be acquired. This is complemented by radioactive xenon gas, which demonstrates lung ventilation. Other radionuclides may be excreted by the kidneys or into the biliary system, allowing visualization of these structures and an assessment of their function.

A "camera" is produced by an array of solid-state detectors, capable of measuring the gamma rays emitted from the patient. A computer reconstructs a two-dimensional image. While spatial resolution is limited, radionuclide studies are able to depict physiology as well as anatomy and so are a very useful tool.

Computed radiography

Computed radiography (CR) is a fairly new technique that is becoming increasingly available. As in conventional radiography, an image is formed on a receptor by attenuation of an x-ray beam by the object under study. Instead of radiographic film, the image is formed as a series of charges on a radiosensitive imaging plate. This receptor is scanned by the CR processor, converting the latent image into a digital image, which may then be displayed on a television monitor, printed on film, or archived on magnetic or optical disk. A digital image such as this may be manipulated to enhance certain structures such as catheters or bony detail. The images are indefinitely retrievable from the storage device, even if the original films are lost.

USE OF PORTABLE EXAMINATIONS

Portable radiographs should only be ordered whenever it is inadvisable to remove the patient from continuous observation in the emergency department or when additional movement, usually of an injured patient, would entail unnecessary risk of further injury.

Any body part can be studied by portable techniques, but the views that can be obtained are limited and the quality of the film and standardization of the radiographic examination may be compromised. The two factors that have to be considered are patient restrictions and operator or equipment limitations. Patients who require portable radiographs are often critically ill or in immobilization devices and unable to cooperate or to be positioned for optimal views. Motion artifact will be more likely.

In the fixed equipment geometry of the radiology department an ionization chamber is located behind the film, sensing the number of photons and automatically terminating the exposure when a preset threshold is achieved. Portable units do not have this phototiming capability and are dependent on operator judgement in the selection of the appropriate exposure based on patient size. This results in a higher likelihood of a suboptimal film. Grids are used to reduce scatter and are essential to obtain a radiograph of comparable image quality to that obtained in the radiology department. However, it is difficult to align the grid perfectly perpendicular to the beam and malalignment seriously compromises the image quality. Many institutions forego the use of grids and sacrifice the potential for higher quality to compensate for less perfect alignment. The use of a grid also requires an x-ray of higher energy, but that is not a problem with modern equipment.

"Fast" film speeds and intensifying screens are standard today and reduce exposure time and hence movement artifact. The only limitation is that the speed of the film is inversely proportional to the amount of detail that can be obtained. In this regard, however, portable radiographs are no different from those exposed with fixed equipment.

Interpretation of portable radiographs must take into consideration differences in technique. Magnification of mediastinal structures is greater because an AP rather than a PA view is obtained, and absolute measurements cannot be used to determine abnormalities. Sharpness and contrast are reduced, leading to a "grayer" film. An "upright" chest radiograph is seldom obtained at 90° and even when the chest is 90° upright, the abdomen may not be, decreasing the sensitivity of the radiograph to detect small amounts of free air. These disadvantages are usually outweighed by the lesser risk of not transporting the patient to the radiology department.

Portable ultrasonographic units are moveable and can be brought to the bedside. The availability of this modality is institution variable. Recently small ultrasonographic units have been developed specifically for emergency department use. The experience of the ultrasonographer and the radiologist and to a lesser extent, the penetration capability of the equipment determine the usefulness of the study. Situations in which portable ultrasonography is very desirable include evaluating suspected ectopic pregnancy, aortic aneurysm, and pericardial effusions. In most other situations, if ultrasonography is indicated, the patient should be transported to the ultrasonography unit.

CONTRAST MATERIAL ADMINISTRATION
Intravascular contrast agents

Water-soluble contrast agents are organic iodides that are radiodense because of their iodine content. These are generally used for pyelography, angiography, myelography, and arthrography. Two types in use today are ionic and non-ionic. Both are primarily excreted via the urinary tract. Ionic agents have generally been salts of iothalamate or diatrizoate. The new low-osmolality nonionic agents include iopamidol, iohexol, and ioxaglate. First introduced in Europe, non-ionic contrast agents appear to cause a lower incidence of adverse reactions in patients. While there have been conflicting studies, the overall reaction rate to nonionic agents appears to be about one fourth that of the ionic agents. Their use appears to be associated with a much lower death rate. On average, their cost is approximately eight times that of ionic agents. The death rate for ionic agents has been reported as 1 in 40,000. The death rate for non-ionic agents may be as low as 1 in 250,000 to 300,000.[1]

American College of Radiology guidelines for the use of non-ionic agents are listed in the box opposite. It must be emphasized that each patient, study, and situation should be individually evaluated. At times the emergency physician may be aware of certain risk considerations and should discuss these with the radiologist so that the most reasonable decision will be made.

Oral and rectal contrast agents

Barium is the standard contrast material for visualization of the gastrointestinal (GI) tract. It highly attenuates x-ray photons and thus allows for visualization of the lumen and mucosa of the GI system. Barium suspensions are commercially available in a wide range of suspension concentrations, designed for specific purposes. Most radiologists use a 200% to 250% weight/volume (w/v) concentration for double-contrast studies of the upper GI tract. (Gas is the 'second' contrast agent in double-contrast studies, introduced by effervescent gas granules or instilled through a catheter.) A thin coating of barium allows for detailed visualization of the mucosal pattern. A much more dilute mixture is used for single-contrast studies.

Small bowel studies use an approximately 45% to 60% w/v concentration. In general it is administered as a meal but may be instilled through a catheter placed into the duodenum under flouroscopy for a more detailed examination. In this case the concentration may be reduced to approximately 30% w/v. Air may also be administered through the catheter, provided a stronger concentration of barium (60% w/v) is used. This allows for exquisitely detailed visualization of the jejunum.

The barium enema is the routine method of examination of the colon. The standard examination is the double-contrast study in which a 60% to 100% w/v suspension is instilled through an enema catheter. This is allowed to coat the bowel, which is then inflated with air to provide detailed visualization of the lumen and mucosa. Single-contrast studies are still used in infants and for the evaluation of obstruction.

Water-soluble contrast materials are available for bowel examinations. The most common is gastrograffin, an organic iodide. Gastrograffin is advisable whenever bowel perforation is suspected. However, improper use can be disastrous. It probably should not be used for the evaluation of colonic obstruction. Being hyperosmolar, if a small amount flows proximal to a site of obstruction, increased pressure may result from the fluid accumulation, possibly leading to bowel perforation. It may also contribute to

---

American College of Radiology guidelines for the use of non-ionic contrast material

Previous adverse reaction to contrast material*
History of asthma or allergy
Recent or imminent cardiac decompensation
Severe dysrhythmias
Unstable angina
Recent myocardial infarction
Pulmonary hypertension
Severe debilitation
Sickle cell disease
Increased risk for aspiration
Inability to obtain a history of risk factors
High anxiety regarding contrast procedures

---

*Other than a sensation of heat, flushing, or a single episode of nausea or vomiting.
Adapted from American College of Radiology: Current criteria for the use of water-soluble contrast agents for intravenous injections, 1990.

bowel necrosis in neonates or to marked electrolyte imbalance. Gastrograffin is injurious to the pulmonary parenchyma and should not be used when aspiration may occur, or when an esophago-bronchial fistula is suspected.

Magnetic resonance imaging contrast agents

Intravascular contrast material agents for use with MRI are available, and the first to be introduced was the N-methylglucamine salt of the gadolinium complex of diethylenetriamine pentaacetic acid. It provides contrast enhancement of those intracranial lesions with abnormal vascularity or those thought to cause an abnormal blood-brain barrier. Several indications are listed for the use of intravascular MRI contrast material agents:

Extra-axial tumors
   Meningiomas
   Neurofibromas
   Metastases
Meningeal processes
   Meningitis
Intra-axial tumors
   Metastases
   Primary tumors
      Detection and definition
Vascular
   Arteriovenous malformations
   Aneurysms
   Infarctions
Infections
   Abscesses
   Encephalitis
Miscellaneous
   Seizure evaluation
   Brain stem syndrome
   Hydrocephalus of unknown origin
   Pituitary studies
   Internal auditory canal studies
   Orbits

Possible contraindications to the use of MRI contrast material agents are:
- Pediatric patients
- Patients with sickle-cell and other hemolytic anemias
- Renal failure
- Hepatic failure
- Pregnant patients
- Breast-feeding mothers

FOREIGN BODY DETECTION

A foreign body may be detected on plain radiographs only if it is large enough and its radio-opacity is sufficiently different than that of the surrounding tissue. Most metals are easily detectable, but the radio-opacity of aluminum is close to that of soft-tissue and can be overlooked. Glass is generally radio-opaque as are most bone fragments. Intracranial foreign bodies may be more easily demonstrated on a CT scan. Intraorbital foreign bodies

may be demonstrated using ultrasonography or a CT scan. Radiolucent foreign bodies in the GI tract may be more readily demonstrated following the ingestion or instillation of contrast material (see Chapter 24).

USE OF OR NEED FOR COMPARISON RADIOGRAPHS

Previous radiographs of the same patient can be some of the most valuable tools for the radiologist and emergency medicine physician, particularly in the assessment of subtle changes. While this may be most useful in the diagnosis of non-emergent cases such as bronchogenic carcinoma, it may also aid in the diagnosis of an early interstitial pneumonitis such as *Pneumocystitis carinii* pneumonia. Previous radiographs can also be useful in assessing the chronicity of a fracture. In general, comparison with previous radiographs should be performed whenever possible.

Another type of comparison that may be valuable is comparing a structure with a contralateral but similar structure. This can be very important in the evaluation of fractures in pediatric cases where there may be confusion identifying ununited epiphyses and accessory ossicles. Most developmental variants are bilateral, so even if the interpreter is unsure of the spectrum of normality, a comparison with the contralateral structure may yield useful information.

RADIATION EXPOSURE

Most imaging methods, with the exception of ultrasonography and magnetic resonance imaging, expose the patient and, potentially, personnel to ionizing radiation. There are two known risks to consider: carcinogenic and genetic. The carcinogenic effects have been extensively studied. Different tissues and organs have individual degrees of sensitivity to radiation-induced cancer. Three fourths of all cancers induced by whole body radiation exposure include leukemia, breast, thyroid, lung, and gastrointestinal cancers. However, these cancers fail to exhibit the same dose-response curve when human data sets are compiled. In addition to tissue-specific sensitivity, susceptibility to the carcinogenic effects of radiation is age related. Except for lung cancer, younger patients are at greater risk than older ones. Girls and women are more likely to develop thyroid and breast cancers.[2] There may well be genetic markers for radiogenic cancer risk, but we have not yet reached the degree of sophistication to identify them.

Exposure is measured as skin, organ (i.e., gonadal), or whole body dose. Doses and exposure are quantified using several different terms that are confusing to the nonradiologist. The *roentgen* is a unit of radiation exposure that can be measured by the charge it releases in air. The roentgen is no longer an official scientific unit, but it is still widely used. From the point of view of the patient, the energy that is absorbed by the body as the x-rays pass through is what is important. The *rad* is the unit of absorbed dose.

Table A-1. Estimates of whole body radiation for commonly ordered radiographic studies

Study	mrem
Chest	10
Skull	40
Cervical spine	50
Intravenous pyelogram (IVP)	120
Lumbar spine	130
Head CT scan	200
Thoracic spine	240

Adapted from Juhl JH, Crummy AB, eds: *Paul and Juhl's essentials of radiologic imaging,* ed 5, Philadelphia, 1987, JB Lippincott.

Table A-2. Radiographic studies that deliver 100 mrad or more to the fetus

Study	mrad
Hip	130
Pelvis	200
KUB	260
Lumbar spine	410
Lumbosacral spine	640
Intravenous pyelogram (IVP)	820
Barium enema	820

Bone absorbs approximately five times more x-rays than soft tissues (which is why bones look white on a radiograph). For soft tissue 1 roentgen is almost equal to 1 rad. A *rem* is a dose equivalent, or a measure of the ability of the beam to damage tissue. For x-rays, gamma rays, or beta particles, a rem equals a rad. When other types of radiation are used, a proton beam for instance, a rem is higher than a rad. International terminology uses the Systeme Internationale (SI), a metric system whereby a *gray* (Gy) equals 100 rad and a *sievert* (SV) equals 100 rem. Estimates of whole body radiation for commonly ordered radiographic studies are given in Table A-1. The estimates are for equipment in use today. The trend over time has been toward a reduction in dose/radiograph due to technologic advances. Whole body dose and dose of radiation delivered to a specific organ (e.g., the uterus) are not the same. This is important when the pregnant patient is considered.

Pregnant patient

In determining levels of safe x-ray exposure in the pregnant patient, there are three issues: carcinogenic risk to the patient, risk of genetic damage to the conceptus, and future carcinogenic risk to the child. There is also risk to the genetic pool whenever significant gonadal doses are delivered to persons with future reproductive potential. However, this risk and the carcinogenic risk to the mother are presumably unaltered by the presence of the pregnancy; therefore the important consideration is the additional risk to the conceptus. Clearly this depends on the dose delivered to the conceptus. Factors that influence the dose to the uterus include the number of films exposed, the center of the beam, and the equipment. Commonly ordered radiographic studies that deliver a fetal dose of 100 mrad or more are listed in Table A-2. It also appears that gestational age is important. Below 14 days the only effect of radiation is lethality. Radiation-induced congenital abnormalities occur mainly in the central nervous system and would be expected to occur during differentiation and development of that organ system, from the 8th to the 15th week. A recent study has shown that the risk of childhood malignancies is greater for equivalent exposures during the

first trimester than for the other trimesters. The types of radiation exposure, however, may not have been equivalent. In the past, most exposures were the result of third trimester radiographs to estimate fetal age or for pelvimetry. With the development of ultrasonography, third trimester radiation exposures have decreased markedly and now early radiation exposures predominate. Using a mathematic model applied to a case control cohort, it is estimated that irradiating 1 million fetuses with 1 mGy would produce 175 extra cases of cancer before age 15 years. It must be remembered that all risk estimates of *low* dose radiation are imprecise because accurate dosimetry data and follow-up are not feasible for the very large epidemiologic studies that are necessary to show small but significant effects at these radiation exposure levels.[3]

When the patient is pregnant the decision to obtain conventional radiographs or to use other imaging modalities that produce ionizing radiation such as a CT scan or radionuclide studies should depend solely on the risk/benefit ratio. If the study results will affect management of the mother, then the relatively small risk to the fetus should not influence the decision except possibly to limit the number of views to those that provide the needed information. If ultrasonography can be substituted that is ideal. The American College of Radiology (ACR) recommends that no pregnancy ever be terminated solely because of diagnostic x-ray exposure.[4]

When to exclude pregnancy

The question arises in patients whose pregnancy status is uncertain as to whether to screen for pregnancy before standard radiographic studies are obtained. Cost-benefit analyses in the past have concluded that the cost far outweighs the "benefit" of reduced excess cancer death.[5] (The risk of genetic malformation should be inconsequential in this group because, presumably, the vast majority of unknown pregnancies would be in the very early stage where lethality is the only effect). Since that analysis, the cost of pregnancy screening has decreased substantially with the introduction of urine semi-quantitative tests for β hCG. These tests are accurate at a level of 50 mIU and so identify pregnancies of 7 to 14 days gestation. Benefits should also include prevention of anxiety and the possible consideration of pregnancy termination (though unwarranted) associated with the subsequent discovery that a pregnancy was present when radiographs were done. We have found in quality assurance studies that a small number of radiographs are ordered for vague abdominal complaints and vomiting, when pregnancy is the source of the symptoms since the patients' menstrual histories are often inaccurate. The value of abdominal radiographs in women of childbearing age who do not have an acute abdomen is limited and the same is undoubtedly true for the value of lumbosacral radiographs for non-traumatic low back pain in this same age group.[6] It seems rational, then, given the frequency with which abdominal and lumbosacral radiographs are over-ordered to establish guidelines for pregnancy screening. Our recommendation for non-urgent patients (i.e., those patients in whom the decision to obtain the radiograph may be modified by the results) is to obtain a urine pregnancy test on women of reproductive potential prior to obtaining radiographs that deliver 100 mrad or more to the conceptus (Table A-2).

Personnel exposure

Exposure of radiologists and radiologic technicians to radiation is well studied, and regulations exist to limit occupational doses. The ALARA concept is the current prevailing doctrine. ALARA is an acronym for "as low as reasonably achievable." The concern among emergency department personnel has chiefly to do with radiation exposure while doing portable radiographs especially when the patient must be held during the radiographic study. Several studies have confirmed by dosimetry badges that radiation exposure from scatter is well under acceptable occupational exposure limits. Scatter is negligible at 6 feet from exposure. Personnel holding the patient should wear a lead-lined apron.

QUALITY ASSURANCE

Emergency department quality assurance affects two aspects of radiography. Traditionally the accuracy of interpretation of radiographs by emergency physicians has been monitored. In fact this has been specifically required in the Joint Commission of Accreditation of Healthcare Organizations' (JCAHO) standard for emergency departments. The responsibility for notifying patients of amended readings that would change management resides with the emergency department, and logs that document the process of monitoring and following up of discrepancies are standard practice. This system is implemented in practices where the initial radiographic interpretation is done by the emergency physician without immediate consultation with the radiologist. Monitoring is usually accomplished by having the emergency physician write the "reading" on a form that remains with the radiographs. When the official interpretation is done by the radiologist, discrepancies are re-

ported to the emergency department, are reviewed by the emergency physician for clinical significance, and notification of the patient or his physician is documented. There are practical situations in which immediate radiologic interpretation of radiographs is available during some or all hours. Even when official readings are done immediately, the emergency physician should review all radiographs rather than accept a written or telephone report. The advantage of the information gathered by patient history or physical examination allows the emergency physician occasionally to note findings missed by the radiologist. Formal methods of amending official reports are rarely used but are generally accomplished by personal communication.

A second type of quality assurance activity involves review of the appropriateness of the use of diagnostic imaging studies. A wide variety of imaging modalities are available in addition to plain radiographs. The risk associated with contrast material administration, invasive procedures, and ionizing radiation as well as the cost involved oblige the emergency physician to select the study that best provides information with the least risk and at the lowest cost. Monitoring of appropriateness can be done in several ways depending on what the problem is perceived to be. The problem may be overuse, underuse, or inappropriate selection among imaging modalities.

The most familiar review of this type concerns the appropriateness of *use* of a particular radiographic study, where overuse is suspected. An example is the use of skull radiographs. The skull radiograph provides limited information and is generally agreed to be widely overused. There are two groups of patients for whom plain skull radiographs are inappropriate. One is the subset of patients in which the incidence of skull fracture is rare and when present is *not* associated with a higher risk of intracranial injury. The second group includes those patients with evidence of possible neurologic emergency in whom skull radiographs would only delay performing an immediate CT scan or obtaining an immediate neurosurgical consultation, thereby leading to a delay in management. There is an intermediate group where the results of skull radiographs may be useful given the higher incidence of intracranial injury with skull fracture or to confirm the presence of a foreign body. Even in this group a CT scan is usually preferable, but, in the individual case, plain skull radiographs may be the appropriate choice (e.g., for an infant with suspected nonaccidental trauma [NAT] and a normal neurologic examination, where evidence of an old fracture may confirm the suspicion of NAT). Table A-3 refers to a practice standard from an FDA panel who defined the management strategy for radiographic imaging in head trauma. It can be used to develop criteria to screen charts for appropriateness of skull radiography and the CT scan. Cases that do not meet one of the criteria are reviewed by a physician for reasonable exception. If an unacceptable number of radiographic studies are being ordered in the initial sam-

Table A-3. Management strategy for radiographic imaging in head trauma

Symptoms	Management
Low-risk group	
Asymptomatic	Observation alone: discharge
Headache	with head sheet to reliable
Dizziness	environment (watch for
Scalp hematoma	signs of high-risk or
Scalp contusion/abrasion	moderate-risk groups)
Absence of moderate-risk or high-risk criteria	
Moderate-risk group	
History of change of consciousness at time of injury or subsequently	Extended close observation (watch for signs of high-risk group); consider
History of progressive headache	for CT scan or plain skull radiography; may require
Alcohol or drug intoxication	neurosurgical consultation
Unreliable or inadequate history of injury	
Age less than 2 years (unless injury very trivial)	
Post-traumatic seizure	
Vomiting	
Post-traumatic amnesia	
Serious facial injury	
Multiple trauma	
Signs of basilar fracture	
Possible skull penetration or depressed fracture	
Suspected physical nonaccidental trauma (child abuse)	
High-risk group	
Depressed level of consciousness not clearly due to alcohol, drugs, or other cause (e.g., metabolic and other disorders)	Candidate for neurosurgical consultation or emergency CT scan
Focal neurologic signs	
Decreasing level of consciousness	
Penetrating skull injury or palpable depressed fracture	

*Physician assessment of the severity of injury may warrant reassignment to a higher risk group. Any single criterion from a higher risk group warrants assignment of the patient to the highest risk group applicable.
Adapted from HHS Publication FDA 86-8263: *The selection of patients for x-ray examination: skull x-ray for trauma.*

ple reviewed, action can be taken to correct the problem. Action should be tailored to the perceived cause. If the overuse of a particular study is by most or all of the physicians, it may be related to the practice of "defensive medicine" or it may result from a misperception of its value. A department meeting, literature review, conference, or discussion of the criteria may solve the problem. The success of the action must be evaluated by subsequent sampling or monitoring to document improvement. Occasionally the results of an audit indicate a problem with one or two physicians. In such cases corrective action may be limited to the physicians involved.

In the practice of emergency medicine it is often an incorrect choice of radiographic studies or the failure to obtain a second radiographic study that causes problems in the quality of care. Criteria can be developed to screen those patients with a high likelihood of needing a particular radiographic study to determine if the study is being used appropriately. One example is the use of CT head scans in patients with acute neurologic findings. This method of assessing appropriate use is more problematic because the screening criteria must often use or indeed may depend upon the presenting complaint. Thus it is harder to select the cases for review. Still, this is the method that must be employed when underuse of a radiographic study is believed to be a problem.

It is becoming increasingly valuable to compare the use of two (or more) radiographic studies that provide similar or overlapping information to determine whether the more appropriate one was selected or that both were not used if only one would have sufficed. Patients suspected of having biliary colic offer an example of how to compare the judicious use of two or more imaging studies. Ultrasonography of the gallbladder offers a far higher probability of providing clinically useful information in a case of biliary colic than plain radiographs of the abdomen, with the additional benefit of avoiding ionizing radiation exposure. Charts of patients who have had either study performed could be reviewed to determine appropriate selection and to identify those who had both.

A third aspect of quality assurance seldom addressed in the Department of Emergency Medicine involves the technical quality of the emergency radiographic studies themselves. This is generally acknowledged to be the responsibility of the Department of Radiology. Emergency physicians, however, should have a general appreciation for which structures should be visible on a properly exposed radiograph as well as those anatomic areas included on standard views.

QUALITY CONTROL

There may be large variations in the technical quality of radiographic studies. This is due to differences in equipment, film and screen type, the skill of the technician, and frequently the condition or cooperativeness of the patient. Technical factors include exposure or film density, image contrast, resolution of the image, noise in the image, and patient positioning. However, the basic principle is that the physician must be able to clearly identify the structures in question. No assumptions may be made if the radiograph is technically inadequate.

In general radiography, several fundamental guidelines may be applied. A chest radiograph must include the entire thorax. The contrast should not be so great as to obscure mediastinal detail in order to see the lung texture. A rule of thumb is that the lung parenchyma or vasculature must be clearly visible at the same time as the thoracic spine and the retrocardiac region are visible.

In skeletal work, proper positioning is highly important. A full complement of views should be obtained whenever possible. Both cortical and trabecular bone detail should be visible as well as the soft tissues. This is especially important in the evaluation of the cervical spine where overlying soft tissues may obscure the lower cervical region.

Another quality assurance issue for Departments of Radiology is monitoring the amount of radiation exposure emergency patients are subjected to. Several studies have found variation in exposure levels for a given diagnostic procedure that differ by factors of 10 to 100 or more.[7] While this may, in part, be equipment related, human factors are far more commonly the cause. A recent study has shown that a quality assurance program can lead to a 50% reduction in whole body dose from diagnostic radiation.[7]

SUMMARY

It is clear that the patient is best served when communication and cooperation between the emergency physician and the radiologist are optimal. The majority of studies indicate that only brief written communication from the ordering physician regarding the clinical findings or diagnostic question to be answered is required. Regularly, however, situations arise in which consultation prior to ordering a study or additional views will allow both specialists to select the best approach with the lowest cost or risk to the patient. It is always advisable for emergency physicians to review the radiographs they order even when immediate interpretation by a radiologist is available. The emergency physician approaches the radiograph with the advantage of clinical information that directs the film interpretation. The radiologist has the advantage of systematic unbiased approach to the entire radiographic study, often identifying unsuspected or additional abnormalities.

Clearly, in emergency medicine the timeliness of interpretation is as important as the accuracy. In many situations an on-site radiologist is not available 24 hours a day. A system for readily available consultation whether for interpretation or performance of special imaging studies must be arranged that meets the need for quality patient care. Recently the development of teleradiography has made immediate consultation more available. With this technology the image to be interpreted is sent using digitized information from a computer terminal at the point of origin via telephone lines to a remote location in another institution or even in the radiologist's home. There it is viewed on a monitor and the interpretation returned by telephone. As technologic improvements continue and costs decrease, this procedure will become more prevalent, enabling even small hospitals with few or no radiologists to obtain prompt consultation.

As new imaging equipment is developed and added to the diagnostic armamentarium of the emergency physician, both specialities need to cooperate to set policies and procedures for the assurance of high quality patient care. A close, mutually helping, and understanding working relationship between the Departments of Radiology and Emergency Medicine is essential to our common purpose—the benefit of the patient.

REFERENCES

1. Juhl JH, Crummy AB, eds: *Paul and Juhl's Essentials of radiologic imaging,* ed 5, Philadelphia, 1987, JB Lippincott.
2. Shore RE: Electromagnetic radiation and cancer, *Cancer* 62:1747, 1988.
3. Bithell JF, Stiller CA: A new calculation of the carcinogenic risk of obstetric x-raying, *Statist Med* 7:857, 1988.
4. American College of Radiology: *Medical radiation—a guide to good practice,* Reston, Virginia, 1985, Committee on Radiological Units, Standards, and Protection.
5. Mossman KL: Medical radiodiagnosis and pregnancy: evaluation of options when pregnancy status is uncertain, *Health Physics* 48:297, 1985.
6. Greene CS: Indications for plain abdominal radiography in the emergency department, *Ann Emerg Med* 15(3):257, 1986.
7. Cohen M: Quality assurance as an optimizing procedure in diagnostic radiology, *Br J Radiol* 18(Suppl):134, 1985.

Additional readings

Brent RL: Radiation teratogenesis, *Teratology* 21:198, 1980.
Curry TS, Dowdey JE, and Murry RC Jr: *Christensen's Introduction to the physics of diagnostic radiology,* ed 3, Philadelphia, 1984, Lea & Febiger.
Kelsey CA: Introduction. In Juhl JH, Crummy AB, eds: *Paul and Juhl's Essentials of radiologic imaging,* ed 5, Philadelphia, 1987, JB Lippincott.
Russell JGB: How dangerous are diagnostic x-rays? *Clin Radiol* 35:347, 1984.

INDEX